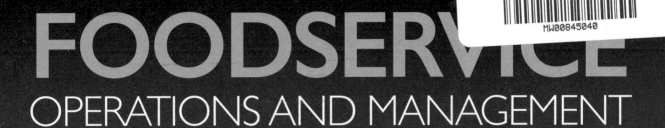

FOODSERVICE
OPERATIONS AND MANAGEMENT

Concepts and Applications

Karen Eich Drummond, EdD, RD, LDN, FAND
Lecturer
Gwynedd Mercy University
Gwynedd Valley, PA

Thomas J. Cooley, MA, RD, LDN
Managing Director
TCB Partners, LLC
Advisors to Dining and Hospitality
Quakertown, PA
Instructor of Food Service Systems Management
Cedar Crest College
Allentown, PA

Mary Cooley, MA, RD, LDN
Director of Dining Services
Pennswood Village CCRC
Newtown, PA
Instructor of Management in Dietetics
Cedar Crest College
Allentown, PA

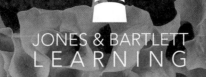

JONES & BARTLETT
LEARNING

World Headquarters
Jones & Bartlett Learning
25 Mall Road, Suite 600
Burlington, MA 01803
978-443-5000
info@jblearning.com
www.jblearning.com

Jones & Bartlett Learning books and products are available through most bookstores and online booksellers. To contact Jones & Bartlett Learning directly, call 800-832-0034, fax 978-443-8000, or visit our website, www.jblearning.com.

Substantial discounts on bulk quantities of Jones & Bartlett Learning publications are available to corporations, professional associations, and other qualified organizations. For details and specific discount information, contact the special sales department at Jones & Bartlett Learning via the above contact information or send an email to specialsales@jblearning.com.

Copyright © 2022 by Jones & Bartlett Learning, LLC, an Ascend Learning Company

All rights reserved. No part of the material protected by this copyright may be reproduced or utilized in any form, electronic or mechanical, including photocopying, recording, or by any information storage and retrieval system, without written permission from the copyright owner.

The content, statements, views, and opinions herein are the sole expression of the respective authors and not that of Jones & Bartlett Learning, LLC. Reference herein to any specific commercial product, process, or service by trade name, trademark, manufacturer, or otherwise does not constitute or imply its endorsement or recommendation by Jones & Bartlett Learning, LLC and such reference shall not be used for advertising or product endorsement purposes. All trademarks displayed are the trademarks of the parties noted herein. *Foodservice Operations and Management: Concepts and Applications* is an independent publication and has not been authorized, sponsored, or otherwise approved by the owners of the trademarks or service marks referenced in this product.

There may be images in this book that feature models; these models do not necessarily endorse, represent, or participate in the activities represented in the images. Any screenshots in this product are for educational and instructive purposes only. Any individuals and scenarios featured in the case studies throughout this product may be real or fictitious but are used for instructional purposes only.

18672-7

Production Credits

VP, Product Development: Christine Emerton
Director of Product Management: Cathy Esperti
Product Manager: Whitney Fekete
Content Strategist: Rachael Souza
Content Coordinator: Elena Sorrentino
Project Manager: Jessica deMartin
Project Specialist: David Wile
Digital Project Specialist: Rachel DiMaggio
Director of Marketing: Andrea DeFronzo
VP, Manufacturing and Inventory Control: Therese Connell

Composition: Exela Technologies
Project Management: Exela Technologies
Cover Design: Scott Moden
Text Design: Scott Moden
Media Development Editor: Faith Brosnan
Rights Specialist: Benjamin Roy
Cover Image, Title Page: © Smspsy/Shutterstock.
 (Part Opener, Chapter Opener): © Denis Val/Shutterstock
Printing and Binding: LSC Communications

Library of Congress Cataloging-in-Publication Data

Names: Drummond, Karen Eich, author. | Cooley, Thomas J., author. | Cooley, Mary, author.
Title: Foodservice operations and management : concepts and applications / Karen Eich Drummond, EdD, RD, LDN, FAND, Thomas J. Cooley, MA, RD, LDN, Mary Cooley, MA, RD, LDN.
Description: Burlington, MA : Jones & Bartlett Learning, [2022] | Includes bibliographical references and index. | Summary: "Foodservice Operations & Management: Concepts and Applications is written for Nutrition and Dietetics students in undergraduate programs to provide the knowledge and learning activities required by ACEND's 2017 Standards in the following areas: Management theories and business principles required to deliver programs and services. Continuous quality management of food and nutrition services. Food science and food systems, environmental sustainability, techniques of food preparation and development and modification and evaluation of recipes, menus, and food products acceptable to diverse populations. (ACEND Accreditation Standards for Nutrition and Dietetics Didactic Programs, 2017) The textbook can also be used to meet the competencies in Unit 3 (Food Systems Management) and Unit 5 (Leadership, Business, Management, and Organization) in the Future Education Model for both bachelor's and graduate degree programs"– Provided by publisher.
Identifiers: LCCN 2020057146 | ISBN 9781284164879 (paperback)
Subjects: LCSH: Food service.
Classification: LCC TX943 .D78 2022 | DDC 647.95068–dc23
LC record available at https://lccn.loc.gov/2020057146

6048

Printed in the United States of America
25 24 23 22 21   10 9 8 7 6 5 4 3 2 1

To the foodservice workers who helped feed Americans during the coronavirus pandemic and especially to those who lost their lives and their families.
KED

To my co-authors: Karen Eich Drummond for the opportunity; and to Mary, who makes the entire journey worthwhile.
TJC

To my ever-supportive husband Tom and our wonderful children, Patrick, Elizabeth, and William, who keep me inspired and moving forward.
MC

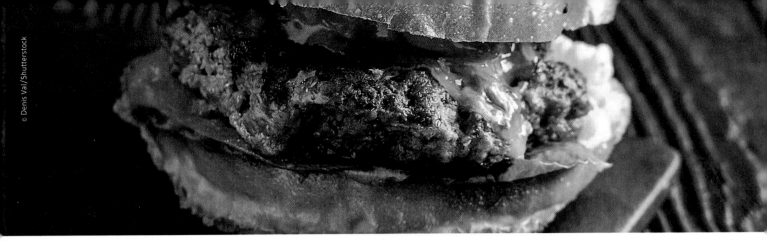

© Denis Val/Shutterstock

BRIEF CONTENTS

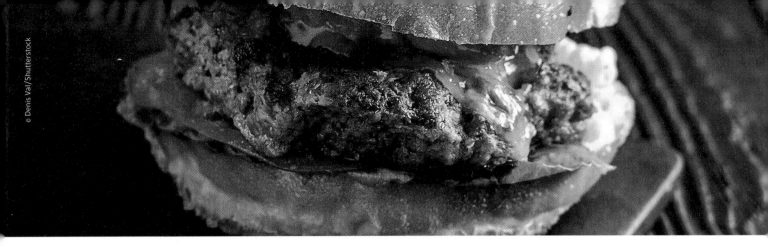

© Denis Val/Shutterstock

CONTENTS

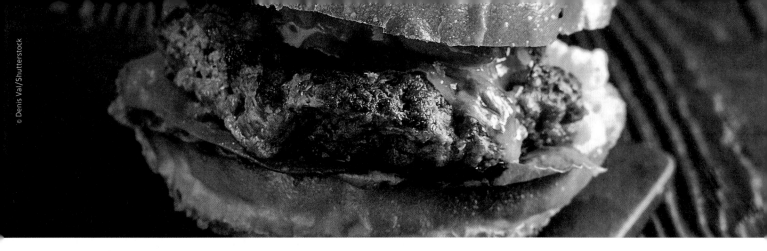

© Denis Val/Shutterstock

PREFACE

Foodservice Operations & Management: Concepts and Applications is written for undergraduate foodservice management and culinary students as well as nutrition and dietetics students. It provides the knowledge and learning activities necessary to be comfortable working in a restaurant or onsite foodservice such as is found in healthcare facilities, schools, colleges, and universities. What makes this textbook different is the variety of ways in which students can practice new skills, such as by completing case studies, creating a foodservice concept, or doing exercises that emphasize real-life applications. Chapter application exercises, organized by learning outcome, are available in the back of the book and can be pulled out for completion by students at home or in class, alone or in a group.

CONTENT AND ORGANIZATION

After the first chapter introducing the foodservice industry, there are nine chapters on operations and seven chapters on management. The content is organized and sequenced so that students build on prior concepts.

Operations

1. Introduction to the Foodservice Industry
2. Sanitation & Safety
3. Menus: The Heart of the Operation
4. Foodservice Equipment
5. Foodservice Design & Layout
6. Standardized Recipes & Food Cost
7. Food Purchasing
8. Food Receiving, Storage, Inventory & Issuing
9. Quantity Food Production
10. Distribution & Service

Management

11. Introduction to Management
12. Planning & Organizing
13. Managing Human Resources
14. Managing Quality & Customer Satisfaction
15. Managing Finances
16. Marketing & Business Plans
17. Being an Effective Leader

Each chapter is organized by numbered learning outcomes. For example, the first section of Chapter 7 on food purchasing is learning outcome 7.1: "Outline the distribution system for food and supplies." Dividing each chapter by learning outcomes helps break the content into chunks for enhanced learning.

Compared with competing books, *Foodservice Operations & Management* offers more coverage on these topics.

1. Culinary math and costing out recipes. Using the bridge method, students are taken step by step through converting measurements within volume or weight and then between volume and weight. They also learn to use yield percent to determine As Purchased (AP) and Edible Portion (EP) quantities. Finally, they take the appropriate steps to calculate ingredient cost for a recipe when there is ingredient waste and when there isn't waste. Using these skills, they can calculate cost of a recipe and a portion.

2. Purchasing. In addition to the usual chapter on purchasing, this textbook includes an equally long "Guide to Writing Specifications for Specific Foods." Students have enough information in this Guide, as well as on the Navigate Companion Website, to write food specifications and prepare a Purchase Order. The Navigate Companion Website includes a "Distributor Catalog" listing products and packaging for foods commonly purchased and students can copy and paste items from the catalog onto a Purchase Order form.

3. Financial management. Students are taken step by step through the process of planning an operating budget for both commercial and noncommercial foodservices, analyzing budget variances, and preparing an income statement. In addition, students learn how a balance sheet is completed, how and when to use three categories of financial analysis tools (such as break-even analysis and ratio analysis), as well as measure productivity.

4. Foodservice equipment. A full chapter on foodservice equipment covers all aspects from choosing major equipment to purchasing smallwares and tabletop supplies. The latest technologies and equipment are explained, such as rapid cook ovens and clamshell griddles. Over 60 photographs and drawings help acquaint students with a variety of equipment.

5. Human resources management. Because most students will not take a course in human resource management, this chapter is very thorough and is designed to give a good foundation. It includes current topics such as violence in the workplace and outsourcing labor.

SKILLS-BASED APPROACH

Learning about foodservice and management should not be boring, in large part because there are actual skills that can be practiced, such as writing a purchase order for produce or role-playing an employee performance appraisal. The approach taken in this text is based on giving the student:

- Step-by-step explanations
- Examples
- Practice, simulations, role-playing, and other methods that require critical thinking skills

The following chart shows opportunities for students to practice skills and interact with the book's content. Although not interactive in nature, students also have access to PowerPoint slides and the book's Appendices on the Navigate Companion Site.

Ways for Students to Practice Skills and Interact with Content	
Book	**Navigate Companion Site**
<u>Review and Discussion Questions</u>: Each chapter provides basic review questions as well as discussion questions for in-class use.	<u>Purchasing Exercise</u>: Students can prepare purchase orders by choosing food and beverage items from the "Distributor's Catalog," then copying and pasting them onto the Purchase Order form.
<u>Small Group Project</u>: Groups choose a foodservice segment and create an idea for a specific foodservice within that segment, such as a fast-casual restaurant or a retirement community foodservice. As they go through each chapter of the book, the group is asked to add different elements—such as menus, job descriptions, or a customer satisfaction survey.	<u>Practice Quiz</u>: Every chapter has a quiz with multiple-choice and true-false questions. Students find out right away whether their answers are correct.
	<u>Flashcards with Glossary Terms</u>: Flashcards are organized by chapter and include over 700 terms.
<u>Application Exercises</u>: Organized by chapter and then by learning outcome, these are placed at the back of the textbook where the student can pull them out (also available online for instructors). They include exercises and critical-thinking questions for use in the classroom or as assignments. Many can be used to start class discussions. Answers are in the Instructor's Manual.	

CHAPTER FEATURES

To enhance student learning, *Foodservice Operations & Management: Concepts and Applications* includes the following features.

- <u>Learning Outcomes.</u> Learning Outcomes can be used by students to help guide and focus study. Each chapter is split up by Learning Outcomes. In other words, each major heading is a learning outcome. For example, in Chapter 11, the second heading (Learning Outcome 11.2) is "Compare and contrast major approaches to management theory."
- <u>Key Terms</u>. All highlighted terms are defined in the Glossary.
- <u>Generous use of bulleted/numbered lists and examples</u>. It is easier to read and understand procedures and guidelines when they are put into a bulleted or numbered list. Examples make concepts easier to grasp.
- <u>Tables and Figures</u>. The textbook uses many tables and illustrations to further explain concepts, show what something looks like, and make it easy for students to find and review information. The textbook includes over 400 tables, photos, and drawings.
- <u>Summary.</u> Designed to help students focus on the important concepts within the chapter, the summary is organized by learning outcome.
- <u>Review and Discussion Questions.</u> These questions check the comprehension of factual material in the chapter. Some of these questions are also good choices for classroom discussion or small group discussion. Answers to these questions are in the Instructor's Manual.
- <u>Small Group Project</u> and <u>Application Exercises</u> (as described in the table).

INSTRUCTOR RESOURCES

Qualified instructors can receive the full suite of Instructor Resources, including the following.

- Slides in PowerPoint format.
- Test Bank, containing more than 500 questions.
- Applications.
- Case Studies.
- Instructor's Manual containing:
  - Outline and Key Terms
  - PowerPoint Guide (for slides containing questions, blanks, or problems to solve)
  - Classroom Activities
  - Answers to End-of-Chapter Review and Discussion Questions
  - Answers to Application Exercises
  - Answers to Case Studies

NAVIGATE COMPANION WEBSITE (FOR STUDENTS)

Using Navigate, students will have these useful resources at their fingertips.

- Purchasing Exercise. This includes the Distributor Catalog and Purchase Order.
- For each chapter, there are the following.
  - Practice Quiz with answers.
  - Powerpoint slides.
  - Flashcards with glossary terms.
- Appendices. These give additional information, such as yield information and resource information on purchasing beef, as well as sanitation inspection and emergency response forms used by foodservices.

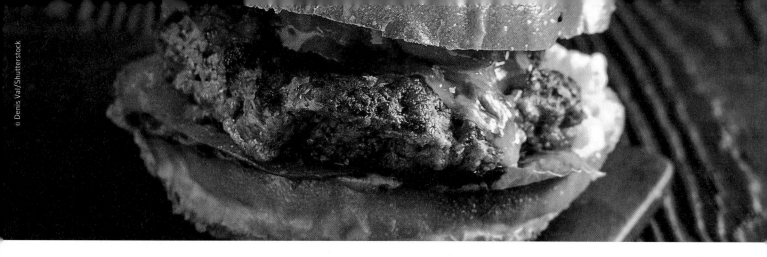
© Denis Val/Shutterstock

ABOUT THE AUTHORS

Karen Eich Drummond, EdD, RD, LDN, has experience managing and consulting in onsite and commercial foodservices. She is currently a lecturer at Gwynedd Mercy University (Gwynedd Valley, PA) and the author of *Nutrition Research: Concepts and Applications*, also published by Jones & Bartlett Learning. In addition, she is the senior coauthor of *Nutrition for Foodservice & Culinary Professionals* (10th edition), published by John Wiley & Sons.

Thomas Cooley MA, RD, is currently the Chairman of the Self-Operations Task Force of the Association for Healthcare Foodservice and an instructor for Foodservice Systems at Cedar Crest College (Allentown, PA). He has over 30 years of experience managing food and nutrition services at three over-400 bed tertiary-care hospitals in the Philadelphia region. He currently does quality improvement, sanitation, and financial performance consulting for healthcare and university dining.

Mary Cooley, MA, RD, LDN, has over 30 years of experience as a manager and administrator in healthcare foodservice and senior dining. She teaches Foodservice Management at Cedar Crest College (Allentown, PA).

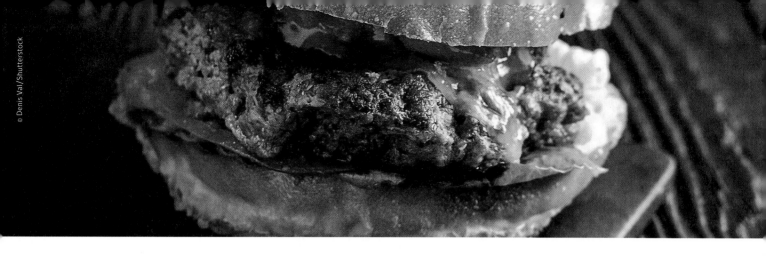
© Denis Val/Shutterstock

REVIEWERS

Brian Bergquist, PhD
Professor
University of Wisconsin-Stout
Menomonie, WI

Kathleen Carozza, MA (in foodservice administration), RDN, FAND
Director Dietetic Internship
College of Saint Elizabeth
Morristown, NJ

Beverley Demetrius, EdD, RDN, LD
Associate Professor
Life University
Marietta, GA

Coila Farrell
Purchasing Systems Administrator
Kansas State University Housing & Dining Services
Manhattan, KS

Charles Feldman, PhD
Professor Food Systems
Montclair State University
Montclair, NJ

Joey Kathleen Freeman, MS, RD, CD
Food and Nutrition Director; Assistant Professor of Nutrition
Seattle Pacific University
Seattle, WA

Avis Graham, PhD, RDN, LD
Assistant Professor
Howard University
Washington, D.C.

Traci Grgich, MS, RD, SNS, CP-FS, FAND
Sr. Lecturer and DPD Director
Arizona State University
Tempe, AZ

Kevin Haubrick, PhD, RD, LD, FAND
Clinical Assistant Professor
University of Houston
Cypress, TX

Laura Horn, MEd, RD, LD
Associate Dean
Cincinnati State Technical and Community College
Cincinnati, OH

Carol Longley, PhD, RD, LD
Associate Professor, Emeritus
Western Illinois University
Macomb, IL

Sarah Martinelli, MS Nutrition, School Nutrition Specialist
Lecturer
Arizona State University
Phoenix, AZ

Cynthia R. Mayo, RDN, MBA, MA, PhD
Retired Professor
Delaware State University
Dover, DE

Katie Miner, PhD, RDN, LD
Senior Instructor, Food and Nutrition
School of Family and Consumer Sciences/University of Idaho
Moscow, ID

Linda M. Mocny, MS, RDN, CDN
Clinical Assistant Professor
D'Youville College, Dietetics Department
Buffalo, NY

Nell E. Robinson, MS, RDN, LD
Adjunct Faculty
University of North Florida
Jacksonville, FL

Danielle M. Torisky, PhD, RDN
Associate Professor
James Madison University
Harrisonburg, VA

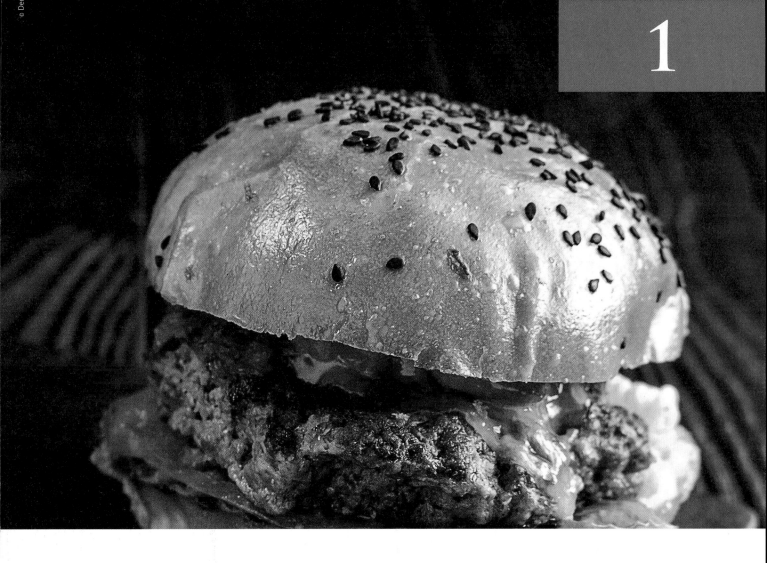

The Foodservice Industry

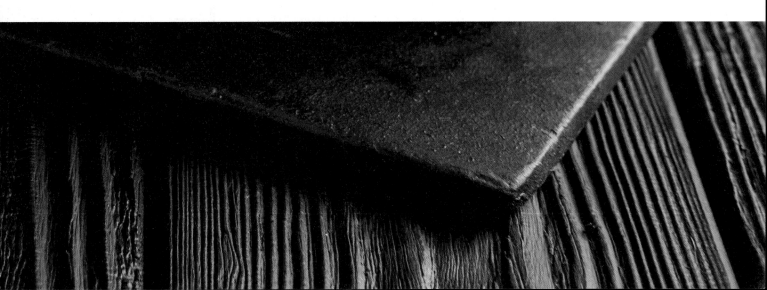

© Denis Val/Shutterstock

Introduction to the Foodservice Industry

LEARNING OUTCOMES

1.1 Describe commercial and noncommercial foodservice segments.

1.2 Discuss the pros and cons of self-operated and contracted foodservices.

1.3 Apply systems theory to a foodservice organization.

1.4 Contrast types of foodservice operations.

1.5 Discuss foodservice trends.

INTRODUCTION

Today's foodservice industry, including restaurants and other foodservices, is an essential part of the American economy. Before the coronavirus pandemic, foodservices employed almost one in 10 American workers (National Restaurant Association, 2017). The foodservice industry was consistently growing for many years as Americans were eating more meals away from home than ever before. In 1970, 26% of all food spending was on food away from home. By 2012, that share rose to 43%. Several different factors contributed to this trend, including more two-earner households, higher incomes, smaller families, more affordable and convenient food outlets and options, and increased advertising and promotion by large foodservice chains (U.S. Department of Agriculture, 2019).

The COVID-19 pandemic had several dramatic effects on commercial and noncommercial foodservice. Both sectors shrank between 28% and 35% and nearly 20% of restaurants in the U.S. closed. A disproportionate number of bankruptcies and closures involved independent restaurant concepts. Well-funded chain restaurants (franchises) performed better because of access to capital and the ability to shift to drive-through, take-out, curbside pick-up, online and mobile ordering, and partnerships with delivery services such as DoorDash (IFMA, 2020). This same access to capital is now allowing chain restaurants to purchase and expand into the best real estate and business traffic locations vacated by the independents.

Prior to the approval of the COVID-19 vaccines, the foodservice industry was expected to grow between 7% and 10% in 2021. This is about 20% slower than pre-pandemic numbers. Virtual or ghost kitchens that specialize in delivery grew by 51%

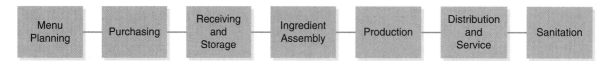

FIGURE 1-1 Operations within a Restaurant/Foodservice

during 2020. The demand for eating out at restaurants will be great when the pandemic subsides, but there will a retrenching and excessive caution exercised in determining which restaurant and foodservice concepts will get investors to back them. It is also unclear how much of the shift to take-out and home delivery will become a permanent part of the American lifestyle. Prototypes of drive-through and take-out-only restaurants are being evaluated along with labor saving technology designed to help businesses cope with the cost of increasing the minimum wage. For those who choose a career in foodservice, getting and maintaining an education in foodservice systems management remains an essential starting point.

The objective of this book is to help the reader understand how foodservices work, as well as the important skills that a manager needs to acquire to face the challenges in this industry. In any industry, the term *operations* refers to how the business's products and/or services are produced. Therefore, foodservice **operations** examine the processes from planning menus to cooking and serving foods and cleaning up. **Figure 1–1** reveals foodservice operations in more detail. Keep in mind that the actual steps involved in producing meals will vary depending on the specific foodservice.

In the foodservice industry, managers rely heavily on how well hourly employees, such as cooks and servers, do their jobs. If the hourly employees consistently do an excellent job of producing and serving good-quality, safe meals, their customers will return over and over again. On the other hand, poor employee performance can drive customers away. How well hourly employees do their jobs is greatly influenced by how well they are managed. **Management** means that the work activities of others are overseen and coordinated so that jobs are completed according to standards and in an efficient way. In this manner, the foodservice's objectives can be realized.

The goal of this chapter is to introduce the reader to numerous aspects of the foodservice industry and to discuss many of the trends that affect foodservices. The chapter also examines foodservices using a systems approach and contrasts the various types of foodservice operations. Whenever the term foodservice is mentioned in this book, it refers to restaurants as well as other foodservices that produce meals.

1.1 DESCRIBE COMMERCIAL AND NONCOMMERCIAL FOODSERVICE SEGMENTS

According to the National Restaurant Association (2016), the foodservice industry includes over 40 segments. A **segment** is a part of the overall market and it has distinguishing characteristics. For example, quick-service restaurants are considered a segment and include restaurants such as McDonald's. A key feature of quick-service restaurants (also called limited-service restaurants) is that customers generally order at a cash register or computer screen and pay before eating. *Each segment fits into one of these three categories.*

1. Commercial foodservices (example: full-service and limited-service restaurants)
2. Noncommercial foodservices (example: hospital that runs its own kitchen and meal services)
3. Military Foodservices (example: feeding the U.S. Army)

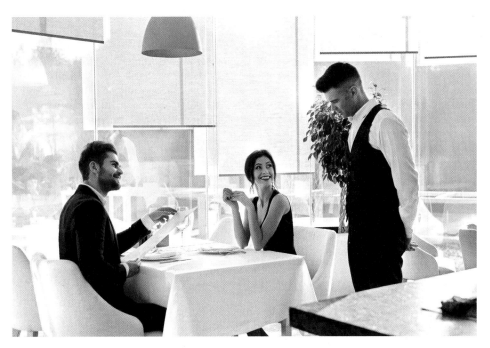

FIGURE 1-2 A Full-Service Restaurant

© Puhhha/Shutterstock

Commercial foodservices, such as restaurants (**Figure 1-2**), are in business to provide meals and make a profit (the term "commercial" refers to profit-making). **Noncommercial foodservices** also provide meals and include many onsite foodservices.

Whereas restaurants provide meals for the public, **onsite foodservices** provide meals and snacks for people who are, for example:

- At work
- At school (preschool or Kindergarten through 12th grade)
- Attending a college or university
- In a hospital or other healthcare facility
- In a childcare center, senior eating program, or community center
- In a correctional facility

As you might understand, food is not the primary purpose of the organization in which the onsite foodservice operates.

The foodservice at your university is an onsite foodservice, and it may be *either* a commercial *or* a noncommercial foodservice depending on *who* operates the foodservice. If your college runs the foodservice itself and the managers and employees all work for the university, it is a **self-operated foodservice**. A self-operated onsite foodservice is noncommercial because its primary purpose is to provide a service, not (typically) to make a profit.

A little more than half of the colleges and universities in the United States hire a foodservice contract company, such as Aramark or Chartwells, to run their foodservice operations. Chartwells is a division of Compass Group and is an example of a **foodservice contract company**. Compass Group manages foodservices in colleges, hospitals, schools, and other locations. When an onsite foodservice is managed by an outside company, that foodservice is considered a commercial foodservice. The foodservice contractor is hired to provide meals for their client, but it also wants to make money, so the onsite foodservice run by an outside company such as Compass is profit driven and commercial in nature.

THE BIG PICTURE

The foodservice industry includes commercial (profit-making) foodservices, noncommercial foodservices, and the military. Commercial foodservices include restaurants, onsite foodservices that are run by foodservice contract companies, foodservices provided at locations providing leisure and sporting activities, caterers, vending, and foodservices in retail operations (such as grocery stores). Noncommercial foodservices include onsite foodservices that are run by the business, school, college, hospital, or other organization in which they operate. Onsite foodservices run by a foodservice contractor are considered commercial in nature.

Each foodservice has its own mission. A **mission statement** is a general statement describing what the foodservice does, why the foodservices exists, and what purpose it serves for its customers. For example, a restaurant's mission may be "to provide a relaxing and enjoyable dining experience with distinctive food, drinks, and service for our guests, as well as offer a cooperative, rewarding environment for our employees." A school foodservice's mission is to "promote good nutrition by providing quality meals while maintaining the highest level of customer satisfaction."

COMMERCIAL FOODSERVICES

Commercial foodservices include restaurants; onsite foodservices run by foodservice contract companies; foodservices provided at locations providing recreation, leisure, and sporting activities; caterers; vending; and foodservices (such as hot food bars) in retail operations such as supermarkets (**Table 1-1**).

Restaurants include the following segments.

- Limited-service restaurants. Also known as quick-service or fast food restaurants, limited-service restaurants provide food quickly and offer good prices and value. Customers order online or at a counter or screen and pay before receiving their food. The food that is served at these establishments go way beyond burgers and includes sandwiches, chicken, tacos and other Tex-Mex foods, gyros, pizza, bagels, coffee, donuts, and ice cream—to name a few. Examples include Burger King, KFC, Chick-fil-A, Taco Bell, Domino's Pizza, Dunkin' Donuts, and Baskin-Robbins.
- Fast-casual restaurants. These restaurants do not offer table service but are more upscale than a limited-service restaurant when it comes to food, service, decor, and atmosphere. For example, Panera Bread uses high-quality, fresh ingredients (from bread to meats to greens), gives customers a pager that buzzes when their order is ready, and offers a warm, comfortable dining area. Other examples of fast-casual restaurants include Starbucks, Chipotle Mexican Grill, Panda Express, Noodles & Company, Jimmy John's Gourmet Sandwiches, Einstein Bros. Bagels, Shake Shack, and Smashburger.

Table 1-1 Foodservice Segments by Category		
	Description	**Examples**
1. Commercial Foodservices		
A. Restaurants		
Limited-Service (Quick Service) Restaurants	Order at the counter (or screen) and pay before eating. Static menu. Known for speed of service, consistency of food, and perceived value.	McDonald's, Subway, Dunkin' Donuts, Pizza Hut, KFC, Dairy Queen
Fast, Casual Dining	Order at the counter (or screen) and pay before eating, but more upscale food, service, and decor.	Firehouse Subs, Five Guys Burgers and Fries, Panera Bread, In-N-Out Burger

Family Restaurants	Table service with a simple menu and low prices designed to appeal to families.	Bob Evans, Waffle House, Cracker Barrel Old Country Store
Casual Dining	Table service along with a casual atmosphere and moderate prices. Alcoholic beverages served.	Red Lobster, Chili's Grill & Bar, Cheesecake Factory, Olive Garden
Fine Dining	Elegant atmosphere, excellent food and beverages, quality service, and high prices.	Ruth's Chris Steak House, The French Laundry (Yountville, CA), Daniel (New York City)
Hotel Restaurants	May include restaurants, room service, coffee shops, bars, and/or catering.	Victoria & Albert's Restaurant at the Grand Floridian Resort, Starbucks at Marriott Hotel (Philadelphia)
B. Foodservice Contract Companies	Includes contractors who manage onsite foodservices at schools, colleges, businesses, hospitals, stadiums, museums, etc.	Sodexo at Children's Hospital of Philadelphia, Aramark at Central Bucks School District, Restaurant Associates at World Bank
C. Recreation, Leisure, and Sports	Food provided at sports stadiums, cruise ships, and other recreation/leisure activities. (Sometimes food is contracted out, such as at many sports stadiums.)	Liberty Tree Tavern (Disney World), Public House at Oracle Park (San Francisco), Celebrity Cruise dining
D. Caterers	May use their own catering hall or be a mobile caterer. Some provide airline meals.	Flying Food Group (airline and nonairline catering—nationwide), Elegant Affairs (New York City)
E. Vending	Offer ready-to-eat foods from chips, candy, soda, to fresh smoothies and salads.	Canteen Vending Services
F. Foodservice in Retail	Includes foodservice in retail such as grocery store, convenience store, or gas station that sells prepared foods such as sandwiches.	Salad bar and hot food bar at Whole Foods, hot and cold sandwiches at Wawa (convenience store chain on the east coast)
2. Noncommercial Foodservices (self-operated onsite foodservices)		
A. Hospitals	Provides meals for patients, employees, and visitors, as well as catering.	Tucson Medical Center (AZ)
B. Long-Term Care	Provides meals for patients. May include employee and visitor meals.	Sunrise Senior Living (nationwide)
C. Colleges and Universities	Provides meals for students, faculty, staff, administrators, and visitors.	Princeton University (NJ)
D. Schools (K-12)	Provides meals for children from Kindergarten through 12th grade.	Greeley-Evans School District 6 (CO)
E. Business and Industry	Provides meals for people at work.	Department of Defense (Washington, D.C.)
F. Correctional Facilities	Provides meals for offenders.	New York State Department of Corrections
G. Transportation	Provides meals for people using planes, trains, and ships.	Amtrak (rail service)
H. Child and Adult Daycare Centers, Senior Meal Programs	Provides meals for government-funded programs for use in daycare centers, daycare programs for older adults and chronically impaired disabled persons, and seniors.	Head Start Child Care Centers (nationwide)
3. Military Foodservices		
Air Force, Army, Coast Guard, Marine Corps, Navy	Provides meals on bases and ships in dining facilities, exchange foodservice, and hospital foodservices. Provides meals for troops on missions and in the field.	King Hall, U.S. Naval Academy (MD), Sodexo, and other contractors operate some military foodservice operations.

- <u>Family restaurants.</u> Family restaurants offer table service, with a simple menu and low prices designed to appeal to families. Examples include Denny's, and Waffle House.
- <u>Casual dining restaurants.</u> Casual dining restaurants offer table service along with a casual atmosphere and moderate prices. Examples include independent restaurants as well as chain restaurants such as Applebee's, the Cheesecake Factory, Olive Garden, Red Lobster, and the Hard Rock Cafe. This category includes many restaurant ideas, and some have a specific focus, as seen here.
  - Cuisines from other countries such as Mexican (On the Border), Italian (Maggiano's Little Italy), or Asian (P.F. Chang's).
  - Food *and* entertainment such as Dave & Buster's or Hard Rock Cafe.
  - Sports theme such as Chickie's & Pete's, Buffalo Wild Wings, and Champps.
  - Steakhouse theme such as Outback Steakhouse, LongHorn Steakhouse, and Texas Roadhouse.
  - Brew pubs such as Iron Hill Brewery and Restaurant and the Appalachian Brewing Company.
- <u>Fine dining restaurants.</u> For the best in food, drinks, service, and surroundings, customers often select a fine dining restaurant where dining is leisurely, the atmosphere is elegant and formal, and prices are quite high. These restaurants tend to be independently owned, often by a chef, and the food is usually unique and creative. For example, Chef Daniel Humm is co-owner of Eleven Madison Park, a fine dining restaurant in New York City that highlights local ingredients and seasonal flavors.
- <u>Hotel foodservice.</u> The foodservice options in hotels vary a great deal depending on size and type of hotel. Hotel foodservice may include restaurants, room service, coffee shops, bars, and/or catering. In large cities like New York or San Francisco where street-level store fronts are pricey, fine dining restaurants can be found in upscale hotel lobbies with street access, such as Allium in the Four Seasons Hotel in Chicago.

There are also many other types of restaurants such as restaurants at golf clubs and other clubs, food trucks, and pop-up restaurants. Food trucks serve food on college campuses, at parks and events, and almost anywhere people are looking for something to eat (**Figure 1-3**).

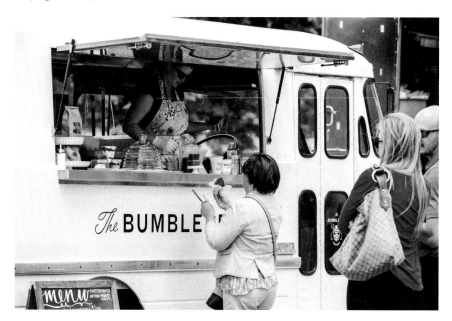

FIGURE 1-3 A Food Truck

© Arina P. Habich/Shutterstock

SPOTLIGHT ON RESTAURANT CONCEPTS

When speaking about restaurants, you will hear about a restaurant's concept. A **restaurant concept** includes everything that affects your customer's perception of the restaurant. A restaurant concept involves more than just what food is served and whether the restaurant is upscale, casual, or quick service. A restaurant concept also looks at the following.

- Which "dayparts" are served: such as breakfast, lunch, dinner, coffee breaks, or snacks.
- How food is served.
- The decor, table settings, tone, and atmosphere.
- The demographics of the customers: age group, disposable income, etc.
- Where the restaurant is located: the neighborhood, its visibility.

To be successful, it is important that your restaurant concept be different from the competition, fit together well, and be profitable (or at least work within certain cost guidelines).

For example, let's look at Harvest Seasonal Grill and Wine Bar, a restaurant with locations in Pennsylvania, New Jersey, and Florida. Their concept is to provide fresh, healthy, and seasonal foods, many of which are from local farms, and also a wide variety of wines, local and organic beers. Although many other restaurants have a similar concept, this restaurant differentiates itself by only using high-quality local ingredients and offering a wider range of menu items including gluten-free, vegetarian, and vegan options. Additionally, many of the menu items contain less than 500 calories. Harvest maintains a serious focus on sustainability, as the restaurant uses organic cleaning products, recycled paper products, and even environmentally friendly ink for all menus. The restaurants are located in areas in which many consumers live a healthy lifestyle, and the atmosphere is casual, yet upscale.

Pop-up restaurants often exist for just a few days in many different settings such as parks, warehouses, and even restaurants (when the restaurant is closed), businesses, and industry foodservices. Pop-up restaurants often have a very specific dining concept or cuisine, which is frequently unusual or experimental and allows chefs and restaurateurs to hone their skills and test menu items. Social media is used to advertise when and where food trucks and pop-up restaurants are open. People operating food trucks or pop-up restaurants do need to obtain the proper permissions and permits to operate in the locations they choose.

Restaurants are either independent or part of a chain. An **independent restaurant** usually has one location (but sometimes a few more). The owner of an independent restaurant is physically present and engaged in the daily operations of the restaurant. Multiunit or **chain restaurants**, such as Ruby Tuesday, have multiple units located in towns and cities across the United States. However, there are also chain restaurants that have multiple units in just one city or region. For example, Federal Donuts is found in the Philadelphia area and Rubio's Coastal Grill has limited itself to Southern California and Florida where there is a "surf culture" and greater demand for seafood (keep in mind that a restaurant concept may work well in one region but not in another).

There are advantages to running an independent restaurant or a chain restaurant. Whereas an independent restaurateur has more flexibility and freedom when making decisions about menus or service and can often provide a more personalized experience for customers, chain restaurants have better marketing, buy food at better prices (because they are buying larger amounts), and have well-developed policies and systems of operation.

You cannot discuss chain restaurants without mentioning franchises. Most chain restaurants are either owned by the chain itself (called "company-owned restaurants"), are **franchise restaurants**, or both. For example, Panda Express is a chain restaurant that owns all of its locations, so all of its freestanding restaurants are company-owned. On the other hand, *all* of the Dunkin' Donuts in the United States are franchise stores. To own and run a Dunkin' Donuts franchise, you (as the **franchisee**) must pay a fee for the right to use the name, design, and operating system from the **franchisor**

SPOTLIGHT ON FRANCHISING

In a franchise contract, each party has different responsibilities. The franchisee must do the following.

- Develop a complete business plan that shows they have considered every possible aspect of the business and are capable of making the franchise successful.
- Provide all of the capital to purchase the franchise license and build the restaurant, as well as reserve capital to get the business up and running well.
- Have the management expertise and experience to successfully manage the business to the exacting standards of the franchise.

The franchisor has the following responsibilities.

- Assist with site selection and development of architectural plans (including checking building codes).
- Provide or assist with equipment specifications, policies and system manuals, purchasing, and inventory specifications.
- Help with opening the restaurant, including marketing campaigns; help with software and access to consult with successful units.

For example, a Panera Bread franchise requires experience as a multiunit operator and net worth of $7.5 million. You also need $3 million in liquid assets in order to qualify to buy a franchise. So this is not exactly a starter franchise. However, with some experience in business, marketing, sales, customer service, or the hospitality business, you can buy a Wok Box franchise license for $30,000 and open a store for between $200,000 and $450,000, depending on the site.

Once a franchise restaurant is up and running, the franchisee usually pays an ongoing royalty fee (based on a percentage—such as 5%—of revenue), as well as a marketing fee to pay for advertising and marketing. Some franchisors also require that a franchisee purchase certain products from the franchisor.

(Dunkin' Donuts) as well as pay royalty, advertising, and possibly other fees once the operation is up and running.

Many chains have *both company-operated restaurants and also franchised restaurants*. For example, over 80% of McDonald's (both in and outside of the United States) are operated by franchisees, and the remaining stores are company-owned (McDonald's, 2018).

Franchise restaurants are not just on Main Street in your town. They are also found in colleges and universities, hospitals, and other onsite foodservices. For example, a typical university food court might have a Papa John's Pizza, Panda Express, Steak N'Shake, and Starbucks. Flexible dining plans allow students to go where they want to eat.

NONCOMMERCIAL FOODSERVICES

Noncommercial foodservices include onsite foodservices that are operated by the healthcare facility, college, school, business, or another organization in which they reside. Many noncommercial foodservices are unique in that their potential customers are consistent day after day, such as employees of a large technology company or university students who live on campus. In these types of venues, foodservice managers need to incorporate more variety into their menus as well as special promotions or theme-day events to keep the customers' interest high.

Compared with commercial foodservice, noncommercial foodservices often have a less-hurried and less-stressful atmosphere and better, shorter working hours. Additionally, managers get some weekends off and don't need to work most Friday and Saturday nights.

For each segment of noncommercial foodservice, there is usually one or more professional associations for foodservice managers to consider joining. Professional

Table 1-2 Professional Associations		
Association	**Members**	**Publication(s)**
National Restaurant Association www.restaurant.org	Restaurants owners and managers.	Newsletters, research
American Culinary Federation www.acfchefs.org	Chefs and cooks.	*The National Culinary Review* magazine
Restaurant Facility Management Association www.rfmaonline.com	Restaurant facility management professionals.	*Facilitator* magazine
American Hotel and Lodging Association www.ahla.com	Hospitality executives and managers	*Lodging* magazine
International Foodservice Executives Association www.ifsea.org	Restaurant owners, chefs, catering directors, food suppliers, and other hospitality professionals.	*IFSEA News*
Association for Healthcare Foodservice connect.healthcarefoodservice.org	Self-operated healthcare food and nutrition management professionals.	*So Connected*
Academy of Nutrition and Dietetics www.eatrightpro.org	Food and nutrition professionals (most are credentialed as Registered Dietitian Nutritionists).	*Journal of the Academy of Nutrition and Dietetics, Food & Nutrition* magazine
Association of Nutrition and Foodservice Professionals www.anfponline.org	Food and nutrition professionals working in healthcare, schools, and other onsite settings (most are Certified Dietary Managers).	*Nutrition & Foodservice Edge* magazine
National Association of College & University Food Services www.nacufs.org	Campus dining professionals.	*Campus Dining Today* magazine
School Nutrition Association https://schoolnutrition.org	Managers and employees working in K–12 foodservice.	Journal of Child Nutrition & Management, *School Nutrition* magazine
Society for Hospitality and Foodservice Management www.shfm-online.org	Executives and managers in corporate foodservice and workplace hospitality industries.	*Food & Hospitality At Work* e-newsletter
Association of Correctional Food Service Affiliates www.acfsa.org	Foodservice personnel working in corrections.	*Insider* magazine

associations help managers keep current with developments in their field, expand their knowledge, encourage networking with other professionals, attend conferences and meetings, and continue to grow professionally. **Table 1-2** lists professional associations for both noncommercial and commercial segments.

Hospitals

According to the American Hospital Association (2020), there are approximately 5,500 registered hospitals in the United States. The hospitals range in size from small to very large and are located in urban and rural areas. About half are not-for-profit community hospitals, which means that they are not operated by federal, state, or county governments.

In addition to feeding patients, hospital foodservices also provide meals and snacks for hospital employees and visitors as well as catering services for meetings and events.

A hospital foodservice does not charge directly for patient meals (which are included as part of the daily patient room rate), but it does charge for employee and visitor meals and often for catering services. For example, if the foodservice caters a lunch for nursing, the nursing department must designate money in its budget to reimburse foodservice for its cost.

In approximately half of the hospitals in the United States, patients order their meals using a room-service menu. A room-service menu is available next to the patient's bed and the patient (or a family member, friend, or nurse) calls to the hospital kitchen to order a meal to be delivered (often within 45 minutes or fewer). Before room-service menus were used, patients received a menu for the next day and were asked to circle their food choices. Then the menus were collected and used the following day. Patient meals are usually prepared in a central kitchen. Some hospital patients receive meals that are modified to meet certain nutritional requirements, such as low sodium for a patient with high blood pressure or cardiovascular disease.

A registered dietitian nutritionist (RDN) ensures that patients with dietary restrictions receive appropriate meals along with education. A RDN is a food and nutrition expert who has met the minimum academic and professional requirements to qualify for the credential RDN. RDNs are what most would consider a "nutritionist," but with the specific credential of RDN, which not all nutritionists possess.

Hospitals also offer meals to hospital employees and visitors, which is the "retail" part of their business, and many hospitals serve a similar number of meals each day to patients as they do to employees and visitors. The old-style hospital "cafeteria" has evolved to a food court format (**Figure 1-4**) featuring a variety of stations, such as pizza and pasta, a grill, a salad bar, and a deli, where diners can select what they want to eat. Food for employees and visitors may also be available from a franchised operation (such as Starbucks or Dunkin' Donuts), an onsite convenience store, and/or vending machines.

Hospital foodservice directors are extremely serious about meal quality. Not only is patient satisfaction monitored very carefully by hospital administration but feedback from employees and visitors about the quality of the retail operations is also collected to improve the operation and the menu. Foodservice directors continue to innovate and provide upscale services despite having to do more with less money.

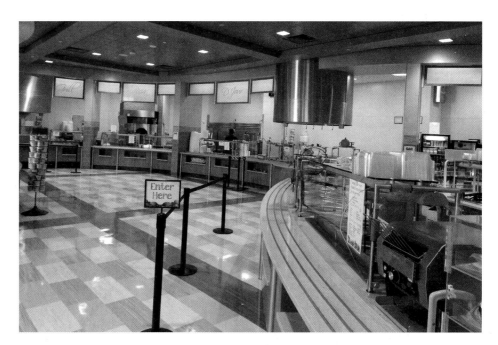

FIGURE 1-4 Hospital Café Entrance. Tower Health Reading Hospital, Reading, PA.

Long-Term Care

Two common long-term care facilities include **residential care facilities** and **skilled nursing facilities**. They are generally used by older adults who are not able to live independently and need assistance and/or medical care. The major difference between them is that only skilled nursing facilities provide 24-hour nursing care and require that a doctor supervise medical care and record treatment for each resident.

Residential care facilities are often referred to as assisted-living facilities or personal care homes. They provide meals in a dining room, housekeeping, supervision, and assistance with activities such as dressing. Some assisted-living facilities do employ nurses, but round-the-clock nursing care is not typical. Overall, assisted-living facilities and personal care homes tend to be more comfortable and home-like than nursing homes.

Skilled nursing facilities (also called nursing homes) offer daily medical assistance to adults. Some nursing homes have staff who also provide physical, speech, and occupational therapy. Nursing homes are often set up like a hospital with a nurses' station on each floor. Other nursing homes try to be more like home. Residents eat together in dining rooms, as this generally improves their eating.

A **continuing care retirement community (CCRC)** offers assisted living and/or skilled nursing along with independent living. Older adults usually enter these communities into apartments, condominiums, or single-family homes and live independently. If their needs change and they need more assistance, most CCRCs have assisted living and skilled nursing available on the same campus.

For example, Pennswood Village is a CCRC located in Newtown, Pennsylvania, and is committed to the provision of residential and healthcare services for those age 65 years and older. As a CCRC, Pennswood Village provides a continuum of care through all stages of life. Residents typically join the community as an independent resident and live in apartments. Healthcare services are available to residents as they need those services through the aging process and include personal care and skilled nursing care residences. The goal is to support the individual's continued independence and engagement within a senior living community.

Colleges and Universities

Foodservices at colleges and universities mainly serve current students but also feed faculty, staff, administrators, and visitors such as alumni and future students. College foodservice has evolved tremendously over the years, just as student tastes have developed and their expectations have increased. Students no longer eat all of their meals in the "dining hall." Nowadays, students have residential dining *and* retail dining options. Retail dining may include micro restaurants, a chain restaurant franchise (such as Starbucks), and retail markets (like convenience stores) with fresh food bars, smoothies, and many other choices. Dining halls offer many stations and concepts using innovative foodservice equipment such as tandoori ovens, display cooking woks, and stone hearth pizza ovens. College menus are dynamic, including healthful foods; global menu items; and fresh, sustainable choices. Many different menu items can be customized by the student.

To illustrate how college foodservice has evolved from dining halls with only two to three choices per meal, let's look at Shippensburg University in south central Pennsylvania. Shippensburg has a total enrollment of about 6,500 students. The dining service is contracted to Chartwells. The University boasts two large dining halls that are "all you can eat" with one "meal swipe" off your meal plan when you eat there. A meal has a value of between seven and eight dollars. Both dining halls offer made-to-order entrées, salad and deli bars, a grill, healthy choices (such as vegetarian), fresh baked desserts, ice cream, and allergy-free items.

Students can also use a "meal swipe" at retail locations on campus, such as Papa John's Pizza, a national chain. Shippensburg features a food court that includes Dunkin'

Donuts and several of Chartwell's branded concepts that mimic national chains. For example, 2.mato is a pizza outlet and mimics California Pizza Kitchen. GrillNation is for burgers, steak sandwiches, and fries. Mondo Subs is a deli concept that makes hoagies, wraps, and paninis like Subway.

Each purchased meal plan also comes with between 250 and 375 flex dollars that can be used at any of the retail food locations, including Starbucks. Some colleges even allow students to use flex dollars downtown in businesses that are not associated with the university. With all of these choices including 24-hour availability, college dining is a vast improvement over what it was.

Schools (K-12)

Schools provide meals for students in high school as well as in lower grades (**Figure 1-5**). Most schools in the United States participate in the National School Lunch Program (founded in 1946), which means that the schools must meet federal nutrition standards (such as reducing sodium in meals) and serve certain amounts of food groups (such as fruits and vegetables) at each meal. Participating school districts and independent schools receive cash subsidies for every meal served that meets the federal requirements. Schools also receive some free foods, such as American cheese, purchased by the U.S. Department of Agriculture. In exchange for cash and food, schools have a responsibility to offer the lunches at a free or reduced price to eligible children (based mostly on income) and meet Federal meal pattern requirements for lunch.

School foodservices can also be reimbursed for snacks served to children who participate in an approved afterschool program and for breakfast if participating in the School Breakfast Program. The School Breakfast Program began as a pilot project in 1966 and was made permanent in 1975. It operates in the same way as the National School Lunch Program. The meal pattern for breakfast includes milk, fruit, and other foods.

Running a school foodservice has unique challenges, especially when dealing with complex government regulations and limited budgets. Other challenges include

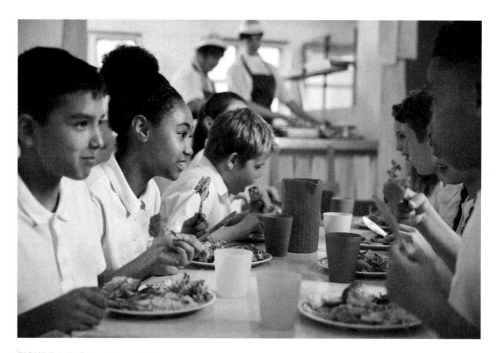

FIGURE 1-5 School Lunch Program

© Monkey Business Images/Shutterstock

providing healthy school meals that students will eat and working with student food allergies and dietary restrictions. Participation in the program by students (called the participation rate) is critical so that the foodservice is not losing money. A majority of school foodservices are self-operated.

Business and Industry

Wherever people work, they will either look for some place to eat in their building or nearby, or bring food with them from home. Larger companies are more likely to provide onsite foodservices for their employees, but a number of smaller companies also provide this employee perk or benefit. Offering an onsite foodservice has some advantages for the company: more productivity (employees don't leave to get meals), a way to connect with employees and reinforce a company's culture, and a perk to attract new employees.

Although some companies, such as Google, provide free food, it is not usually the case. However, the company may keep menu prices moderate or low (another benefit for the employees) and, as a result, the foodservice revenue may not cover all of the costs. In this case, the company pays for *some* of the cost of the foodservice—which is referred to as a subsidized foodservice. The exact amount of the **foodservice subsidy** varies.

Foodservice directors in business and industry (B & I) oversee all aspects of corporate foodservice, including their retail operations, catering, vending, and even conference planning and support. The corporate "cafeteria" has been replaced with a café operation with innovative menus and multiple food stations, giving employees the freedom to make their own selections. Food stations may include salad bars, entrée stations, grills, delis, and pizza/Italian stations. Food in this segment tends to be quite upscale, with an emphasis on fresh, healthy, and local foods and beverages. Foodservice directors like to use theme-day meals, chef demonstrations and tastings, and even pop-up food stations to increase interest and participation. Corporate catering manages onsite catering for business meetings and may also provide off-site catering of company events such as annual employee picnics.

Many foodservices also offer online ordering as well as a convenience store or micro-market so that employees can just grab a meal or a snack. **Micro markets** are a recent innovation found in workplaces, colleges and universities, healthcare facilities, and other locations. Micro markets are small, self-service retail stores in a secure area where customers can choose foods and beverages and pay at self-checkout kiosks. Vending companies sometimes replace a bank of vending machines with micro markets to give customers more choices and an opportunity to examine items more carefully before service. Security is maintained through webcams and/or closed-circuit television.

Business and industry foodservices have the highest rate of foodservice contract companies—over 80%. Some foodservice contract companies that work in this arena include Guckenheimer Corporate Foodservice and Sodexo.

Correctional Facilities

Foodservices in correctional facilities offer meals for offenders and often provide employee meals and foodservice training for offenders. Food is essential to maintaining a peaceful atmosphere. Undoubtedly, correctional foodservices are unique in many ways. For example, every cabinet, refrigerator, and storage unit in the kitchens are locked. Offenders are often given preselected meals, or feeding may be more in the cafeteria style in which the offenders can refuse food items they don't want or perhaps choose their meal from a salad bar. Also, offenders are often trained to work foodservice jobs in the facility.

Each correctional foodservice is unique, partly depending on the type of facility, governing agency (county, state, or federal), and accreditations for the facility. Many facilities are accredited by the American Correctional Association and/or the National Commission on Correctional Health Care. These associations provide standards that must be met throughout all areas of the facility, including foodservice.

Menus in correctional foodservice are responsible for meeting these regulations as well as accommodating regional food preferences and diets with medical and/or religious restrictions, all while staying within budget. RDNs are employed in this segment to perform a nutrient analysis of menus to ensure that they meet the regulations. Sometimes, RDNs also write the menu. In addition to a regular menu, there may be other menus such as kosher, halal, or vegan. RDNs also develop modified diets and provide medical nutrition therapy as needed.

Transportation

Whereas many airline meals are prepared by caterers such as LSG Sky Chefs (a commercial foodservice), meals on trains and cruise ships are generally self-operated and, therefore, noncommercial in nature. As with any foodservice, a great deal of time is spent on planning and preparing quality meals, but in transportation, a lot of time is also devoted to the logistics of serving safe meals.

There can be many challenges with airline food. It is usually made at a commissary kitchen near the airport and then blast-chilled. Next, the meals are transported to the airplane, placed on board, and reheated at the appropriate time. Serving meals on planes, as well as trains or ships, can also be challenging because of turbulence in an airplane or sudden jerks and movement on trains or on ships.

Additional Examples of Noncommercial Foodservices

The Child and Adult Care Food Program, a federally funded program, provides nutritious meals and snacks for infants and children in many daycare centers across the United States. The program also provides nutritious meals and snacks for daycare programs for older adults and permanently disabled persons. Another federally funded program, the Elderly Nutrition Program, provides congregate and home-delivered meals. Congregate meals are often provided at local community centers. For seniors who are unable to leave their homes, nutritious meals can be delivered by one of 5,000 Meals on Wheels programs in the United States. These programs also provide companionship for seniors.

Military Foodservices

In addition to commercial and noncommercial foodservices, there are the foodservices associated with all five branches of the military (Army, Marine Corps, Navy, Air Force, Coast Guard and Space Force). Foodservices can be found on U.S. military bases such as dining facilities, exchange foodservice, and hospital foodservices. Military foodservices are also found in the field. For example, when troops are out training or in a war zone. Many military foodservices are self-operated, but some are run by contract companies.

Most often, troops eat regular food. However, during maneuvers or a mission, it is not always practical to spend a lot of time preparing and eating food. That is where the Meal, Ready-to-Eat (MRE) comes in. It is a prepackaged meal that can be heated or can also be eaten unheated. MREs are nutritionally balanced and generally include an entrée, side dish, cracker or bread, spread, dessert, candy, and beverage mixes. A MRE tastes much better when heated with the supplied ration heater and powdered drinks are mixed with water. Instructions that come with each meal explain how to heat them up. The contents can be eaten out of the wrappers with the plastic utensils that are provided.

1.2 DISCUSS THE PROS AND CONS OF SELF-OPERATED AND CONTRACTED FOODSERVICES

A self-operated foodservice (also called in-house) is run by people who work for the organization in which the foodservice operates. As a self-operated foodservice professional, you work to meet the needs and demands of your organization, using identical tools to other departments. You have one supervisor (boss) who has the same organizational mission and vision that you have. This helps explain why in-house foodservice directors have a greater commitment to their organizations and appreciate the flexibility to develop programs and initiatives that are aligned with and support the needs of those they serve. They are allowed greater creativity to meet the needs of the operation and describe a greater sense of being empowered to improve programs, services, and customer satisfaction.

Although a self-operated foodservice might have a budget based on a profit and loss model, it is generally run on a not-for-profit basis as it exists to serve as a convenience and benefit to its customers—which might be college students or hospital employees. Most businesses are willing to "break even" on the cost of foodservice in order to increase the productivity of their workers who don't have to leave the building to eat. Also, the dining area often serves as the centerpiece for social interaction and the exchange of current events and company news.

Numerous healthcare, school, university, and business and industry foodservices have outstanding operations and have been awarded the Silver Plate by the International Foodservice Manufacturers Association. The winning organizations took the time to hire and develop excellent foodservice staff and implement systems and budgets that allowed the foodservice to flourish and meet or exceed the expectations of customers.

Self-operated foodservices have a great advantage when it comes to cost and flexibility but an in-house foodservice will only be as effective as the leadership of the organization it serves. If the organization has poor leadership, poor human resources, poor employee engagement, and tight budget restrictions, there is a good chance that it will have a poor foodservice. In a competitive atmosphere of limited budget resources, a not-for-profit foodservice will often lose the battle for money and resources to other departments that make money for the organization.

Contracted foodservice is a $46 billion industry (IBISWorld, 2020). The major corporations involved are Compass Group, Sodexo, Aramark, Delaware North, and Elior North America. They provide foodservice for businesses, stadiums, universities, theme parks and resorts, hospitals and nursing homes, K–12 schools, prisons, museums, and the military. There is intense competition and a lot of expertise involved in the contract foodservice market.

Foodservice contract companies are typically found in business and industry settings and colleges and universities, where well over half of the foodservices are operated by contract companies. Many not-for-profit healthcare organizations and some universities hesitate to outsource foodservice to a for-profit contract company because of their own tax-exempt status.

Outsourcing foodservice to a foodservice contract company is common because many organizations do not have the knowledge or experience to do foodservice well or the desire to take time away from the core functions of the healthcare entity, university, school, or other organization. Here are some of the main reasons that organizations outsource their foodservice.

- The existing foodservice is mismanaged or heavily subsidized.
- The existing foodservice lacks the vision or expertise to improve service or keep up with industry trends.
- There is low dining participation or poor customer satisfaction with the current foodservice.

- The organization needs to spend money but cannot afford to do so.
- The organization wishes to reduce its total workforce or at least reduce the cost of employee benefits.
- No foodservice currently exists and there is employee demand.

A foodservice contract company is composed of people who have all of the expertise to run a foodservice. Not only can they manage your foodservice but they can also design kitchen and dining area upgrades and introduce new menu concepts. They can also provide cash register systems, recipes, holiday specials, theme meals, catering, office coffee service, vending, and even run your daycare, wellness, and recycling programs.

When you sign a contract with one of these providers, you become one of the contractor's accounts, and the contractor applies their proprietary systems approach to running the foodservice. It is important to remember that while providing the management expertise, purchasing power, and marketing skills to run the foodservice operation, their primary goal is to make a profit for themselves. The facility will pay a management fee for the service that the contract company provides. The contract may also contain incentives for customer satisfaction and profit-sharing based on the volume of food sold or meals provided.

Foodservice contract companies buy food for their accounts through contracts with approved vendors. By purchasing in large volume, they get competitive prices and good service. However, depending on the contract, this may limit the accessibility to purchase certain products and may limit variety for a foodservice director running an account.

A contract company is often able to provide additional dollars to make capital improvements for the foodservice operation if the client agrees to the terms of the contract. The capital improvement could be, for example, updating kitchen equipment or implementing a room service menu in a hospital. These dollars are ultimately funded by profits that are generated by the foodservice operation (nothing is free).

The foodservice contract company generally employs the management team, meaning the foodservice director, managers and supervisors, and dietitians (when appropriate). However, they may also employ the cooks, servers, receivers, dishwashers, and other hourly personnel—it depends on the contract.

Most of these companies have top-quality training programs for the management team that are focused on financial management and controls, such as methods to control inventory, how to complete a profit-and-loss statement, implement standardized recipes and menus, and other useful management tools. Managers will also have access to marketing programs and training programs that can be implemented.

As an employee of a contract company, you may feel that you have two bosses and in reality, you do: the client and the contract management company. This can become a balancing act that will present many challenges. Because the contract employee is not an employee of the organization for which they provide service, they may feel like outsiders within the organization. Some foodservice managers describe the relationship as complicated, especially if the client and contractor want different things.

On the positive side, contract companies often promote from within their ranks. They can offer young professionals many opportunities to move up through the ranks, although sometimes this may involve relocating. If your company loses the contract for your account, you may be relocated, but you will still have a job. This can be challenging for managers who seek to establish solid working relationships with staff members and workplace trust, if the contract runs out in the future.

Many foodservice managers and RDNs start their careers with foodservice contract companies and hone their financial management skills and cost-control techniques. As they develop their management expertise, they eventually switch to self-operated foodservice operations, which give them more control and flexibility and also often pay more. Others find that their skills mesh nicely with corporate culture and move up the ranks within the contract company. **Table 1-3** lists advantages and disadvantages of using a foodservice contracting company.

Table 1-3 Advantages and Disadvantages of Using a Foodservice Contracting Company
Advantages
• The contractor's purchasing power and purchasing/inventory systems can decrease costs.
• The contractor provides business and financial accountability systems, including business tools such as weekly and monthly profit and loss statements.
• The contractor provides menu ideas and ready-to-use standardized recipes with nutrition information that have been successful in other similar facilities.
• By providing resources such as policy and procedure manuals and training, the contractor helps the account comply with regulatory requirements such as sanitation inspections.
• The contractor's marketing and sales expertise and programs can help increase sales and revenue.
• By outsourcing, the facility hopes to find something it lacks, such as expertise, increased sales, or funding to make needed capital improvements.
Disadvantages
• The mission and goals of the foodservice contract company may be too different from the mission and goals of the facility.
• The foodservice management team may feel conflicted in their loyalties to the contractor and the facility, resulting in lower levels of commitment than found in self-operated foodservices.
• If the foodservice includes employees paid by the facility and employees paid by the contractor, divisions can grow between these groups.
• The foodservice director will probably not have the freedom to buy food from any vendor.
• The facility must pay for the services of the foodservice contract company.
• Although the facility has outsourced foodservices, oversight of the contractor (such as checking food quality, food pricing, cleaning, etc.) is necessary to make sure the contract is being honored.

1.3 APPLY SYSTEMS THEORY TO A FOODSERVICE ORGANIZATION

Systems theory is a contemporary approach to management. Systems theory was originally developed by Ludwig von Bertalanffy (1968), a biologist, for the sciences. von Bertalanffy called for the study of living things by looking at the interactions among the parts of an organism. You can't understand a bacterium, for example, by just looking at its isolated parts; instead, what is important is how the parts interact and are interdependent.

According to management experts Robbins and Coulter (2018), a **system** is a "set of interrelated and interdependent parts arranged in a manner that produces a unified whole." A systems approach can be used to describe how an organization (such as a foodservice company) operates. Using this approach, you can analyze interactions within the organization as well as the relationships between an organization and its environment. An organization is an example of an **open system**, meaning that it interacts with the environment outside of the organization. (There are also closed systems that don't interact with the environment.)

For example, let's take a look at a chef in charge of food purchasing and production in a restaurant kitchen. Using a systems approach, the chef not only thinks about how a cook is preparing fish, the special at dinner tonight. She also considers if the fish will be ready at just the right time to serve with the pasta from another station, the quality of the fish when it was delivered this morning, making more decisions on sustainable fish choices for the restaurant, and the climate's impact on local fisheries. Being a chef requires a systems approach for the many processes that occur in and out of the kitchen, and how they all interact to produce meals.

Certain characteristics are found in all systems (Kast & Rosenzweig, 1985; Luchsinger & Dock, 1976). Each characteristic is discussed here as related to a foodservice organization.

1. *A system is organized and its parts are interdependent.* In order to meet the goals of an organization, systems have parts (or components, also called subsystems) that are organized and interact in a significant manner. A **subsystem** is a group of interactive components that perform an important job as a system itself. For example, in a foodservice, you have a subsystem, such as purchasing foods and supplies, which is part of operations. In foodservices, **operations** refers to the process from menu planning to purchasing food to cooking and serving meals. A foodservice also has subsystems that deal with management processes, such as planning or evaluating. There is interaction between the subsystems in a foodservice—just as a restaurant's food, service, and setting interact to give the customer an overall impression. The subsystems are interdependent, so a change in one subsystem affects other subsystems. For example, a new menu affects purchasing, marketing, and more. When the parts or subsystems work well together to meet the organization's goals, they are considered integrated. Because integrated subsystems can produce a combined effect greater than the sum of their parts, they are synergistic.

2. *An open system, such as an organization, receives various inputs and transforms them in different ways to generate outputs.* Inputs, transformation, and outputs are the major parts of the system. In the foodservice industry, **inputs** include, for example, people, materials (such as food), and facilities. The work of an organization is **transformation**—meaning that it uses the inputs to create the outputs. In foodservice, the operations and management subsystems are used to transform inputs to **outputs**, such as quality meals (tangible) and customer satisfaction (intangible). The outputs will vary depending on the goal of the organization.

3. *Outputs are examined to provide* **feedback** *on how well the system is reaching its objective(s).* Feedback, which can also come from outside of the organization, is filtered through the system's **controls**, meaning that managers use feedback to monitor, evaluate, and compare results with the objectives of the organization, its standards, and policies and procedures. Feedback can be positive or negative. An example of positive feedback could be that an onsite foodservice is staying within its budget. Negative feedback, such as low satisfaction of patient meals, shows that adjustments (corrective actions) need to be taken to inputs or subsystems.

4. *Each system exists within a larger setting, the* **environment**, *which is relied upon for securing inputs into the system and finding outlets for outputs (in other words, customers).* In an open system, the boundary between the organization and its environment is considered permeable, meaning that information, raw materials, products, services, and more can flow freely to and from the environment. Organizations certainly can't respond to everything going on in the environment, but a foodservice company would certainly want to concentrate on regulatory agencies, competitors, suppliers, and customers, as examples. Other environmental factors, such as economic conditions, also affect the organization.

5. *When an open system is steadily transforming inputs into outputs and responding to feedback from internal and external environments, it is said to be in a state of* **dynamic equilibrium** *(or steady state).* Foodservice managers must continually evaluate how the system is working, such as assessing the cost of food (inputs) or quality of meals (outputs), and make appropriate changes and adjustments in order for the organization to remain in a steady state and be sustainable. Management

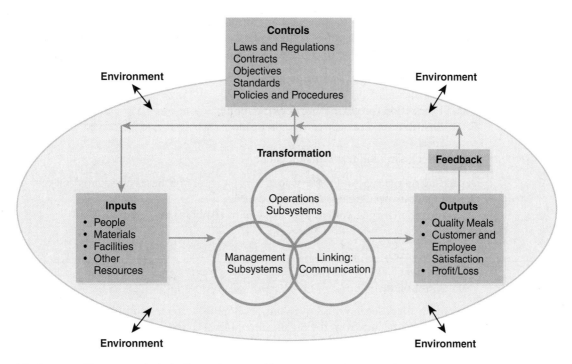

*Environmental factors may include: Competitors, suppliers, customers, future employees, unions, climate, laws and regulations, economic picture, political climate, social changes, and technology.

FIGURE 1-6 A Foodservice Systems Model

is responsible for maintaining balance while reacting to changes and forces in the internal and external environments. Over time, organizations change and evolve.

Figure 1-6 shows an example of a foodservice systems model. Several foodservice systems models have been developed and published (Livingston, 1968; Martin, 1999; Vaden, 1980). Inside the circle is the organization or system, and outside the circle lies the environment. You will notice the arrows to and from the environment, showing how the environment influences the organization and vice versa.

Keep in mind that foodservices, such as a foodservice in a hospital or a chain restaurant, exist within a larger system. For a hospital foodservice, the larger system is the hospital. From the hospital perspective, foodservice is one system alongside other subsystems such as pharmacy and nursing. For a chain restaurant, the larger system is the corporation. All foodservice organizations exist as part of larger systems (called **suprasystems**). For example, independent restaurants are part of all independent restaurants in their regions and in the restaurant industry.

Inputs for a foodservice include the following.

- People (who provide their time, skills and abilities, and ideas)
- Materials (food, supplies)
- Facilities (space, equipment, utilities)
- Other Resources (time, money, information, technology)

Most inputs are brought into the organization, such as food purchased from a distributor or an employee who is interviewed and then hired. The specific inputs that are required will depend on the type of foodservice and its goals. Consider the differences, for example, between what a white tablecloth restaurant requires to what a quick-service donut shop needs. The white tablecloth restaurant will need more space for both food production and service, as well as a skilled executive chef and waitstaff. The donut shop needs a lot less space and fewer employees, mostly with basic skills.

Next, inputs will be transformed into meals and other outputs. In foodservice, the operations and management subsystems work interdependently to transform inputs to outputs. Operations have four subsystems (Gregoire, 2017).

1. Procurement (purchasing, receiving, and storing food/supplies and inventory management)
2. Production (preparing and cooking food)
3. Distribution and service (moving food to where it will be served and serving meals)
4. Safety, sanitation, and maintenance

Depending on the type of foodservice, the exact nature of these subsystems will vary to meet the unique needs and goals of a foodservice.

Likewise, management has four subsystems (Robbins and Coulter, 2018).

1. Planning
2. Organizing
3. Leading
4. Controlling

Planning involves setting objectives and developing strategies and plans to meet those goals. Planning occurs from the organizational level to the employee level. Organizing involves structuring work to accomplish the organization's goals as well as managing human resources. There are many aspects to leading, but overall, it involves influencing others and creating an organizational culture to achieve goals. Controlling involves monitoring and comparing performance against the plans and standards so that corrections can be made when necessary.

In order to coordinate the subsystems, communication is also part of the transformation process. Communications (oral and written) are considered a linking process because it links together, or coordinates, the subsystems to produce outputs.

A foodservice has outputs that generally include quality meals, customer satisfaction, employee satisfaction, and profit or loss. Customer satisfaction is related to the customer's expectations for both the food quality and dining experience. Expectations will likely be different for an evening out at an expensive restaurant compared with picking up lunch at a convenience store. Employee satisfaction is also important, and while employees must work toward meeting the foodservice's goals, managers should also encourage them to work toward some personal goals, such as improving specific skills. Not all foodservices are profit-making. For example, a hospital café may be run to break even—meaning that it neither makes nor loses money. The hospital administration may want to break even to keep prices low. Meanwhile, patient meals are provided without direct reimbursement to the foodservice department (although the hospital gets reimbursed for the daily room rate, which includes meals, housekeeping, laundry, etc.), so patient meals are run at a loss.

In Figure 1-6, arrows show the flow of feedback from the outputs to the controls and other parts of the system. Managers use feedback to compare results with the objectives of the organization, its standards, and policies and procedures. A **policy** is a guideline for making decisions, such as a policy on safe food handling, and **procedures** describe how each policy will be put into action. Examples of feedback include taste testing, temperature monitoring, results of customer satisfaction surveys, employee turnover, and profit margins (for profit-making operations). Feedback plays an important part in gauging customer satisfaction and other quality issues. Using social media, managers can get "real time" feedback.

Managers working for foodservice contract companies also use feedback to make sure they are honoring the terms of the contract that they have with their client such as a university or nursing home. When feedback is filtered through the controls, it helps ensure that resources are used effectively and efficiently to achieve the organization's objectives and ensure that the organization is compliant with regulatory and legal standards.

Factors in the environment can influence the organization, such as the organization's competitors, suppliers, customers, future employees, and labor unions. These factors are indeed outside of the environment, but they are more local than broad environmental factors such as the political environment. Another local environmental factor is the climate. Foodservice managers know that the weather affects how many customers walk in the door, with good weather (warmth and sunshine) bringing in more business. Even in a hospital foodservice, climate (especially cold winters when people get hit with colds and flus) affects how many patients are in the hospital at different times of the year.

Additional environmental factors are broader in scope: laws and regulations, the economic environment, the political climate, social changes, and technology. For example, economic factors include how the economy is doing, how many people are looking for jobs, and how much it costs to take out a business loan. Political factors can especially influence government-funded programs, such as the School Lunch Program. Social factors can affect employees and customers. For example, a manager has a problem with employees who are using their cell phones for personal use when they are supposed to be working. Changes in technology may help a restaurateur increase productivity or improve the customer experience.

Using the systems approach has advantages in the workplace. First, it pushes managers to communicate and problem solve from a broad perspective. It also puts an emphasis on coordinating activities in various parts of the organization because managers know that actions in one area can affect another area. This helps to ensure that subsystems are working together to accomplish the organization's objectives. A systems approach also encourages managers to consider the environment, whether it be considering what to do because of a lack of skilled personnel, how to incorporate new food trends into the menu, or how climate change affects the availability of menu items.

1.4 CONTRAST TYPES OF FOODSERVICE OPERATIONS

Running a foodservice operation has unique challenges that are not experienced in other industries. For example, the quality of fresh food can decrease quickly because it is very perishable, and food can give someone foodborne illness if not handled properly. Operationally, demand for meals can vary significantly from day to day. Perhaps poor weather has decreased a restaurant's sales or the number of patients in a hospital is high due to flu season. Also, demand for meals peaks at breakfast, lunch, and dinner. Preparing and serving food is labor intensive, and the higher the skills needed, the more an employee is paid. Finally, our customers all have different food tastes, and even if the chef makes what you think is a delicious lasagna, your customers will not always agree with you. Each customer has his or her own idea of what makes a top-notch lasagna.

Unklesbay et al. (1977) described four types of foodservice operations: conventional, ready-prepared, assembly/serve, and commissary. Each type of operation works a little differently to meet foodservice challenges. Let's see how each type works and differs from the others.

CONVENTIONAL

In a **conventional operation**, meals are prepared and served in the same facility. Some of the menu items (or most of them—it varies) are cooked from scratch—meaning that they are prepared from basic ingredients using a recipe. Some convenience items, such as frozen lasagna or rolls, are also purchased. Conventional kitchens have a long history, and in the past many included bakeries, butchers, and vegetable preparation areas. However, each of these areas required more kitchen space, specialized equipment, and skilled employees with higher salaries were sometimes in short supply. Currently, foodservice managers save time and money by buying bakery items such as muffins from a commercial baker, meats that are ready to cook, and some vegetables (as well as fruits) that are already washed, trimmed, and/or cut to specification for a type or style of cooking.

The conventional foodservice is the most common, and is seen in restaurants, the military, and many onsite foodservices such as hospitals and business and industry. After food production, meals will be assembled and then served as soon as possible. In a table service restaurant, meals are assembled in the kitchen and a server brings the meal to the customer. In a hospital café, customers assemble their own meals and pay before sitting down to eat. For example, a customer may have a sandwich made to order at the sandwich station, make a small salad with dressing at the self-service salad bar, then pick up a bottle of iced tea from a refrigerator and head to a cash register.

Meals for hospital patients are different. They are assembled in the kitchen and placed on trays, then trays are placed on carts and transported to the patient floors (**Figure 1-7**). Each tray is delivered directly to the patient's bedside. This is called **centralized service**, as the trays are assembled close to the production area and then delivered. In some hospitals, the main kitchen where food is cooked and trays are assembled is quite a distance away from some of the patient floors, so by the time a tray is delivered, the food is no longer hot. When that happens, a hospital may decide to use decentralized service.

In **decentralized service**, food is moved in bulk from the main or central kitchen to a **galley** or **satellite kitchen**, where it is kept at proper temperatures and trays are then assembled and transported to the patient. A galley or satellite kitchen basically receives food from another location and assembles and serves meals. For example, one of the patient units at Rhode Island Hospital was a distance from the main kitchen and food from the main kitchen would never arrive hot in patient's rooms. So hot foods, such as eggs and oatmeal for breakfast, were put into a steam table to stay hot, and rolled

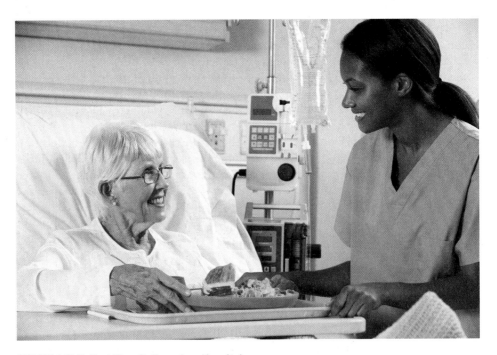

FIGURE 1-7 Patient Tray Delivery in a Hospital

© Monkey Business Images/Shutterstock

over to a galley kitchen located directly in this unit just prior to meal service time. Cold foods were also brought over in carts. Employees in the galley kitchen usually do a small amount of preparation, such as making coffee and toast, just before assembling and delivering meals.

Advantages of Conventional Operations:

1. Food is fresh and often made from scratch, which equates to a quality product that customers want.
2. Food costs are lower when preparing foods from scratch.
3. Menus can feature a wide variety of recipes that meet the preferences of your customers.
4. Menu changes are easier to implement when seasons change or food prices are lower, such as berries and peaches during the summer months.

Disadvantages of Conventional Operations:

1. Conventional operations are quite labor-intensive as you need cooks and other food production personnel whenever the operation is open to prepare and assemble fresh meals. Labor costs in conventional operations can be quite expensive.
2. In any conventional operation serving two or three meals a day, the workload tends to peak at mealtimes, when everyone is very busy and declines between meals. Although cooking staff are kept busy between meals, sometimes their tasks could be performed by lower-level employees.

READY-PREPARED

As just mentioned, conventional operations are labor-intensive with cooking personnel working days, evenings, and weekends. Now, imagine a situation in which most of the cooks work from 9:00 AM to 5:00 PM, Monday through Friday. That is possible in a **ready-prepared operation** because most menu items are prepared and then either chilled or frozen *for later (not immediate) use*. A ready-prepared foodservice is like a home cook who prepares entrées on the weekend, and has an inventory of chilled and frozen foods that will be reheated during the week as needed. However, in a foodservice that serves hundreds of meals each day, you can't cook and reheat without using special procedures to reduce the risk of foodborne illness.

Two methods used in this type of operation are cook-chill and cook-freeze. As their names imply, initially, foods are cooked and then either chilled or frozen.

First, let's look at cook-chill. Here are the steps for one **cook-chill system**.

1. *Cooked food* (while still hot) is placed into impermeable plastic bags, which causes the air to be pushed out of the bags. The bags are then sealed or crimped closed.
2. It is not a good idea to put these hot bags into a refrigerator or freezer—it will take too long to cool and endanger other food that is being stored there. So a **blast chiller** (**Figure 1-8**) or tumbler chiller is used to reduce the temperature quickly. Chilling the food quickly also preserves its flavor, texture, and nutritional value.
3. Chilled foods are often stored in a dedicated refrigerator, which is kept at a lower-than-normal temperature. All foods in the refrigerator have a "use by" date on them. Because the bags of food have had the air expelled, they are considered "reduced oxygen packaging" and may stay fresh for only seven days when held at or below 41°F (5°C)—but can be held longer if the food is kept at 34°F (1°C) (2017 Food Code, p. 104).
4. Finally, foods are reheated and portioned.

Reduced oxygen packaging (ROP) results in a reduced oxygen level in the sealed food package. By reducing the oxygen normally found in the package, the number of bacteria that cause food spoilage are reduced and fat oxidation is also reduced

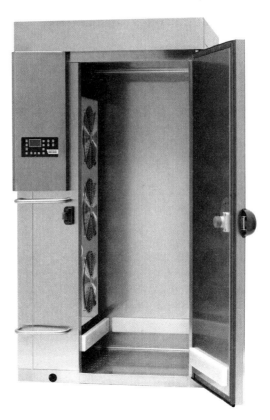

FIGURE 1-8 Blast Chiller
Courtesy of Victory Refrigeration.

so there is less possibility of rancidity. ROP has the unique advantage of extending the shelf life of cooked foods and improving quality retention, but food safety is still most important because ROP can allow growth of several important pathogens, such as *Listeria monocytogenes* and *Clostridium botulinum*. Following an appropriate Hazard Analysis and Critical Control Points plan (discussed in Chapter 2) can reduce these food safety risks.

In a different type of cook-chill method, food is cooked and then put into hotel pans or preplated before being blast chilled. These foods can be stored in a refrigerator for five days before they have to be used (Alto-Shaam, 2018).

In a **cook-freeze system**, foods are cooked and then frozen rapidly (also called flash frozen), using a blast chiller or blast freezer, and stored at −10°F (−23°C). Foods are usually thawed before reheating, which can be done quickly in the blast chiller. Then a combi-oven (which also has moisture) can be used to reheat the food. A combi-oven, in addition to being able to roast or steam, rethermalizes frozen or chilled items very evenly so the outside of the food does not cook faster than the inside. To take advantage of cook-freeze, some recipes, such as thickened sauces, will need to be altered.

Flash freezing (freezing rapidly to prevent the formation of ice crystals) is a very effective way to maintain a quality product and retain its nutrient value without having issues with texture changes or freezer burn. It can be very useful to flash freeze fruits and vegetables, for example, when they are at their cheapest and peak freshness, so that you can use them at times of the year when they are more expensive or their quality is not as good.

A ready-prepared operation may also be using **sous vide**. In sous vide, raw food is vacuum packaged in an impermeable bag, cooked in the bag, rapidly chilled, and refrigerated. Similar to the first cook-chill method just discussed, sous vide also uses reduced oxygen packaging, and a HACCP plan will be needed to obtain a variance from your local regulatory authority to use sous vide in your establishment.

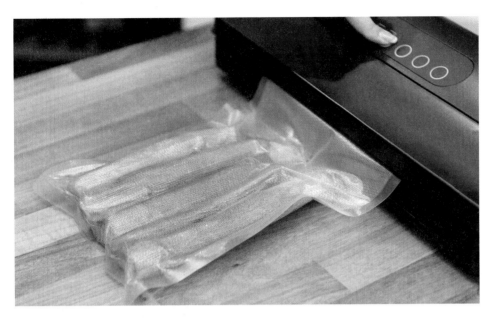

FIGURE 1-9 Using a Vacuum Sealer for Sous Vide Cooking

© FotoCuisinette/Shutterstock

Sous vide is a cooking method that originated in France. Using sous vide effectively is a complex process that, when followed properly, can produce good-quality, safe foods. The following is a *basic* introduction to the steps in the process.

1. Using a chamber vacuum packager (**Figure 1-9**), you vacuum-pack a *raw food* in impermeable plastic pouches so that air is removed and the package is hermetically sealed (meaning no air can enter until the vacuum seal is broken). Removing the air from the cooking pouch ensures that the food will cook evenly.

2. Next, you cook the food in an immersion circulator at below simmering temperatures. An immersion circulator moves the water to ensure an even temperature throughout the bath. The beauty of sous vide cooking is that foods are cooked evenly, with the same doneness from the outside to the center. This is very useful for meats, because when they are cooked in an oven, the center will be at a lower temperature than the outside.

3. Once cooked, the food may be finished before serving. For example, a steak may be seared and then served.

4. When the food is not immediately served, it is placed in equipment (such as an ice bath or blast chiller) to bring down the temperature to 37°F within two hours (Gisslen, 2015). Now the food is ready to be refrigerated or frozen.

5. To reheat a portion at a time, the bag may be reheated in the immersion circulator at a temperature below its original cooking temperature so there is no chance to overcook it.

Sous vide foods can sit in the refrigerator for two days, some for up to one week. Sous vide cooking is particularly effective at tenderizing meats and bringing out their flavor. Sous vide is also used for some proteins, soups, sauces, pasta dishes, and more. However, it is not a particularly good cooking method for ground meats or green vegetables.

Cook-chill and cook-freeze systems are used in the catering industry, restaurants, hospitals, universities, the military, and other foodservices. Sous vide is quite popular and used in a wide array of restaurants (such as Panera and Chipotle) and other foodservices. Keep in mind that foodservices may use cook-chill, cook-freeze, or sous vide to prepare just *some* of their menu items—and use conventional systems for everything else.

Advantages of Ready-Prepared:

1. The ready-prepared method saves labor time and money because large amounts of food can be prepared at one time and the peaks and valleys of a conventional operation are eliminated. Another way to say this is that more food can be produced per labor hour.
2. There is more flexibility in scheduling food production because you are not serving right after preparing the foods.
3. In foodservices that use cook-chill, cook-freeze, or sous vide for just some of their menu items (and otherwise use a conventional system), it is a real time saver for the production crew to have some items that are already prepared.
4. Cooks can maintain high quality and consistency in the finished product, and nutrients are maintained as well.

Disadvantages of Ready-Prepared:

1. Attention to detail is imperative to retain the quality, safety, and nutrition in foods that are cook-chilled, cook-frozen, or undergo the sous vide process.
2. Recipes for a conventional operation may not necessarily work in cook-chill, cook-freeze, or sous vide. Some may need to be modified and some are just not good candidates for these methods.
3. Depending on the system you use, you will need to purchase equipment, which, of course, increases energy and maintenance costs. Possible purchases could be for vacuum packaging equipment, blast chiller, cold storage or freezer units, or equipment to rethermalize (reheat) foods, such as combi-ovens.

ASSEMBLY/SERVE

An **assembly-serve operation** is similar in most respects to a conventional operation, *except that the assembly-serve operation does no cooking from scratch*. Most purchased foods are either ready-to-heat or ready-to-serve. Many foods are also portion controlled, such as 4-ounce portions of grilled chicken. The rationale behind an assembly-serve operation is that it can be operated with minimally skilled personnel who use equipment such as convection ovens and microwave ovens to heat foods as needed and then serve.

Many quick-service restaurants use a lot of convenient, portion-controlled items. For example, some coffee chains receive portion-controlled baked items, sandwiches, salads, and ready-to-heat breakfast sandwiches.

Assembly-serve may also be used in some healthcare settings. For example, frozen entrées are sometimes paired with frozen vegetables that, once heated up, can provide hot meal service without using skilled cooking staff. Some manufacturers offer several versions of an entrée to meet the requirements of modified diets (such as low sodium) in healthcare.

Advantages of Assembly/Serve:

1. Because foods do not require much preparation, labor costs are lower. Lower skilled personnel can be used, which is cheaper.
2. Assembly-serve foodservices do not need as much space and equipment as one that will be cooked from scratch. That also saves money.

Disadvantages of Assembly/Serve:

1. Buying mostly prepared foods costs more than cooking from scratch. Foodservice managers have to really examine whether the higher cost of prepared items is offset by the lower labor cost.
2. Menu variety will be more limited because you have to use convenience foods.
3. Many customers today value freshly made menu items, not premade foods.
4. The quality of some of the convenience foods used may not be acceptable to customers, and some frozen entrées may be low in protein/serving.

5. If a foodservice is switching to assembly/serve, it will likely require more refrigeration/freezer space and reheating equipment.

COMMISSARY

In a **commissary operation**, food is prepared in a central kitchen and then transported (by truck or van) to external satellite kitchens where the meals are then served. A commissary operation is most effective when there are many meals to be served at several different locations—such as meals required on airplanes or school lunches for a large school district. Because most commissary kitchens prepare very large quantities of food, they usually have some equipment that wouldn't be seen in a conventional operation, such as very large kettles or pumping stations. Foods prepared in commissaries may be distributed in bulk (such as in steam table pans), preportioned, or preplated—hot, cold, or frozen.

In the case of airline food, the central kitchen preplates and seals the hot food (which has been chilled or frozen), which will be transported to the plane. The trays with the cold items are assembled and also transported to the plane. At the appropriate time, the plates are reheated onboard in convection ovens and the airline personnel places each passenger's choice of hot entrée on the tray with the cold items.

Now let's look at a school foodservice. The foodservice at Greeley-Evans School District 6 in Colorado uses locally sourced foods whenever possible and tries hard to provide meals that students like (there are over 20,000 students in the district). Meals start in a 12,000 square foot central production facility where nearly all meals are prepared from scratch and transported in bulk to each school. After receiving daily deliveries, each school gets set up to serve meals. In some school districts, one school may be used as the commissary kitchen.

A number of chain restaurants also use commissary kitchens to supply some of their menu items to individual stores. For example, Chipotle uses centralized kitchens to prepare some bulk ingredients that are then transported to area restaurants so workers can assemble tacos, burritos, and other menu items. Be aware that some centralized kitchens use cook-chill, cook-freeze, and/or sous vide technology to prepare some of their menu items.

Advantages of a Commissary:

1. Overall, commissary operations are very efficient and save money. Large centralized operations have more purchasing power and, therefore, lower food costs. Instead of having cooks prepare menu items in half a dozen kitchens, a commissary kitchen is more efficient, resulting in lower labor costs. Of course, it costs quite a bit of money to build or outfit a commissary kitchen, but the facility allows for better space and equipment utilization compared with preparation and cooking equipment in satellite kitchens. It also allows satellite kitchens to be smaller in size. Finally, there is less waste and better inventory control when there is only one kitchen involved in most of the food preparation.
2. A centralized kitchen allows for more consistent food quality and nutritional quality for all of the satellite kitchens being served, because it is easier to supervise one operation than many. Consistent taste, appearance, and texture of foods are very important, especially for specific brands and chain operations.
3. A centralized kitchen also lends itself to more control over the food safety aspects of food production.

Disadvantages of a Commissary:

1. Transporting food is expensive and special attention must be paid to food safety during transportation. The cost of trucks or vans, drivers (who may need a Commercial Drivers license and/or be unionized), delivery equipment,

THE BIG PICTURE

In a conventional operation, meals are prepared and served in the same facility, and many of the menu items are made from scratch (with some convenience items used). In an assembly/serve operation, no scratch cooking is done and many convenience foods are used so meals are assembled (some heating may be needed) and served without using a lot of labor time. In a ready-prepared operation, most menu items are prepared ahead of time and then either chilled or frozen for later (not immediate) use. Finally, in a commissary operation, food is prepared in a central kitchen and then transported (by truck or van) to external satellite kitchens where the meals are then served.

insurance, and gas all add up. Additionally, most transporters must comply with the U.S. Food and Drug Administration's Food Safety Modernization Act (2011), which requires food transporters to ensure that food is properly refrigerated and protected during transport and that trucks and equipment are properly cleaned and sanitized. There may also be other state and local regulations.

2. Specialized personnel with higher-level skills and higher salaries are needed in many central food production facilities to oversee sanitation, specialized equipment, and quality.

3. If something goes wrong with the equipment or the food-safety procedures, the impact would affect *all* of the satellite kitchens and customers. If the trucks or vans run into weather or breakdown, that will also affect customers.

4. The people making the food are not the ones serving the customer, so they don't receive direct feedback from customers unless they visit the satellite operations.

1.5 DISCUSS FOODSERVICE TRENDS

Trends in foodservice are a more recent innovation than you might suspect. In the past, foodservice trends were often driven by huge technological innovations like refrigeration replacing the ice box or from scientific breakthroughs like pasteurization that extended the life of milk. When practically all meals were prepared and consumed in the home in the past, you could go 20 years between trends. Today, trends seem to come and go like Instagram photos. While there is a lot to keep up with in the foodservice industry, you don't want to ignore new menu ideas, cooking, equipment, and other trends because you could be missing out on something that will eventually become mainstream. What if you had ignored microwave ovens, vegetarian meals, or Asian foods?

Now, let's look at restaurants. Baby boomers, now in their 60s and 70s, saw the fast food chains grow in popularity in the 1960s and visited restaurants such as McDonald's, Burger King, Kentucky Fried Chicken, Arthur Treacher's Fish & Chips, Dunkin' Donuts, and Dairy Queen. The 1970s brought the drive-through window and people got used to eating in the car. The 1980s went ethnic with Taco Bell, Popeye's Louisiana Kitchen, Papa John's Pizza, as well as growth in Irish pubs and Chinese buffet restaurants. In the 1990s, dramatic improvements in quality were made with Starbucks's exceptional coffee drinks, Boston Market's rotisserie chicken with vegetables, Chi-Chi's taco salads, Chili's Baby Back Ribs, Olive Garden's freshly made pasta, and Subway sandwiches on freshly baked rolls. In other words, trends started to escalate.

As a New York Times's headline stated in 1985, "New American Eating Pattern: Dine Out, Carry In," two-paycheck families were cooking less and eating out more.

Food continued to be produced faster and to be made more portable. When standard grills became too slow to keep up with hamburgers, clam shell griddles and flame broilers that cooked both sides of the burger at the same time were introduced. When fryers got too slow for French fries, pressure fryers were born. When pizza took too long, pizza ovens that go up to 675°F (357°C) were born, and that led to the customized fresh hot pizza in 30 minutes or less promise. This arguably may be humanity's greatest accomplishment of the 21st Century.

Since then, the Internet was born, everyone has a smart phone, DVRs and Netflix have stimulated binge watching, and foodie apps (such as Grubhub) allow you to order any kind of food you want. There are pilot programs with drones and driverless vehicles delivering your food and robots making your pizza. For now, let's deal with trends that are having an impact on commercial foodservice.

According to foodservice industry experts and data miners like the National Restaurant Association, the Deloitte Center for Industry Insights, and industry publications such as *Nation's Restaurant News*, some of the drivers of foodservice trends include the following.

1. The economic and business environment (consider how increased competition or rising labor costs could affect menu prices).
2. Societal trends (such as how the increased awareness of the environment has encouraged farm-to-table and farm-to-counter eating).
3. Customer demographics (think about how the millennial generation prefers fresh ingredients and freshly prepared menu items).
4. Customer demands (consider how more consumers want healthy foods and/or convenient meals).
5. Technology and big data (such as the expansion of online options for ordering).

Foodservice operators have to successfully juggle these forces in order to remain relevant in the foodservice industry.

Keeping these drivers in mind, let's explore some trends affecting most foodservice segments.

1. **Increase in Foodservice Options**. A household's disposable income influences where Americans go out to eat. In turn, a household's disposable income is also influenced by economic and political factors such as if the overall economy is doing well with increasing wages or how big of a bite healthcare and taxes are taking out of paychecks. Money increasingly drives consumers to different foodservice options. For example, chain restaurants often differentiate themselves as the $15, $10, or $5 lunch. Then there are variations such as the McDonald's Dollar Menu or the 2-for-$10 options at some sit-down eateries, which are seen as a good value. With Asian food, middle income workers might seek Panda Express or P.F. Chang's, while lower income workers may buy take-out at the best local Chinese restaurant. When available, many consumers go directly to the supermarket and get food from the salad bar or hot display case. There is no longer a universal "something for everyone" cafeteria, lunch counter, or diner. Instead, the number of options and price points have increased.

2. **Focus on Increasing Convenience.** With many Americans reporting "busy" lifestyles, it comes as no surprise that demand for convenient ordering, payment, pick-up, and delivery options are growing. Mobile apps make this process more convenient and also help customers earn rewards and loyalty points, receive specials, and look up menu items. In addition, some people can pick up a dinner meal from their corporate foodservice as they are leaving work, while others will stop by Whole Foods or Wegmans and pick up hot meals or cold items from a salad bar. Still other adults will go home and use a preordered meal kit (such as from Blue Apron) with portioned ingredients to make dinner using the supplied instructions.

3. **Focus on Sustainable Practices.** Sustainable practices in a restaurant means operating in ways that protect the natural environment.

   a. *As the emphasis on sustainability expands, locally sourced foods, such as meat and produce, are in greater demand.* Hyper-local restaurants will grow their own food using traditional gardening methods or soil-less gardens through the use of hydroponic or aquaponics cultivation (**Figure 1-10**) if land is scarce. These methods incorporate mineral nutrient solutions in water without the use of soil and work well without the land or climate required for traditional gardening techniques. Growing vegetables, herbs, and fruits in onsite or nearby land is also more common now in hospitals, schools, universities, and retirement communities. Artisan and farm-branded produce, as well as heritage breeds of grass-fed livestock, are other examples of locally sourced sustainable foods.

   b. *Buying sustainable fish is also growing.* Fishing practices worldwide are depleting fish populations, destroying habitats, and polluting the water. Sustainable seafood comes from species of fish that are managed in ways that provides for today's needs without damaging the availability to future generations. The FishChoice website helps seafood buyers source sustainable seafood.

   c. *The popularity of organic foods continues to grow.* Organic food is produced by farmers who emphasize the use of renewable resources and the conservation of soil and water to enhance environmental quality for future generations. Organic foods are free of genetically modified organisms (GMOs) and antibiotics.

   d. *Reducing food waste and improving resource management, especially water and energy management, has become a growing trend among conscientious foodservice operators.* Finding ways to minimize food waste through improved food production methods, eliminating overproduction, and enlisting more effective food tracking and monitoring systems can yield significant reductions in food waste and increase profits. Reducing the amount of paper, plastic, and glass is also helpful.

   e. *Incorporating plant-based proteins with a smaller carbon footprint into the menu also supports the increasing focus on health and nutrition.* Vegetarian and vegan options are commonplace and expected to be offered as part of a standard menu.

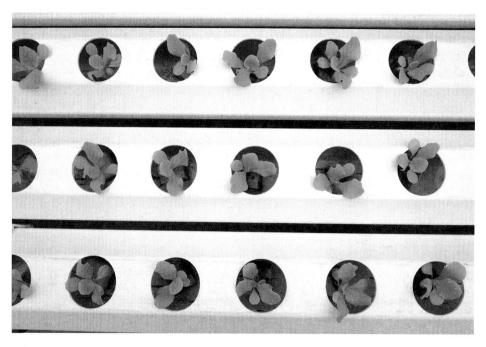

FIGURE 1-10 Using Hydroponics to Grow Lettuce

© Dewiness/Shutterstock

4. **Capture and Conquer by Cohort**. Marketing foodservice to the three major age cohorts of Baby Boomers (born 1946–1964), Generation X (born 1965–1980), and Millennials (born 1981–1994) is an art and a science. Generation Z (born starting in 1995) have grown up with the Internet from a very young age and are very tech savvy. Each group gets advertising from different sources, uses technology differently, and has varying expectations of what makes a food experience good. For example, millennials use social media a lot to get reviews and information on a restaurant. Many consumers from each of these cohorts are looking for some of the same things when they go out to eat: healthy and fresh ingredients with an interest in new flavors, such as ethnic cuisine.

5. **Offer Healthy Options.** The desire to be fit and healthy cuts across all demographic groups. The link between obesity and the increased incidence of heart disease, diabetes, stroke, certain cancers, and depression make a compelling case to practice healthy eating and maintain a healthy weight. The old adage, "you are what you eat" rings true among modern consumers who understand and appreciate the impact of food on their health and well-being. The "clean food" trend focuses on whole foods like fruits, vegetables, and whole grains, plus healthy proteins, fat, and dairy, while avoiding processed foods, additives, preservatives, and too much sugar or sodium. As consumers' demand for healthy food increases, so too does their demand for greater transparency from food companies, including complete, accurate, and easy-to-understand product information (such as a full list of ingredients).

6. **Offer Authentic Ethnic Dishes.** Today's consumer is seeking ethnic cuisines with bold flavors from around the world. As our economy becomes more global, and indeed the American population becomes more diverse, so too does the food we eat. With ready access to international ingredients, chefs can produce authentic global cuisines that accurately reflect the flavors of diverse cultures. Ethnic dishes are no longer limited to lunch and dinner entrées as more ethnic-inspired breakfast items and kid's meals are hitting the menu.

7. **Use Technology and Big Data.** These factors very much influence a number of different aspects of the restaurant business.
   a. *Options for ordering food have greatly expanded.* From using an app on your phone or a touchscreen kiosk or tablet in the store, new ordering options are faster and more convenient. With apps like Grubhub or Seamless, you can order from a selection of restaurants and get meals delivered.
   b. *Foodservice equipment has also benefited from new technology, allowing innovations such as combi-ovens and rapid-cook ovens that use air impingement.* A combi-oven has moisture so you can roast, bake, steam, or rethermalize frozen or chilled items using the same piece of equipment. Ovens using air impingement, such as a TurboChef oven, use forced air movement at much higher rates than in convection ovens to reduce baking time. Also, the airflow in an air impingement oven is highly focused on the product so heat penetrates more and the product cooks really rapidly.
   c. *New technology has also helped foodservice equipment manufacturers to produce equipment that saves labor, water, energy, and space.* Saving space has been important for smaller operators.
   d. *The use of software that enables the user to gather and organize all sorts of restaurant data to help answer marketing and other questions is continuing to grow.* The use of big data will impact what's on the menu, how menu items are priced, how the kitchen forecasts production needs, and which marketing approach is used.

Although menu trends tend to get the most publicity, keep an eye on other trends too!

SUMMARY

1.1 Describe commercial and noncommercial foodservice segments.

- The foodservice industry includes over 40 segments (Table 1-1). Each segment fits into commercial, noncommercial, or military foodservice.
- Commercial foodservices include restaurants, onsite foodservices that are run by foodservice contract companies, foodservices provided at locations providing leisure and sporting activities, caterers, vending, and foodservices in retail operations (such as convenience stores).
- Many restaurants fall into these segments: limited-service, fast-casual, casual dining, fine dining, and hotel foodservice. There are other types of restaurants, such as club restaurants, food trucks, and pop-up restaurants.
- An independent restaurant usually has one location while chain restaurants have multiple units in a city, region, or nationwide.
- Whereas an independent restaurateur has more flexibility and freedom when making decisions about menus or service and can often provide a more personalized experience, chain restaurants are generally well advertised, purchase food at better prices due to quantity, and have well-developed operations.
- Many chain restaurants have both company-operated restaurants and franchised restaurants.
- Noncommercial foodservices include onsite foodservices that are run by the hospital, long-term care facility, college, school, business, correctional facility, or other organization in which they operate. Food is not the primary purpose of the organization in which the onsite foodservice operates.

1.2 Discuss the pros and cons of self-operated and contracted foodservices.

- You are most likely to find foodservice contract companies in business and industry settings and colleges and universities, where well over half of the foodservices are run by contract companies.
- Outsourcing foodservice to a foodservice contract company is common because many organizations lack the expertise to do foodservice well or the desire to take time away from the core functions of the organization.
- A foodservice contract company is made up of people who have all the expertise and systems to run a foodservice. Typically, the company is paid a fee to run a facility's foodservice.
- Table 1-3 gives the advantages and disadvantages of using a foodservice contract company.

1.3 Apply systems theory to a foodservice organization.

- A systems approach can be used to describe how an organization (such as a foodservice company) operates. Using this approach, you can analyze interactions within the organization as well as the relationships between an organization and its environment. An organization is an example of an open system.
- A system is organized and its parts (called subsystems) are interdependent. Foodservice organizations receive inputs (such as food), which are transformed to generate outputs (such as meals and customer satisfaction). Outputs provide feedback on how well the system is reaching its objectives. When an open system is steadily transforming inputs into outputs and responding to feedback from internal and external environments, it is said to be in a state of dynamic equilibrium (or steady state).
- Figure 1-6 is an example of a foodservice systems model. Transformation includes operations subsystems (procurement, production, distribution and service, and safety, sanitation, and maintenance), and management subsystems (planning, organizing, leading, and controlling). To coordinate the subsystems, communications is also part of the transformation process.
- Using a systems approach pushes the manager to communicate and problem solve from a broad perspective, coordinate activities in different parts of the organization, and consider the environment.

1.4 Contrast types of foodservice operations.

- In a conventional operation, meals are prepared and served in the same facility. Some of the menu items (or most of them—it varies) are cooked from scratch.

Conventional foodservice is very common as food costs are generally lower and a variety of dishes can be made fresh daily. However, this type of operation is quite labor-intensive and because the workload peaks at mealtimes, productivity between meals may not be that high.

- In centralized service in a healthcare facility, trays are assembled close to the production area and then delivered. In decentralized service, food is moved in bulk from the main or central kitchen to a galley or satellite kitchen, where it is kept at proper temperatures and trays are then assembled and transported to the patient.
- In a ready-prepared operation, most menu items are prepared, and then either chilled or frozen for later (not immediate) use using cook-chill or cook-freeze technology. A ready-prepared operation may also be using sous vide, a reduced-oxygen packaging technique, which extends the shelf life of cooked foods and improves quality retention. In sous vide, raw foods are first vacuum packed before being cooked very evenly in an immersion circulator. Using sous vide properly is a complex process.
- Ready-prepared saves labor time and money because large amounts of food can be prepared at one time and the peaks and valleys of a conventional operation are eliminated. Cooks must pay attention to detail to retain the quality, safety, and nutrition in foods prepared using cook-chill, cook-freeze, or sous vide. Some equipment will need to be purchased.
- An assembly-serve operation is similar in most respects to a conventional operation, except that the assembly-serve operation does no cooking from scratch and, instead, uses mostly convenience foods. Labor costs are lower but food costs are higher. Also, menu variety will be limited and customers prefer freshly made foods.
- In a commissary operation, food is prepared in a central kitchen and then transported (by truck or van) to external satellite kitchens where the meals are then served. Foods may be distributed in bulk (such as in steam table pans), preportioned, or preplated—hot, cold, or frozen.
- Although commissary operations require some specialized personnel and equipment, as well as the costs of transporting, overall, these operations are efficient, save money, and allow for consistent food quality. However, if something goes wrong with the equipment or the food safety procedures, the impact would affect *all* of the satellite kitchens and customers.

1.5 Discuss foodservice trends.

- Trends discussed include: increase in foodservice options, focusing on increasing convenience and sustainable practices, marketing to each age cohort, offering healthy options and authentic ethnic dishes, and using technology and big data.

REVIEW AND DISCUSSION QUESTIONS

1. Compare and contrast onsite foodservices that are commercial in nature from those that are noncommercial.
2. List two restaurants you have been to. Which segment of the restaurant industry does each one fall into? Was each restaurant independently owned or part of a chain?
3. How would a job in a commercial foodservice be different from working in an onsite foodservice, such as working for a hospital or school? Consider hours, benefits, responsibilities, menu, customers, and so on.
4. If you were to get a job in an onsite foodservice, which type would interest you and why? Would you rather work for a foodservice contract company or work directly for the foodservice? Explain why you choose your answer.
5. If you worked in a university foodservice, belonging to the National Association of College and University Food Services could bring you what types of benefits?
6. Find the name of a skilled nursing facility or continuing care retirement community in your area.
7. How is school (K–12) foodservice different from a restaurant?
8. Why do some onsite foodservices, such as a university foodservice, use a foodservice contract company such as Compass Group?

9. In one or two paragraphs, describe the food-service systems model.

10. Make a table of the four types of foodservice operations including a basic description and advantages/disadvantages for each type.

11. Use the following two publications online to identify and briefly describe three trends in foodservice: FoodService Director (covers noncommercial) and Nation's Restaurant News (covers restaurant industry). Include only one menu-related trend.

SMALL GROUP PROJECT

Choose a foodservice segment (commercial or non-commercial) that is of interest to you. Next, create an idea for a specific foodservice in that segment, such as a continuing care retirement community. When creating your foodservice, make sure you include the following information.

1. Type of facility/institution (such as restaurant, continuing care retirement facility, hospital, etc.) and location.

2. Mission statement.

3. Description of your customers and foodservices available to them.

4. Size of facility/institution (such as number of seats in a restaurant dining room; number of beds in independent living/assisted living/nursing home/hospital; number of students in school or college.)

REFERENCES

Alto-Shaam. (2018). *Quickchillers*. Retrieved from https://www.alto-shaam.com/en/quickchillers

American Hospital Association. (2020). *Fast Facts on U.S. Hospitals, 2020*. Retrieved from https://www.aha.org/research/rc/stat-studies/fast-facts.shtml

Gisslen, W. (2015). *Professional Cooking*. Hoboken (NJ): John Wiley and Sons, Inc.

Gregoire, M. B. (2017). *Foodservice Organizations: A Managerial and Systems Approach* (9th ed.). Pearson Education Inc.: New York.

IBISWorld. (2020). *Foodservice Contractors Industry in the US - US Market Research Report*. Retrieved from https://www.ibisworld.com/industry-trends/market-research-reports/accommodation-food-services/food-service-contractors.html

IFMA (2020) IFMA Scope: IFMA Publishes 2021 Foodservice Industry Forecasts, Projecting 7.3% Growth in Next Calendar Year. International Foodservice Manufacturers Association August 19, 2020. Retrieved from: https://www.ifmaworld.com/fresh-on-ifma/ifma-publishes-2021-foodservice-industry-forecasts/

Kast, F. E., & Rosenzweig, J. (1985). *Organization and management: A systems and contingency Approach* (4th ed.). New York: McGraw-Hill.

Livingston, G. E. (1968) Design of a foodservice system. *Food Technology, 22*(1), 35–39.

Luchsinger, V. P., & Dock, V. T. (1975). *The Systems Approach: A Primer*. Dubuque (IA): Kendall/Hunt Publishing.

Martin, J. (1999). Perspectives on managing child nutrition programs. In Martin, J. & Conklin, M. (eds.), *Managing Child Nutrition Programs*. Gaithersburg (MD): Aspen.

McDonald's. (2018). *Franchising Overview*. Retrieved from http://corporate.mcdonalds.com/mcd/franchising.html

National Restaurant Association. (2016). *National Restaurant Association Restaurant Industry Outlook*.

National Restaurant Association. (2017). *Industry Impact: Jobs and Careers Powerhouse*.

North Central Regional Research Publication No. 245. Columbia: University of Missouri-Columbia Agriculture Experiment Station.

Reproduced from Mt. Lebanon School District.

Robbins, S. P., & Coulter, M. (2018). *Management* (14th ed.). New York: Pearson Education Inc.

Unklesbay, N., Maxcy, R., Knickrehm, M., Stevenson, K., Cremer, M., & Matthews, M. (1977). *Foodservice systems: Product flow and microbial quality and safety of foods*.

U.S. Department of Agriculture. (2019). *Food Away from Home*. Retrieved from https://www.ers.usda.gov/topics/food-choices-health/food-consumption-demand/food-away-from-home.aspx

U.S. Public Health Service and U.S. Food and Drug Administration. (2017). *Food Code 2017*. Retrieved from https://www.fda.gov/Food/GuidanceRegulation/RetailFoodProtection/FoodCode/ucm595139.htm

Vaden, A. G. (1980). A foodservice systems model. *A Model for Evaluating the Foodservice System*. Manhattan (KS): Kansas State University.

von Bertalanffy, L. (1968). *General System Theory: Foundations, Development, Applications*. New York: George Braziller.

© Denis Val/Shutterstock

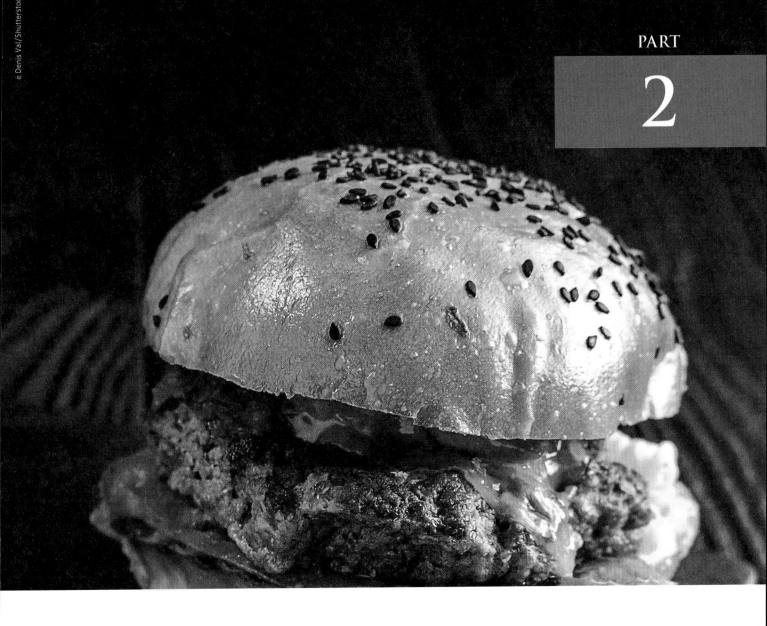

Foodservice Operations

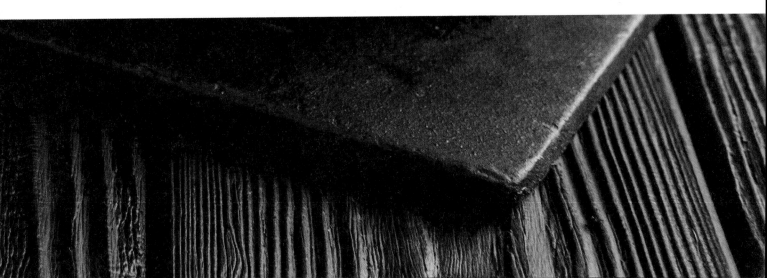

© Denis Val/Shutterstock

Sanitation and Safety

LEARNING OUTCOMES

2.1 Discuss causes and prevention of foodborne illness.

2.2 Describe safe personal hygiene practices.

2.3 Apply food safety principles.

2.4 Manage food safety.

2.5 Explain how to have a successful sanitation inspection.

2.6 Maintain an accident-free workplace.

INTRODUCTION

The Centers for Disease Control and Prevention estimate that 48 million people get sick from a foodborne illness each year, and 3,000 of those people die (Centers for Disease Control and Prevention, 2020; Scallan et al., 2011a, b). **Foodborne illness** encompasses a wide spectrum of illnesses resulting from eating food contaminated in one of three ways.

1. *Biological contamination:* Foodborne illness is most likely from this category. Biological contamination most often refers to very small, living organisms (called **microorganisms**) such as bacteria and viruses that find their way into food. Most microorganisms are harmless, but some can cause disease, and they are called **pathogens**. Pathogens can make you sick in one of two ways: either the pathogen itself makes you sick or the pathogen produces a **toxin** (a poisonous substance) and the toxin makes you sick. Pathogens are killed during proper cooking, but toxins are not usually destroyed by the cooking process.

2. *Chemical contamination:* This happens, for example, when an employee sprays a cleaning solution or pest control product and it accidentally gets into a pan of food. Products used in foodservices to clean and sanitize may, when not used properly, be introduced to foods and cause sickness and death.

3. *Physical contamination:* Physical items, such as metal shavings from a can opener or a bandage from someone's hand, can also accidentally find their way into foods. Physical contaminants range from papers clips to earrings and broken pieces of a scouring pad.

Common symptoms of foodborne illness are gastrointestinal in nature and include nausea, vomiting, stomach cramps, and diarrhea. A fever may also be present. The exact symptoms vary depending on the type of contamination and the exact pathogen (when biological).

Certain groups of people are at an increased risk of getting foodborne illness, and these groups are also more likely to get seriously ill and require hospitalization. Groups at high risk for foodborne illness include young children (under 5 years old), older adults, pregnant women, and people with their immune systems weakened by disease or medical treatment (such as cancer, chemotherapy, or HIV/AIDS).

Although requirements vary, most foodservice operations are required to have someone certified as a Food Protection Manager—often on every shift. There are several programs across the country that offer this certification, such as the National Restaurant Association that offers the ServSafe Food Manager program (as well as tools for training staff). Foodservice operators should have all certificates on display for the public to see.

2.1 DISCUSS CAUSES AND PREVENTION OF FOODBORNE ILLNESS

Pathogens causing foodborne illness include bacteria, viruses, parasites, and fungi. Fungi (such as molds) and some parasites are the only pathogens that are visible; the others are microscopic. First, we will look at bacteria: the microbes that cause most cases of foodborne illness.

BACTERIA

Bacteria are one-celled organisms that are invisible to the eye. Here's some basic facts about them.

- Bacteria are found normally on your skin such as your hands and face, under your fingernails, in cuts and infections, and in your digestive tract.
- Bacteria also exist in the soil, air, and water.
- Refrigeration or freezing does not kill bacteria.
- Adequate cooking does not always prevent foodborne illness. Toxins produced by certain bacteria are not destroyed by heat.

When conditions are right, the number of bacteria can increase rapidly to the point where they cause foodborne illness. To grow, bacteria need the following conditions.

1. *Food*: Certain foods are more likely than others to become unsafe. They are referred to as **Time and Temperature Control for Safety (TCS)) foods** because they require time and temperature controls to prevent the growth of bacteria. **Table 2-1** is a list of TCS foods. You will notice that high protein foods (meat, poultry, seafood, and dairy) are on the list. Bacteria use nutrients, such as protein and also carbohydrates, to survive. You may see that cut melons, leafy greens, and tomatoes are also TCS foods. These foods are protected from outside contaminants until they have been cut. Cutting these foods encourages growth of microorganisms, so refrigeration is essential.
2. *Temperature*: Because bacteria grow rapidly between 41°F and 135°F (5°C and 57°C), this is called the **temperature danger zone** (**Figure 2-1**). This is why it is so important for food to be stored correctly, cooked to the right temperature, and cooked and reheated properly.
3. *Time*: The more time bacteria spend in the temperature danger zone, the more likely they reproduce and grow to unsafe levels.
4. *Moisture and little or no acid*: Bacteria grow better in foods that contain some moisture. For example, they are much more likely to grow in meat than dried rice.

Table 2-1 TCS Foods
Meat (beef, pork, lamb, game)
Poultry
Seafood
Milk and other dairy products
Eggs
Cut leafy greens or cut tomatoes
Cut melon
Raw seed sprouts
Heat-treated plant food (such as cooked rice, baked potatoes, or soy protein such as tofu)
Garlic-in-oil (not treated)

2017 Food Code, p 22, by the U.S. Public Health Service and Food & Drug Administration, 2017. Retrieved from https://www.fda.gov/Food/GuidanceRegulation/Retail Food Protection/FoodCode/ucm595139.htm

They also grow better in food that is neutral to slightly acidic, which includes a lot of foods. Highly acidic foods such as lemons, limes, and tomatoes are not going to provide a place for bacteria to reproduce.

In addition, most bacteria need oxygen, but some bacteria (called anaerobic bacteria) thrive without oxygen and can do well in a garlic-and-oil mixture that has not been treated with an acid (like vinegar) or cooked to 140°F (60°C).

The following are the four ways to prevent foodborne illness.

1. *Practice good personal hygiene*, such as washing hands frequently and wearing clean uniforms and single-use gloves.
2. *Purchase food and beverages from approved, reputable vendors.* Approved suppliers are frequently inspected and meet all local, state, and federal laws. You may want to review copies of inspections, which may be completed by the U.S. Department of Agriculture, the U.S. Food and Drug Administration, or a third-party inspector.
3. *Control time and temperature.* A leading cause of foodborne illness is time and temperature abuse of TCS foods. This occurs when these foods are not cooked to the recommended minimum internal temperature, not held at the proper temperature, or not cooked or reheated properly. The goal is to reduce the amount of time TCS foods are left at temperatures between 41°F and 135°F (5°C and 57°C). In recent years, sanitation inspections have been zeroing in on the cooling of foods prepared a day or more in advance of being served.

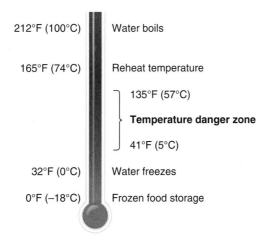

FIGURE 2-1 The Temperature Danger Zone

4.   *Prevent cross-contamination.* **Cross contamination** is the transfer of harmful bacteria from uncooked foods, people, and equipment/surfaces to ready-to-eat foods and cooked foods. For example, if an employee places meat to thaw on the top shelf in the walk-in cooler, some of the juices from the meat may later splatter onto cooked foods on a lower shelf. This is why raw foods are always placed on the bottom shelves. Also, employees should always wash hands before and after handling different foods, because they can transfer harmful bacteria to food.

The predominant bacteria that cause foodborne illness include the following (Centers for Disease Control and Prevention, 2020).

1.   *Salmonella* (nontyphoidal): Poultry and eggs are the typical foods in which *Salmonella* is found, but sometimes it appears in meat and cheese. To prevent foodborne illness, poultry, eggs, and meat should be cooked to proper temperatures, and employees should prevent cross-contamination between raw poultry and cooked or ready-to-eat food.
2.   *Campylobacter jejuni*- Like *Salmonella*, *Campylobacter* is found in chicken. Illness is associated with eating undercooked poultry or from contamination of other foods by raw poultry. Foodborne illness caused by this bug results in diarrhea, and it is one of the most common causes of diarrhea in the United States. To prevent this illness, poultry must be cooked to required temperatures and cross-contamination avoided.
3.   *Clostridium perfringens:* These bacteria are commonly found on raw meat and poultry, and they grow rapidly in the temperature danger zone so they are more likely to cause problems when foods are held for periods of time. Beef, poultry, gravies, and precooked foods are the foods most likely to cause *C. perfringens* infections. To prevent illness, foods must be held at proper temperatures and if not served, they must be cooled and reheated correctly.
4.   *Staphylococcus aureus:* Approximately 20% of healthy adults have this bacteria on their skin and about 30% have it in their nose (Bush, 2018). Problems start when, for example, an employee touches his skin, nose, or an infected cut, and then handles foods without washing his hands. Although these bacteria are killed by heat, they produce heat-stable toxins when the bacteria are allowed to grow to large numbers. Foods associated with transmitting *Staphylococcus* toxins are not usually cooked but require some minimal handling. Examples include sliced meats, tuna salad, and similar salads containing TCS foods and cream pastries. Handwashing, using waterproof bandages, and holding food correctly will all help prevent this illness.

The following bacteria don't cause as many cases of foodborne illness as the bacteria just discussed but are usually more serious and more likely to result in hospitalizations.

1.   *Clostridium botulinum:* This bacterium is unique in that it grows in low oxygen conditions and forms a deadly toxin that can damage your nervous system, causing paralysis and death if not treated. The toxin is made when food is improperly canned. Botulism has also been linked to foods including temperature-abused vegetables (such as baked potatoes wrapped in foil), reduced-oxygen packaged food (such as sous vide meat), and untreated garlic-and-oil mixtures. Canned foods should always be checked for leaking, dents, and bulging before opening, as these are signs of *C. botulinum*. Also, cooked foods need to be held, cooled, and reheated correctly.
2.   *Listeria monocytogenes: Listeria* is unique because it can grow at colder temperatures, such as in the cooler. It causes a disease, called listeriosis, which occurs mostly in pregnant women, newborn babies, people over 65, and people with weakened immune systems. Listeriosis can cause major problems for pregnant women, including miscarriage or fetal death. *Listeria* outbreaks are often linked

to ready-to-eat foods such as lunch and deli meats, frankfurters, ice cream, soft cheeses made with unpasteurized milk, raw sprouts, and smoked seafood.

3. *Escherichia coli* (shiga toxin-producing): *E. coli* are bacteria found in the intestines of animals. Most *E. coli* are harmless, but some strains cause disease when they make a toxin, called Shiga toxin, after the bacteria has entered the human intestine. In most cases, the disease involves diarrhea and vomiting and lasts about five days. However, approximately 5 to 10% of people with the disease develop a life-threatening complication involving the kidneys. The main culprit is raw or undercooked ground beef, although produce may also be contaminated with these bacteria. To prevent disease, ground beef must be cooked to minimum internal temperatures and cross-contamination must be avoided. In addition, employees with diarrhea should not be working with food.

VIRUSES

Viruses are smaller than bacteria and need to live in another living cell to reproduce. While viruses do not grow in food like bacteria, they are transferred through food to another human. People can get viruses from food, water, or air contaminated with viruses. To keep viruses out of the foodservice, employees who are sick need to stay home. Also, employees need to observe proper personal hygiene guidelines, and foods must be purchased from reputable vendors.

The leading cause of foodborne illness is a virus called **norovirus**, which is highly contagious. It causes what is often called the stomach flu, with symptoms including stomach pain, vomiting, and diarrhea. Outbreaks of norovirus illness occur on cruise ships, restaurants, schools, catering facilities, and at home.

You can get norovirus from an infected person, food, or water contaminated with the virus, or by touching contaminated surfaces such as a door knob. Sometimes, a food may be contaminated at its source, such as oysters harvested from contaminated water, or fruits and vegetables contaminated in the field.

Norovirus is primarily spread through food or water contaminated by an infected employee. Employees with norovirus can not only shed billions of noroviruses when they are sick but also during the early stages of recovery. If an infected employee, for example, touches ready-to-eat foods (such as apples) with bare hands or coughs over cooked food, the norovirus will spread to the customers. It takes less than 20 noroviruses to get someone sick.

Following are ways to prevent foodborne norovirus outbreaks.

1. Employees should stay home when sick with vomiting or diarrhea, and for at least 48 hours after symptoms stop.
2. Employees should wash their hands frequently and avoid touching food with bare hands.
3. Fruits and vegetables should be carefully rinsed.
4. Shellfish should be cooked to appropriate temperatures.
5. Clean and sanitize surfaces and utensils.

If an employee becomes sick with norovirus at work, clean and sanitize any affected surfaces and send the employee home immediately.

The hepatitis A virus causes a type of liver disease called hepatitis A. This virus is spread primarily through food or water contaminated by feces from an infected person. It can also be spread by eating shellfish from contaminated waters. Therefore, good personal hygiene and purchasing shellfish from approved, reputable vendors are the two ways to prevent hepatitis A.

Foodborne gastrointestinal viruses such as norovirus can make people ill through contaminated food. There is no evidence of food or food packaging being associated with transmission of COVID-19, the virus that took center stage in early 2020. COVID-19 is a respiratory illness that can spread from person to person. The outbreak first started

BE HEALTHY, BE CLEAN

- Employees - Stay home or leave work if sick; consult doctor if sick, and contact supervisor
- Employers - Instruct sick employees to stay home and send home immediately if sick
- Employers - Pre-screen employees exposed to COVID-19 for temperature and other symptoms

- Wash your hands often with soap and water for at least 20 seconds
- If soap and water are not available, use a 60% alcohol-based hand sanitizer per CDC
- Avoid touching your eyes, nose, and mouth with unwashed hands
- Wear mask/face covering per CDC and FDA

- Never touch Ready-to-Eat foods with bare hands
- Use single service gloves, deli tissue, or suitable utensils
- Wrap food containers to prevent cross contamination
- Follow 4 steps to food safety Clean, Separate, Cook, and Chill

CLEAN AND DISINFECT

- Train employees on cleaning and disinfecting procedures, and protective measures, per CDC and FDA
- Have and use cleaning products and supplies
- Follow protective measures

- Disinfect high-touch surfaces frequently
- Use EPA-registered disinfectant
- Ensure food containers and utensils are cleaned and sanitized

- Prepare and use sanitizers according to label instructions
- Offer sanitizers and wipes to customers to clean grocery cart/basket handles, or utilize store personnel to conduct cleaning/sanitizing

SOCIAL DISTANCE

- Help educate employees and customers on importance of social distancing:
  - Signs
  - Audio messages
  - Consider using every other check-out lane to aid in distancing

- Avoid displays that may result in customer gatherings; discontinue self-serve buffets and salad bars; discourage employee gatherings
- Place floor markings and signs to encourage social distancing

- Shorten customer time in store by encouraging them to:
  - Use shopping lists
  - Order ahead of time, if offered
- Set up designated pick-up areas inside or outside retail establishments

PICK-UP AND DELIVERY

- If offering delivery options:
  - Ensure coolers and transport containers are cleaned and sanitized
  - Maintain time and temperature controls
  - Avoid cross contamination; for example, wrap food during transport

- Encourage customers to use "no touch" deliveries
- Notify customers as the delivery is arriving by text message or phone call

- Establish designated pick-up zones for customers
- Offer curb-side pick-up
- Practice social distancing by offering to place orders in vehicle trunks

FIGURE 2-2 Summary of Best Practices for Foodservices During the COVID-19 Pandemic
U.S. Food and Drug Administration.

in China, but the virus spread internationally and in the United States. Foodservices can prevent and slow the spread of COVID-19 in the workplace by coordinating with state and local health officials. **Figure 2-2** summarizes best practices for foodservices.

In addition to resources at the U.S. Food and Drug Administration (FDA), the following are additional resources from the Centers for Disease Control and Prevention (CDC) on COVID-19.

- For additional information when employees may have been exposed to COVID-19, refer to "CDC's Interim Guidance for Implementing Safety Practices for Critical Infrastructure Workers Who May Have Had Exposure to a Person with Suspected or Confirmed COVID-19."
- For additional information on employee health and hygiene and recommendations to help prevent worker transmission of foodborne illness, refer to "FDA's Employee Health and Personal Hygiene Handbook."
  - If FDA recommendations differ from CDC's regarding employee health and COVID-19, follow the CDC's recommendations.
- For returning previously sick employees to work, refer to "CDC's Guidance for Discontinuation of Home Isolation for Persons with COVID-19."
- Follow CDC and FDA information on **personal protective equipment** (i.e., gloves, face masks/coverings, and protective gear).
- Understand risk at the workplace—use "OSHA's Guidance on Preparing Workplaces for COVID-19."

Other Pathogens

Two additional groups of pathogens include parasites and fungi, which are less common causes of foodborne illness. **Parasites** are organisms that can be transmitted to humans by consumption of contaminated food and water. Like viruses, parasites don't grow in food but need a host to live and reproduce. Parasites are most commonly associated with:

- Seafood (especially sushi that has not been handled properly)
- Wild game
- Contaminated water
- Foods such as chopped lettuce and other fresh produce that are processed with contaminated water
- Employees who have a parasite and contaminate food or water due to poor handwashing

To prevent problems with parasites, good personal hygiene as well as purchasing from approved, reputable suppliers is vital. Also, all seafood should be cooked to minimum internal temperatures.

Fungi are more likely to spoil food than to make people sick, and they are often visible. Fungi include mold and yeast. **Molds** are made of many cells and can sometimes be seen with the naked eye, such as mold on bread. Mold can grow on plant or animal food and growth is encouraged by warm and humid conditions. Unlike bacteria, molds can grow under other conditions as well, including in acidic foods (such as jams and jellies) and in foods with little moisture content (such as cured meats). Refrigeration does not kill them—they can continue to grow there. Although molds are used to make certain kinds of cheeses (such as Roquefort), some molds can cause illness.

A few molds, under the right conditions, produce **mycotoxins**, which are poisonous and may cause allergic reactions. There are different kinds of mycotoxins, and depending on which one, they can cause damage to the nervous system or liver. They occur in foods such as grains; tree nuts such as almonds, peanuts, spices, milk; and sometimes apple and grape juice. Of particular importance is **aflatoxin**—a group of toxins found on crops such as peanuts and tree nuts. Aflatoxin-producing fungi can contaminate crops in the field, at harvest, and during storage. Aflatoxins cause liver damage and increase the risk of liver cancer.

To avoid problems with mold, you should throw out foods with visible mold. The only foods that are okay to eat after cutting away moldy areas include hard cheese and hard salami. When cutting out moldy areas in these foods, cut out an area at least one inch from the visible mold. Reduce your aflatoxin exposure by buying only major commercial brands of nuts and nut butters and by discarding nuts that look moldy, discolored, or shriveled.

Yeast also belongs to the fungus family, but they are single-celled organisms. Yeast break down carbohydrates in foods such as jellies, jams, syrup, and fruit juice. Most yeast spoilage is detected as an off smell or taste, which can taste like alcohol. If there are any signs of yeast, such as white or pink slime, the food should be discarded.

Seafood and Plant Toxins

Up to this point, we have looked at microorganisms that cause foodborne illness. It is also possible to get foodborne illness from shellfish or fin fish that contain toxins. For example, **ciguatoxin** may be found in fin fish, such as red snapper and grouper that ate smaller fish that, in turn, ate toxic algae containing this toxin. Ciguatoxin is not destroyed through cooking and can cause nervous system symptoms that persist for months.

Scombroid poisoning is due to a combination of substances, most often histamine, that form when certain fish aren't properly refrigerated before being processed or cooked. Examples of fish that can form the toxin if they start to spoil include tuna,

THE BIG PICTURE

In most cases, unsafe food has been contaminated with harmful substances. Although food can become contaminated for chemical reasons (perhaps a pesticide was sprayed in an area with food that wasn't covered) or physical reasons (perhaps a paper clip fell into a bowl of mashed potatoes), the greatest threat to food safety is biological.

Biological hazards include these three groups.

1. Pathogenic microbes:
   a. Bacteria—When conditions are right, the number of bacteria can increase rapidly to the point where they cause foodborne illness. To grow best, bacteria like TCS foods, time to grow, and a temperature in the danger zone (41°–135°F or 5°–57°C). Bacteria cause many cases of foodborne illness.
   b. Viruses—Viruses do not grow in food like bacteria, they simply use food to get to their next victim. To keep viruses out of the foodservice, employees who are sick need to stay home. Also, employees need to observe proper personal hygiene guidelines and foods must be purchased from reputable vendors. Norovirus causes many cases of foodborne illness and is spread by infected employees.
   c. Fungi—Fungi includes molds and they are more likely to spoil food than cause foodborne illness, except in the case of nuts.
2. Parasites—Parasites are associated with seafood, wild game, and contaminated water.
3. Toxins—Toxins can occur in these foods: fin fish, shellfish, and plants such as wild mushrooms. Toxins are not destroyed when foods are cooked.

mackerel, and mahi-mahi. The fish might not look or smell bad, but it can cause illness. What sets it apart from all other seafood poisonings is that it is totally preventable if the fish are handled and refrigerated correctly. Along with ciguatoxin, it is one of the most common illnesses caused by seafood. The symptoms, which are treated with antihistamines by a health professional, usually are mild and start within minutes or hours after eating. They may include tingling or burning of the mouth or throat, rash or hives, dizziness, nausea, low blood pressure, and itching.

In addition, toxins are possible in shellfish. **Shellfish poisoning** is caused when shellfish feed on algae that produce toxins. Eating these shellfish results in a wide variety of symptoms, depending on which toxin is present; its concentration in the shellfish; and how much shellfish is eaten. For example, Neurotoxic Shellfish Poisoning (NSP) is a disease caused by eating oysters, clams, mussels, or scallops contaminated with brevetoxins, compounds that are tasteless and cause neurological and gastrointestinal symptoms in humans.

Certain plant foods may also contain toxins. For example, some wild mushrooms contain poisonous toxins that are not likely to be destroyed by washing, cooking, or freezing. Many poisonous wild mushrooms are almost impossible to tell apart from those that aren't poisonous.

To avoid toxins in seafood or plants, the most important step to take is to purchase only from approved, reputable vendors. Also, in the case of scombroid poisoning, it is important to prevent time and temperature abuse from the moment it is received until it is served. In general, seafood has to be handled very carefully to prevent foodborne illness.

2.2 DESCRIBE SAFE PERSONAL HYGIENE PRACTICES

When foodservice employees pay attention to good personal hygiene, it is a step in preventing foodborne illness. Employees who are sick can contaminate food in many ways, such as by coughing, sneezing, and touching foods without gloves (especially after using the bathroom and not washing hands). Employees who are not outwardly sick can also cause foodborne illness. Consider an employee with an infected cut that is not properly covered or an employee who is a carrier. A **carrier** is someone who carries a pathogen but has no symptoms. Unfortunately, a carrier can pass the pathogen to others. For example, some healthy adults carry *Staphylococcus aureus* on their skin, which can easily be transferred to food if, for example, an employee mixes up tuna salad with his bare hands.

This section will discuss the essentials of personal hygiene. Handwashing is the most important component of personal hygiene, and employees should wash hands in a sink dedicated solely to handwashing (not in a sink used for food preparation or washing pots and pans). Here are the steps for washing hands (**Figure 2-3**).

1. Wet your hands and wrists with running, warm water.
2. Apply soap and lather your hands by rubbing them together with the soap. Be sure to lather the backs of your hands, between your fingers, under your nails, and your wrists.
3. Scrub your hands for at least 20 seconds.
4. Rinse your hands well under running, warm water.
5. Dry your hands and wrists by using a clean towel or air dryer.

If you use a paper towel, you can use the towel to turn off the faucet or open the restroom door to prevent contamination.

When employees have to use their hands to make a cold sandwich, for example, they must use single-use (or disposable) gloves. The reason is that the sandwich will not be cooked any further and is, therefore, considered a ready-to-eat food. Gloves are used primarily to protect the food from pathogens on an employee's hands. Like their name implies, single-use gloves are used for one task only and must be changed often. Here are some rules for using gloves.

- Always wash hands before putting on gloves.
- Change gloves between tasks, especially between handling raw products and ready-to-eat products.

Be a Germ-Buster...
WASH YOUR HANDS!

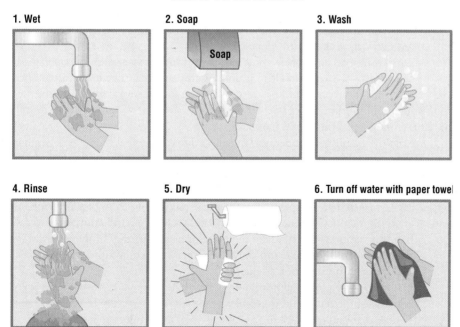

FIGURE 2-3 How to Wash Hands

Reproduced with permission from the Washington State Department of Health.

- Discard torn or damaged gloves. In any case, gloves should always be removed after four hours of continuous use.
- Do not wash or reuse gloves.

Also, employees should not blow into gloves or roll them to make them easier to put on, as that introduces microbes inside the gloves. Disposable gloves must be the type that are "approved" for use in foodservice.

The following is additional guidance on employee personal hygiene.

1. Before Going to Work
   - Employees who are not feeling well must call in to their supervisor, especially if there are any gastrointestinal symptoms such as vomiting or diarrhea, fever, or signs of jaundice (yellowing of the skin), which is a sign of hepatitis A. Employees who have typical cold symptoms are generally not allowed to work with food or equipment. Employees with vomiting, diarrhea, or jaundice cannot work at all. Neither can employees who have been diagnosed with norovirus, hepatitis A, *Salmonella* (typhoidal or nontyphoidal), *Shigella spp.*, or *E. coli* that produce shiga toxins. When an employee reports one of these diagnoses or jaundice, the manager must also notify the regulatory authority.
   - Employees should shower or bathe before work.
2. At Work: Dress Code
   - If possible, employees should change from street clothes into clean work clothes in an employee locker room just prior to starting work. Don't wear anything knit or fuzzy like sweaters or velour as they cause static electricity and attract dust, hair, and lint. Keep street clothes and jackets in lockers, not food preparation areas.
   - Employees should wear only jewelry that is permitted in the dress code, such as a plain ring. Jewelry can collect and spread harmful pathogens and also fall into the food.
   - Fingernails should be short and clean without nail polish or false fingernails.
   - Many employees will have to wear a hair covering, such as a hat or hairnet, to keep hairs from falling into the food or onto food-contact surfaces. Beard guards should be worn by anyone with facial hair (**Figure 2-4**).
   - Any cuts, wounds, or boils should be completely covered with a waterproof bandage. If the wound or boil is located on the hand or wrist, it should also be covered with a single-use glove.
   - Dirty uniforms and aprons can carry bacteria and other pathogens, so employees need to change into clean uniforms and aprons as needed. Aprons should be removed before handling trash or using the rest room, and also when leaving food preparation areas.
3. At Work: Preventing Food Contamination
   - Employees must be trained and monitored to ensure that they wash their hands after using the restroom, eating, drinking, handling raw proteins (meat, poultry, seafood), touching their body or clothing, coughing or sneezing, using a tissue, touching money or an electronic device (such as a cell phone), taking out trash, handling cleaning chemicals, returning from break, or touching anything that may contaminate their hands. Using a hand sanitizer, also called hand antiseptics, does not take the place of handwashing. Only use hand sanitizers *after* handwashing, and only use sanitizers that comply with U.S. Food and Drug Administration standards.
   - Use single-use gloves appropriately when handling ready-to-eat food (except when washing fruits and vegetables).
   - Eating, drinking, or smoking are not allowed in areas where food is prepared or served or where there are clean utensils and equipment. This is because these activities can result in saliva being transferred from mouth to hands. Eating, drinking or smoking should only be in designated areas, with one exception.

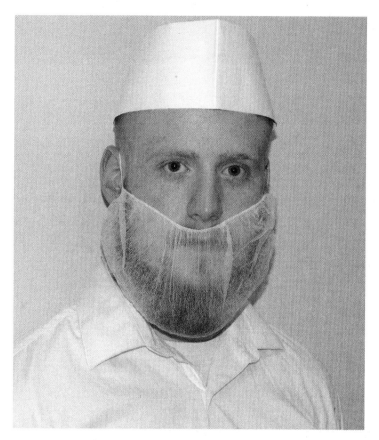

FIGURE 2-4 Beard Guard

Employees may drink from a closed beverage container (such as cup with lid and straw) as long it is handled to prevent contamination of the employee's hands, the container, and any exposed food, equipment, etc., in the area.

2.3 APPLY FOOD SAFETY PRINCIPLES

Before looking at good food safety practices for each area of a foodservice operation, we need to look at an important piece of equipment: thermometers. Using a thermometer is the only reliable way to know that a food is cooked to the right temperature or that foods are being held at correct temperatures. Thermometers in storage areas also help us ensure that foods in storage are safe. **Figure 2-5** shows various types of thermometers.

The most inexpensive food thermometer is the **instant read thermometer**, also known as the **bimetal thermometer**. This thermometer takes about 15 to 20 seconds to measure temperature. For accurate measurement, the probe of the thermometer must be inserted *up to the dimple on the stem*—about two to three inches. This thermometer needs to be calibrated regularly to maintain accuracy. Just under the head of the thermometer where you read the temperature, there is a calibration nut that can be used to keep the thermometer accurate. Use the ice-point method to calibrate this thermometer (**Figure 2-6**).

Thermocouple thermometers and **thermistor thermometers** are more expensive but have a faster response time (2 to 10 seconds), high accuracy, and digital display. In both thermometers, the temperature is sensed at the tip of the probe so you don't have to insert it as deep into food as the instant read thermometers.

Thermocouples and thermistors are different types of technology. Thermistor technology is often used in **digital instant-read thermometers**, and thermocouple

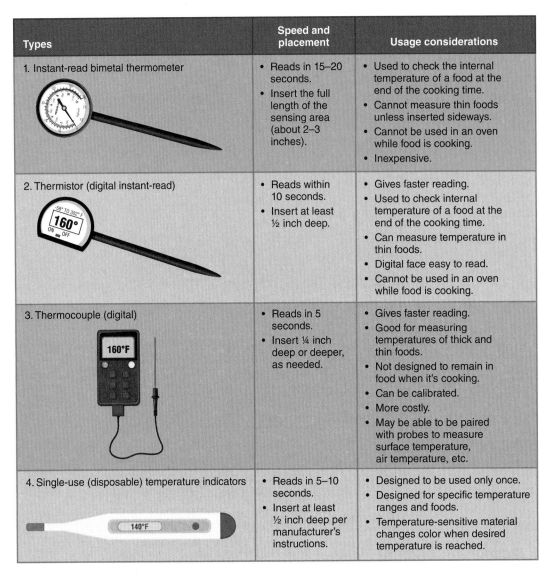

Types	Speed and placement	Usage considerations
1. Instant-read bimetal thermometer	• Reads in 15–20 seconds. • Insert the full length of the sensing area (about 2–3 inches).	• Used to check the internal temperature of a food at the end of the cooking time. • Cannot measure thin foods unless inserted sideways. • Cannot be used in an oven while food is cooking. • Inexpensive.
2. Thermistor (digital instant-read)	• Reads within 10 seconds. • Insert at least ½ inch deep.	• Gives faster reading. • Used to check internal temperature of a food at the end of the cooking time. • Can measure temperature in thin foods. • Digital face easy to read. • Cannot be used in an oven while food is cooking.
3. Thermocouple (digital)	• Reads in 5 seconds. • Insert ¼ inch deep or deeper, as needed.	• Gives faster reading. • Good for measuring temperatures of thick and thin foods. • Not designed to remain in food when it's cooking. • Can be calibrated. • More costly. • May be able to be paired with probes to measure surface temperature, air temperature, etc.
4. Single-use (disposable) temperature indicators	• Reads in 5–10 seconds. • Insert at least ½ inch deep per manufacturer's instructions.	• Designed to be used only once. • Designed for specific temperature ranges and foods. • Temperature-sensitive material changes color when desired temperature is reached.

FIGURE 2-5 Types and Uses of Food Thermometers

Data from "Thermy: Types of Food Thermometers," by the United States Department of Agriculture, 2013. Retrieved from https://www.fsis.usda.gov/wps/portal/fsis/topics/food-safety-education/teach-others/fsis-educational-campaigns/thermy/types-of-food-thermometers

technology is seen in the larger thermometers. Thermocouple thermometers can often be paired with a variety of probes for different applications.

- An immersion probe measures the temperature of liquids, such as frying oil.
- A penetration probe measures the internal temperatures of food and are really useful for thin foods such as a fish fillet or hamburger patty.
- A surface probe measures surface temperature, such as that of a griddle.
- An air probe can measure the air temperature inside a cooler, freezer, or oven.

Single-use (or disposable) temperature indicators may be used for foods and to test the water temperature for dishwashers. They are accurate, easy to use, and read temperatures quickly (within 5 to 10 seconds). They are designed to be used within specific temperature ranges and for specific foods—such as to determine if beef has been cooked to 165°F (74°C). The sensor is inserted into a food and when the food reaches the safe temperature, the sensor changes color. The sensor is designed to be used once.

1. Fill a large glass or measuring cup with finely crushed ice. Add cold water so glass is full. Stir well.

2. Submerge the stem of the bimetal thermometer in the ice water so that the stem does not touch or get close to the sides or bottom of the glass. In the photo, the thermometer is clipped to its case which rests on the top of the glass so the thermometer stays in place properly.

3. Wait at least one minute or until the needle stops moving before reading the dial. If the thermometer reads 32°F (0 °C), the thermometer is correctly calibrated. If not, use a small hex wrench to adjust the hex nut under the head of the thermometer until the needle points to 32°F (0 °C).

Note: If using a digital thermometer with a reset button, adjust the thermometer to read 32°F (0 °C) while the thermometer is sitting in the ice water if needed.

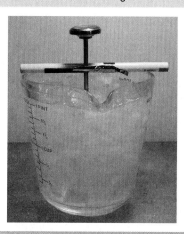

FIGURE 2-6 How to Calibrate a Bimetal Thermometer

Infrared thermometers do not measure internal temperatures. Instead, they only measure surface temperatures from up to four feet away and can provide a quick check of temperatures of food at receiving and storage. Because there is no need to touch food, there is less chance for cross-contamination.

Whichever thermometer you are using, there are some general guidelines to follow.

1. After using a thermometer, clean and sanitize it. Individually wrapped thermometer wipes can be purchased to sanitize a thermometer. Then let it air dry. If the thermometer fits into a case, keep the case clean as well.

2. Using the manufacturer's instructions, calibrate a thermometer as recommended. Bimetal thermometers tend to lose accuracy after they have been bumped or dropped, so they must be calibrated regularly. Thermometers must be accurate to within ±2°F or 1°C.

3. Bimetal thermometers should be inserted into food up to the dimple on the stem and for 15 seconds in order to get an accurate temperature. Thermocouple and thermistor thermometers don't need to be pushed in as far and the temperature can generally be read within 5 seconds.

4. Always insert the thermometer into the thickest part of food and take at least one additional reading in a different spot.

PURCHASING AND RECEIVING

Food and beverages must be purchased from approved, reputable vendors. Approved suppliers have met all local, state, and federal laws, and have been inspected. You can request a recent inspection report and review it to see how well the vendor performs in food safety and quality. Inspections may be completed by the U.S. Department of Agriculture, the FDA, or a third-party inspector.

Receiving clerks are responsible for inspecting foods as they are delivered and also for putting goods into storage. Guidelines to keep food safe during receiving include the following.

1. Because many of the goods being delivered need to be kept cold or frozen, it is important to *schedule deliveries* so the receiving clerks have the time to inspect them properly and put them into storage in a timely manner. Also, receiving clerks should have the loading dock(s) clear and all storage areas in good order before deliveries come in.

2. When delivery trucks pull up to the loading dock, the *inspection process* begins. The receiver should look inside the truck to make sure it is clean and free of bad odors and pests. The receiver should also check that refrigerated foods are delivered on a refrigerated truck. The clerk should check frozen goods for signs of thawing and refreezing such as fluid leakage or damp packaging. While counting items and checking the delivery against the invoice, the receiver can also look for damaged or spoiled goods. For example, the clerk may find mold on strawberries, rusty #10 cans, slimy fresh beef, smelly fresh fish, warm milk, or fresh bread past the sell-by date. The clerk may also find that fresh produce or canned goods that traveled in a freezer truck under an insulated blanket may have frozen precut salads or canned goods that split or exploded because of the cold. Rejected items should be set aside and reasons for rejection noted on the invoice and/or receiving log.

3. Take *sample temperatures* of all TCS foods, being sure to sanitize the thermometer after each use. When taking temperatures, insert the thermometer into the thickest part of the food and make sure the stem does not touch the package. To test the temperature of reduced-oxygen packaging food, place the thermometer stem between two packages—do not puncture the packaging. **Table 2-2** shows temperature requirements for receiving foods.

4. Check for U.S. Department of Agriculture *inspection stamps* on meat, poultry, and egg cartons.

5. Shellfish (including oysters, mussels, scallops, and clams) must be delivered with a *shellfish identification tag* (**Figure 2-7**) on the container that identifies where the shellfish were harvested and when. Once the shellfish are used up, the date should be put on the tag and the tag must be removed and held for 90 days. This is done in case a foodborne illness related to these shellfish occurs so that the source of the problem can be identified. This is especially critical if you serve raw oysters.

Table 2-2 Temperature Requirements When Receiving Foods	
Fresh meat, poultry, fish	Receive at 41°F (5°C) or lower.
Shellfish	Shucked shellfish: Receive at 45°F (7°C) or lower. Then cool to 41°F (5°C) or lower within four hours.
	Live shellfish: Receive at air temperature of 45°F (7°C) or lower and internal temperature no higher than 50°F (10°C). Then cool to 41°F (5°C) or lower within four hours.
Milk	Receive at 45°F (7°C) or lower. Then cool to 41°F (5°C) or lower within four hours.
Raw (shell) eggs	Receive in refrigerated equipment that maintains an air temperature of 45°F (7°C) or lower.
Hot TCS foods	Receive at 135°F (57°C) or higher.

Data from *2017 Food Code*, p. 62, by the U.S. Public Health Service and Food & Drug Administration, 2017. *National Shellfish Sanitation Program Guide for the Control of Molluscan Shellfish*, p. 108, by the Interstate Shellfish Sanitation Conference, 2015.

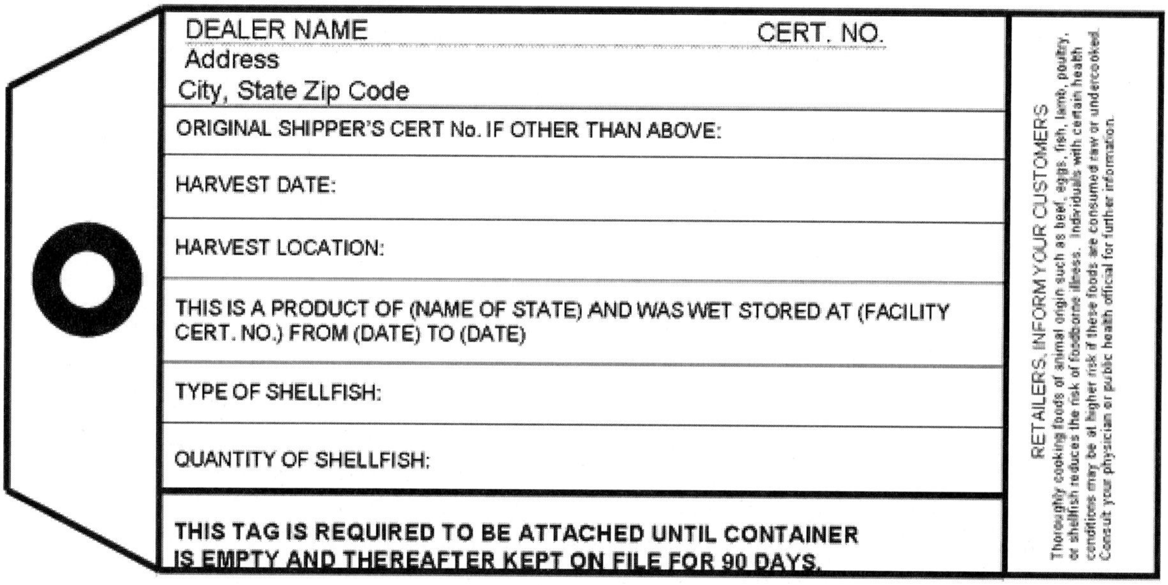

FIGURE 2-7 Example of a Shellfish Identification Tag with Minimum Required Information

National Shellfish Sanitation Program Guide for the Control of Molluscan Shellfish, p. 335. by the Interstate Shellfish Sanitation Conference, 2015. Retrieved from https://www.fda.gov/downloads/Food/GuidanceRegulation/FederalStateFoodPrograms/UCM505093.pdf

STORING FOODS

Once the paperwork is completed, cold and frozen foods should be put away as soon as possible. Use the following guidelines when putting away and storing foods.

1. *When receiving clerks put foods into storage, they must use the first-in, first-out (FIFO) method of stock rotation.* Using the FIFO system, foods are shelved based on use-by or expiration dates, so older foods are used first. For example, if the boxes of cereal you just received in April have a use-by date of 7/18 of the current year, and the cereal in stock has a use-by date of 6/1 of the current year, the employee should put the cereals with the 6/1 date in front of the cereals with the 7/18 date. When putting foods away, employees must regularly check use-by and expiration dates and discard food that is beyond either date.

2. *All foods need to be labeled with product names, and many operations put receiving dates on all incoming food.* Any food not in its original container, such as flour that has been put in a bin, must be labeled with the name of the food. Any ready-to-eat TCS food that will be held for more than 24 hours must be marked with a use-by date that is no more than seven days beyond when it was received. The same rule applies to TCS foods, such as egg salad, that are prepared in the foodservice. Once prepared, many foodservices label them with both the date the food was made (such as February 7) and the use-by or discard date (such as February 14). If an employee combines two TCS foods with different discard dates, the new discard date should be the earliest of the two.

3. *All foods need to be stored at appropriate temperatures.* Dry storage areas should be maintained between 50°F (10°C) and 70°F (21°C). Cold pipes and air conditioning ducts should be wrapped with insulation so that liquid condensate is not dripping on food or floors. Higher temperatures may shorten the shelf life of dry goods. High humidity in dry storage areas (over 60%) can cause cans to rust and grains (such as crackers) to get moldy. TCS foods must be kept at an internal temperature of 41°F (5°C) or lower, and it is best to store meat, poultry, seafood,

and dairy in the coldest part of the cooler or freezer. Shelving should be open to allow for air circulation. If you overload a cooler or freezer, it prevents good air circulation necessary to maintain proper temperatures. Moisture forming on the refrigerator ceiling and black mold indicate poor air circulation and temperature inconsistencies. Storage areas must have at least one thermometer that measures air temperature and it must be accurate to within ± 3°F (± 1.5°C). Thermometers are placed in the warmest part of cold storage areas (generally by the door). Temperatures in all storage areas are checked often and documented on forms such as seen in **Table 2-3**. Higher humidity helps fruits and vegetables stay fresh, so keep the relative humidity at 85 to 95% if you have a cooler containing just fruits and vegetables.

4. *Food storage areas must be kept clean and dry.* To keep floors clean and reduce cross contamination and pests, food is always stored at least six inches above the ground and six inches away from the wall. Any spills should be mopped up quickly. Upper shelving should be wire mesh or slotted to allow air circulation, but bottom shelves should be solid to prevent food from being exposed to mop spray when floors are cleaned.

5. *Food has to be stored properly to avoid cross-contamination.* Never store food near dirty linens, cleaning chemicals or pesticides, exposed waste or sewer lines, or under anything that could drip moisture. Also, never store food in a room such as a locker room or garbage room. If food is put into a container, the container should be approved for food use, leakproof, sanitized, covered, and labeled. Live shellfish should always be stored in their original container. Due to splash contamination from handwashing, sanitation inspectors are beginning to recommend splash protection on the sides of the sink (**Figure 2–8**).

6. *Store raw meat, poultry, and seafood separately or away from ready-to-eat foods,* because you don't want poultry juices, for example, to accidentally contaminate a food that won't get any further cooking. If you must store these raw foods on the same shelving with ready-to-eat foods, always store the ready-to-eat foods

Table 2-3 Refrigerator Temperature Log			
Daily Temperature Log for Walk-In Refrigerator #1			
Instructions: Every day, the designated employee(s) will record the time and temperature using the thermometer in the rear of the refrigerator. The employee must also initial the log. If the refrigerator is not between 36°F and 41°F, circle the date and inform your supervisor immediately. The corrective action must then be noted on the back of this form. Month/Year: _____			
Date	**Time Temperature Taken**	**Temperature**	**Employee Initials**
1			
2			
3			
4			
5			
6			
7			
8			
9			
10			

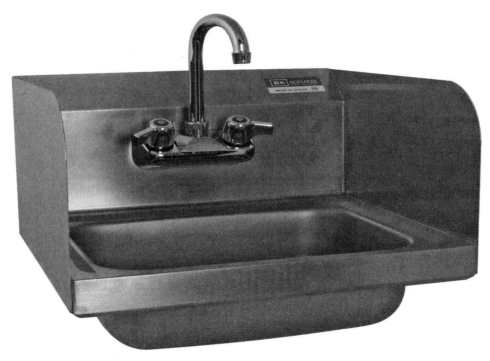

FIGURE 2-8 Hand Sink with Side Splashes
Courtesy of Franklin Machine Products.

above raw meat, poultry, or seafood. When storing these raw protein foods in the same rack, they should be stored in the following top-to-bottom order: seafood, whole cuts of beef and pork, ground meats and ground fish, and whole or ground poultry on the very bottom shelf. This order is based on the fact that the minimum internal temperature of each food (once cooked) increases as you move down the rack from seafood to poultry. The food requiring the highest internal cooked temperature (whole or ground poultry) is at the bottom.

7. *Store cut melons, cut tomatoes, and cut leafy greens at 41°F (5°C) or lower*, as they are considered to be TCS foods.

FOOD PREPARATION

Food preparation includes all the steps taken in a kitchen from pulling foods from storage areas to preparing and cooking foods for service. Thawing foods, especially frozen meats, poultry, and seafood, must be done safely and in a timely manner. There are several ways to defrost foods. The easiest method is to move foods from the freezer to the refrigerator, but this method can also take a number of days before large pieces of meat, for example, are thawed. If a schedule is developed so that cooks know when to pull meats out of the freezer, this method can work well. A faster thawing method is to place the food in a pan and submerge it under running water that is 70°F (21°C) or lower. The food should not go over 41°F (5°C) for more than four hours. Food can be thawed in the microwave only if it will be cooked immediately after thawing. Some thin foods, such as hamburger patties, are thawed as part of the cooking process.

Additional guidelines for preparation and cooking follow.

1. *Prepare raw meat, poultry, and seafood separately from fresh fruits and vegetables*. Many foodservices use color-coded cutting boards, such as green cutting boards for fruits and vegetables, red cutting boards for raw meat, yellow for raw poultry,

and blue cutting boards for cooked foods. This decreases the chances of cross-contamination. In addition, to decrease cross-contamination of foods with peanuts or other foods associated with food allergies, purple cutting boards are used, along with purple-handled chefs' knives and serving utensils (**Figure 2-9**). Approximately 90% of food allergy reactions are due to the "Big 8" foods: milk, eggs, peanuts, tree nuts, fish, crustacean shellfish, wheat, and soy.

2. *Clean and sanitize work areas and equipment between uses*, such as after working with TCS foods. Cleaning removes food, grease, and other soil from a surface. *To sanitize* means to reduce the number of bacteria and other pathogens on a surface to safe levels. Dishes and other equipment are sanitized through either high heat (171°F or 77°C for at least 30 seconds) or chemical sanitizers with ingredients like chlorine, iodine, or quaternary ammonium compounds. Recent research shows that *Listeria monocytogenes* may be tolerant to quaternary ammonium compounds, so chlorine sanitizers are recommended for sanitizing equipment, etc., used for foods that could contain *Listeria* (Kovacevic et al., 2016)

3. *During preparation, remove only enough food from the cooler that can be prepared within a short period of time.* Prepare food in small batches, especially when handling raw meat, poultry, or seafood; making cold salads such as chicken salad that contain TCS foods; cracking eggs into a bowl with other eggs (called pooled eggs); or coating foods with breading or batters. Once preparation is complete, either cook the foods or return to the cooler. Also, clean and sanitize all surfaces and equipment.

4. *Wash fresh produce vigorously under cold running water or by using chemicals that comply with the FDA Food Code or your local health department.* Always wash produce *before* cutting or combining with another ingredient and pull apart produce (such as lettuce) to wash all surfaces. Effective commercial fruit and vegetable washes are available and normally consist of a 60 ppm (parts per million) peracetic acid solution (Cornell University Cooperative Extension, 2015). Packaged fruits and vegetables that have already been washed do *not* need to be washed again.

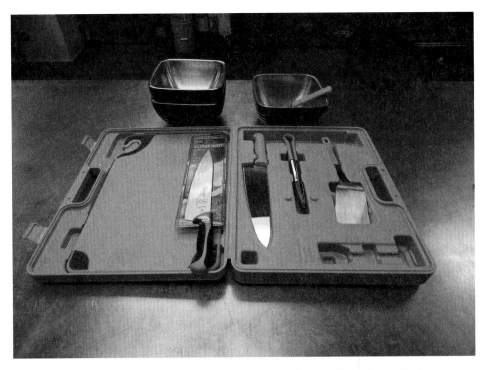

FIGURE 2-9 Big 8 Allergen-Free Zones are Commonly Designated Using Purple Tools

5. *When using ice in the kitchen, use sanitized ice scoops to pick up and transfer ice—no hands allowed!* Store the ice scoop outside of the ice machine. If raw meat, poultry, or fish are held on ice, dispose of the ice after use and clean and sanitize the container.

6. *Cook food to required minimum internal temperatures* (**Table 2-4**). The guidelines in Table 2-4 are mostly from the 2017 *Food Code* (2017), which is released every four years by the FDA. Cooking temperatures may vary in your operation depending on the local regulations. When cooking, avoid putting too much food into an oven, fryer, or other equipment, as it makes it hard to get everything fully cooked. Keep in mind that cooking to required temperatures will destroy pathogens, but it neither eliminates their toxins nor seafood or plant toxins.

7. *If your operation serves raw or undercooked TCS items, you must disclose this and include a warning on your menu* such as: "This item is served raw or undercooked. Consuming raw or undercooked meats, poultry, seafood, shellfish, or eggs may increase your risk of foodborne illness." Raw or undercooked TCS items are not recommended for children, the elderly, or anyone with a compromised immune system.

8. *Follow safe procedures when partially cooking foods to be finished just before service.* During the initial cooking, do not heat the food for more than 60 minutes. Cool the food immediately, then hold cold or frozen and keep away from ready-to-eat food. Be sure to label the food as "partially cooked" with the date. Finally, heat the food to its required minimum internal temperature and serve. When splitting up the cooking of foods like this, you are required to have written procedures and cooling logs to show the local regulatory authority, including how the operation will monitor and document the process.

Table 2-4 Minimum Internal Cooking Temperatures*

165°F (74°C) for 1 second

- Poultry (whole or ground)
- Stuffed meat, stuffed poultry, stuffed seafood, or stuffed pasta
- Stuffing containing meat, poultry, fish
- Wild game animals

155°F (68°C) for 17 seconds

- Ground meat (such as ground beef or ground pork)
- Ground, chopped, or minced seafood
- Injected meats (such as flavor-injected meat or brined ham)
- Shell eggs that will be held in steam table for service
- Ratites (such as ostrich and emu)

145°F (63°C) for 4 minutes

- Whole meat roasts (beef, veal, lamb, pork, cured pork such as ham)
  (Alternate cooking temperature and times are given such as 155°F for 22 seconds, 149°F for 85 seconds, 140°F for 12 minutes, or 135°F for 36 minutes.)

145°F (63°C) for 15 seconds

- Steaks/chops of beef, veal, pork, lamb
- Seafood (shellfish, fin fish, crustaceans)
- Shell eggs cracked and cooked for immediate service
- Game animals (commercially raised)

135°F (57°C)

- Plant foods (grains, legumes, vegetables, fruits) that are cooked for hot holding

*If using a microwave oven, raw animal foods should be cooked to at least 165°F (74°C) in all parts and the food should be rotated or stirred during cooking to more evenly distribute the heat.

2017 Food Code, p 84-91, by the U.S. Public Health Service and Food & Drug Administration, 2017. Retrieved from https://www.fda.gov/Food/GuidanceRegulation/Retail Food Protection/FoodCode/ucm595139.htm

9. *When hot food is not going to be served immediately, you must cool and reheat foods properly.* To cool hot foods, first cool from 135°F to 70°F (57°C to 21°C) within two hours. Then cool it from 70°F to 41°F (21°C to 5°C) or lower in the next four hours. Therefore, the cooling process must get hot TCS foods to 41°F (5°C) or lower within six hours. Proper cooling methods include using rapid cooling equipment (such as a blast chiller) or placing food in small metal pans in an ice bath. Stirring the food often helps cool it faster. Using an ice paddle (a plastic paddle filled with ice) for stirring quickens the process even more.

10. *When reheating food for immediate service, you can reheat to any temperature with one exception. If reheating a TCS food that will then be held hot (as in a steam table) before service, the food must be reheated to 165°F (74°C) for 15 seconds.*

SERVICE

There are a range of guidelines for service, keeping in mind the many ways in which food is served. In some cases, foods are made to order and served immediately. In other cases, food is held, such as on a steam table where an employee will serve the food. Many foodservices also have self-service food bars such as a salad bar. The following are guidelines for different service situations.

1. *When foods are not served immediately, you must hold hot foods at an internal temperature of 135°F (57°C) or higher and cold foods at an internal temperature of 41°F (5°C) or lower.* Temperatures must be checked at least every four hours. If you check temperatures every four hours and a hot food is now below 135°F (57°C), you have to throw out the food. However, if you check the temperature every two hours and find that a hot food is below 135°F (57°C), you can reheat it up to 135°F (57°C) and put it back into the hot-holding unit. Every operation must have a policy about how often temperatures are taken, how they are documented, and when food will be thrown out.

2. *Hot-holding equipment is not to be used to warm food up to 135°F (57°C), unless the equipment was designed to do so.*

3. *Some operations can hold TCS foods without temperature controls when using certain guidelines.* Operations that serve mostly high-risk populations are not allowed to do this. High-risk populations include preschool-age children, elderly people, and people with compromised immune systems. Cold foods must have an initial temperature of 41°F (5°C) or lower, and time must be marked so employees know when the food must be removed. After 6 hours, or if the food temperature gets higher than 70°F (21°C), the food must be thrown away. Hot foods must have an initial temperature of 135°F (57°C) or higher and may be held for four hours before being thrown away. The time must also be noted. Written policies and procedures should be maintained when holding TCS foods without temperature control.

4. *Food that is being held for service must have sneeze guards installed to prevent contamination* (**Figure 2-10**).

5. *Servers and others who handle dishes, glasses, and flatware should avoid touching the food-contact surfaces of these items.* For example, employees should pick up flatware by the handle or dishes by the bottom or edge.

6. *Instead of using a drinking glass to scoop ice (which may chip the glass), employees should use tongs or a scoop to get ice out of the ice machine.*

7. *Employees should use single-use gloves; deli sheets; a spatula, tong, or other equipment when touching ready-to-eat food, such as placing a roll on a plate.*

8. *Servers who put flatware on tables before service starts must cover the flatware* (such as with the napkin) unless the excess flatware is either removed when guests are seated or will be cleaned and sanitized after service.

9. *Any food or condiment on a customer's table cannot be reused, unless it is prepackaged, unopened, and in good condition (such as a condiment packet).*

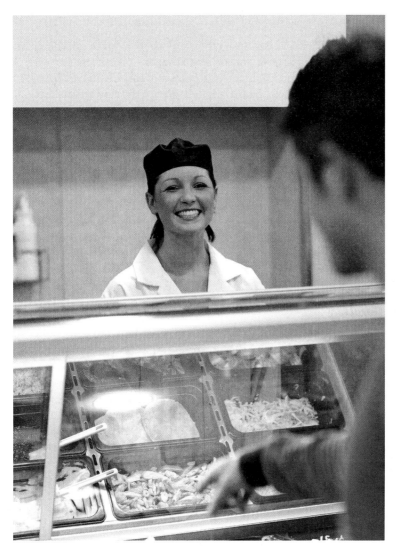

FIGURE 2-10 Sneeze Guards Prevent Contamination of Food Being Served
© Wavebreakmedia/Shutterstock

10. *If food spills when a server is placing dishes in front of guests, the server may use a dry, clean cloth to wipe up these spills. To wipe food spills on a steam table, employees should use a wet wiping cloth that is kept in a sanitizing solution between uses.*

11. *In self-service areas (such as salad bars), observe the following rules.*
   - Food must be protected with sneeze guards or other devices that keep food from being contaminated.
   - Each food item must have a clean and sanitary utensil, such as tongs. The handle of the utensil should be above the edge of the container so that customers can easily grab it without touching the food. Utensils may also be placed on a sanitized surface. If the utensils are used throughout a longer period of time, they must be removed, cleaned, and sanitized every four hours.
   - Foods for self-service must be labeled.
   - Foods must be monitored for proper temperature control at least every four hours.
   - When customers use a self-service bar and finish eating, they must get a new plate and utensils if they return to get more from the self-service bar. Signs should be posted so customers know to do this, and employees should make sure customers don't refill their dirty plates.

CLEANING AND SANITIZING

Cleaning removes food, grease, and other soil from a surface, whereas sanitizing reduces the number of bacteria and other pathogens on a surface to safe levels. In order to sanitize dishes, for instance, you need to clean the dishes first for the sanitizing to be the most effective. Sanitizing is accomplished by either heat or chemical sanitizers.

Cleaning requires hot water, scrubbing, and a detergent that penetrates into soil and softens it so it can be easily washed away. Different detergent products are made to wash a variety of surfaces, such as floors, food preparation tables, equipment, or utensils. There are also special purpose cleaners, such as abrasive cleaners (to help clean pots and pans with baked-on food), degreasers (to help remove oil and grease), and delimers (to remove mineral deposits in dishwashers or other equipment).

When cleaning, employees should choose the appropriate cleaner for the job, and read and follow its instructions carefully. Also, cleaning chemicals should never be mixed together as that can cause poisonous, even deadly, gases.

There is lots to clean and sanitize in a kitchen, so a **master cleaning schedule** should be developed and used. A master cleaning schedule includes what should be cleaned and when it should be cleaned, as well as who is responsible and who checks that the work is done properly. Keep in mind that surfaces that don't come into contact with food, such as floors and walls, only need to be cleaned (not sanitized).

First, let's look at dishes and utensils. Plates, cups, bowls, and utensils are washed and sanitized in a dishwasher. There are several types of commercial dishwashers available, but chances are you will be using either a door-type dishwasher (also called a stationary rack dishwasher) or a conveyor dishwasher. The **door-type dishwasher** accommodates one rack full of dishes as seen in **Figure 2-11**. A dishwashing rack is 19 inches by 19 inches. Once the rack is placed in the door-type dishwasher, the door is closed, and the cleaning cycle starts. In just minutes, you have clean, sanitized dishes. For larger foodservices with more dishes, **conveyor-type dishwashers** are larger machines and they move full racks of dishes through regular wash, power rinse, and

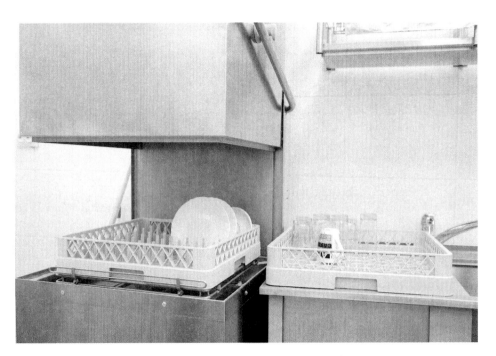

FIGURE 2-11 A Door-Type Dishwasher Accommodates One Rack of Dishes
© Vereshchagin Dmitry/Shutterstock

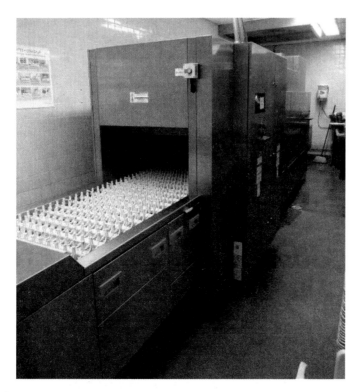

FIGURE 2-12 Flight-Type Dishwasher
Courtesy of MEIKO International.

sanitizing rinse cycles. Some machines also feature prewash and/or airdry cycles. For very high-volume operations, a **flight-type dishwasher** does not use racks. Instead, dishes are put on a moving belt (**Figure 2-12**).

Dishwashers are usually available as either high-temperature or low-temperature machines. A high-temperature machine uses very hot water to sanitize, while low-temperature machines use chemical sanitizers and a minimum water temperature that varies depending on the sanitizer used. For heat sanitizing, the FDA (Food Code, 2017) requires a minimum of 180°F (82°C) for all dishwashers except stationary rack machines, for which the required minimum is 165°F (74°C). Dishwashers that use heat to sanitize have a built-in thermometer that displays the sanitizing temperature. To confirm that the sanitizing temperature is high enough, employees can also put a maximum registering thermometer in a rack, put it through the dishwasher, and the thermometer will show the highest temperature reached.

Guidelines for using a commercial dishwasher follow.

1. Before starting the dishwasher, check its cleanliness and make sure the spray nozzles are clear. Keep an eye on mineral deposits in the machine (from hard water), which have to be removed from time to time using an acidic descaling solution.
2. Fill the tank(s) with clean water and check that dispensers (such as for detergent) are full.
3. Employees must scrape food off dishes before putting into dishwasher.
4. Dishes and flatware are loaded into racks so the dishwasher spray hits all surfaces. The racks should not be overloaded.
5. Once the cycle is complete, let all items air-dry.
6. When handling clean items, an employee's hands should be clean and gloves should be worn. Employees should not touch the food-contact surfaces of dishes or flatware.
7. Water temperatures, pressure, and chemical levels need to be monitored.

While dishwashers are used mostly for dishes and flatware, manual warewashing refers to washing pots, pans, etc., by hand using a sink with three compartments (**Figure 2-13**). Space for manual warewashing is normally kept separate from the dishwashing area. A typical three-compartment sink has drainboards on each side and three compartments: one each for washing, rinsing, and sanitizing. The drainboard on the left side of the sink is where dirty pots, pans, and so forth are placed. The drainboard on the right is where cleaned and sanitized items are initially placed.

To set up a three-compartment sink for use, the drainboards and sinks must first be cleaned and sanitized. Next, the first sink is filled with detergent and water that must be maintained at no less than 110°F (43°C) *or* the temperature recommended by the manufacturer of the detergent. The second sink needs clean water for rinsing off the soap and any residue. The temperature of the rinse water is determined by the chemical sanitizer being used. The third sink will be used to sanitize—usually using water containing a chemical sanitizer. Very hot water (minimum of 171°F or 77°C for 30 seconds) can also be used to sanitize, but a booster heater will likely be needed to get water that hot, and 171°F (77°C) water is not comfortable for the employee's hands. Instead, one of these chemical sanitizers are often used: chlorine, iodine, or a quaternary ammonium compound. Once the sink is set up, guidelines for washing and sanitizing pots and pans are given below.

1.   Scrape items so that residue goes into a trash pail or garbage disposal, not the wash sink.
2.   Scrub and wash in the first compartment, using nylon scrub pads or brush to loosen up soil. When the water looks dirty or the suds are gone, it's time to empty and refill this sink with water and detergent.
3.   Rinse in the second compartment and place rinsed items in the next compartment once free of detergent and soil. When the rinse water looks dirty or full of soap suds, it should be emptied and replaced. In some kitchens, items are rinsed with a sprayer-hose in the rinse sink.
4.   Sanitize in the third compartment by using a chemical sanitizer and appropriate water temperature *or* by heating the water to a minimum of 171°F (77°C) for 30 seconds. For the chemical method, use a chemical test kit with test strips (**Figure 2-14**) to confirm that the sanitizer is active and use a clock to make sure the items have sufficient contact time. The sanitizing solution must be changed when the concentration becomes low or the temperature goes below the minimum. The required contact time and water temperature vary depending on a number of factors. See **Table 2-5**.
5.   Place sanitized items upside down (so water runs off) on a clean, sanitized surface and let them air-dry completely before nesting. Don't use towels for drying as this may contaminate them.

How well a chemical sanitizer works depends on several factors including the concentration of the sanitizer as well as the water temperature, pH, and hardness. The

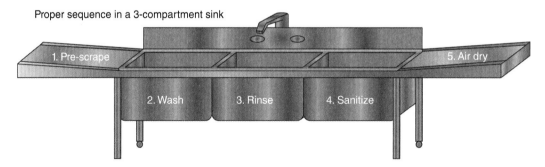

FIGURE 2-13 How to Clean Pots, Pans, and More in a Three-Compartment Sink

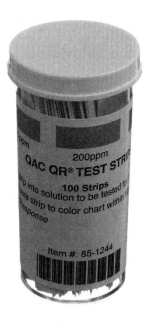

FIGURE 2-14 Test Strips for Testing Sanitizing Concentration
Courtesy of Franklin Machine Products.

concentration of the sanitizer is measured in parts per million (ppm) and employees have to use test strips to check sanitizer concentration. Test kits, including test strips, are usually sold by the company who supplies your cleaning chemicals. If the sanitizer concentration is too high, the solution may be unsafe. If the concentration is too low, it won't effectively sanitize pots, pans, etc. Guidelines for using different chemical sanitizers are summarized in Table 2–5.

So far, we have looked at cleaning and sanitizing using a dishwasher or three-compartment sink. Employees also need to wash and sanitize stationary equipment, such as a slicer. The following are guidelines for cleaning this type of equipment.

1. Unplug the equipment.
2. Disassemble the equipment.
3. Wash, rinse, and sanitize the removable parts in a three-compartment sink or run them through a dishwasher if appropriate.
4. Wash the stationary parts with a cleaning solution with detergent and appropriate tool, such as a cloth towel or brush. Rinse with clean water.

Table 2-5 Guidelines for Using Chemical Sanitizers in a Three-Compartment Sink
• When using a chlorine solution, the water must be kept at a minimum temperature based on the concentration and pH of the solution. For example, if the pH is 10 or fewer, the temperature must be at least 100°F (38°C) when the sanitizer concentration is 50 to 99 ppm. If the pH is 8 or fewer, the temperature must be at least 75°F (24°C) when the sanitizer concentration is 50 to 99 ppm. In either case, the items being sanitized must be in contact with the sanitizing solution for at least seven seconds and staff must wear gloves.
• When using an iodine solution, the water must be kept at a minimum temperature of 68°F (20°C), the pH must be 5.0 or lower, and the concentration kept at 12.5–25 ppm. The contact time must be at least 30 seconds.
• When using a quaternary ammonium compound solution, the water must be kept at a minimum temperature of 75°F (24°C), the water hardness must be less than 500 mg/L, and the concentration must be at the level recommended by the manufacturer. The contact time must be at least 30 seconds.

Data from *2017 Food Code*, p 43, by the U.S. Public Health Service and Food & Drug Administration, 2017. Retrieved from https://www.fda.gov/Food /GuidanceRegulation/Retail Food Protection/FoodCode/ucm595139.htm

5. Sanitize the food-contact surfaces of the stationary parts with a sanitizing solution.
6. Allow all surfaces to air-dry before reassembling.

Some stationary equipment, such as a soft-serve ice cream or yogurt machine, are designed so that water or a sanitizing solution can be poured in and then pumped through the machine for cleaning and sanitizing. Since ice cream and frozen yogurt are TCS foods, these machines are usually cleaned and sanitized daily.

Of course, there's still more that needs to be cleaned, such as tables, floors, and walls. Any surfaces that come into contact with food, such as food preparation tables, must be cleaned, rinsed, and sanitized. Surfaces that don't come into contact with food, such as floors and the exterior of equipment, just need to be cleaned and rinsed.

To clean food–contact surfaces such as a food preparation table, remove any soil first, then wash the surface with a detergent and water solution. Next, rinse the surface with clean water and sanitize the surface with a nontoxic sanitizing solution. Don't dry the surface with a towel—let it air-dry to prevent contamination. Today's foodservice sanitizers do not leave a chemical residue and should be allowed to evaporate on their own. Food-contact surfaces are cleaned and sanitized after each use, such as when food preparation employees switch from trimming meat to cutting melons, or switch from working with any food to something different. Surfaces also need to be cleaned and sanitized any time they have been in use for four hours.

2.4 MANAGE FOOD SAFETY

As mentioned earlier in this chapter, the major risk factors for foodborne illness include the following:

1. Purchasing food and beverages from unsafe sources.
2. Poor personal hygiene.
3. Poor control of time and temperature.
4. Cross-contamination of food, equipment, or prep surfaces.

If managers and employees work together to decrease these risks, a lot can be done to prevent foodborne illness.

Foodservice operations use various methods to ensure food safety, such as these.

- *Standard operating procedures (SOPs):* SOPs are written instructions for a specific task such as how to wash pots and pans in the three-compartment sink or how to receive refrigerated foods. SOPs for the operation are usually put into a binder and used in training new and current employees.
- *Employee training program:* Employees need periodic training sessions on food safety and personal hygiene. Don't just tell employees what to do, tell them *why* to do it. Also, managers and supervisors need to be excellent role models for food safety.
- *Hazard Analysis Critical Control Point (HACCP) system:* The HACCP system is a prevention-based food safety system discussed in a moment.
- *Vendor selection program:* A vendor selection program includes the criteria and process used to select vendors. The process is used when looking for new suppliers or evaluating current suppliers. Performing a site visit on a vendor is not uncommon.
- *Food specifications:* For each food or beverage that a foodservice orders, purchasing has a product specification. A product specification describes the quality and size, weight, or count of each item purchased.
- *Quality management:* There are many different approaches to improve quality and performance, such as Six Sigma, that a foodservice may use (this is discussed in Chapter 14).

- *Master cleaning schedule:* A master cleaning schedule includes what should be cleaned in the kitchen and other parts of the operation. It details when each item should be cleaned and who is responsible.
- *Pest control program:* By working with a licensed pest control operator and denying pests access to the operation, you can help keep pests out of your operation.
- *Disaster plans:* In any kitchen, you have to plan for emergencies, such as being flooded during a hurricane or losing power. Disaster planning is discussed in Chapter 12.

When you put all of these together, you have a **food safety management system**, which greatly increases your ability to serve safe food.

The **Hazard Analysis Critical Control Point (HACCP)** system is a prevention-based food safety system. The seven steps in the HACCP process are designed to prevent the occurrence of foodborne illness. First, you use menus and recipes to identify the preparation steps when certain foods could be mishandled. Control procedures are then established to prevent mishandling and these procedures are monitored. When control procedures are not properly followed, corrective action is taken. The following are the steps.

1. *Conduct a hazard analysis.* Review your menu to identify which items present the highest risks. Most menu items fall into one of these categories: no cook, cook and serve on same day, or more complex food preparation. An example of a menu item with more complex food preparation may be a dish that is heated, cooled, and then reheated. Because this menu item requires three trips through the danger zone, it presents more risks than an item that is cooked and served immediately.

2. *Determine* **critical control points (CCPs)**. A critical control point is any point, step, or procedure in which a food safety hazard can be prevented, eliminated, or reduced to an acceptable level. For example, if a menu item, such as bone-in chicken, is cooked and held on a steam table for meal service, there are two critical control points: cooking to the required minimum internal temperature and holding it at the correct temperature. If your chicken is delivered fresh, you may add another critical control point at the time of receiving.

3. *Establish control procedures and critical limits.* For each CCP, you have to determine the best control measures to prevent the introduction of hazards. Critical limits are the time and/or temperature that must be achieved or maintained to control a hazard. When critical limits are not met, the food may not be safe. An example of critical limits is minimum internal cooking temperatures. Sanitation inspectors like to see the critical control points listed in the recipe (**Table 2-6**).

Table 2-6 Recipe with Critical Control Points

Tuna Salad

Prep Process: No Cook   Yield: 14 lbs (75–3 oz. portions)

Store in: Full-size polycarbonate deep pan

Ingredient	Weight	Measure
Tuna, canned or pouch, water pack, drained, refrigerated	10.75 lbs	5.4 qt
Celery, fresh, chopped fine (¼ dice), refrigerated	2.0 lbs	4 cups
Onion, green (scallion) chopped fine, refrigerated	1.0 lbs	2 cups
Mayonnaise, heavy-duty, refrigerated	2.5 lbs	5 cups
Lemon juice, reconstituted, refrigerated	8 oz.	1 cup
Salt, Kosher, fine	1 oz.	2 T
Pepper, black, fine	½ oz.	1 T

(continues)

Table 2-6 Recipe with Critical Control Points (continued)

Preparation Method

1. Chill a 5-gallon mixing bowl and appropriate pans for draining tuna.
2. Open tuna into a cold perforated 6" pan inside solid 8" pan to drain. Keep in refrigerator.
3. Once tuna is drained (15 minutes), transfer to mixing bowl. Take and record temperature. **CCP**—Tuna must be at or below 41°F (5°C) —otherwise return to refrigerator.
4. Add salt, black pepper, celery, green onions, and lemon juice and stir well with a gloved hand or spatula to incorporate seasoning.
5. Add chilled mayonnaise and mix until well blended.
6. Transfer to clean deep, full-size polycarbonate container with tight-fitting lid or film.
7. Label and date to include production and expiration dates (within five days of expiration date) on label.
8. **CCP** - Record the temperature and store under refrigeration at 40° (4°C) or below.

4. *Establish monitoring procedures, such as taking temperature of cooked chicken.* Of course, you will also need to determine when and how often temperatures will be taken, and who will be doing it.

5. *Establish corrective actions to be taken when monitoring indicates, for instance, that the chicken has not reached the minimum internal temperature.* In this case, the corrective action would be to continue cooking until time and temperature requirements are met. In other situations, food may be discarded.

6. *Verify that the system works.* Look at your records, perhaps on a daily or weekly basis, to see if the monitoring and corrective actions are going as planned.

7. *Establish documentation procedures including how long to keep records.* In order to perform steps 4–6, forms should be developed so that employee actions are documented or written down. **Table 2–7** is an example of a documentation form used by a foodservice when cooling foods.

In addition to documenting cooking and cooling processes, foodservices should also keep records of food invoices and food specifications as part of the HACCP plan.

Table 2-7 Cooling Log

Cooling Log

Instructions: Record temperatures every hour during the cooling cycle. Record corrective actions, if applicable. If no foods are cooled on any working day. Indicate "No foods Cooled" in the **Food Item** column. Foodservice manager will verify that foodservice employees are cooling food properly by visually monitoring foodservice employees during the shift and reviewing, initiating, and dating this log each working day. Maintain this log for a minimum of one year.

Date	Food Item	Time/ Temp	Time/ Temp	Time/ Temp	Time/ Temp	Time/ Temp	Corrective Actions Taken	Initials	Verified by/Date

Guidance for School Food Authorities: Developing a School Food Safety Program Based on the Process Approach to HACCP Principles, p. 76, by the United States Department of Agriculture, Food and Nutrition Service, 2005. Retrieved from https://fns-prod.azureedge.net/sites/default/files/Food_Safety _HACCPGuidance.pdf

2.5 EXPLAIN HOW TO HAVE A SUCCESSFUL SANITATION INSPECTION

A number of federal agencies have active roles in food safety.

- The U.S. Food and Drug Administration (FDA) has two major roles: issuing the *Food Code* and inspecting all foods except meat, poultry, and eggs.
- The Food Safety and Inspection Service (FSIS) is the agency in the U.S. Department of Agriculture responsible for ensuring that the nation's supply of meat, poultry, and egg products is safe, wholesome, and correctly labeled and packaged.
- The Centers for Disease Control and Prevention (CDC) leads federal efforts to gather data on foodborne illnesses, investigate outbreaks of foodborne illness, and monitor the effectiveness of prevention and control efforts in reducing foodborne illnesses.
- The Public Health Service (PHS) also investigates outbreaks and researches the causes of outbreaks.

In addition, state and local authorities have food safety roles.

The *Food Code* (2017), released every four years by the FDA, provides scientifically sound guidance on food safety and sanitation. It is comprehensive and includes, for example, sections on employee health and hygiene, preventing contamination of foods, temperature and time control, and sanitization of equipment and utensils. It is referred as a model code because it acts as a guide for local, state, and other jurisdictions in developing or updating their own codes. The *Food Code* (2017) can also be adopted by any jurisdiction.

Wherever a foodservice operates, managers must know which regulatory authority comes in to do inspections and be familiar with their regulations. The inspector may come, for instance, from the county or city health department. In addition, some operations get their kitchen inspected by more than one regulatory authority. For example, in addition to the local health authority, healthcare foodservices are also often inspected by the Centers for Medicare and Medicaid Services (usually through the state department of health) as well as an accrediting agency, such as the Joint Commission.

It is also important to know how often health inspectors come into the operation and the inspection report form they use. Health inspectors, also called sanitarians or environmental health specialists, generally visit operations with previous problems or violations more often. They may also make more frequent visits to large foodservices and foodservices serving groups at high risk for foodborne illness such as the young and the elderly.

Figure 2-15 is an example of an inspection report form found in the *Food Code* (2017) that is used by a number of health departments across the United States. Appendix B contains two additional foodservice inspection forms. One is used in New York City and the other is used by the Centers for Medicare and Medicaid Services when they inspect kitchens of healthcare facilities. Most inspections are risk-based, meaning that violations more likely to result in foodborne illness are more important. For example, cooking food to minimum internal temperature is more consequential than covering a trash pail.

Health inspectors almost always show up without warning to do a foodservice inspection. They will normally enter your operation and ask the nearest employee to direct them to who is in charge (so employees need to know how to respond). Once you meet the inspector, it is appropriate to ask for identification and also the reason for the visit. The inspector may simply be doing a routine inspection or may have come in response to a customer complaint. The following are tips for inspections.

1. *Be professional and courteous.* Good communication is important for a successful inspection.

FORM 3-A

Food Establishment Inspection Report

Page _____ of _____

As Governed by State Code Section XXX.XXX	No. of Risk Factor/Intervention Violations	Date
Do Good County	No. of Repeat Risk Factor/Intervention Violations	Time In
12344 Any Street, Our Town, State 11111	Score (optional)	Time Out

Establishment	Address	City/State	Zip Code	Telephone

License/Permit #	Permit Holder	Purpose of Inspection	Est. Type	Risk Category

FOODBORNE ILLNESS RISK FACTORS AND PUBLIC HEALTH INTERVENTIONS

Circle designated compliance status (IN, OUT, N/O, N/A) for each numbered item   Mark "X" in appropriate box for COS and/or R

IN=in compliance   OUT=not in compliance   N/O=not observed   N/A=not applicable   COS=corrected on-site during inspection   R=repeat violation

Compliance Status			COS	R	Compliance Status			COS	R
Supervision					17	IN OUT	Proper disposition of returned, previously served, reconditioned & unsafe food		
1	IN OUT	Person in charge present, demonstrates knowledge, and performs duties			**Time/Temperature Control for Safety**				
2	IN OUT N/A	Certified Food Protection Manager			18	IN OUT N/A N/O	Proper cooking time & temperatures		
Employee Health					19	IN OUT N/A N/O	Proper reheating procedures for hot holding		
3	IN OUT	Management, food employee and conditional employee; knowledge, responsibilities and reporting			20	IN OUT N/A N/O	Proper cooling time and temperature		
4	IN OUT	Proper use of restriction and exclusion			21	IN OUT N/A N/O	Proper hot holding temperatures		
5	IN OUT	Procedures for responding to vomiting and diarrheal events			22	IN OUT N/A N/O	Proper cold holding temperatures		
Good Hygienic Practices					23	IN OUT N/A N/O	Proper date marking and disposition		
6	IN OUT N/O	Proper eating, tasting, drinking, or tobacco use			24	IN OUT N/A N/O	Time as a Public Health Control; procedures & records		
7	IN OUT N/O	No discharge from eyes, nose, and mouth			**Consumer Advisory**				
Preventing Contamination by Hands					25	IN OUT N/A	Consumer advisory provided for raw/undercooked food		
8	IN OUT N/O	Hands clean & properly washed			**Highly Susceptible Populations**				
9	IN OUT N/A N/O	No bare hand contact with RTE food or a pre-approved alternative procedure properly allowed			26	IN OUT N/A	Pasteurized foods used; prohibited foods not offered		
10	IN OUT	Adequate handwashing sinks properly supplied and accessible			**Food/Color Additives and Toxic Substances**				
Approved Source					27	IN OUT N/A	Food additives: approved & properly used		
11	IN OUT	Food obtained from approved source			28	IN OUT N/A	Toxic substances properly identified, stored, & used		
12	IN OUT N/A N/O	Food received at proper temperature			**Conformance with Approved Procedures**				
13	IN OUT	Food in good condition, safe, & unadulterated			29	IN OUT N/A	Compliance with variance/specialized process/HACCP		
14	IN OUT N/A N/O	Required records available: shellstock tags, parasite destruction							
Protection from Contamination									
15	IN OUT N/A N/O	Food separated and protected							
16	IN OUT N/A	Food-contact surfaces; cleaned & sanitized							

Risk factors are important practices or procedures identified as the most prevalent contributing factors of foodborne illness or injury. Public health interventions are control measures to prevent foodborne illness or injury.

GOOD RETAIL PRACTICES

Good Retail Practices are preventative measures to control the addition of pathogens, chemicals, and physical objects into foods.

Mark "X" in box if numbered item is not in compliance   Mark "X" in appropriate box for COS and/or R   COS=corrected on-site during inspection   R=repeat violation

		COS	R			COS	R
Safe Food and Water				**Proper Use of Utensils**			
30	Pasteurized eggs used where required			43	In-use utensils: properly stored		
31	Water & ice from approved source			44	Utensils, equipment & linens: properly stored, dried, & handled		
32	Variance obtained for specialized processing methods			45	Single-use/single-service articles: properly stored & used		
Food Temperature Control				46	Gloves used properly		
33	Proper cooling methods used; adequate equipment for temperature control			**Utensils, Equipment and Vending**			
34	Plant food properly cooked for hot holding			47	Food & non-food contact surfaces cleanable, properly designed, constructed, & used		
35	Approved thawing methods used			48	Warewashing facilities: installed, maintained, & used; test strips		
36	Thermometers provided & accurate			49	Non-food contact surfaces clean		
Food Identification				**Physical Facilities**			
37	Food properly labeled; original container			50	Hot & cold water available; adequate pressure		
Prevention of Food Contamination				51	Plumbing installed; proper backflow devices		
38	Insects, rodents, & animals not present			52	Sewage & waste water properly disposed		
39	Contamination prevented during food preparation, storage & display			53	Toilet facilities: properly constructed, supplied, & cleaned		
40	Personal cleanliness			54	Garbage & refuse properly disposed; facilities maintained		
41	Wiping cloths: properly used & stored			55	Physical facilities installed, maintained, & clean		
42	Washing fruits & vegetables			56	Adequate ventilation & lighting; designated areas used		

Person in Charge (Signature)	Date:
Inspector (Signature)	Follow-up: YES NO (Circle one) Follow-up Date:

FIGURE 2-15 Food Establishment Inspection Report

2017 Food Code, p 717, by the U.S. Public Health Service and Food & Drug Administration, 2017. Retrieved from https://www.fda.gov/media/110822/download

2. *It's expected that you will accompany the inspector during the inspection*, and you are allowed to make your own notes as you do so.

3. *Be honest and thorough in answering questions from the inspector. If the inspector finds a violation that you can immediately correct, be sure to do so.* If you can't correct the violation right away, be honest. If you are not clear about any part of the inspection, ask questions.

4. *Ahead of time, make sure various records are easy to find if you need to show them to the inspector.* Examples include temperature logs (refrigerator and freezer, hot food cooling, dish machine temperatures, pot sink sanitizer titration, food receiving log), food protection manager certificates, and purchasing records.

5. *When the inspection is completed, the inspector will go through the results with you, including any violations, and ask for a signature.* You need to understand exactly why each violation was noted and discuss with the inspector how to correct each situation, the timeframe for correction, and if and when the inspector will be returning to check on compliance. By signing the inspection form, you acknowledge that you have received the report. The inspector will give you a copy of the report, which should be used to talk to other managers and employees about designing and implementing corrections. All inspection reports must be kept on file. Repeat violations are noted and subject to fines or closures.

Inspectors normally ask operators to suspend operation only if there is a problem, such as sewer backup in the kitchen, that presents an imminent health hazard to customers.

Effective managers perform periodic self-inspections of the kitchen that mimic what the health inspector does. Appendix B includes an example of a self-inspection form.

2.6 MAINTAIN AN ACCIDENT-FREE WORKPLACE

Kitchens present a lot of hazards: sharp knives; wet floors; steam; hot pots and pans; electrical equipment, some with moving blades, and more. Typical foodservice accidents include slipping or falling, getting cut or burned, or getting hurt while lifting heavy boxes. Accidents can occur for many reasons, but often, employees are rushing around or don't know the right procedure to follow, so they end up getting hurt. Whatever the reason may be, accidents are painful and costly and may lead to lost work time and lowered morale. The following are tips so employees can prevent cuts, burns, falls, back strain, fires, and electric shock.

How to Use Knives Safely

1. Keep your knives sharp—you are more likely to cut yourself with a dull knife.
2. When using a knife, slice away from your hand and keep your fingertips curled under and out of the way of the blade.
3. Put a damp towel under your cutting board so it stays in place when cutting.
4. Carry a knife with the blade pointing downward.
5. Don't put a dirty knife into a sink of sudsy water—lay it on a sideboard.
6. To wash and dry a knife, wipe both sides at once with the sharp edge away from your hand and the towel.
7. Store knives securely after being washed and sanitized.
8. Don't use a knife to open cans.

More Ways to Prevent Cuts

1. Pay attention when using sharp equipment. Make sure that safety guards are attached and used properly on slicers, blenders, food processors, and specialized handheld food-chopping equipment.
2. Turn equipment off before adjusting.

3.   Never touch food in a machine, even with a utensil, when the machine is in motion.
4.   Do not use equipment when wearing loose sleeves or dangling jewelry that may accidentally be pulled into a machine. Identification badges hanging loosely from lanyards around the neck are also dangerous around moving equipment.
5.   Sweep up broken glass; don't use your hands. Use a special container to dispose of broken glass, dishes, and other sharp objects.
6.   Remove can lids entirely from cans and put back into the empty cans for disposal.

How to Prevent Burns

1.   Pay attention when working around hot equipment.
2.   Use dry potholders (wet potholders conduct heat to your hands).
3.   Keep pot handles turned in away from the edge of the range and away from open flames.
4.   Get help lifting heavy pots of food.
5.   Open lids of pots and doors of steamers away from you.
6.   Warn others (including customers) about hot surfaces.
7.   Put foods into the fryer slowly and stand back.
8.   Let equipment cool before cleaning.

How to Prevent Fires and What to Do in Case of a Fire

1.   Do not turn your back on hot fat.
2.   Keep equipment and hoods free from grease buildup.
3.   Keep fire hazards, such as paper products, away from heat.
4.   Know where the nearest fire extinguisher is and how to use it. Also know where the fire suppression pull-stations for ventilation hoods are located.
5.   Never throw water on a grease or electrical fire.
6.   Report damaged and worn plugs and frayed cords to your supervisor.
7.   Flammable substances like Sterno (canned heat) or other chafing fuel must be stored in fireproof metal boxes designed for such items. Canned butane used for torches (for flaming lemon meringue, for example) must also be stored in fireproof boxes.

How to Prevent Falls

1.   Wipe up spills immediately and use "Wet Floor" signs.
2.   Wear slip-resistant shoes.
3.   Keep aisles and stairs clear.
4.   Walk, do not run.
5.   Do not carry anything that blocks your vision.
6.   Use ladders properly. Do not stand on a table, chair, or box

How to Prevent Electrical Shock

1.   Never touch electrical equipment or outlets with wet hands or while standing in water.
2.   Unplug equipment before disassembling or cleaning.
3.   Report damaged and worn plugs and cords to your supervisor.

How to Prevent Head Trauma from Pressurized Tanks

1.   Pressurized carbon dioxide tanks for soft drink carbonation can fail and explode, so they must be chained or in an approved, locked container. They should be stored at or below 70°F (21°C).
2.   Pressurized tanks of helium for balloons or nitrogen for beer and wine should also be locked in place or chained.

In addition, employees who have to lift heavy boxes need to lift correctly to prevent back strain and other injuries. **Figure 2-16** shows the right way to lift. The secret

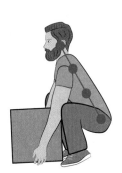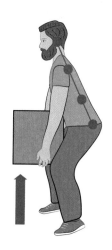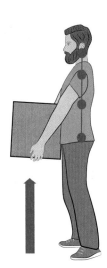

FIGURE 2-16 How to Lift Properly
© Lemurik/Shutterstock

to lifting is to use your leg and stomach muscles instead of your back muscles. Always kneel down in front of the box and keep your back rounded as you lift. To set the box down, slowly resume the original position. To carry a heavy load, keep your knees bent and your back rounded, with your load at waist level or below. To avoid carrying heavy things long distances, use a cart.

Many foodservice employees use cleaning chemicals in their jobs. Because cleaning chemicals can pose a wide range of health hazards (such as irritation) and physical hazards (such as corrosion), employers are required to do the following.

1. All chemicals must be labeled with safety information.
2. **Material safety data sheets (MSDS)** for each product must be provided to the foodservice by the vendor that conveys each chemical's potential hazards (health, reactivity with other chemicals, fire, environment) and how to use the product safely.
3. Employees must be trained on the hazards of the chemicals in their work area and how each chemical is to be handled to protect themselves, including the use of any personal protective equipment such as special gloves.

The **Occupational Safety and Health Administration (OSHA)** is a federal agency charged with keeping employees safe and healthy at work. Many employers with more than 10 employees are required to keep a record of serious work-related injuries and illnesses using OHSA Form 300. A recordable injury or illness includes any work-related injury or illness that results in loss of consciousness, days away from work, restricted work, or transfer to another job. It also includes any work-related injury or illness requiring medical treatment beyond first aid or fractured or cracked bones or teeth (Occupational Safety and Health Administration, 2018).

This information helps employers, employees, and OSHA evaluate the safety of a workplace and implement worker protections to reduce and eliminate hazards. The records must be maintained for at least five years and each February through April, employers must post a summary of the injuries and illnesses recorded the previous year (Occupational Safety and Health Administration, 2018).

Finally, employees should be trained to deal with emergencies, such as choking and possible heart attacks. Emergency contact numbers should be posted and readily available on bulletin boards and near phones. If a portable defibrillator or AED is available, someone on each shift should be trained on its use and in CPR. Training should be provided for dealing with a choking customer, and choking posters showing how to use the Heimlich maneuver should be placed in proximity to eating areas.

SUMMARY

2.1 Discuss causes and prevention of foodborne illness.

- Foodborne illness results from eating food contaminated through biological, chemical, or physical contamination.
- Common symptoms of foodborne illness are nausea, vomiting, stomach cramps, and diarrhea.
- Groups at high risk for foodborne illness include young children, older adults, pregnant women, and people with weakened immune systems.
- Pathogens causing foodborne illness include bacteria, viruses, parasites, and fungi. Fungi (such as molds) are the only pathogens that are visible—the others are microscopic.
- When conditions are right, the number of bacteria can increase rapidly to the point where they cause foodborne illness. To grow, bacteria need food (see 2-1 for TCS foods), temperature between 41°F and 135°F (5°C and 57°C)—the temperature danger zone, time to grow, moisture, and little or no acid.
- The top bacteria that cause foodborne illness include *Salmonella* (nontyphoidal) and *Campylobacter jejuni*, both found in chicken, as well as *Clostridium perfringens* (found in raw meat and poultry) and *Staphylococcus aureus* (found on human skin and nose).
- The four major ways to prevent foodborne illness include: practice good personal hygiene, purchase food and beverages from approved vendors, control time and temperature, and prevent cross contamination.
- Viruses do not grow in food like bacteria do. To keep viruses out of food, employees who are sick must not work with food. The leading cause of foodborne illness is norovirus, which is highly contagious and causes what is often called the stomach flu. You can get norovirus from an infected person, food or water contaminated with the virus, or by touching a contaminated surface such as a door knob.
- Additional pathogens include parasites (such as sometimes found in water and seafood) and fungi (includes mold and yeast). To prevent problems with parasites, good personal hygiene as well as purchasing from approved, reputable suppliers is vital. Also, all seafood should be cooked to minimum internal temperatures. To avoid problems with mold, you should throw out foods with visible mold. The only foods that are okay to eat after cutting away moldy areas include hard cheese and hard salami. Reduce your aflatoxin exposure by buying only major commercial brands of nuts and nut butters and discarding nuts that look moldy, discolored, or shriveled.
- Because some shellfish or fin fish contain toxins, purchase only from approved, reputable vendors. Also, in the case of scombroid poisoning, it is important to prevent time and temperature abuse from the moment it is received until it is served.
- Appendix A gives information on bacteria, viruses, parasites, and mycotoxins.

2.2 Describe safe personal hygiene practices.

- Employees who are sick can contaminate food in many ways, such as by coughing, sneezing, and touching foods without gloves (especially after using the bathroom and not washing hands). Employees who are not outwardly sick can also cause foodborne illness. Consider an employee with an infected cut that is not properly covered or an employee who is a carrier.
- Guidelines are given for washing hands. Single-use gloves are used to protect the food from pathogens on an employee's hand and must be used for one task only, as well as changed often.
- Basics of good personal hygiene are listed.

2.3 Apply food safety principles.

- Figure 2-5 shows various types of thermometers. Always insert the thermometer into the thickest part of the food and be sure that bimetallic thermometers go in up to the dimple on the stem. Clean and sanitize after each use and calibrate as needed.
- Guidelines are listed for purchasing and receiving, storing foods, and preparing and serving foods.
- Cleaning involves using a detergent to remove food, grease, and other soil from a surface, whereas sanitizing reduces the number of bacteria and other pathogens on a surface to safe levels.
- A master cleaning schedule includes what should be cleaned and when it should be cleaned, as well as who is responsible and

how items are cleaned and sanitized. Surfaces that don't come into contact with food, such as floors and walls, only need to be cleaned.

- Guidelines are listed to clean dishes and flatware using the dishwasher, pots and pans using a three-compartment sink, and stationary equipment.
- To clean food-contact surfaces such as a food preparation table, remove any soil first, then wash the surface with a detergent and water solution. Next, rinse the surface with clean water and then sanitize the surface with a correct sanitizing solution. Don't dry the surface with a towel—let it air dry to prevent contamination. Food contact surfaces are cleaned and sanitized after each use such as when food preparation employees switch from trimming meat to cutting melons, or switch from working with any food to something different. Surfaces also need to be cleaned and sanitized any time they have been in use for four hours.

2.4 Manage food safety.

- Components of a food safety management system may include standard operating procedures, employee training program, HACCP system, vendor selection program, food specifications, quality management, master cleaning schedule, pest control program, and disaster planning.
- HACCP is a prevention-based food safety system with seven steps: conduct a hazard analysis, determine critical control points, establish control procedures and critical limits, establish monitoring procedures and corrective actions, verify that the system works, and establish documentation procedures.

2.5 Explain how to have a successful sanitation inspection.

- The 2017 *Food Code*, released every four years by the FDA, provides scientifically sound guidance on food safety and sanitation and is adopted for use by some health departments.
- Wherever a foodservice operates, managers must know which regulatory authority comes in to do inspections and be familiar with their regulations. Figure 2-15 is an example of an inspection report form found in the *Food Code* (2017). Most inspections are risk-based.
- When a health inspector enters your establishment, be professional and courteous and accompany the inspector during the inspection. Be honest when answering questions from the inspector and ask questions when needed. If the inspector identifies a violation that you can immediately correct, try to do so. Make sure necessary records are available to show the inspector. When the inspector goes through the report with you, be sure you understand exactly why each violation was noted and discuss with the inspector how to correct each situation, the timeframe for correction, and if and when the inspector will be returning to check on compliance.

2.6 Maintain an accident-free workplace.

- Guidelines are listed for using knives safely and preventing cuts, burns, fires, falls, electrical shock, and head trauma.
- Figure 2-16 shows how to use your legs to lift (not your back).
- Employees should be trained on the Heimlich maneuver for choking and some should also be trained in cardiopulmonary resuscitation and using a portable defibrillator.
- The Occupational Safety and Health Administration is a federal agency charged with keeping employees safe and healthy at work. Many employers with more than 10 employees are required to keep a record of serious work-related injuries and illnesses using OHSA Form 300.

REVIEW AND DISCUSSION QUESTIONS

1. Describe which foods are most likely to cause foodborne illness and the different ways they can become contaminated.
2. What is the temperature danger zone? What are four ways to prevent foodborne illness?
3. Compare bacteria to viruses and seafood toxins in terms of how they cause foodborne illness.
4. Describe a situation when it would be best to use an instant read thermometer, a

thermocouple thermometer with an immersion probe, an infrared thermometer, and a disposable temperature indicator.

5. Describe how FIFO works.

6. Describe three ways to defrost frozen foods safely and when each method is best used.

7. Describe how to cool hot foods and then reheat them.

8. Why are raw meat, poultry, and fish stored on the lowest rack in the refrigerator?

9. Why isn't the steam table used to heat up cold foods? What is the required minimum temperature for hot foods that are being held hot?

10. What is the difference between a clean plate and a sanitized plate?

11. Discuss how pots and pans are sanitized in a three-compartment sink.

12. Find a recipe and determine where there are critical control points (CCP). Briefly describe each CCP you found.

13. Which are better to use to avoid cuts—a sharp or dull knife? Explain your answer.

14. How do you avoid steam burns and grease fires?

15. How do you lift properly to avoid back injury?

16. How do employees use a material safety data sheet?

17. Name the federal agency charged with keeping employees safe at work.

18. How does a manager ensure a safe workplace and safe food to eat?

SMALL GROUP PROJECT

For the foodservice concept that you created in Chapter 1, develop the following.

1. An attractive poster (using a PowerPoint slide) to encourage safe food handling in food production areas.

2. An attractive trifold handout for employees to help them prevent accidents (cuts, burns, etc.) in the kitchen and serving areas.

3. A HACCP plan for one recipe.

REFERENCES

Bush, L.M. (2018). Staphylococcus infections. In *Merck Manual Consumer Version*. Retrieved from https://www.merckmanuals.com/professional/infectious-diseases/gram-positive-cocci/staphylococcal-infections

Centers for Disease Control and Prevention. (2020). *Foodborne germs and illnesses*. Retrieved from https://www.cdc.gov/foodsafety/foodborne-germs.html

Cornell University Cooperative Extension. (2015). *Standard operating procedure for washing produce with a peracetic acid solution*. Retrieved from https://rvpadmin.cce.cornell.edu/uploads/doc_451.pdf

Kovacevic, J., Ziegler, J., Walecka-Zacharska, E., Reimer, A., Kitts, D. D., & Gilmour, M.W. (2016). Tolerance of *listeria monocytogenes* to quaternary ammonium sanitizers is mediated by a novel efflux pump encoded by *emrE*. *Applied and Environmental Microbiology*, 82, 939–953. doi:10.1128/AEM.03741-15

National Restaurant Association. (2017). *SERVSAFE coursebook (7th ed.)*. Chicago, IL: National Restaurant Association.

Occupational Safety and Health Administration. (2018). *OSHA injury and illness recordkeeping and reporting requirements*. Retrieved from https://www.osha.gov/recordkeeping/index.html

Scallan, E., Hoekstra, R. M., Angulo, F. J., Tauxe, R. V., Widdowson, M.-A., Roy, S. L., & Griffin, P. M. (2011). Foodborne illness acquired in the United States—major pathogens. *Emerging Infectious Diseases, 17(1)*, 7–15. doi: 10.3201/eid1701.P11101

Scallan, E., Griffin, P. M., Angulo, F. J., Tauxe, R. V., & Hoekstra, R. M. (2011). Foodborne illness acquired in the United States—unspecified agents. *Emerging Infectious Diseases, 17(1)*, 16–22. doi: 10.3201/eid1701.P21101

U.S. Public Health Service and U.S. Food and Drug Administration. (2017). *Food Code 2017*. Retrieved from https://www.fda.gov/food/fda-food-code/food-code-2017

© Denis Val/Shutterstock

Menus: The Heart of the Operation

LEARNING OUTCOMES

3.1 Identify menu type.

3.2 Plan menus.

3.3 Design a printed menu.

3.4 Set menu prices.

INTRODUCTION

When thinking about going to a new restaurant, the first thing most people do is look for the menu on the restaurant's website. The online menu will tell you if they serve food that you would enjoy and whether the prices are within your budget. At this point, the menu becomes the key sales tool for an operation as it serves to entice and keep customers. The menu also determines what happens as inputs are transformed into outputs using the systems approach. The employees who are in charge of purchasing, storage, food production, and service will all use the menu to do their jobs. This chapter covers all of the work involved in planning menus, designing the printed menus, and setting menu prices. However, it first discusses the many types of menus in varied foodservice settings.

3.1 IDENTIFY MENU TYPE

Menus can vary in a number of ways such as by:

- How often the menu changes
- How the pricing works
- The degree of choice a customer has to select foods

When you think of a chain restaurant menu, for example, the menu only changes occasionally, customers usually pay for each item they order, and customers choose exactly what they want to eat. But if you are at a university dining hall menu, the menu can be quite different, so let's take a look at different *types* of menus.

When a menu is the same from day-to-day, it is known as a **static menu**, also called a restaurant-style menu. Your typical restaurant uses a static menu format but incorporates changes as needed. Most restaurant menus are updated *at least* once or twice a year to remove items that are not selling well or that have dramatically increased in cost, or to take advantage of seasonal items or new food trends. Prices can then be adjusted so they better reflect food and labor costs. In addition, restaurant menus are kept fresh and interesting through the use of specials, meaning menu items that rotate and appear seasonally or weekly or for just one meal or one day. A list of specials may appear on its own menu, clipped onto the regular menu, written on black or white boards, or simply spoken by the server. **Figure 3-1** shows a restaurant menu.

Now, imagine that you had to eat one or more meals every day at the same restaurant, and this restaurant used a static menu with two special items each day. In time, the menu would become boring. When college students live on campus, the dining hall menu changes *daily to keep the food choices interesting*. Similar onsite foodservices serving meals to people at work or in a nursing home are more likely to use a cycle menu rather than a static menu. A **cycle menu** (**Table 3-1** and **Figure 3-2**) changes daily for a certain length of time, such as one week or even up to eight weeks. At the end of a two-week cycle menu, for instance, the menu returns to Day 1 of Week 1 after the final day of Week 2 (Day 14). Many cycle menus, such as a university menu, change entrées and other foods daily, but do keep certain items, such as burgers, pizza, and a salad bar, on the menu every day.

The length of the cycle is influenced by a number of factors, but probably the most important factor is having the cycle long enough to incorporate much variety and maintain interest. Shorter cycle menus (such as one to two weeks) work well in hospitals where patients normally stay for less than one week. A 3- or 4-week cycle menu is not unusual for high school students. Longer cycles, such as four or five weeks, are designed for operations that serve customers for an extended period of time, such as long-term care facilities or businesses.

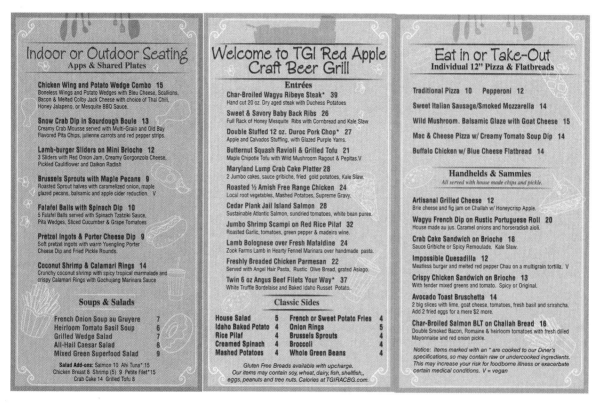

FIGURE 3-1 Restaurant Menu

Table 3-1 Week One of a Four-Week Cycle Menu for Assisted Living Facility

BREAKFAST

Category	Sunday 1	Monday 1	Tuesday 1	Wednesday 1	Thursday 1	Friday 1	Saturday 1
Fruits & Yogurts	Orange or apple juice (½ cup)	Orange or grape juice (½ cup)	Orange or cranberry juice (½ cup)	Orange or apple juice (½ cup)	Orange or grape juice (½ cup)	Orange or cranberry juice (½ cup)	Orange or apple juice (½ cup)
	Banana (1 small)	Banana (1 small)	Banana (1 small)	Banana (1 small)	Banana (1 small)	Banana (1 small)	Banana (1 small)
	Fresh fruit cup (½ cup)	Fresh fruit cup (½ cup)	Fresh fruit cup (½ cup)	Fresh fruit cup (½ cup)	Fresh fruit cup (½ cup)	Fresh fruit cup (½ cup)	Fresh fruit cup (½ cup)
	Applesauce (½ cup)	Applesauce (½ cup)	Applesauce (½ cup)	Applesauce (½ cup)	Applesauce (½ cup)	Applesauce (½ cup)	Applesauce (½ cup)
	Vanilla yogurt (1 cup)	Vanilla yogurt (1 cup)	Vanilla yogurt (1 cup)	Vanilla yogurt (1 cup)	Vanilla yogurt (1 cup)	Vanilla yogurt (1 cup)	Vanilla yogurt (1 cup)
	Low-fat fruit yogurt (1 cup)	Low-fat fruit yogurt (1 cup)	Low-fat fruit yogurt (1 cup)	Low-fat fruit yogurt (1 cup)	Low-fat fruit yogurt (1 cup)	Low-fat fruit yogurt (1 cup)	Low-fat fruit yogurt (1 cup)
	Raisins (2 T)	Raisins (2 T)	Raisins (2 T)	Raisins (2 T)	Raisins (2 T)	Raisins (2 T)	Raisins (2 T)
Entrées	Eggs, any style (2)	Cheese Omelet (2 eggs, 1 oz cheese)	Eggs, any style (2)	Vegetable Omelet (2 eggs, ¼ cup bell pepper)	Eggs, any style (2)	Cheese Omelet (2 eggs, 1 oz cheese)	Eggs, any style (2)
	Pancakes (2)	French Toast (2)	Waffles (2)	Pancakes (2)	French Toast (2)	Waffles (2)	Pancakes (2)
Sides	Bacon strips (2)	Bacon strips (2)	Bacon strips (2)	Bacon strips (2)	Bacon strips (2)	Bacon strips (2)	Bacon strips (2)
	Sausage links (2)	Sausage links (2)	Sausage links (2)	Sausage links (2)	Sausage links (2)	Sausage links (2)	Sausage links (2)
Cereals	Oatmeal (½ cup)	Oatmeal (½ cup)	Oatmeal (½ cup)	Oatmeal (½ cup)	Oatmeal (½ cup)	Oatmeal (½ cup)	Oatmeal (½ cup)
	Cheerios (¾ cup)	Cheerios (¾ cup)	Cheerios (¾ cup)	Cheerios (¾ cup)	Cheerios (¾ cup)	Cheerios (¾ cup)	Cheerios (¾ cup)
	Frosted Flakes (¾ cup)	Frosted Flakes (¾ cup)	Frosted Flakes (¾ cup)	Frosted Flakes (¾ cup)	Frosted Flakes (¾ cup)	Frosted Flakes (¾ cup)	Frosted Flakes (¾ cup)
	Raisin Bran (½ cup)	Raisin Bran (½ cup)	Raisin Bran (½ cup)	Raisin Bran (½ cup)	Raisin Bran (½ cup)	Raisin Bran (½ cup)	Raisin Bran (½ cup)

(continues)

Table 3-1 Week One of a Four-Week Cycle Menu for Assisted Living Facility (continued)

Category	Sunday 1	Monday 1	Tuesday 1	Wednesday 1	Thursday 1	Friday 1	Saturday 1
Toast & Baked Goods	Toast—white or multigrain (2 sl.) English muffin Corn muffin	Toast—white or multigrain (2 sl.) English muffin Blueberry muffin	Toast—white or multigrain (2 sl.) English muffin Danish pastry	Toast—white or multigrain (2 sl.) English muffin Banana muffin	Toast—white or multigrain (2 sl.) English muffin Blueberry muffin	Toast—white or multigrain (2 sl.) English muffin Danish pastry	Toast—white or multigrain (2 sl.) English muffin Corn muffin
Beverages	Reduced-fat milk, low-fat milk, nonfat milk, soy milk, coffee, decaf coffee, hot tea, decaf hot tea, hot chocolate.						
LUNCH							
Appetizers (soups are all 1 cup)	Tomato rice soup White bean salad (½ cup)	Cream of Broccoli Soup Tossed garden salad (1 cup)	Minestrone soup Greek salad (1 cup)	Chicken orzo soup Tossed garden salad (1 cup)	Beef barley soup Chopped caprese salad (1 cup)	Creamy tomato soup Tossed garden salad (1 cup)	Cream of mushroom soup Pasta salad (½ cup)
Entrées (1 hot, 1 sandwich, 1 salad)	Roast sliced chicken (3 oz.) with herbed butter (2 tablespoons) Turkey sandwich (3 oz. turkey + ½ oz. cheddar cheese) Chef's salad (2 cups)	Soft dough cheese pizza (1 slice) Roast beef sandwich (3 oz. meat + ½ oz. American cheese) Egg salad with salad greens (½ cup egg salad with 1 cup greens)	Beef pot pie (1) Grilled cheese w/ tomato (1.5 oz cheese) Turkey Waldorf salad (1 cup with ½ cup greens)	Cheese Ravioli w/ marinara (1 cup with 1/4 cup sauce) Tuna salad sandwich (½ cup tuna) Cranberry chicken salad with salad greens (½ cup chicken salad with 1 cup greens)	Hamburger on bun (3 oz.) Ham and Swiss sandwich (3 oz. ham + ½ oz. Swiss cheese) Cobb salad (2 cups)	Meatloaf (4 oz.) with gravy (2 tablespoons) Egg salad sandwich (½ cup egg salad) Honey Grilled Chicken with Citrus Salad (1.5 cups)	BBQ Pork (4 oz.) Chicken caesar wrap (3 oz. chicken) Cottage cheese and fruit plate (½ cup cottage cheese, ½ cup fruit, lettuce)
Sides (all ½ cup)	French-cut green beans Mashed maple sweet potatoes	Peas and pearl onions	Cauliflower	Italian vegetable medley	Baked French fries Broccoli	Corn Mashed potatoes	Cole slaw Potato salad
Bread	Soft roll	Popover	Biscuit	Plain muffin	Soft roll	Cheese biscuit	Cornbread

Dessert (all are ½ cup except bakery items)	Jelly roll (1 sl.) Ice cream/Italian ice Canned fruit	Snickerdoodle cookies (2) Ice cream/Italian ice Canned fruit	Brownie (1) Ice cream/Italian ice Canned fruit	Frosted white cake (1 sl.) Ice cream/Italian ice Canned fruit	Chocolate pudding Ice cream/Italian ice Canned fruit	Oatmeal cookies (2) Ice cream/Italian ice Canned fruit	Red velvet cake (1 sl.) Ice cream/Italian ice Canned fruit

Beverages: Same as breakfast and add: cola, diet cola, ginger ale, diet ginger ale, sweetened iced tea, unsweetened iced tea, apple juice, lemonade.

DINNER

Appetizer (soups are all 1 cup)	Chicken noodle soup Tossed garden salad (1 cup)	Butternut squash soup Spinach mushroom salad (1 cup)	Vegetable soup Tossed garden salad (1 cup)	Broccoli cheddar soup Caesar salad (1 cup)	Split pea soup Tossed garden salad (1 cup)	Italian wedding soup 7 vegetable salad (1 cup)	Chicken gnocchi soup Tossed garden salad (1 cup)
Entrées (2 hot *plus* sandwich and entrée salad from lunch)	Roast beef w/ gravy (3 oz. + 2 tablespoons gravy) Stir-fried chicken with vegetables (3 oz chicken, 1/2 cup vegetables)	Penne Pasta w/ meatballs and sauce (1 cup penne, 2 oz. meat, ¼ cup sauce) Crumb crusted salmon (4 oz.)	Honey mustard chicken (3 oz.) Macaroni and cheese (1¼ cups)	Salisbury steak (4 oz.) Battered fish of the day (4 oz.)	Baked honey ham (3 oz.) Oven fried chicken (1 each)	Sautéed chicken w/creamy lemon sauce (3 oz. chicken, ¼ cup sauce) Parmesan crusted flounder (4 oz.)	Beef stroganoff (1 cup + ½ cup noodles) Baked meaty rigatoni (1 cup)
Sides (all 1/2 cup)	Glazed carrots Rice	California mixed vegetables Penne pasta with tomatoes	Sautéed spinach Quinoa w/pine nuts	Carrots Mashed potatoes	Green beans Scalloped potatoes	Roasted tomatoes Herbed rice	Peas Buttered noodles
Bread	Soft roll	Popover	Biscuit	Plain muffin	Soft roll	Cheese biscuit	Cornbread
Dessert (all are ½ cup except bakery items)	Apple pie (1 sl.) Ice cream/Italian ice Sliced fresh fruit	Strawberry shortcake (1) Ice cream/Italian ice Sliced fresh fruit	Vanilla pudding Ice cream/Italian ice Sliced fresh fruit	Chocolate chip cookies (2) Ice cream/Italian ice Sliced fresh fruit	Frosted chocolate cake (1 sl.) Ice cream/Italian ice Sliced fresh fruit	Peach crisp (1 sl.) Ice cream/Italian ice Chocolate pudding Sliced fresh fruit	Butterscotch pudding Ice cream/Italian ice Sliced fresh fruit

Beverages: Same as breakfast and add: cola, diet cola, ginger ale, diet ginger ale, sweetened iced tea, unsweetened iced tea, apple juice, lemonade.

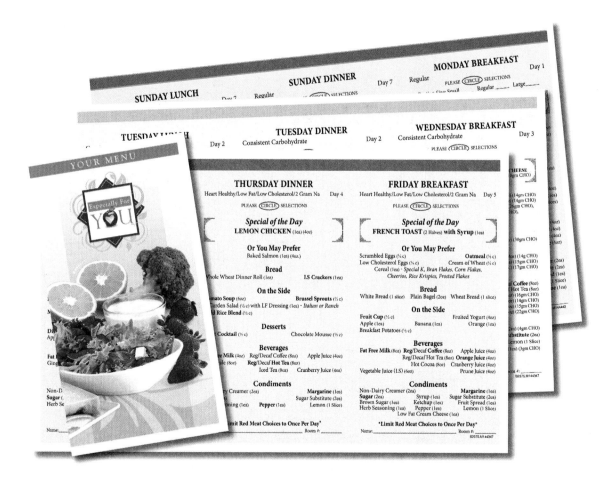

FIGURE 3-2 Three Days of a One-Week Cycle Menu for a Hospital

Courtesy of MedFare LLC.

Like a static menu, cycle menus are also updated on a regular basis to get rid of menu items that just do not fit for various reasons or to incorporate new and seasonal items. In many parts of the United States, winter menus feature more hearty soups and stews, for example, while summer menus offer more fresh fruits and salads, including fresh, locally sourced products.

Whereas the use of a cycle menu adds variety to meals (an advantage), a cycle menu does make food production more complicated than a static menu (a disadvantage). When managers, cooks, and others prepare the same menu items daily, they are quite knowledgeable about how much food to purchase and are efficient at preparing the foods. However, since the cycle menu changes daily for one week or longer, more food items will need to be purchased and stored. Also, cooks and food preparation workers will be preparing different items on most days and will need some time to become fully acquainted with the demands of each day of the cycle.

When looking at how often a menu changes, you have seen a static and a cycle menu. There is also a **single-use or event menu**, which is a menu designed and used for only one meal or occasion. For example, a catering menu is developed for a retirement dinner and is used only for that event. Caterers do have menus but they are usually customized for each client and event. Some onsite foodservices, such as hospital and business and industry foodservices, offer catering for meetings or special functions, and some of their menus are also single-use menus.

Another way that menus vary is by how the pricing works. Most menus are **à la carte**, meaning that each individual item on the menu has its own price. Some

THE BIG PICTURE

Menus can vary in a number of ways.

- By how often the menu changes: Static (like a restaurant menu—it may change a few times a year), cycle (such as a one-week cycle in a hospital or a four-week cycle in a school cafeteria), or single-use (used a lot in catering).
- By how the pricing works: À la carte (each item is priced separately) or table d'hôte (one price for a full meal).
- By the degree of choice a customer has to select foods: Selective, semi-selective, or nonselective (possibly with write-ins).

Whereas the use of a cycle menu adds variety to meals in foodservices that serve a "captive clientele," a cycle menu does make food production more complicated than a static menu.

Within one foodservice, such as a hospital, there be may several different types of menus used. For example, the patients may choose meals from a static, restaurant-style menu (**Figure 3-3**); the employees of the facility who eat in the cafeteria choose meals from a four-week cycle menu that is à la carte; and the catering manager uses single-use menus. Also, the hospital-owned nursing home uses a semi-selective cycle menu.

---

foodservices offer a complete meal for a stated price—such as a three-course meal for $25. This is referred to as a **table d'hôte menu**.

The final way in which menus can vary is by the degree of choice the customer has. You can look at the degree of choice from two perspectives. First, you can look at the *total number of menu items offered*—it can go anywhere from a limited selection (such as McDonald's) to an extensive selection (such as Cheesecake Factory with over 250 menu items). Of course, an extensive menu appeals to a broader range of customers but also requires a bigger kitchen, and more cooks, equipment, and storage space for ingredients. Operations (including purchasing, storing, preparing and serving food) are simpler in foodservices with fewer menu items.

The second way to look at degree of choice is to examine *the number of choices the customer gets in each menu category* such as appetizers or desserts.

- A **selective menu** offers at least two choices in each menu category.
- A **semi-selective menu** offers at least two choices in some categories, while other categories have only one choice. For example, there may be two choices for entrée and dessert, but just one appetizer or one vegetable offered.
- A **nonselective menu** (also called a preselective menu) does not offer any choices.

Most restaurant menus are selective and offer choices in all menu categories.

So who uses semiselective or nonselective menus? They are generally found in certain onsite foodservices such as long-term care facilities (nursing homes and assisted living facilities) and most correctional facilities and federally-funded child and adult care programs. Offering fewer selections is very cost-effective and generally used where food costs/meal are strictly budgeted. When a nursing home or correctional facility use a nonselective menu, alternate items must be available for taste, allergies, and cultural or religious preferences. For example, if a nursing home is serving fish for dinner, a resident who doesn't eat fish can pick an alternate item such as a hamburger or grilled cheese. The alternate items are often referred to as **write-ins** because they are written onto that patient's menu to replace the preselected item. A facility often maintains a list of write-ins or approved substitutions that are allowed at certain meal periods, such as a turkey sandwich at lunch or a cheeseburger at dinner.

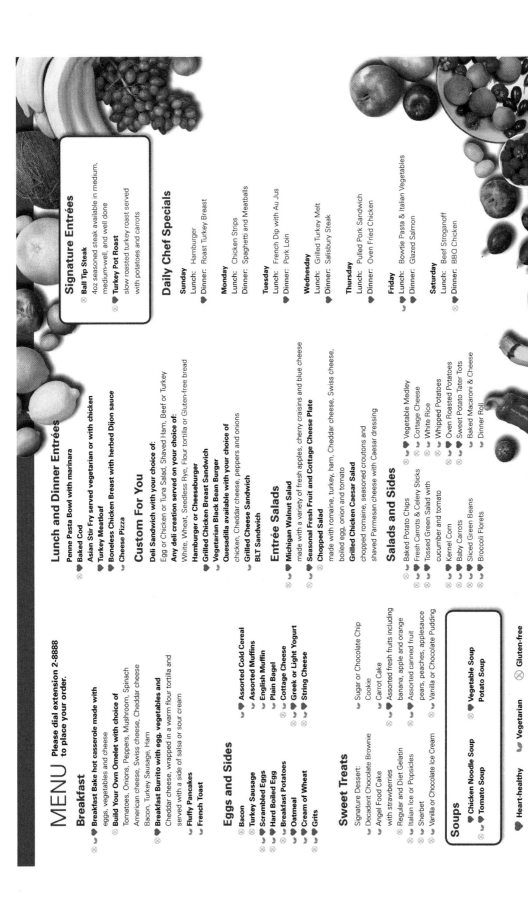

MENU Please dial extension 2-8888 to place your order.

Breakfast

⊗ ↳ ♥ **Breakfast Bake hot casserole made with** eggs, vegetables and cheese

⊗ **Build Your Own Omelet with choice of** Tomatoes, Onions, Peppers, Mushroom, Spinach American cheese, Swiss cheese, Cheddar cheese Bacon, Turkey Sausage, Ham

⊗ **Breakfast Burrito with egg, vegetables and** Cheddar cheese, wrapped in a warm flour tortilla and served with a side of salsa or sour cream

↳ ♥ **Fluffy Pancakes**

↳ ♥ **French Toast**

Eggs and Sides

⊗ **Bacon**

⊗ **Turkey Sausage**

⊗ ↳ ♥ **Scrambled Eggs**

⊗ ↳ ♥ **Hard Boiled Egg**

⊗ ↳ **Breakfast Potatoes**

↳ ♥ **Oatmeal**

↳ ♥ **Cream of Wheat**

⊗ ↳ ♥ **Grits**

↳ ♥ **Assorted Cold Cereal**

↳ **Assorted Muffins**

↳ **English Muffin**

↳ **Plain Bagel**

⊗ ↳ **Cottage Cheese**

⊗ ↳ ♥ **Greek or Light Yogurt**

⊗ ↳ ♥ **String Cheese**

Sweet Treats

Signature Dessert:

↳ **Sugar or Chocolate Chip** Cookie

↳ **Decadent Chocolate Brownie**

↳ **Carrot Cake**

↳ **Angel Food Cake** with strawberries

↳ ♥ **Assorted fresh fruits including** banana, apple and orange

⊗ ↳ **Regular and Diet Gelatin**

⊗ **Assorted canned fruit** pears, peaches, applesauce

⊗ ↳ **Italian Ice or Popsicles**

⊗ **Sherbet**

⊗ ↳ **Vanilla or Chocolate Pudding**

⊗ ↳ **Vanilla or Chocolate Ice Cream**

Soups

⊗ ↳ ♥ **Chicken Noodle Soup**

↳ ♥ **Tomato Soup**

⊗ ↳ ♥ **Vegetable Soup**

↳ **Potato Soup**

♥ **Heart-healthy**   ↳ **Vegetarian**   ⊗ **Gluten-free**

Lunch and Dinner Entrées

↳ ♥ **Penne Pasta Bowl with marinara**

⊗ ♥ **Baked Cod**

↳ **Asian Stir Fry served vegetarian or with chicken**

♥ **Turkey Meatloaf**

♥ **Boneless Chicken Breast with herbed Dijon sauce**

↳ **Cheese Pizza**

Custom For You

Deli Sandwich with your choice of:
Egg or Chicken or Tuna Salad, Shaved Ham, Beef or Turkey

Any deli creation served on your choice of:
White, Wheat, Seedless Rye, Flour tortilla or Gluten-free bread

♥ **Hamburger or Cheeseburger**

♥ **Grilled Chicken Breast Sandwich**

↳ **Vegetarian Black Bean Burger**

Quesadilla available with your choice of chicken, Cheddar cheese, peppers and onions

⊗ ↳ **Grilled Cheese Sandwich**

BLT Sandwich

Entrée Salads

⊗ ↳ ♥ **Michigan Walnut Salad** made with a variety of fresh apples, cherry craisins and blue cheese

⊗ ↳ **Seasonal Fresh Fruit and Cottage Cheese Plate**

⊗ **Chopped Salad** made with romaine, turkey, ham, Cheddar cheese, Swiss cheese, boiled egg, onion and tomato

Grilled Chicken Caesar Salad chopped romaine, seasoned croutons and shaved Parmesan cheese with Caesar dressing

Salads and Sides

⊗ ↳ **Baked Potato Chips**

⊗ ↳ **Fresh Carrots & Celery Sticks**

⊗ ↳ **Tossed Green Salad with** cucumber and tomato

⊗ ↳ **Kernel Corn**

⊗ ↳ **Baby Carrots**

⊗ ↳ ♥ **Sliced Green Beans**

⊗ ↳ ♥ **Broccoli Florets**

↳ ♥ **Vegetable Medley**

⊗ ↳ **Cottage Cheese**

⊗ ↳ **White Rice**

⊗ ↳ **Whipped Potatoes**

⊗ ↳ **Oven Roasted Potatoes**

⊗ ↳ **Sweet Potato Tater Tots**

↳ **Baked Macaroni & Cheese**

↳ **Dinner Roll**

Signature Entrées

⊗ **Ball Tip Steak** 4oz seasoned steak available in medium, medium-well, and well done

♥ **Turkey Pot Roast** slow roasted turkey roast served with potatoes and carrots

Daily Chef Specials

Sunday
Lunch: Hamburger
♥ Dinner: Roast Turkey Breast

Monday
Lunch: Chicken Strips
Dinner: Spaghetti and Meatballs

Tuesday
Lunch: French Dip with Au Jus
♥ Dinner: Pork Loin

Wednesday
Lunch: Grilled Turkey Melt
♥ Dinner: Salisbury Steak

Thursday
Lunch: Pulled Pork Sandwich
♥ Dinner: Oven Fried Chicken

Friday
♥ Lunch: Bowtie Pasta & Italian Vegetables
♥ Dinner: Glazed Salmon

Saturday
Lunch: Beef Stroganoff
⊗ Dinner: BBQ Chicken

FIGURE 3-3 Restaurant-Style Room Service Menu for Hospital Patients

Courtesy of MedFare LLC.

3.2 PLAN MENUS

Menu planning is the process of considering and deciding which dishes to offer on the menu. Many operators will keep an eye on competitors' menus to see what they are offering. To look for menu ideas, there are lots of resources, such as restaurant and food-service trade journals (*FoodService Director, Food Management, Plate, Restaurant Business, FSR*), the food section in newspapers, as well as food magazines (*Cooking Light, Cook's Illustrated, Bon Appétit, Food and Wine*) and food shows on television (Food Network).

CONSIDERATIONS WHEN PLANNING MENUS

Since the menu is the heart of a foodservice, there are a number of considerations to keep in mind when planning the menu.

1. <u>Is the menu consistent with the foodservice's concept and mission?</u> For example, part of the mission of the chain Panda Express is to offer an "exceptional Asian dining experience." When you look at their menu full of dishes such as Kung Pao chicken and veggie spring rolls, the menu is certainly consistent with their mission. If the mission of a retirement facility foodservice is to provide nutritious, healthy meals using fresh ingredients, you would expect the menu to feature chicken, fish, lean beef, meatless entrées, whole grains, and lots of fresh fruits and vegetables.

2. <u>Does the menu reflect the food habits and preferences and sociocultural backgrounds of your target market?</u> In short, the menu needs to offer foods that your target market loves to eat at prices they find reasonable. A **target market** represents the groups of customers you have identified as most likely to come in to eat. Members of a group share certain characteristics, such as age, income level, education, lifestyle preferences (such as vegetarian), and geographic location. For example, a foodservice looking to attract millennials (someone born generally between 1981 and 1996) would offer fresh ingredients and authentic, tasty food at moderate prices. Millennials are also looking for variety, customization of meals, and eating places that are environmentally conscious and offer nutritious options. **Table 3-2** gives characteristics of a nutritionally balanced menu, and **Table 3-3** summarizes the *Dietary Guidelines for Americans (2020–2025)*. Keep in mind that cultural and ethnic backgrounds also influence food preferences and habits. For information on cultural and ethnic food habits, consult a textbook such as *Food and Culture* (2017).

3. <u>Does the menu offer a variety of flavorful and visually appealing meals with different textures, colors, shapes, sizes, and cooking methods?</u> The most important

---

Table 3-2 Characteristics of a Nutritionally Balanced Menu

1. Portion sizes are moderate, with three to four oz. for center-of-the-plate proteins.
2. Most of the menu items are nutrient dense with no or very little salt, sugar, or solid fat added.
3. Whole-grain breads and grains are available at each meal.
4. Most meat and poultry items are lean. Fish, beans, nuts, and other meat alternates are offered at lunch and dinner.
5. A wide variety of vegetables and fruits are available, and most vegetables and fruits have their skins and seeds (baked potatoes with skin or apples or pears with peels).
6. Flavorful vinaigrette salad dressings using high-quality vegetable oils are available.
7. Low-fat or fat-free milk, yogurt, and other dairy choices are offered.
8. Desserts high in fat and sugar are balanced with more nutritious choices such as fruit-based desserts.
9. A soft margarine that does not contain trans fat is available.
10. Unsweetened beverages and a variety of waters are offered.

Data from Drummond, Karen & Brefere, Lisa. (2017). *Nutrition for foodservice and culinary professionals.* Hoboken, NJ: John Wiley & Sons, Inc.

Table 3-3 Dietary Guidelines for Americans (2020–2025)

Key Recommendations.

Guideline 1. Follow a healthy dietary pattern at every life stage.

At every life stage - infancy, toddlerhood, childhood, adolescence, adulthood, pregnancy, lactation, and older adulthood - it is never too early or too late to eat healthfully. Establishing a healthy dietary pattern early in life may have a beneficial impact on preventing disease over the course of decades. A dietary pattern represents everything you habitually eat and drink - meaning the quantities, proportions, and variety or combination of different foods and drinks.

Guideline 2. Customize and enjoy nutrient-dense food and beverage choices to reflect personal preferences, cultural traditions, and budgetary considerations.

A healthy dietary pattern can benefit all individuals regardless of age, race, or ethnicity, or current health status. The **Dietary Guidelines** provides a framework intended to be customized to individual needs and preferences, as well as the foodways of the diverse cultures in the United States.

Guideline 3. Focus on meeting food group needs with nutrient-dense foods and beverages, and stay within calorie limits.

An underlying premise of the **Dietary Guidelines** is that nutritional needs should be met primarily from foods and beverages - specifically, nutrient-dense foods and beverages. Nutrient-dense foods provide vitamins, minerals, and other health-promoting components and have no or little added sugars, saturated fat, and sodium. A healthy dietary pattern consists of nutrient-dense forms of foods and beverages across all food groups, in recommended amounts, and within calorie limits.

The core elements that make up a healthy dietary pattern include:

- Vegetables - of all types.
- Fruits - especially whole fruit.
- Grains - at least half of which are whole grain.
- Dairy - including fat-free or low-fat milk, yogurt, and cheese, and/or lactose-free versions and fortified soy beverages and yogurt as alternatives.
- Protein foods - including lean meats, poultry, and eggs; seafood; beans, peas and lentil; and nuts, seeds, and soy products.
- Oils - including vegetable oils and oils in food, such as seafood and nuts.

Guideline 4. Limit foods and beverages higher in added sugars, saturated fat, and sodium, and limit alcoholic beverages.

At every life stage, meeting food group recommendations - even with nutrient-dense choices - requires most of a person's daily calorie needs and sodium limits. A healthy dietary pattern doesn't have much room for extra added sugars, saturated fat, or sodium - or for alcoholic beverages. Small amounts of added sugars, saturated fat, or sodium can be added to nutrient-dense foods and beverages to help meet food group recommendations, but foods and beverages high in these components should be limited. **Limits are**:

- **Added sugars** - Less than 10 percent of calories per day, starting at age 2. Avoid foods and beverages with added sugars for those younger than age 2.
- **Saturated fat** - Less than 10 percent of calories per day starting at age 2.
- **Sodium** - Less than 2,300 milligrams per day - and even less for children younger than age 14.
- **Alcoholic beverages** - Adults of legal drinking age can choose not to drink or to drink in moderation by limiting intake to 2 drinks or less in a day for man and 1 drink or less in a day for women, when alcohol is consumed. Drinking less is better for health than drinking more. There are some adults who should not drink alcohol, such as women who are pregnant.

Data from U.S. Department of Agriculture and U.S. Department of Health and Human Services. *Dietary Guidelines for Americans, 2020–2025.* 9th Edition, December 2020. Available at DietaryGuidelines.gov.

consideration when choosing something to eat is the **taste** of the food. Taste happens mostly on the tongue, where you taste sweet, salty, sour, bitter, and umami (savory). You may think that taste and flavor are the same thing, but taste is actually a component of flavor. **Flavor** also includes aroma, texture, and temperature. Much of what we perceive as flavor comes from smell, so when your nose is clogged up, food is less flavorful. Food **texture** is how a food feels in your mouth. Textures that most people enjoy include crispy, crunchy, juicy, creamy, tender, and firm. Customers generally don't like foods that are tough, crumbly, lumpy, soggy, or watery. The temperature of foods and beverages are also important—no one wants to finish a latte once it has turned cold. In addition to flavor, you also need to consider qualities that contribute to eye appeal—colors, shapes, and sizes. Serve foods with a variety of colors, shapes, and sizes to create balanced, attractive plates. When you pair side dishes with an entrée, colorful vegetables look great next to meats, poultry, fish, and grains, which tend to be white, off-white, or brown. Cutting vegetables into different shapes and sizes gives food a caring, home-made look and can add interest to items such as salads. Also offer dishes that use different cooking methods, such as roasted, grilled, sautéed, or simmered. *In summary, make sure your menu offers a variety of flavors, textures, colors, shapes, sizes, and cooking methods, as well as hot and cold food choices.*

4. Are there enough low-cost menu items to balance those with higher costs so the overall menu is cost-effective in terms of food and labor costs? Food and labor costs vary with the type of operation, the **sales mix** (proportion of total sales that each menu item generates), pricing, and other factors. Operators monitor their food-cost percentage and labor-cost percentage to control costs. **Food cost percentage** is the cost of food divided by total sales, so if a foodservice had sales of $45,000 last week and food and beverages cost $15,000, the food-cost percentage is 33%.

$$\frac{\text{Food and beverage cost}}{\text{Total sales}} = \text{Food-cost percentage} = \frac{\$15,000}{\$45,000}$$

Labor cost percentage is calculated similarly. In restaurants, food cost percentage is usually close to 33% and labor cost percentage close to 35% (Reynolds & McClusky, 2013), although some restaurants keep food cost and/or labor cost percentages down a bit lower, such as 25%. Food and labor costs vary a great deal due to different concepts, menus, and other considerations. Certain onsite foodservices, such as schools and correctional facilities, have very tight budgets so their menus rarely utilize expensive foods, such as grass-fed beef or fresh wild-caught fish. Many onsite foodservices have a budget that is based on a daily food cost per person. Labor costs are also important and every time you add another item to your menu, you are increasing your labor costs. In the cycle menu in Table 3-1 for an assisted living facility, you will notice that the sandwich and entrée salad offered at lunch each day (along with a hot entrée) are also available at dinner. That is one way to increase variety without a corresponding increase in workload.

5. Can each menu item be effectively purchased, produced, and served? If a menu item requires an ingredient that is out of season and very expensive to buy, is difficult to find, or has to be purchased in a large amount when only a little will be used, these are problems that may require dropping the menu item. You also have to consider production and if you have enough equipment capacity and trained employees to produce the menu items. If all the menu items for Tuesday lunch on a one-week cycle menu have to be cooked or finished in the oven, is there enough oven space? If foods are held in a steam table and/or transported hot before being served, certain menu items will lose quality. For instance, fried foods lose their crispness, sliced meats dry out, and grilled cheese gets soggy, so better choices might be meat loaf, chicken stew, or a cheeseburger. Chefs and cooks can be very helpful in pointing out potential issues with cooking and transportation.

6. If the menu falls under governmental regulations, does the menu meet those regulations? For example, school lunch programs that participate in the National School Lunch Program must include the food components and meet the nutritional requirements for lunches shown in **Table 3-4**. In addition, hospitals and long-term care facilities that accept Medicare must demonstrate how their menus meet the nutritional needs of patients. The *State Operations Manual* published by the Centers for Medicare and Medicaid Services (CMS) gives guidelines for meals and snacks served to patients. A registered dietitian nutritionist (RDN) performs a nutrient analysis of each menu to verify that there are sufficient calories and nutrients using the Recommended Dietary Allowances (RDA).

Whereas a school lunch program has different menus and requirements for elementary, middle, and high schools, hospitals and long-term care facilities

Table 3-4 National School Lunch Program Five-Day Lunch Meal Pattern and Nutrition Requirements

National School Lunch Meal Pattern

Food Components	Grade K–5	Grade 6–8	Grade 9–12
Milk	5 cups/week (1 cup daily)	5 cups/week (1 cup daily)	5 cups/week (1 cup daily)
Meat or Meat Alternatives -Weekly minimum	8 oz equivalent/week (1 oz daily minimum)	9 oz equivalent/week (1 oz daily minimum)	10 oz equivalent/week (2 oz daily minimum)
Vegetables (total) -Weekly minimum	3¾ cups/week (3/4 cup daily minimum)	3¾ cups/week (3/4 cup daily minimum	5 cups/week (1 cup daily minimum)
Dark Green Subgroup	½ cup/wk	½ cup/wk	½ cup/wk
Red/Orange Subgroup	¾ cup/wk	¾ cup/wk	1 ¼ cup/wk
Legumes Subgroup	½ cup/wk	½ cup/wk	½ cup/wk
Starchy Subgroup	½ cup/wk	½ cup/wk	½ cup/wk
Other Subgroup	½ cup/wk	½ cup/wk	¾ cup/wk
Fruits -Weekly minimum	2 ½ cups/week (½ cup daily minimum)	2 ½ cups/week (½ cup daily minimum)	5 cups/week (1 cup daily minimum)
Grains / Breads -Weekly minimum -At least half whole grain beginning School Year 2012–13 -All whole grain beginning School Year 2014–2015	8 oz equivalent/week (1 oz daily minimum)	8 oz equivalent/week (1 oz daily minimum)	10 oz equivalent/week (2 oz daily minimum)
Minimum – Maximum Calories (kcal) -Weekly average	550–650	600–700	750–850
Saturated Fat (% of total calories) -Weekly average	<10%	<10%	<10%
Sodium** -Weekly average	≤1230 mg*	≤1360 mg*	≤1420 mg*
Trans fat	0 grams / serving	0 grams / serving	0 grams / serving

*Effective School Year 2014–2015.
**Increasingly restrictive targets in School Year 2017–2018 and School Year 2022–2023.
U.S. Department of Agriculture, National School Lunch Program chart. Retrieved from https://www.fns.usda.gov/nslp/national-school-lunch
-program-meal-pattern-chart

have a regular (or "house") diet for patients without any dietary restrictions and also diets that have been modified to meet individual medical nutrition therapy needs. For instance, a patient with high blood pressure may be on a low-sodium diet that restricts foods high in salt (sodium chloride). An RDN makes sure that patients with dietary restrictions receive appropriate meals along with education.

Calorie labeling is required for restaurants and similar retail food establishments that are part of a chain of 20 or more locations. For standard menu items, calories are listed clearly and prominently on menus and menu boards, next to the name or price of the food or beverage. For self-service foods

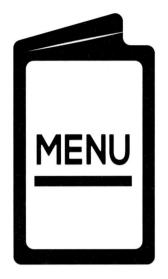

Factors to Consider from the Customers' Point of View:

1. Food habits and preferences (including for healthy and/or sustainable choices).
2. Sociocultural backgrounds.
3. Prices.
4. Flavorful, visually appealing meals using different flavors, textures, colors, shapes, sizes, and cooking methods.

Factors to Consider from the Managers' Point of View:

1. Consistency of menu with the concept/mission.
2. Cost-effectiveness in terms of food and labor costs.
3. Ease of purchasing, preparation, and serving.
4. Consistent with pertinent government regulations.
5. Environmental responsibility.

FIGURE 3-4 Factors to Be Considered in Menu Planning

© Flatvector/Shutterstock

(like a salad bar), calories are shown on signs that are near the foods. In addition to calorie information, restaurants are also required to provide written nutrition information on their menu items (such as grams of fat and sodium) on posters, computers, or other means. Most vending machines must also include calorie information.

7. <u>Is the menu environmentally responsible?</u> For example, a foodservice may source some items locally and serve several meatless entrées. See the following "Spotlight on Sustainable Menus" for more on this topic.

Figure 3–4 summarizes the factors to be considered in menu planning.

SPOTLIGHT ON SUSTAINABLE MENUS

The term "sustainable" is not always defined in the same way. At a professional symposium in 2010 organized by the Food and Agriculture Organization of the United Nations and Biodiversity International, the following definition of sustainable diets was developed and agreed upon (FAO, 2010).

> "those diets with low environmental impacts which contribute to food and nutrition security and to healthy life for present and future generations. Sustainable diets are protective and respectful of biodiversity and ecosystems; culturally acceptable; accessible; economically fair and affordable; nutritionally adequate, safe, and healthy; while optimizing natural and human resources."

This definition considers not only the environment, but other factors such as safety and nutrition.

To discuss principles of sustainable menus, we will first look at ingredients that are appropriate for sustainable diets. In general, reducing animal foods and increasing plant foods results in less environmental impact. We will also discuss general guidelines that affect purchasing, operations, and menu choices (Culinary Institute of America and Harvard T.H. Chan School of Public Health, 2018; Drummond & Brefere, 2017; Fischer & Garnett, 2016).

1. <u>Consider plant foods first: fruits, vegetables, whole grains, legumes, nuts, and seeds; and use legumes, nuts, seeds, and whole grains to replace animal protein.</u> An animal-based diet requires more fertilizer, water, energy, and pesticides than a plant-based diet. Therefore, menus should feature a variety of fruits and vegetables daily, fresh whenever possible but frozen or preserved without added sugar or salt is acceptable. Whole grains that have not been milled, such as wheat berries or steel-cut oatmeal, can be

used in a main course, appetizer, salad, side dish, or breakfast selection. Legumes contain even more fiber and protein per serving than grains. Both legumes and grains are extremely cost-effective and add color, flavor, and texture to a variety of dishes. Nuts and seeds are versatile and nutritious ingredients. Most are rich in monounsaturated fats and good protein sources. Nuts and seeds play many roles in the kitchen such as being ground in hot and cold sauces, dips and spreads, appetizers, and side dishes.

2. <u>Focus on recipes using whole foods or minimally processed foods, such as canned low-sodium navy beans</u>. Whole foods are close to how we find them in nature. Foods, such as milk, are minimally processed to make it safe to drink. Processed foods, like canned soup, contain parts of whole foods and often have added ingredients such as sugar and salt. That's the beauty of whole foods—no sugar, salt, or fat is added.

3. <u>Choose menu items using healthy oils (such as in salad dressings) and ingredients with healthy oils such as seafood, nuts, seeds, and avocadoes</u>. Most vegetable oils (except coconut oil, palm kernel, or palm oil) are good sources of healthy monounsaturated and polyunsaturated fats and can be used in cooking such as to sauté vegetables. Flavorful fats that are high in saturated fats (such as the fat in beef, cheese, butter, and cream) are not heart-healthy but can be used in small amounts in the kitchen. Partially hydrogenated vegetable oils should be avoided as they contain trans fats, which are also not heart-healthy.

4. <u>Serve more seafood and different kinds of seafood from responsibly managed sources</u>. Fishing practices worldwide are depleting fish populations, destroying habitats, and polluting the water. Sustainable seafood comes from species of fish that are managed in a way that provides for today's needs without damaging the availability of the species to future generations. Fish and shellfish are excellent sources of protein, contain healthy fats including omega-3 fatty acids, and are relatively low in calories. Most Americans do not eat the recommended two servings per week of seafood. There are programs, such as FishChoice and Seafood Watch, that help foodservices find sustainable seafood choices.

5. <u>Red meats (especially beef), poultry, and eggs are harder on the environment than plant foods, so serve in moderation</u>. Fresh poultry raised without antibiotics has less of an environmental footprint than red meat and is a healthy protein. Fresh is best as processed chicken products are high in sodium. Most people can eat one egg a day, so use vegetables in omelets and other egg dishes to add plant foods. Beef and other red meats can be used occasionally as entrées and otherwise used in supporting roles with plant foods. When using red meats, choose grass-fed animals raised without the use of antibiotics. Pork is a better choice than beef using some environmental gauges (Culinary Institute of America and Harvard T.H. Chan School of Public Health, 2018).

6. <u>Use a variety of techniques to add flavor to food without using salt (or using very small amounts)</u>. Use fresh foods for maximum natural taste along with flavorful cooking techniques such as marinating, toasting, grilling, and searing. Slow cooking of meats and vegetables (such as tomatoes) that are high in glutamate cause the development of umami, which increases savory flavors. Ingredients such as herbs, spices, vinegars, oils, aromatic vegetables, glazes, citrus fruits, and condiments (low-sodium soy sauce, sriracha, mustard) enhance and build flavor profiles. Look to various ethnic cuisines for lower-in-sodium recipes as many rely on a variety of herbs, spices, and other flavorings.

7. <u>Reduce sugar in desserts and beverages</u>. Newly composed sweet endings with less sugar incorporate ingredients such as fruit (fresh or dried), nuts, dark chocolate, whole grains, healthy oils, low-fat dairy such as yogurt, and eggs. When fruits are at their peak of ripeness, chefs can make a sorbet without sugar. Compote is an additional way to serve fruit. Phyllo dough can be stuffed with strawberries and house-made granola, baked, then served with maple Greek yogurt and spiced apples. Bake a chocolate ricotta flan or oatmeal-crusted peach cobbler. The best beverage choice is filtered tap water (no bottle) which can be dressed up with sliced fruit or other flavorings.

8. <u>Buy your ingredients fresh and local when possible</u>. For optimal flavor, get fresh fruits and vegetables locally when they are at their peak of ripeness. Local fruits and vegetables are allowed to ripen longer before harvesting so they are bursting with flavor and nutrition. During the colder seasons, try to find a grower with heated greenhouses or in warmer regions. Also, feature menu items using root vegetables such as carrots, beets, yams, or other vegetables that keep well.

9. <u>Buy from purveyors/farms with more sustainable practices</u>. Chefs should look at the environmental cost of how the food is produced. The better producers will use little or no synthetic pesticides or fertilizers, avoid using valuable groundwater for irrigation, or in the case of livestock, avoid antibiotics and give outdoor access. In some cases, chefs may specify organic-certified foods. To be certified as organic, meat, poultry, eggs, and dairy products must come from animals with outdoor access that are given no antibiotics or growth hormones. Organic fruits and vegetables are produced without using most conventional pesticides or fertilizers made with synthetic ingredients. It is not always necessary or possible to buy only organic products, so chefs need to look at how the food was produced.

10. It's often easier to introduce new items that are healthier and more sustainably produced than to modify a current menu item. Some menu items just can't be modified without losing flavor or something else. Look to cuisines from other cultures and countries to find new menu ideas.

11. Use moderate portion sizes so your operation does not contribute to obesity and food waste. Emphasize the quality of the calories, not the quantity of the calories or the amount of food.

12. Talk about flavor and local sources on the menu. Customers are much more likely to pick a menu item that sounds really delicious than one that sounds healthy, so you need to describe and emphasize the *flavors*. Also be transparent about where foods came from, such as chicken from a local, well-known organic farm, as this adds value for your customers.

STEPS FOR PLANNING MENUS

When developing a menu, first you must decide on the **meal pattern**, meaning which menu categories (such as appetizer) will be used for a meal, and approximately how many choices to offer in each menu category. For instance, the left side of **Table 3–5** shows a meal pattern for lunch and dinner for meals served in a national-assisted living chain. Whereas this meal pattern and number of choices works well for a three-week cycle menu in assisted living, it is quite different from a restaurant-style menu. The right side of Table 3–5 shows an example of a meal pattern for a restaurant-style menu used in a hospital foodservice for lunch and dinner meals. Since the restaurant-style menu is a static menu, there are more categories and also choices within each category because a patient will be using the same menu every day until discharged from the hospital.

Menus in quick-service and fast casual restaurants vary from other types of restaurants. First, they don't usually have a paper menu. Instead, menu items are displayed on a menu board, often above the ordering area. Menus in quick-service and fast casual

Table 3-5 Comparison of Meal Patterns and Number of Choices for a Cycle Menu and a Restaurant-Style Menu	
Cycle Menu for Assisted Living—*Lunch*	**Restaurant-Style Hospital Menu—***Lunch or Dinner*
Appetizer (1 choice)	Appetizers (6 choices)
Soup and Salad (1 choice each)	Deli Sandwiches (6 fillings with choice of cheese and bread/wrap)
Entrées (1 hot, 1 sandwich, 1 salad)	Grill Choices (9 choices)
Side Dishes (2 choices)	Pizza (3 choices)
Breads (2 choices)	Hot Entrées (10 choices)
Desserts (3 choices)	Entrée Salads (3 choices)
Beverages	Side Dishes (12 choices)
Cycle Menu for Assisted Living – *Dinner*	Desserts (15 choices including fruit, ice cream, ices, pudding, sweets)
Appetizer (1 choice)	Beverages
Soup and Salad (1 choice each)	
Entrées (2 hot, 1 salad)	
Side Dishes (2 choices)	
Breads (2 choices)	
Desserts (3 choices)	
Beverages	

Table 3-6 Blank Form for Planning a Cycle Menu							
Week Number: _____ Breakfast/Lunch/Dinner (circle one) Dates: _____							
	Sunday Day 1	Monday Day 2	Tuesday Day 3	Wednesday Day 4	Thursday Day 5	Friday Day 6	Saturday Day 7
Appetizers							
Entrées							
Side Dishes							
Salads							
Breads							
Desserts							

restaurants tend to contain fewer menu choices, omit an appetizer section, and are the same for lunch and dinner. Other restaurants, such as family dining or casual restaurants, offer larger menus including appetizers and often alcoholic beverages.

To start writing a menu, you can use a blank form that lists each category. If you are writing a cycle menu, you can use the form found in **Table 3-6** and just fill in the category names. To make the process of writing a menu a little bit easier, there are logical steps to follow.

1. Plan the dinner entrées first. Since a meal is usually built around the entrée, and the entrée is the most expensive part of a meal, this is where to start. This is known as the Center-of-the-Plate. Within the entrée category, you have many choices: meat (beef, pork, lamb, and game animals), poultry (chicken, turkey, duck, and game birds), seafood, pasta entrées, meatless and other mixed dishes, and so on. For a dinner meal, portions of meat, poultry, or seafood may be cooked in their solid form (such as a chicken breast or pork chop), ground and cooked (such as a meatloaf), cut up and featured in a mixed dish (such as stir-fried chicken or fish tacos), or added to an entrée salad. Within the categories of meat, poultry, and seafood, you need to vary your offerings so they are not all steaks, grilled chicken breasts, and fish fillets. Any animal protein can be offered in mixed dishes, which also varies the cooking methods represented on your menu. Keep in mind that meatless dishes generally have a lower food cost and will be welcomed by customers who won't eat animal protein for religious or other reasons, such as being vegetarian. It can be very useful to create a list of entrée recipes or potential entrée names when you start to plan a menu. An artist's color wheel is a good thing to have in front of you to remind you to contrast and complement the colors of your food choices. Also, don't forget to balance high-cost entrées with some that are lower in cost.

2. Plan the lunch entrées next. Some foodservices offer several dinner entrées at lunch (sometimes using a smaller portion and price) along with more traditional lunch items including a variety of sandwiches (hot and cold), grilled items, pizza, soups, and salads. Other foodservices offer pretty much the same menu at lunch and dinner.

If planning a cycle menu, you should avoid offering any of the dinner entrées at lunch because that would be redundant. For example, if the dinner menu offered meat loaf, breaded fish, and baked ziti, you might consider a chicken dish and red beans and rice at lunch along with sandwiches, soups, and salads. If you look at the cycle menu in Table 3-1, examine how the entrées vary from meal to meal and day to day.

When planning sandwiches, soups, and salads, be sure to offer a variety of colors, textures, shapes, and hot and cold choices. Avoiding repetition should be easy when you consider the huge number of ingredients to choose from just to make a sandwich—different breads, fillings, spreads, toppings, and condiments. You can also choose from cold sandwiches (consider club sandwiches, open-faced sandwiches, tea sandwiches, wraps) or hot sandwiches (consider simple, open-faced, grilled, panini).

3. <u>Plan the side dishes for lunch and dinner</u>. Depending on the operation, you may want to include side dishes with each entrée or offer side dishes separately. Traditional side dishes include vegetables, potatoes in their many forms, legumes, grains (such as rice), pasta (such as macaroni and cheese), noodles, and other starches. If you have specific side dishes for each entrée, try to picture them all together on the plate to make sure it will have visual appeal. Due to dietary restrictions, most healthcare menus will offer side dishes *separately* from the entrée.

4. <u>Plan the menu items that will be offered as appetizers (eaten before the entrée)</u>. Appetizers are meant to be small in size and stimulate the appetite. Appetizers generally include salads, soups, dips with vegetables or chips, and many other options, some of which are really main dishes that have been reduced in size (like mini-burgers or mini-quiche). Most operations offer at least a basic tossed salad, which can then be the base for entrée salads. Because a cycle menu has fewer entrée choices than a restaurant-style menu, avoid repetitive foods or flavors in appetizers and entrées. For example, don't serve tomato soup at the same meal with spaghetti with marinara sauce. Use appetizers to add more color and creative flavor combinations to meals.

5. <u>Plan desserts for lunch and dinner</u>. Desserts mostly fall into these categories: cakes, pies, pastries, cookies, puddings and mousses, fruit-based desserts, and frozen desserts such as ice cream, sherbet, water ices, and sorbet. Healthcare and school foodservices using cycle menus may offer only a few desserts at each meal, so it's important to avoid repetitive foods or flavors. Frozen desserts (such as ice cream) are easy to store and serve, so they can be easily added on any menu.

6. <u>Plan beverages and condiments for all meals, and bread(s) for lunch and dinner</u>. Most foodservices offer some type of bread and/or cracker choice at lunch and dinner. For some foodservices, their bread is one of their "signature" items, such as Boston Market's cornbread or Red Lobster's Cheddar Bay Biscuits. Onsite foodservices using a cycle menu may rotate a selection of breads on the menu as seen in Table 3-1. Beverage choices are both hot (coffee, decaf coffee, tea, decaf tea, hot chocolate, specialty coffee drinks) and cold (soft drinks, iced tea, lemonade, juices, milkshakes, fruit smoothies, milk). Appropriate condiments must be taking into consideration for each menu item.

7. <u>Plan breakfast (if served)</u>. Breakfast is often split up into these categories: entrées (such as egg dishes, pancakes, French toast, or breakfast sandwiches), sides (such as sausage, bacon, breakfast potatoes, fruit, or yogurt), cereals (hot and cold), breads and pastries (such as muffins, bagels, toast, Danish pastry), and beverages. On a cycle menu, it is not unusual to serve breakfast favorites (such as scrambled eggs, oatmeal, cold cereals like Cheerios, bananas, toast, muffins, and sausage) every day. The cycle menu may rotate pancakes with French toast and waffles, for example, as well as rotate a type of hot cereal and type of muffin each day. Overall on a cycle menu, the breakfast menu may not change a lot from day to day.

8. <u>If you haven't already done so, decide on portion sizes for each item</u>. Portion size largely depends on the type of foodservice operation and age of the clientele. Obviously, the portion size in an elementary school will be much smaller than you would find in a restaurant. A range of portion sizes for many menu items is shown in **Table 3-7**, with smaller portion sizes generally used in healthcare and schools (K–12).

9. <u>For foodservice operations with modified diets to meet individual medical nutrition therapy needs, the regular diet must be "extended" to create the modified diets</u>. What this means is that the RDN will use as much of the regular diet as

Table 3-7 Examples of Moderate Portions	
Meat, fish, poultry	3–6 oz.
Casseroles	6–10 oz. (includes protein such as chicken, vegetable, and sauce)
Soup	6–8 fluid oz.
Gravy, jus	1–2 fluid oz. (1 fluid oz. = 2 tablespoons)
Pasta (entrée)	1–1.5 cups (2 oz. dried pasta makes about 1 cup)
Sauce	1–3 fluid oz.
Vegetables, cooked	3–5 oz. (about ½-¾ cup)
Grains (such as rice)	4–5 oz.
Sandwich	3–5 oz. meat, 1-oz. cheese
Mixed green/garden salad	2–3 oz.
Vegetable, grain, legumes and pasta salads	3–4 oz.
Salad dressing	0.5–2 fluid oz. (1 fluid oz. = 2 tablespoons)
Pudding	4–5 oz.
Ice cream	0.5–1 cup
Eggs, scrambled or omelet	2–3 eggs
Dry cereal	1 cup
Yogurt	6 oz. (¾ cup)
Milk	8 fluid oz. (1 cup)
Butter, margarine	1–2 teaspoons

possible for each modified diet, but some changes will have to be made to meet the requirements of each modified diet. For instance, if chocolate cake is offered as dessert on the regular diet, it will be changed to an item like fruit for the carbohydrate-controlled diet. **Table 3-8** gives an example of extending out a dinner meal.

10. <u>If needed to meet regulations, do a nutrient analysis of the menu.</u> For restaurants required to put calories on their menus, they must also have a nutrient analysis

Table 3-8 Extending a Breakfast and Lunch Menu for Modified Diets						
Waterford Health Center Menu Cycle: <u>Week 2, Day 3 (Wednesday)</u>						
Regular Menu	Portion Size	Mechan. Soft	Puree	2 gram Sodium	Carbohydrate Controlled	Fat Controlled
Breakfast						
Apple juice	½ cup	✓	✓	✓	✓	✓
Scrambled eggs	½ cup	✓	✓	Salt Free	✓	✓
Oatmeal	½ cup	✓	✓	✓	✓	✓
Whole wheat toast	2 sl.	✓	---	✓	1 slice	✓
Margarine	2 pats	✓	---	✓	1 pat	✓
Jelly	1 ea.	✓	---	✓	Sugar Free	✓
Milk - low-fat	1 cup	✓	✓	✓	½ cup	Nonfat

(continues)

Table 3-8 Extending a Breakfast and Lunch Menu for Modified Diets (continued)						
Regular Menu	Portion Size	Mechan. Soft	Puree	2 gram Sodium	Carbohydrate Controlled	Fat Controlled
Lunch						
Vegetable soup	6 fl. oz.	✓	Puree	Salt Free	✓	✓
Baked chicken	3 oz.	Ground	Puree	✓	✓	✓
Mashed potatoes	½ cup	✓	✓	✓	✓	✓
Green beans	½ cup	✓	Puree	✓	✓	✓
Gravy	1 fl. oz.	✓	✓	Salt Free	Fat Free	Fat Free
Soft Roll	1 ea.	✓	---	✓	---	✓
Margarine	1 pat	✓	✓	✓	✓	✓
Strawberry Shortcake	1 ea.	✓	Puree	✓	½ C berries	½ C berries
Milk –low-fat	1 cup	✓	✓	✓	½ cup	Nonfat

for each menu item. Most healthcare foodservices must show that their menus meet the nutritional needs of patients for calories and nutrients, so a nutrient analysis is done of at least one week of the menu for the regular or house diet as well as the modified diets. School foodservices must also analyze nutrients in the foods offered over a school week to determine if specific levels for a set of key nutrients and calories are met for each age/grade group.

Once the menu is written, you need to put it aside for a while before doing a final evaluation. Use the seven considerations of planning menus to evaluate the menu.

3.3 DESIGN A PRINTED MENU

A quality menu is attractive, well-organized, easy-to-read, and persuasive. Foodservices typically place the menu categories in the order in which they are eaten. Menu expert Dave Pavesic (2005) advises you to "think of your menu as your restaurant business card—it introduces the customer to your restaurant, and its design should complement the decor, service, food quality, and price range of the restaurant (p. 37)." Indeed, many customers look at menus online to help them decide where to eat.

USE PSYCHOLOGY OF MENU DESIGN

The design of your menu can affect what customers will order, and this is referred to as the **psychology of menu design**. For example, a menu may be designed to draw attention to dishes with a high profit (and low food and labor costs), which can help a foodservice achieve its profit goals. You can draw attention to certain dishes using any of these techniques.

1. When listing menu items, place the items you want to sell at the top or bottom of the list (Dittmer & Griffin, 1994, Pavesic, 2005). This is because people tend to remember the first and the last item in a list better than any other items on the list (McCrary & Hunter, 1953).
2. Pavesic (2005) recommends using eye magnets—an attention-getter that attracts the eye to an item. An eye magnet could be a colored or shaded box, a border or frame perhaps set in a different color, arrows, highlighted text, or graphic. You can also simply increase the font or use a bolder font.

3.   Gregg Rapp, a menu engineer, recommends avoiding the Paradox of Choice (too many choices) as it causes anxiety in diners and to, therefore, limit selections to six or seven in each category (Hullinger, 2016).

4.   Other menu engineers use "decoys," deliberately overpriced items to lead you to choose more profitable entrées (Hullinger, 2016).

Using any of these techniques involves **merchandising**, the process of presenting products for sale in ways that influence a shopper's purchasing decision. For instance, retail stores build eye-catching displays and signs to draw attention to items they want to move.

Although many authors (Miller & Pavesic, 1996; National Restaurant Association, 2007; Pavesic, 2005) recommend placing high-profit items on the upper right-hand page of a two-page menu (because the eye supposedly gravitates to this spot), more recent research shows otherwise (Yang, 2011, p. 1022). Yang (2011) performed an eye-tracker study in which participants looked at a two-page folded menu (made of 8-1/2 x 11-inch sheets) and were asked to review the menu, then order a meal. Once the menu was opened, foods were listed by category on the interior two pages. When participants opened the menu, they read it like a book—from the top of the left-hand page down to the bottom, and then to the top of the right-hand page and down to the bottom. On the first pass, participants checked out the menu items in each category, especially the entrées, and then on the second pass, they continued to read the menu like a book as they decided on other items to eat with the entrée.

Another example of the psychology of menu design is how prices are put on menus. When menu prices are listed in a column, it is easier for customers to see which items are cheapest. The use of the dollar sign may also lead customers to pick cheaper items and spend less money (Yang, Kimes, & Sessarego, 2009). Therefore, some menus don't use dollar signs or put prices in a column. Instead, prices are placed beneath item descriptions. Sometimes, prices are even spelled out.

DESCRIBE MENU ITEMS

How a menu item is described on the menu can really tempt a customer to order it, so writing good descriptive copy is quite useful. Before discussing how to write good descriptions, you must first know everything about each menu item, such as how big the portion size is or how it is cooked. To misrepresent menu items (such as "prime" quality beef when it is only "choice" quality beef) violates federal, state, and local **Truth in Menu laws**. Truth in menu means being honest and accurate when you describe attributes of ingredients such as these.

- Portion size. When you order McDonald's Quarter-Pounder® sandwich, do you expect it to be 4 oz. before or after being cooked? If you look at their menu, it says it is 4 oz. *after* being cooked. When the portion size is given for a menu item, make sure it is accurate.
- Preparation and cooking methods. Cooking methods and preparation techniques must also be accurately described, when used on the menu. For example, if a steak was pan-broiled, you can't advertise that it is flame grilled. Likewise, if your menu says the hamburger is "fresh," it cannot be made from previously frozen ground beef.
- Name and quality of ingredients. If you advertise "Boar's Head" roast beef on your deli menu, you shouldn't use another brand. Many foods have quality grades, such as U.S.D.A. Choice beef or U.S. Fancy apples, so be sure you know which grade is being used. Other foods have to meet federal identity standards. For example, mayonnaise must contain at least 65% vegetable oil by weight in order to be called mayonnaise. If you advertise mayonnaise, you can't use Miracle Whip. If you use the term "organic" on the menu, be sure the vendor has organic certification. Before a product can be labeled organic, a government-approved certifier must inspect the farm where the food is grown to make sure

the farmer is following all the rules necessary to meet USDA organic standards, such as produce must be grown without using most conventional pesticides and fertilizers. Organic meat, poultry, eggs, and dairy products must come from animals that are given no antibiotics or growth hormones.

- Point of origin. If the point of origin of an item, such as a Kansas City steak, is indicative of quality, it may be useful to put on the menu as long as it is accurate. You may use geographic terms to describe styles of cooking such as Caribbean style.
- Nutrient claims or health claims. Just as a box of cereal may contain a nutrient claim (such as low in sodium) or health claim (such as whole grains reduces risk of heart disease), menus sometimes include these types of claims. Nutrient claims can only be used on menus if the claims meet definitions set by the U.S. Food and Drug Administration (FDA). For instance, a low-sodium menu item may contain 140 milligrams of sodium or less. Health claims are also regulated by the FDA.

In addition, if the menu includes photographs of any menu items, they must accurately reflect the appearance and serving size of the actual menu item.

If you look at a variety of menus, you will find that some menus simply list major ingredients in each of their dishes while other menus give more information such as this description of Chicken Florentine.

> Sautéed chicken breast topped with spinach and mozzarella cheese, served on top of sautéed mushrooms and spinach in a white wine sauce.

When writing descriptions for menu items, use the following guidelines.

1. Keep it simple, brief, and to the point. Most customers are looking for information about the main ingredients and cooking methods as they may be trying to avoid certain ingredients they don't like or are allergic to, and/or they may be searching for healthier cooking methods such as grilling as opposed to frying. If a foodservice emphasizes sustainability or Farm to Table, descriptions are often longer due to listing the farms and orchards where ingredients were obtained.
2. Mouthwatering descriptions are fine but don't overdescribe and oversell with statements such as "drenched with olive oil" or "cooked to perfection." Take a more moderate approach and avoid wording that is too flowery.
3. Be sure the descriptions reflect the personality of the foodservice. Use descriptors that your customers are looking for, such as "freshly made" or "spicy."
4. Be personal and friendly in your writing style.
5. Be very clear about what accompanies each menu item (when applicable). For example, if a sandwich comes with chips or an entrée comes with sides, make sure that will it will be easy for the customer to know exactly what they will get.

While writing menu item descriptions, you should also look at the name of each dish and decide whether it is appropriate as is or should be revised.

DECIDE ON MENU SIZE

The size of the physical menu is determined by factors such as:

- The number of menu categories and number of items in each category
- The length of descriptions for each menu item
- Whether wine, alcoholic beverages, breakfast, or desserts are listed on separate menus
- What will be easy for the guest to hold and read
- What is the cost to produce the menu.

Figure 3-5 gives examples of some menu sizes, from a single page to folding menus with two or three panels. With a double panel, single-fold menu, the interior panels display most of the menu items, with beverages and desserts often appearing on one of the back panels or on a separate menu. Double-panel, single-fold menus are the most

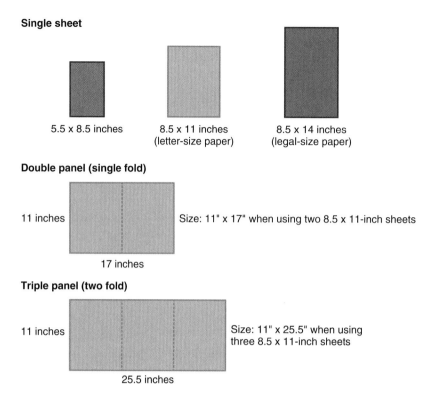

FIGURE 3-5 Examples of Menu Sizes

popular, and they often use standard letter-size paper (8.5 x 11 inches) or legal-size paper (8.5 x 14 inches), although any size paper can be used. Restaurants such as the Cheese-cake Factory with an exceptionally large menu use a booklet with over 20 pages, but that is the exception rather than the rule. A double-panel menu offers more than enough room for most operations.

LAY OUT THE MENU

Before laying out the actual menu that customers will use, get some ideas by looking at different menus, either by looking at restaurant websites or menu templates at a website such as canva.com. When laying out or arranging a menu, keep in mind that most customers will read the menu for just a few minutes. Here are additional guidelines to use.

1. Keep in mind that the customer will read your menu like a book.
2. **White space** is important to create a balanced, professional menu that is easy for customers to navigate and read. White space is the blank space surrounding and in between the content/graphics of the menu. At least half of the physical menu should be white space (Miller & Pavesic, 1996). White space can also be used to give focus and emphasis.
3. For text, use a font size of at least 12 points (larger for older adults). Use a sans serif font such as Arial or Helvetica, because they are easier to read. Sans serif letters don't have the little flourishes or lines that serif letters have.
4. Avoid using more than two or three different fonts.
5. Avoid long blocks of text as customers don't want to read it.
6. Use headings (such as "Appetizers") consistently as they help the customer navigate the menu. Do not spell out "Appetizers" in all capital letters—they are harder to read. Put headings in a larger font than the menu items.
7. For optimum readability, be sure there is a sharp contrast between the font color and the color of the paper.

8. Do not overdo color. Stick to about two to three colors that match the character of the foodservice and use complementary colors. Too much color is distracting and makes the menu harder to read.

9. Any artwork should be consistent with the foodservice concept and of high enough quality to print. Artwork cannot be "borrowed" from websites. Instead, purchase stock photography and illustrations from websites such as Shutterstock.

10. When selecting a paper for the menu, consider the image you want to project, the size and shape of the menu, and how often the menu changes.

3.4 SET MENU PRICES

Many factors affect menu prices. Food and labor costs are of course major factors, as are competitors' prices and the level of demand. If you charge higher prices than similar foodservices for common menu items, you may lose customers and sales. On the other hand, if you charge a little more for signature items and demand is good for those items, this will increase your sales. Of course, economic conditions (local and national) also affect how much money people have to spend on meals away from home. The bottom line when establishing menu prices is to find prices that keep your customers satisfied, demand high, and also achieves a profit (although for some onsite foodservices, breaking even—meaning taking in as much money as is used—is acceptable).

Before discussing how to set menu prices, let's look at the costs that a typical food-service has to cover from their sales dollars before showing a profit.

1. <u>Food and Beverage Costs</u>. This includes all food/beverage costs as well as the cost of paper goods (such as a soda cup or napkins) and condiments (such as bottles of ketchup on each table) that accompany meals.

2. <u>Labor Costs</u>. This includes salaries/wages paid to employees and the cost of providing employee benefits (when available). In addition to withholding each employee's social security and Medicare taxes, *employers also pay a matching amount.*

3. <u>Operating expenses</u>. There are many operating expenses, such as rent, utilities, depreciation of equipment, insurance, administrative costs, and marketing.

4. <u>Income taxes</u>. Just like individuals, businesses pay taxes on their income.

The two *biggest* costs in this list are food/beverage costs and labor costs, which together are referred to as **prime costs**. Many foodservices try to keep their prime costs at or below two-thirds of their sales, so remaining sales will pay for operating expenses, incomes taxes, and hopefully a profit (Deutsch, 2013).

A foodservice could keep prime costs at 66% by, for example, maintaining a food cost percentage of 31% and labor cost percentage of 35%. Therefore, when a customer spends $15 on a lunch of a classic cheeseburger with fries, dessert, and soft drink, this is approximately where the money would go.

- About 31%, or $4.65, would pay for the food and drink. The actual food cost for the soft drink would be much lower than for the other items. When a foodservice owner says their food cost percentage is 31%, *it's an average for all items sold.*
- About 35%, or $5.25, would pay for the labor.
- The remaining $5.10 would pay for operating expenses for the foodservice, taxes, and profit.

Each operation has different operating expenses and profit objectives. For example, a restaurant may be paying off a mortgage on its building and aiming for at least 5% net profit, whereas an onsite hospital cafeteria is not likely to pay rent and is only supposed to break even.

There are various ways to give estimates that are used to help set menu prices. Whichever method you use, the selling prices you get should be regarded as ballpark estimates. You still need to consider how the prices work together in each menu cat-egory as well as what the competition is charging.

FOOD COST PERCENTAGE (OR FACTOR) PRICING METHOD

To apply this commonly used pricing method, management must agree on a desired food cost percentage. For instance, if a foodservice wants to keep its food cost percentage at 33.3% (one-third of sales) and a menu item costs $1.00, the selling price should be about $3.00. The formula to estimate the selling price is as follows.

$$\underline{Formula:} \frac{Food\ cost}{Desire\ food\ cost\ percentage} = Selling\ price$$

$$\underline{Example:} \frac{\$1.00}{0.333} = \$3.00\ (Selling\ price)$$

To get the selling price, divide the food cost by the desired food cost percentage. In the example, the food cost is $1.00, so when you divide the food cost by the food cost percentage of 33.3% (move the decimal left 2 places—0.333—because this is a percent), the selling price should be around $3.00. If that item sold for $3.00, a 33.3% food cost would be achieved for that item.

A quicker way to use the food cost percentage method is to multiply the food cost by a factor or multiplier that is assigned to each desired food cost percentage. For example, when the food cost percentage is 33.3%, you use a factor of 3 as shown in **Table 3–9**. Now you can use this formula to get the same answer of $3.00.

$$\underline{Formula:}\ Food\ cost \times Factor = Selling\ price$$

$$\underline{Example:}\ \$1.00 \times 3 = \$3.00\ (selling\ price)$$

Table 3-9 gives markup factors for different food cost percentages. For example, if food cost percentage is 25%, the markup factor is 4. **Markup** refers to the difference between the selling price and the actual cost of an item. (Markup factors are calculated by dividing 1.0 by the desired food cost percentage.)

It does not matter which formula you use to get an estimated selling price. It is up to you whether to use division or multiplication, as you will get the same results.

Table 3-9 Markup Factors for Menu Pricing	
Food Cost Percentage Desired	**Factor or Multiplier**
20%	5.00
23%	4.35
25%	4.00
28%	3.57
30%	3.33
33.3%	3.00
35%	2.86
38%	2.63
40%	2.50
43%	2.33
45%	2.22
50%	2.00
60%	1.67
66.6%	1.50

This method of menu pricing ignores the cost of labor. Scratch products, which require much labor, may be priced too low, and products that require little labor may be priced too high. It is also not advantageous to use a flat factor, such as 3.0, across the board when you have a variety of food costs. When using the same factor, the higher food cost items may be priced beyond what the customer is willing to pay, and the lower food cost items may be priced too low. This is why any pricing method gives ballpark estimates at best, and prices should be set only after evaluating all menu prices together and comparing prices with competitors.

PRIME COST PRICING METHOD

The prime cost pricing method goes one step further than the food cost percentage method. It is based on adding labor cost to food cost, then dividing the sum by the desired prime cost percentage. The **prime cost percentage** is the sum of the desired food cost percentage and labor cost percentage. As mentioned, many foodservices try to keep their prime costs at or below two-thirds (66% or less) of their sales. The formula for menu pricing using this approach is as follows.

$$Formula: \frac{Food\ cost + labor\ cost}{Desire\ food\ cost\ percentage} = Selling\ price$$

$$Example: \frac{\$1.00 + 1.25}{0.60} = \$3.75\ (Selling\ price)$$

The example shows that for an item with a food cost of $1 and labor cost of $1.25, the selling price will be somewhere around $3.75 when the desired prime cost percentage is 60%.

An advantage of prime cost is that it takes into account the cost of labor on a product's selling price and corrects the problems brought about when only using a desired food cost percentage. Because it is more accurate, it decreases the price spread in a menu category compared with just using the food cost percentage. A disadvantage is that you have to estimate a labor cost, which at times can be inaccurate or vary depending on the volume produced.

CONTRIBUTION MARGIN PRICING METHOD

Contribution margin is the amount of money left over when you subtract the food cost from the selling price. For example, if an item sells for $5.00 and its food cost is $2.00, it has a contribution margin of $3.00 (which pays for labor, operating expenses, and profit). This method of menu pricing *is designed to determine a specific amount of money that each customer must pay in order for the operation to meet all of its expenses and profit goal.*

Management can determine the desired contribution margin for each menu category by looking at sales records to see how much sold and the gross profit. **Gross profit** is calculated by subtracting the food cost from the sales, so gross profit is the same as contribution margin. To get an idea of how much contribution margin you want each customer to pay, you can divide the gross profit by the number of customers served, as shown here.

$$\frac{\$150,000\ (gross\ profit)}{25,000\ customers} = \$6.00\ Contribution\ Margin$$

So each entrée should contribute $6.00 toward all non-food costs.

This pricing method is based on adding the desired contribution margin, such as $5.00 for entrées, to the food cost for each item. So if the salmon entrée has a food cost of $7.50, add $5.00 to get a ballpark selling price of $12.50. Desserts and appetizers often have lower contribution margins than entrées because they are priced lower.

EXAMPLE: HOW TO SET MENU PRICES

We will use three methods to come up with estimated selling prices for a chicken and smoked mozzarella panini served with chips.

Actual Food Cost: $3.15
Actual Labor Cost: $3.29
Desired Food Cost Percentage: 30%
Desired Prime Cost (Food Cost + Labor Cost): 65%
Contribution Margin for Sandwiches: $5.75

Food Cost Percentage (or Factor) Pricing Method

$$Formula: \frac{Food\ cost}{Desired\ food\ cost\ percentage} = Selling\ price$$

$$\frac{\$3.15}{0.30} = \$10.50\ (Selling\ price)$$

Or you can use the factor of 3.33
$3.15 x 3.33 = $10.50 (selling price)

Prime Cost Pricing Method

$$Formula: \frac{Food\ cost + labor\ cost}{Desired\ food\ cost\ percentage} = Selling\ price$$

$$\frac{\$3.15 + 3.29}{0.65} = \$9.91\ (Selling\ price)$$

Contribution Margin Pricing Method

Formula: Food cost + contribution margin = Selling price
$3.15 + $5.75 = $8.90 (selling price)

Consider the contribution margin, as well as the food cost percentage, for the menu items listed in **Table 3–10**. As you can see, the steak has the highest contribution margin and brings in more cash every time it is sold. Meanwhile, the chicken entrée salad has a higher percentage profit than the steak due to its lower food cost percentage. *The key to a profitable menu is to have items with high contribution margins (like the steak) on the menu along with items with low food cost percentages (like the salad).*

GENERAL GUIDELINES

When setting prices, managers must also decide whether to use odds-cents or even-cents pricing. Odd-cents pricing suggests that customers are attracted to prices that end with an odd number just under a round number, such as $4.99 or $4.95, or that the price ends in a number other than zero (Kreul & Scott, 1982). Ending a price in $0.99 or $0.95 is based on the theory that because we read from left to right, the first digit of the price is most important, so we think $4.99 is a bit cheaper than $5.00 when it is only one penny apart. Even-cents pricing suggests that prices end in a whole number (such

Table 3-10 Comparison of Food Cost Percentage and Contribution Margin of Menu Items				
Menu Item	**Food Cost**	**Selling Price**	**Food Cost %**	**Contribution Margin**
Grilled Chicken Entrée Salad	$4.75	$17.00	28%	$12.25
New York Strip Steak	$9.00	$24.50	37%	$15.50

as $25) or in tenths (such as $4.50). Odd-cents pricing tends to be more useful when a foodservice wants to convey value, whereas even-cents pricing is generally used in higher-price operations that want to convey quality (Naipaul & Parsa, 2001).

In the example given of the chicken and smoked mozzarella panini served with chips, there are three estimates of selling prices from $8.90 to $10.50. If management decides that a price under $10 would be appropriate (given other items on the menu and competitors' prices), they might decide on $9.49, $9.95, or $9.99 if using odd-cents pricing. If using even-cents pricing, they may decide on $9.50.

In addition to setting prices for individual menu items, it is important to consider whether to bundle certain items together to make a meal and set a price for them as well. Meal bundles (such as the ever-popular burger, fries, and drink) are sold for less than when ordering separately, so customers often see them as a good value.

In addition, these guidelines are useful when setting prices.

- Customers will not pay for menu items that are far above a competitor's price.
- Customers should be offered good value for their money. Sales volume increases through the customer's satisfaction and perception of value.
- Excessive price spread among entrées encourages customers to order lower-priced items. If the most expensive entrée is more than twice the price of the least expensive item, or if there are more choices of less expensive items, excessive price spread probably exists.
- The selling prices must allow for a predetermined level of profit.

Of course, menus and prices should be analyzed regularly, a process that requires insight, skill, and experience. One popular way to analyze menus is referred to as **menu engineering**. In menu engineering, you place each menu item into one of these categories based on its popularity and contribution margin.

1. High popularity and high contribution margin
2. High popularity and low contribution margin
3. Low popularity and high contribution margin
4. Low popularity and low contribution margin

A menu item is often considered "high popularity" if it reaches at least 70% of the average number sold (Dopson & Hayes, p. 326). Although this method may be useful in some ways, such as to identify items that should either be removed or improved, it is rather simplistic and does not include labor costs. Menu engineering has some usefulness, but as Reynolds and McClusky (2013) have stated, it "should be supported or replaced by newer, more sophisticated approaches. These new approaches make it possible to leverage technology in testing a host of variables such as profit, labor cost in terms of the complexity of menu-item preparation, and the sources of ingredients" (p. 107). New software for foodservices will be available soon to do a better job of analyzing prices.

SUMMARY

3.1 Identify type of menu.

- Menus can vary by how often the menu changes: static like a restaurant menu, cycle menu like a two-week cycle that changes daily for two weeks, or a single-use menu.
- Menus also vary by the amount of choices a customer has. First, each foodservice varies from offering a limited selection of menu items to an extensive selection. Second, look at the number of choices in each menu category: selective (at least two choices), semi-selective (two choices in most categories), and nonselective (no choices—although write-in items are usually available).
- Menus items are often priced individually (à la carte) or as a complete meal (table d'hôte).

3.2　Plan menus.

- Menus should be consistent with the food-service's concept and mission.
- Menus should reflect the food habits and preferences (including for healthy foods) and socio-cultural backgrounds of the target market and offer prices the target market finds reasonable.
- Menus should offer a variety of flavors, textures, colors, shapes, sizes, and cooking methods, as well as hot and cold food choices. Meals should be visually appealing.
- Menus should be cost-effective in terms of food and labor costs. Food cost percentage is the cost of food divided by total sales, and labor cost percentage is calculated by the cost of labor divided by total sales. Food cost percentage is usually close to 33% and labor cost percentage close to 35%. Many onsite foodservices have a budget based on daily food cost per customer.
- Each menu item should be relatively easy to purchase, produce, and serve.
- Foodservices, such as those providing school lunches and meals in hospitals and many long-term care facilities, must perform a nutrient analysis of their menus to show that they are meeting governmental food and nutrition regulations.
- Calorie labeling is required for restaurants and similar retail food establishments that are part of a chain of 20 or more locations.
- More menu items are being developed to be environmentally responsible (this chapter's *Spotlight* discusses sustainable menus in detail).
- When developing a menu, first you must decide on the meal pattern, meaning which menu categories (such as appetizer) will be used for a meal, and approximately how many choices to offer in each menu category.
- Follow these steps when planning a menu: plan dinner entrées first; plan lunch entrées next; plan side dishes for lunch and dinner; plan appetizers; plan desserts; plan bread, beverages, and condiments for lunch and dinner; plan breakfast; and make sure every item has a portion size. For foodservices with modified diets, extend the regular diet to create the modified diets. Also, do a nutrient analysis of the menu if required.

3.3　Design a printed menu.

- A quality menu is attractive, well-organized, easy-to-read, and persuasive.
- The psychology of menu design recommends techniques to draw attention to high-profit dishes by using eye magnets on the menu or listing those items at the top or bottom of a list. Most customers read a menu like a book.
- When menu prices are listed in a column or dollar signs are used, customers may pick the cheaper items. Instead, some foodservices place prices below the item description.
- Truth in Menu laws mean you must accurately describe attributes of menu items such as: portion size, preparation and cooking methods, name and quality of ingredients, point of origin, and nutrient or health claims.
- When writing descriptions for menu items, keep it simple, brief, and to the point. Don't overdescribe items and be sure the descriptions reflect the personality of the foodservice. Be personal and friendly in your writing style and be clear about what accompanies each menu item (as applicable).
- The size of the physical menu is determined by factors such as the number of menu items and length of their descriptions, what will be easy for a guest to hold and read, and cost.
- Double-panel, single-fold menus are the most popular, and they often use standard letter-size paper (8.5 x 11 inches) or legal-size paper (8.5 x 14 inches).
- When laying out a menu, be sure to allow for plenty of white space. Use a font size of at least 12 points—preferably sans serif—and avoid using more than two or three different fonts. Use headings consistently. Avoid long blocks of text. Use color but stick to about two to three colors that match the character of the restaurant. Any artwork should also be consistent with the foodservice concept.

3.4　Set menu prices.

- The following are the typical costs a restaurant or foodservice has to cover from their sales dollars before showing a profit: food and beverage costs, labor costs, operating expenses, and income taxes.
- The two biggest costs are food/beverage costs and labor costs, which together are referred to as prime costs. Many foodservices try to keep their prime costs at or below two-thirds of their sales.
- There are various ways to give estimates that are used to help set menu prices. Whichever method you use, the selling prices you get

should be regarded as ballpark estimates. You still need to consider how the prices work together in each menu category as well as what the competition is charging.

- The *Example* box shows how these three formulas are used: food cost percentage (or factor) pricing method, prime cost pricing method, and contribution margin pricing method.
- The key to a profitable menu is to have items with high contribution margins on the menu along with items with low food cost percentages.
- Odd-cents pricing suggests that customers are attracted to prices that end with an odd number just under a round number, such as $4.99 or $4.95. Even-cents pricing suggests that prices end in a whole number (such as $25) or in tenths (such as $4.50). Odd-cents pricing tends to be more useful when a foodservice wants to convey value, whereas even-cents pricing is generally used in higher-price operations that want to convey quality.
- Other guidelines for setting prices include offering good value to your customers, avoiding excessive price spread among entrées, and setting prices to allow for a predetermined level of profit.

REVIEW AND DISCUSSION QUESTIONS

1. Compare and contrast a static, cycle, and single-use menu.
2. What does à la carte mean?
3. Which type of foodservice is more likely to have a nonselective menu?
4. What do managers want in their menu? What do customers want in a menu? Can the needs of both managers and customers be met?
5. List the steps in planning a menu and why it makes sense to use that order.
6. Describe two menu design tips using the psychology of menu design.
7. Write a menu description for a tuna fish sandwich that makes an ordinary sandwich sound delicious.
8. Make a copy of a restaurant menu from a website, bring to class, and critique its design.
9. What is markup and how are markup factors used to price menus?
10. If a dessert costs $0.90, what would you charge to achieve a 45% food cost percentage?
11. Describe three guidelines when setting menu prices.
12. Why does the menu have such a huge effect on the inputs, operations, and outputs of a foodservice?
13. Why and how does a menu with many menu items present more of a challenge for employees and managers than a smaller menu?

SMALL GROUP PROJECT

For the foodservice concept that you created in Chapter 1, do the following.

1. Develop a *selective* menu that is appropriate for your customers. The menu may be either a static or cycle menu. If you plan a cycle menu, do a one-week menu. All menus must include at least two meals/day and the following types of items at a minimum.
   a. Breakfast: Entrées, side dishes, cereals, bakery items, hot and cold beverages.
   b. Lunch: Appetizers, hot entrées, sandwiches (hot and cold), salads, sides, desserts, hot and cold beverages.
   c. Dinner: Appetizers, hot and cold entrées (such as entrée salads), side dishes, desserts, hot and cold beverages.

2. Include portion sizes for all items on your menu.
3. Include recipes for all items on the menu for one day if writing a cycle menu and for at least 25% of menu items on a restaurant-style menu. The recipes will be used later to do costing out and purchasing.
4. If you wrote a restaurant-style menu, develop an attractive printed menu. If you have a one-week cycle menu, fit it onto an 8.5 x 14-inch legal sheet and add a few graphic images to make it visually appealing.
5. Evaluate your menu using the seven considerations of planning menus in the chapter. Write up a justification for how you met each consideration (except #6).

REFERENCES

The Culinary Institute of America (CIA) and Harvard T.H. Chan School of Public Health, Department of Nutrition. (2018). *Menus of change: The business of healthy, sustainable, delicious food choices* (2018 Annual Report). Retrieved from http://www.menusofchange.org/images/uploads/pages/2018_Menus_of_Change_Annual_Report_FINAL.pdf

Deutsch, J. (2013). A guideline for payroll costs. *Restaurant Business Magazine*, July 16. Retrieved from http://www.restaurantbusinessonline.com/advice-guy/guideline-payroll-costs

Dittmer, P. R., Griffin, G. G. (1994). *Principles of food, beverage, and labor cost controls for hotels and restaurants.* New York, NY: Van Nostrand Reinhold.

Dopson, L. R., & Hayes, D. K. (2017). *Food & beverage cost control* (6th ed.). Hoboken, NJ: John Wiley & Sons, Inc.

Drummond, K. (1998). *Cafeteria cashiering and menu pricing.* Chicago: American Society for Healthcare Foodservice Administrators.

Drummond, K. E., Brefere, L. M. (2017). *Nutrition for foodservice and culinary professionals.* (9th ed.). Hoboken, NJ: John Wiley & Sons, Inc.

FAO. (2010). *Sustainable diets and biodiversity: Directions and solutions for policy, research, and action.* (Proceedings of the International Scientific Symposium: Biodiversity and sustainable diets against hunger) Rome, Italy: FAO.

Fischer, C. G., & Garnett. T. (2016). *Plates, pyramid, and planets: Developments in national healthy and sustainable dietary guidelines: A state of play assessment.* Rome: Food and Agriculture Organization of the United Nations and the Food Climate Research Network at the University of Oxford.

Hullinger, J. (2016). 8 psychological tricks of restaurant menus. *Mental Floss*. Retrieved from http://mentalfloss.com/article/63443/8-psychological-tricks-restaurant menus

Kreul, L. M. (1982). Magic numbers: Psychological aspects of menu pricing. *Cornell Hospitality Quarterly, 23*(2), 70–75. doi: 10.1177/001088048202300223

McCrary, J. W., & Hunter, W. S. (1953). Serial position curves in verbal learning. *Science*, 117, 131–134.

Miller, J. E., & Pavesic, D. V. (1996). *Menu Pricing & Strategy* (4th ed.). New York: John Wiley & Sons, Inc.

Naipaul, S., & Parsa, H. G. (2001). Menu price endings that communicate value and quality. *Cornell Hospitality Quarterly, 42*(1), 26–37. doi: 10.1177/0010880401421003

National Restaurant Association. (2007). *Menu marketing and management: Competency guide.* Chicago: National Restaurant Association Educational Foundation.

Pavesic, D. (2005). The psychology of menu design: Reinvent your 'silent salesperson' to increase check averages and guest loyalty. *Hospitality Faculty Publication.* Paper 5. Retrieved from http://scholarworks.gsu.edu/hospitality_facpub/5

Reynolds, D., & McClusky, K. W. (2013). *Foodservice management fundamentals.* Hoboken, NJ: John Wiley & Sons, Inc.

Sucher, K. P., Kittler, P. G., & Nelms, M. N. (2017). *Food and culture* (7th ed.). Stamford, CT: Cengage Learning.

Yang, S. S., Kimes, S. E., & Sessarego, M. M. (2009). Menu price presentation influences on consumer purchase behavior in restaurants. Retrieved from Cornell University, SHA School site: http://scholarship.sha.cornell.edu/articles/756

© Denis Val/Shutterstock

Foodservice Equipment

LEARNING OUTCOMES

4.1 Explain how to select foodservice equipment.

4.2 Choose an appropriate power source.

4.3 Describe features of common kitchen equipment.

4.4 Describe considerations to select dinnerware, beverageware, and flatware.

4.5 Write equipment specifications.

4.6 Develop an equipment maintenance program.

INTRODUCTION

Your foodservice equipment transforms your raw ingredients and labor (input) into meals (output). The equipment you need is determined by the menu, the type or style of food that you intend to serve, the cooking space (in square feet), and the ventilation hood systems that you have to work with. Also important is whether you are cooking to serve or cooking to inventory (as in cook–chill or cook–freeze).

This chapter discusses many pieces of equipment used in the kitchen—from 200-gallon steam kettles to measuring cups. Some equipment is simple to use, like a measuring cup, but for most equipment, you need training and practice to operate it correctly and safely. In addition to the equipment discussed here, there are many specialized pieces of equipment available, such as rice cookers, portion steamers, and donut glazers. The chapter also examines purchasing dishes, glasses, and flatware; selecting and writing equipment specifications; and developing equipment maintenance programs so your fryer doesn't break in the middle of lunch service.

4.1 EXPLAIN HOW TO SELECT FOODSERVICE EQUIPMENT

When buying a new piece of equipment, consider the following.

1. Look for equipment with proven performance from manufacturers with a good reputation.

2.　Depending on which source of energy you will use (gas, electric, steam), compare how energy efficient the equipment will be with similar pieces from other manufacturers.

3.　Consider what the equipment is made of. Most foodservice equipment uses stainless steel, aluminum, and galvanized steel (see **Table 4–1**). Stainless steel is most commonly used in large equipment as it is very durable and cleanable, resists dents, and does not react with foods. Aluminum is more so used in pots and pans as it is lightweight, strong, and transmits heat well. Galvanized steel has a support role in some equipment.

4.　Each piece should be easy, comfortable, and safe to use. Ask a sales representative to demonstrate how to use and clean the equipment, and ask about safety features.

5.　Equipment should be easy to maintain and keep in top condition without spending too much time or money. Consider whether service for the equipment is available locally and if you can get competent service quickly when needed.

6.　If the equipment you need comes in different sizes, such as fryers, pick the appropriate size to meet your needs based on your portion sizes and how many customers you are serving over a specific period of time. You also have to consider how the size of the equipment will fit into the space you have in the kitchen. Sometimes, a custom piece of equipment will be necessary to either match the size or function that you need. Of course, custom equipment is more expensive.

7.　Consider equipment and tables/shelves that are multifunctional and movable to give you more flexibility.

8.　Consider equipment that will save labor. For example, combination oven-steamers provide speed, ease of cleaning, and ability to cook more than one food at a time.

Table 4-1 Comparison of Stainless Steel, Galvanized Steel, and Aluminum	
Material	**Characteristics**
Stainless Steel	• Most commonly used material yet more expensive than most other metals. • Very durable: resists rust, scratching, and denting. • Easy to clean. • Good appearance. • Stainproof. • Does not react with foods (also good for storage containers and holding pans). • Poor conductor of heat. Small amounts of aluminum may be added to pots and pans to help conduct heat. • 18–8 stainless steel (18% chromium and 8% nickel) is the most corrosion resistant. Also called Type 304—it is considered the industry standard for foodservice uses. • Finishes (degree of shine) are assigned numbers—from 1 to 7 with 7 like a mirror. A finish of 3 to 4 (brushed or matte finish) is good to prevent glare from lights.
Galvanized Steel	• Made of iron or steel that is coated with zinc. • Coating will eventually wear away and iron or steel will then corrode, pit, and rust. • Emits toxic fumes in case of fire. • Sometimes used for bottom panels, legs, or support components of cooking equipment or tables.
Aluminum	• Lightweight. • Strong (but not as durable as stainless steel). • Conducts heat well. • Commonly used for pots and pans. • Will react chemically with some foods such as acidic foods. • Anodized aluminum has been treated to give the surface extra hardness, make it more resistant to corrosion, and foods are less likely to stick to it. • Aluminum pots/pans can't be used on induction cooktops.

9. Purchase price, freight charges, and installation costs are factors, as well as how much it will cost to operate during its useful life (energy, maintenance, repair, cost of supplies to operate it such as filters, etc.).

10. Several organizations, such as NSF International, work with manufacturers to certify that foodservice equipment meet specific requirements. Consider whether you want one of these certifications (see **Table 4-2**).

11. The quality of the warranty, which often covers defects in materials and workmanship for one year, is important to consider.

When buying equipment, most operators purchase from full-service equipment dealers, manufacturers, independent manufacturers' representatives, full-service food distributors, or dealers on the Internet. Full-service equipment dealers, such as TriMark USA, sell a broad range of equipment from a number of manufacturers. One advantage of working with a full-service dealer is that they can make recommendations based on equipment from several manufacturers. Working directly with a manufacturer is also helpful, as they are truly experts on their products, but you should speak with more than one manufacturer to get the best fit for what you need. Whereas a manufacturer's salesperson or representative works directly for one manufacturer, an **independent manufacturers' representative** represents a number of product lines from more than one manufacturer. However, since they can only represent *noncompetitive* product lines, they are not able to show you, for example, a steam kettle from different manufacturers.

Table 4-2 Equipment Certification Programs	
Symbol	**Certification Organization**
 Courtesy of NSF International.	NSF International is an organization that creates standards for foodservice equipment. Equipment with the **NSF certification mark** means that it has met the industry's food safety and sanitation standards, such as being easy to clean, durable, and corrosion resistant.
	UL (originally called Underwriters Laboratories) tests electrical and gas-fired foodservice equipment for safety issues. A **UL certification mark** means that the product has met national safety standards for fire, electric shock, and other safety hazards. UL also has a separate sanitation certification for foodservice equipment that shows compliance with NSF standards.
	Edison Testing Laboratories (ETL Intertek) tests gas and electrical equipment for safety. The **ETL Intertek certification** verifies that safety standards have been met.
 United States Department of Energy.	**ENERGY STAR certified equipment** is energy-efficient and offers energy savings of 10 to 70% over standard models (depending on the product category) without sacrificing features, quality, or style (Environmental Protection Agency, 2016).

However, they do have a broad background in foodservice equipment. Their salaries are based on commissions set by the manufacturer. Many independent manufacturers' representatives are members of the Manufacturers' Agents Association for the Foodservice Industry (MAFSI). Full-service food distributors, such as US Foods, offer some equipment. Companies on the Internet also sell equipment, typically with low pricing but fewer support services.

The decision of whom to purchase from varies depending on what you need. When planning new construction or a major renovation, full-service dealers and manufacturers' representatives are especially helpful. If looking for smallwares, such as steam-table pans or equipment that doesn't need installation (just needs to be plugged in), you may find a better price from your food distributor or a company online, such as WebstaurantStore. com or Katom.com. Either way, you want to deal with a reputable company.

4.2 CHOOSE AN APPROPRIATE POWER SOURCE

When you choose your equipment, you also need to consider what utilities you have, e.g., gas, electric, direct steam, and water. But it does not stop there. Much of today's advanced cooking equipment has very specific requirements and limited tolerances. Examples will follow.

1. Cooking with Electrical Energy. Here are some considerations for cooking with electricity.
   - Each kitchen will be supplied with electricity through an electric panel that contains circuit breakers and fuses. Each panel has a limit as to how much power it can supply. The panel will be rated in Amps (amperes of electricity). Circuit breakers and fuses are also rated in Amps.
   - The actual kitchen equipment draws electricity in kilowatts (kW). You or your electrician can convert kW to Amps (there are online calculators) and determine how many pieces of equipment can be associated with each circuit breaker.
   - Electrical equipment is also specified in voltages and phases and requires special "grounding" to prevent electrical shocks. You need to know if you have the correct power available for each piece of equipment in voltage (v) and whether it is 115v, 208v, 220 or 240v, or 480v. Then you need to know if it is Single Phase or Three Phase. Phase is a measure of electrical force (the pressure multiplied by the flow of electricity). Three Phase is more powerful than Single Phase.
   - Equipment can be wired directly to a power source (also called hard wired), or can require a cord and plug connection. The National Electrical Manufacturers Association (NEMA) configurations determine the types of plugs and outlets to be used.
2. Cooking with Natural Gas or Propane. When you choose gas-fired equipment, you will need to know some specifics.
   - Heat produced by gas is measured in BTUs or British Thermal Units. Gas cooking equipment is rated in BTUs and each piece of gas equipment is also given an efficiency rating. For example, a 100,000 BTU oven with 25% baseline efficiency indicates that you have 100,000 BTUs produced by the oven, multiplied by 0.25 efficiency. This means that 25,000 BTUs go into the food and 75,000 BTUs are wasted.
   - Natural gas and propane produce heat at different rates; therefore, they require different pressures, gas valves, and manifolds.
   - Because of the inefficiency of gas-fired burners and pilot lights, all natural gas and liquid propane cooking equipment must be placed under the ventilation hood so that unburned gases are drawn out of the kitchen. Electric starters or

spark ignitions are preferred over pilot lights (which are always burning) for most burners and can cut energy use.

- There should be an individual shut-off valve for each piece of gas equipment for maintenance. Most fire codes require that gas be automatically shut off in the event of a fire or fire alarm activation.
- Modern cooking equipment is sensitive to gas pressure fluctuations and require a guaranteed steady "working pressure." This will be listed on the equipment specification sheet.
- You need to know if the gas-fired equipment can be lit manually and operate when the electricity is off. This is important for disaster planning.

3. <u>Cooking with Steam</u>. Many large buildings, hospitals, prisons, schools, and colleges have their own power plants and centralized heating and, therefore, have steam available that is quite inexpensive. Steam that is generated from clean/sanitary water can then be used directly on food in a steamer or steam cabinet. Dirty or unsanitary steam can be used to heat the interior walls of equipment like steam jacketed kettles, steam tables, and booster heaters, because the steam does not contact food or food contact surfaces. Here are some considerations:
   - Steam needs to be consistently available year-round and at a consistent pressure in order for steam cooking equipment to perform.
   - Steam lines are larger than regular pipes and must be wrapped in an approved insulation to prevent burns to employees.
   - Steam can be used for cooking in low pressure or high pressure cabinets. High-pressure cabinets reduce cooking time but require pressure-sensitive doors and time to relieve the pressure before the door can be opened.
   - Some electrical and gas equipment use internal boilers to self-generate steam for cooking. This application does not require the building to have centralized steam, but it does require soft or distilled water.

Which source of heat (gas, electric, or steam) you decide to use will be determined by the following.

- The local availability of natural gas, liquid propane, and steam.
- The current and future cost of gas versus electric in your area.
- The size and capabilities of your hood ventilation systems and what will fit beneath it.
- What the chef and production staff have always dreamed of having.
- The expected life of the item and the cost or regular maintenance.
- The possibility of rebates from local power companies for energy-efficient cookware.
- How you structure your disaster plan based on emergency power and water availability.

4.3 DESCRIBE FEATURES OF COMMON KITCHEN EQUIPMENT

This section discusses key features of kitchen equipment. Because there are so many different types of equipment in a kitchen, this section looks separately at each of these categories: cooking equipment; food preparation equipment; work tables, racks, and carts; smallwares (such as pots and knives); holding and serving equipment; refrigeration equipment; and warewashing equipment.

COOKING EQUIPMENT

Here are the most common and essential tools for cooking, from ranges to fryers.

Ranges

A commercial **range** may be the most widely used piece of cooking equipment. The most common ranges have burners on top and ovens (including convection ovens) under them for roasting and baking. Ranges can be purchased with different types of burners. Open gas burners, where the flames are applied directly to the bottom of the pot, are the most common. Instead of individual burners, the surface may be flat and the gas heats up the surface in zones. Called a hot top, the smooth surface makes it easier to heat large stockpots as well as move pots around. Electric ranges have open burners, sealed individual heating elements, or hot tops.

In addition to having burners, an electric or gas range may have a griddle top (to make eggs, pancakes, and burgers). Gas ranges may also include a broiler (heat from above) or a charbroiler (heat from below). The gas range shown in **Figure 4-1** has griddle on the right, and underneath the griddle is a broiler that pulls out so you can put the food on it.

Electric induction cooktops are becoming popular as induction heats the pot, not the cooktop. When you turn on the burner, electricity produces a magnetic field, which excites the molecules in steel or iron cookware (not aluminum) so only the cookware gets hot. These require specialized cookware, but are more efficient when using electricity and also easier on the kitchen environment as excess heat is not produced.

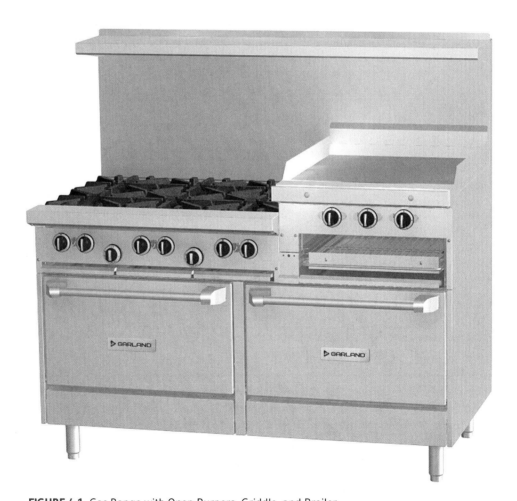

FIGURE 4-1 Gas Range with Open Burners, Griddle, and Broiler

Courtesy of Garland.

A **wok range** is popular for Chinese, Vietnamese, and Thai food as well as stir-fry and noodle bars. They use gas-fired rings to heat round or cone shaped pots. They are not energy efficient but are trending none the less.

Ovens

Ovens have always been the backbone of the kitchen and with improvements in technology and global competition, the variety and capabilities are truly astounding.

1. Range ovens. Range ovens (Figure 4-1) use dry radiant heat from a burner below the central oven cavity. Range ovens are good for roasting and some baking and are the least expensive of the ovens. However, they are generally small and the heat distribution can be uneven when the racks are covered with pans of food that block the normal flow of air. They are not a good choice for busy operations.
2. Convection Ovens. **Convection ovens** (**Figure 4-2**) use radiant heat and forced air (from a fan or blower). The moving air keeps the heat evenly distributed and speeds cooking time but can also dry out foods with little moisture, although the drying action can be used to crisp the coating of breaded or oven-fried products like chicken and fish. Convection ovens cook food faster than standard ovens and are more energy efficient, in part because you need to set the temperature at 25°–50°F (15°–30°C) lower than for a conventional oven for most foods (Gisslen, 2015).
3. Deck Ovens. The **deck oven** (**Figure 4-3**) works like a standard oven but the oven door is not very tall so food is placed directly on the metal, ceramic, or cementitious floor or deck of the oven. Placing food on the floor of the oven allows conducted heat as well as heat from the hot air in the oven cavity to bake or cook the food. Some are equipped with steam injection in order to make crusty breads and rolls. Deck ovens are used in a bakery or pizzeria.
4. Conveyor Oven. **Conveyor ovens** are what you see in most high-volume pizza restaurants like Pizza Hut and Dominos. Food is placed directly onto a wire conveyor or onto a pan on the conveyor, and the conveyor carries foods through a space where hot air hits the food from all angles to cook it. Some conveyor ovens use hot air "impingement," meaning that high-speed air blows through baffles directly onto the food. This focuses the heat and speeds cooking. The

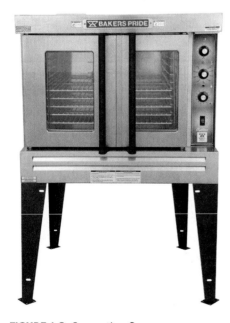

FIGURE 4-2 Convection Oven

Courtesy of Bakers Pride.

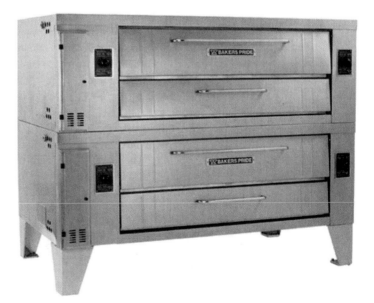

FIGURE 4-3 Deck Oven

Courtesy of Bakers Pride.

high temperature and forced air are great for pizza, calzones, and bread sticks, and also for chicken wings, which are fast baked rather than fried. Other food-services, such as schools, use conveyor ovens to produce items like hamburgers, grilled cheese, fries, and brownies (Foodservice Equipment & Supplies, 2017).

5.   Microwave Ovens. Microwave radiation activates water molecules and when these vibrate, the resulting friction causes heat and heats up the food. This is an excellent way to heat high-moisture foods such as vegetables. However, there are several disadvantages: foods of varying density tend to cook unevenly, most metal pans cannot be used in microwaves, and browning of surfaces is not possible. **Convection microwaves** add forced hot circulating air to help brown or crisp food surfaces (Sherer, 2015a).

6.   Combination Steamer Oven (Combi-Oven). **Combination steamer ovens** combine a convection oven with a steamer. They can be used in one of three ways: convected heat, pressureless steam, or a combination of both. They are perfect for cooking proteins (meat, poultry, etc.) because the dry heat will do the cooking while the moisture from the steam will prevent drying out and shrinkage. When your food shrinks (especially proteins), you lose money. You can program combi-ovens to change temperature and humidity during product cooking, as well as use temperature probes in the food to switch the oven to hold mode or turn it off. Because of their versatility, these ovens are in high demand and are replacing traditional ovens and convection ovens. Manufacturers are building their ovens with additional capabilities like self-cleaning, cook and hold, dry or wet smoking, onboard computers with recipe storage, wireless control and monitoring, and automatically emailing for service when there is a problem. One of the latest innovations is Δ T (Change Temperature) cooking. The Delta (Δ) is the chemical symbol for change. In Δ T, food is not placed in a hot oven. Instead, a probe is placed in the food and the temperature and humidity of the oven cavity rises at a steady rate above the temperature of the food. This prevents the outside of the food from cooking faster than the inside of the food and gives you a uniformly cooked product with minimal drying or shrinkage.

7.   Rapid Cook/High Speed Hybrid Ovens. Starbucks and most quick-serve restaurants, convenience stores, and sandwich shops that offer heated sandwiches or need to quickly melt cheese would be lost without **rapid cook ovens,** which easily fit on a countertop. The oven works extremely fast and generally does not require hood venting. The most popular heating source for hybrid ovens is a microwave combined with impinged convection (meaning that high velocities of hot air are directed at the top and bottom of the food). You can also buy a high-speed oven that uses impingement convection only. Convection microwaves also fit into the rapid cook category. As fast as this technology cooks food, it can also burn and destroy food very quickly. As a result, all of these ovens are programmable and can hold many recipes. Some of these ovens offer three to six-stage cooking to give more control with browning occurring in the last phase after the food has already been heated (Sherer, 2015a).

8.   Specialty Ovens. Rack ovens are used for high volumes of similar products like bread and rolls that the oven actually can fit entire roll-in racks of products. Cook-and-hold ovens are for slow or overnight cooking to tenderize meats and minimize moisture loss. Cold-and-hold smoker ovens are similar except that they add smoke for flavor. Display or rotisserie ovens have clear glass doors, interior lights, and rotating spits to allow customers to see the food (such as chicken) cooking in various stages of doneness and browning.

Steam Kettles and Steamers

Steam-jacketed kettles (**Figure 4-4**) are the workhorses of any kitchen as they are used to make soups, stews, chili, casseroles, sauces, and pasta. They are ideal for blanching, boiling, simmering, rethermalizing, and stewing. When you look at a kettle, the

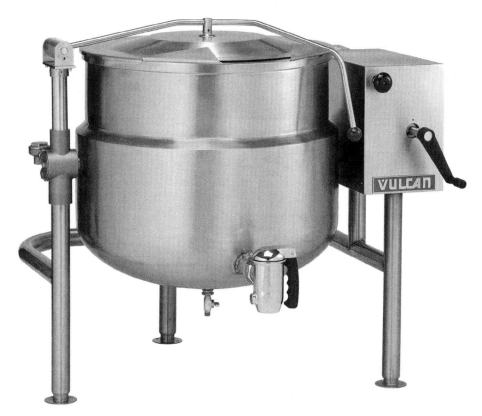

FIGURE 4-4 Steam Kettle

Courtesy of Vulcan.

sides are not solid steel. Steam is actually pumped into a space between the inner and outer walls of the kettle to produce heat. In many kettles, the steam "jacket" only extends two-thirds of the way up the kettle. In other kettles, the steam jacket extends all the way up.

Kettles heat up faster and heat foods more evenly than pots on the range, so they do not need constant monitoring by cooks. They can be used for cooking or reheating and are often used to thaw and reheat sous vide food that is sealed in plastic. Kettles come in many sizes from a three-quart countertop model to over 200 gallons (mounted on the floor). Tilt or trunnion kettles can be tilted to pour cooked foods into serving pans, while larger kettles have draw-off valves on the bottom to drain foods. Foods with large chunks like beef stew are usually scooped or ladled out of the kettle. Kettles can be purchased to use direct steam (supplied within the foodservice) or with a boiler to produce its own steam supply.

Steamers are handy for moist, moderate-temperature cooking and defrosting items. Steam circulates in a closed cavity and when it condenses on the food, it transfers heat energy directly onto the food. Steamers cook foods fast and are an excellent cooking method for nutrient retention. Most steamers use either pressure or convection to speed up the cooking process even more. Pressure steamers use pressure (from 5 to 15 pounds per square inch), which allows steam to reach a temperature higher than the boiling point of 212°F (100°C). Pressure steamers cook faster than convection steamers but require locking doors for safety and can use up to 40 gallons of water per hour (Food Service Technology Center, 2018). Convection steamers cook food at 212°F (100°C) and often produce higher-quality products with better texture and nutrient retention than pressure steamers (**Figure 4-5**). Taste transfer from one pan to another is more likely using a pressure steamer than a convection steamer (Foodservice Equipment & Supplies, 2016).

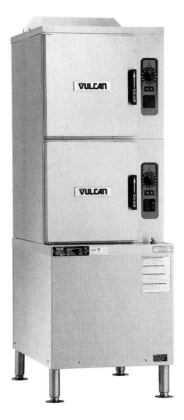

FIGURE 4-5 Convection Steamer

Courtesy of Vulcan.

All steamers hold steam table pans. Boilers will have maintenance problems if you have hard water, so boilerless, convection models are recommended. A boiler-less steamer produces steam by heating water in a compartment and works well for low-volume foodservices.

Tilt Skillet/Braising Pan

Tilt skillets (**Figure 4-6**) are one of the most versatile of all pieces of kitchen equipment, and they can save money and space by performing the jobs of several pieces of equipment. They are like large flat griddles, but with sides to hold liquids, a lid to maintain moisture, and a tilt function so that cooked product can be poured into pans. They can be gas or electric. Like a griddle or frying pan, you can cook breakfast eggs, pancakes, and French toast. For lunch, you can cook hamburgers, grilled cheese, or cheese steaks. For supper, you can make stir-fry, paella, or risotto. They are also ideal for braising. Braising is the simmering of tough cuts of meat in their own juices, with vegetables, broth, beer, wine or vinegars to tenderize and bring out savory flavors. Examples of braised dishes include pot roast, corned beef and cabbage, and braised short ribs. You can also fill it with oil to use it as a fryer or fill it with water to use it as a bain-maire.

Griddles (Flat Grills)

Griddles are polished, flat cooking surfaces that you find at the center of most commercial cooking lines. A griddle can be built into a range-top or a table, or it may be a countertop unit or freestanding. They can be gas or electric, with or without grooves for adding grill lines on foods. **Clamshell griddles** (**Figure 4-7**) speed cooking by applying heat to both sides of the product when the upper griddle plates swing down to touch the food.

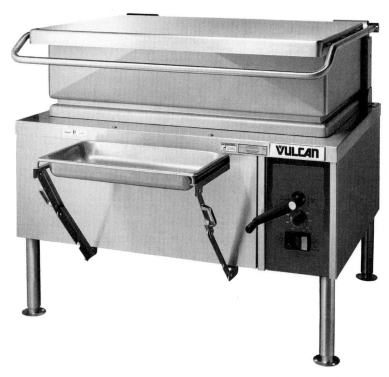

FIGURE 4-6 Tilt Skillet/Braising Pan

Courtesy of Vulcan.

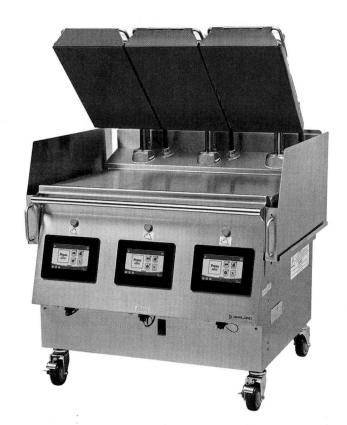

FIGURE 4-7 Clamshell Griddle

Courtesy of Garland.

Griddles vary in price based on size, the amount of heat produced (measured in BTUs), and the thickness and type of griddle plate. Polished steel plates are the most common, least expensive, and most difficult to clean because of the metal's porosity. Chrome is the most expensive material but heats up faster and has better heat retention. However, chrome is not a good choice if your cooks use the griddle surface for chopping with the side edge of a metal spatula as with cheesesteaks, chopped onions, or home fries. For heavy duty chopping and grilling, you are best to go with a low–porosity stainless steel surface, which is also easier to clean. Thicker griddle plates, such as one inch, are more heavy duty and can hold onto more heat, which is useful when cooking frozen hamburgers throughout a lunch period. Splash guards help reduce grease splatter and keep hot dogs and sausages from rolling off. The controls are either manual, which let you set the griddle to low, medium, or high; or thermostatic, which allow you to set an exact temperature for a certain width of the plate.

Cleaning griddles properly takes times but helps the equipment last longer and function better. For polished steel or steel griddles, employees need to coat the griddle surface with oil while the surface is still warm and then use a grill brick to clean it (always working with the grain). This procedure is done again and again until the surface is clean, then it can be rinsed and wiped clean. For griddles with chrome or polished-stainless surfaces, employees can clean with water and mild detergent, while the griddle is warm, and scrub with a palmetto brush. Once clean, wipe with a dry cloth. No metal brushes or scouring pads should be used on chrome (Sherer, 2015b). Griddles also need to be conditioned or seasoned with oil according to the manufacturer's instructions. This helps to maintain a nonstick surface and prevent rusting.

A recent addition to the griddle market is the **plancha** (**Figure 4-8**). The plancha is a griddle that heats up to 800°, that is 150 to 300 degrees hotter than a normal griddle (Culliton, 2018). It gets very hot, very fast, and has a short recovery time. It is great for

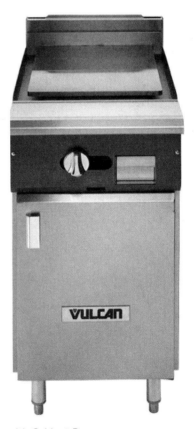

FIGURE 4-8 Plancha Range with Cabinet Base

Courtesy of Vulcan.

browning, searing, caramelizing, or blackening foods, and is ideal for getting a uniform sear or a flavorful crust. The plancha is good for high-production operations.

Char-Broilers and Broilers

A **char-broiler** is like a griddle, but with an open grate, which, when it is hot enough, puts the tell-tale grill marks on your food. Char-broilers are under-fired, meaning the flames come from below the grill. Like your outdoor barbeque grill at home, they have a very basic design and are inexpensive to purchase. Charbroilers produce more flames and smoke than most kitchen appliances because anything cooking drips on the burners. Because they are heating into an open grate, heat retention is poor so the char-broiler is the least efficient appliance in the kitchen. One broiler can use more energy than six fryers. They typically use gas as the power source. Most char-broilers are either radiant charbroilers (transmit radiant heat waves up into the food) or lava rock charbroilers (lava rocks above the burners heat up and radiate heat up). Because lava rocks hold some of the drippings, they impart a smoky flavor. However, lava rocks need more cleaning and maintenance.

Regular **broilers** use heat from above the product. These feature a grate that holds the food and can be pulled in and out of the broiling unit. Broilers cook very fast and are ideal for broiling items such as steaks and chops. Cooks adjust the cooking temperature by raising or lowering the grate holding the food. Adding infrared technology (ceramic or glass plates that glow red) makes the heat more intense and also more even.

There are two categories of smaller broilers called salamanders and cheese melters. A **salamander** (**Figure 4-9**) is a *small* broiler that can melt cheese or cook a steak. A salamander may be a countertop unit or be mounted on the wall or above the range. A cook can top brown a casserole or broil salmon in a range salamander while cooking foods on the range top. Salamanders are also used on a serving line to keep plates hot so that an entire table at a restaurant can be served entrées simultaneously. **Cheese melters** look like salamanders but they provide a more gentle heat and can be used to finish off dishes topped with cheese, toast bread, or brown the top of a casserole. They are not designed to *cook* foods (Katom Restaurant Supply, 2018a).

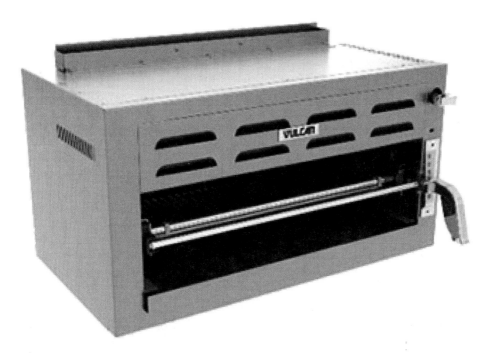

FIGURE 4-9 Salamander Broiler

Courtesy of Vulcan.

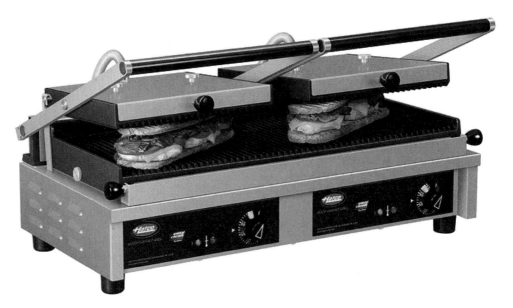

FIGURE 4-10 Panini Press

Courtesy of Hatco Corporation.

Panini Presses

Grilled sandwiches like paninis, Reubens, Cubans, and all types of grilled cheese or wraps are extremely popular. On a tradional grill, they can take over five minutes to make. Double-sided **panini presses** (**Figure 4–10**) cut that time in half. The plates in a panini press may be nonstick or more often they are made of cast iron, which retains heat well and is best for continuous use. The plates can be either grooved or smooth. Nonstick plates are more easily damaged and must be carefully cleaned according to the manufacturer's directions. Some plates, such as cast iron, will need to be seasoned regularly.

Fryers

Commercial **fryers** (**Figure 4–11**) are often referred to by how much fryer oil they can hold, such as a 50-pound fryer. Electric fryers have their heating elements submersed in the oil itself, whereas gas fryers have infrared gas burners under the kettle or they can have hot fired tubes that actually run through the tank of oil. A fryer purposely has a "cold zone," an area designed to capture breading crumbs and food debris. This lower temperature zone keeps the crumbs from carbonizing, which gives the oil a burnt flavor and darkens the oil so that it needs to be replaced more often. Some fryers have built-in filters to remove debris.

Most large operations will use a bank of fryers (two or more side-by-side) with food warmers (dump stations) next to them. Since oil holds heat well, a 100,000 BTU unit will only use about 20,000 BTUs per hour when idling (not having frozen product added to it). High efficiency or EnergyStar® models will save operators about 30%. If you fry a lot of fish, it is good to have a dedicated fryer for seafood. The fish flavor will get into the frying oil and affect the flavor of chicken, mozzarella sticks, vegetables, and French fries.

Newer fryer models contain features such as built-in filtration systems to improve oil quality, oil sensors that alert when oil needs to be replaced, and heat exchangers to improve efficiency. **Pressure fryers** cook faster, make food extra crispy, use less oil, and because they are lidded, they put less grease into the air and onto your hood filters.

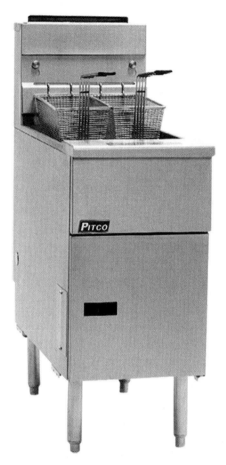

FIGURE 4-11 Basket Fryer

Courtesy of Pitco.

Food Preparation Equipment

Given that food can now be purchased in any form including salad and vegetables already chopped and washed, potatoes peeled, or meats cooked and sliced, it is a great help to really evaluate your needs before buying food preparation equipment. Good general rules to follow are that speed is important in today's labor market, stainless steel lasts longer than plastic, and if you really want your food prepared fresh in small batches, don't buy the largest capacity items (such as a floor mixer when a countertop mixer will suffice).

Slicers

If you serve meats or make sandwiches, electric **slicers** are crucial. They can be purchased as manual or automatically driven. With **manual slicers**, the operator's right arm moves the carriage holding the meat past the rotating blade to slice (**Figure 4-12A**). With **automatic slicers**, a separate motor moves the carriage holding the food being sliced, back and forth over the blade, which is useful when slicing large amounts of product. Automatic slicers can also be operated manually. Fully automatic slicers can be programmed to slice and are only used in high-volume operations. A good automatic slicer can give you 20 to 60 slices per minute. (Foodservice Equipment & Supplies, 2018a). Some slicers, often manual slicers, are described as "gravity feed slicers" because they have a 25° to 50° angle to keep the food hitting the blade during slicing. Other slicers, often automatic slicers, may be vertical slicers because the blade is positioned upright at a 90° angle, which allows the operator an optimal view of the slicing result.

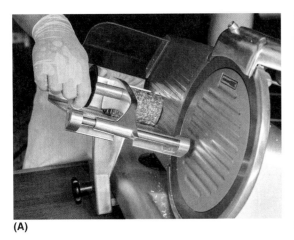

(A)

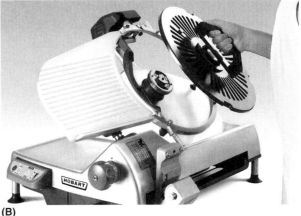

(B)

FIGURE 4-12 (A) Slicer, **(B)** Knife Ring Blade Guard Being Removed from Automatic Slicer

A: © TaraPatta/Shutterstock; B: Courtesy of Hobart.

The more expensive slicers have higher horsepower, slightly larger blades, and often more safety and convenience features. Slicing cheese requires a good bit more horsepower than slicing meat. The most common blades are carbon steel, but stainless steel blades are more durable. Stainless steel blades do need to be sharpened more often and may need to be sharpened once or twice a day or more when in constant use (Sherer, 2018).

Employee safety is a major concern with slicers. Full-knife ring guards (**Figure 4-12B**) are available for most models, and they protect the employee because the knife edge is not exposed. Also available are color-coded parts that indicate safe-to-touch areas while the blade is moving. Employees also have to pay strict attention when the slicer is taken apart to be washed. Knife removal tools keep the sharp edges covered when an employee removes the blade for cleaning.

Food Processing Equipment

Just like with other equipment you purchase, you need to consider your volume and what you desire your food to look like when looking at food processing equipment. High-volume commercial kitchens use buffalo choppers (**Figure 4-13A**) and vertical cutter/mixers. A **buffalo chopper** uses an S-shaped blade and rotating bowl to turn large pieces of vegetables into small pieces and to finely chop meats. This is ideal for salads, soups, and for texture-modified diets. The classic buffalo chopper comes with a slicer attachment, which includes an adjustable slicing blade and a blade for grating (**Figure 4-13B**). **Vertical cutter mixers** process large volumes of food. Some models are able to process 88 pounds of food per minute. However, all 88 pounds will look the same.

So, if you are going for fancier food with a signature look, neither the buffalo chopper nor the vertical cutter mixer are a good choice. If you want a machine to do various cuts and shapes for each of your signature dishes, you are looking for a **commercial food processor**. In a typical batch bowl processor, the employee drops the food into a bowl. As the food drops down, it enters a pillar inside the bowl that contains an S blade or a disc that cuts the food into the desired shape and size. Bowl size varies from about one to six quarts. A wide variety of cutting discs (**Figure 4-14**) allow you to accomplish grating, slicing, ripple cutting, brunoises, waffle-cut, shredding, sticks, julienne, French fries, and strips. Some batch bowl processors allow you to continuously feed food into them.

Continuous-feed food processors (Figure 4-14) are more heavy duty than batch bowl processors and are excellent when you have large quantities of food that need to be chopped, diced, sliced, and more. Other ways to compare food processors are to examine sturdiness, horsepower, and blade speed (measured in revolutions or rotations per minute, RPMs).

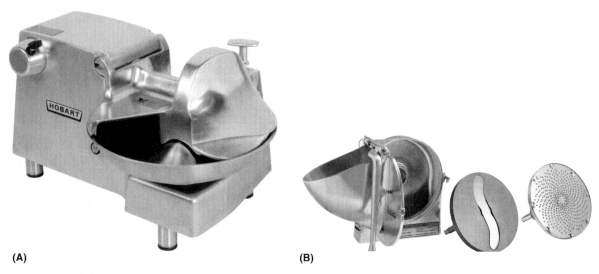

(A)   **(B)**

FIGURE 4-13 (A) Buffalo Chopper, **(B)** Slicer Attachment for Buffalo Chopper with Adjustable Slicing Blade and Grater Blade

A & B: Courtesy of Hobart.

Mixers

Not many operations bake from scratch any longer so large mixers that sit on the floor are not as common. Exceptions are large kitchens that make mashed potatoes, use box mixes for cakes, make their own sauces and dressings, and make pizza dough from scratch (Foodservice Equipment & Supplies, 2018b). Large floor mixers can hold up to 200+ pounds of product but many operations would be fine with a 20-quart stand mixer that can handle 10 to 20 pounds at a time and fits on a counter (**Figure 4–15**). Most mixers are referred to as **planetary mixers**, meaning that the beater (also called the

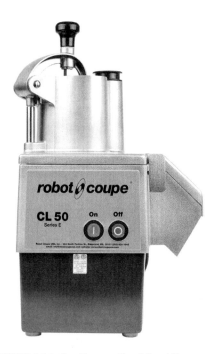

FIGURE 4-14 Continuous-Feed Food Processor

Courtesty of Robot Coupe.

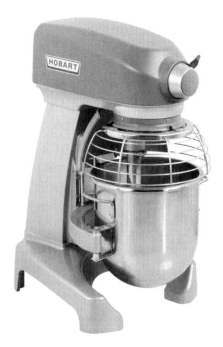

FIGURE 4-15 Stand Mixer with Safety Guard

Courtesy of Hobart.

agitator) moves around the bowl (which is stationary) during operation. Some heavy-duty dough mixers actually have the agitator stay still while the bowl revolves around it, which is called a **spiral mixer**. Dough mixers can process large amounts of dough at once and are useful when making large volumes of bread or pizza dough.

All mixers are electric and most models have three speeds, with speed ranging from about 50 RPM (rotations per minute) to 300 RPM, which is used to incorporate air into egg whites or other items. Most models come with a beater (called a **paddle**) for doing most mixing, a wire whip for making whipped cream, and a dough hook for mixing doughs such as pizza dough. Safety guards look like a cage at the top of the bowl and they help make sure employees don't get near the moving beater (Sherer, 2012). In the United States, the Occupational Safety and Health Administration (OSHA) requires use of a bowl safety guard when using a commercial mixer.

Blenders

Commercial blenders and immersion blenders are also important because they give your cooking staff speed. This is crucial in display cooking operations and anywhere you want a freshly made appearance. **Commercial blenders** have a blade at the bottom of the container in which the ingredients sit (also called the blender jar), and are especially good at blending thick drinks like smoothies, crushing ice or frozen fruit, and whipping up milkshakes. Commercial blenders usually have a clear polycarbonate jar so you can see how well mixing is progressing; however, stainless steel jars are more durable and easier to clean.

Immersion blenders (**Figure 4–16**), which range in size from seven inches to over two feet long, can be placed directly into a pot of food to blend, puree, or emulsify. It is especially useful for pureeing vegetables, soups, or sauces; mashing potatoes;

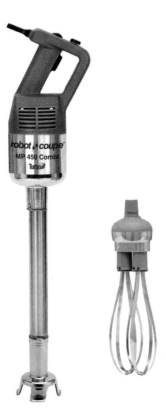

FIGURE 4-16 Commercial Immersion Blender with Blending Arm and Whisk

Courtesty of Robot Coupe.

or chopping soft foods. With a whisk attachment, it can be used to whip up eggs, cream, and frostings. The standard attachment for an immersion blender is called a blending arm, but you can buy blenders that also come with a whisk. Immersion blenders come in a variety of lengths, numbers of speeds, and motor sizes to meet many different needs.

WORK TABLES, RACKS, AND CARTS

Work tables are usually made of stainless steel to ensure durability, corrosion resistance, and cleanability. The typical work table is five to six feet long and 30 inches wide. It has a flat top with four legs and a storage shelf underneath the work surface. Many tables have a four-inch backsplash at the back of the table to protect the area behind it. Work tables are also in longer lengths (in whole feet) and from 18 to 48 inches wide. They can be outfitted with built-in sinks, wheels at the bottom of the legs, a poly-top surface (like a cutting board), and pot racks. Heavy-duty work tables are made of 14-gauge stainless steel and are needed if you are putting equipment such as a mixer or slicer on the table. Standard duty work tables are made with 16-gauge stainless steel, which is not as strong, so these tables are better for hand cutting and other cook's work.

Racks are designed to hold sheet pans and/or steam table pans. They are on wheels so they can be moved around the kitchen and can also roll into a refrigerator. When a rack is enclosed, it is often called a cabinet.

The typical **cart** is about the size of a large supermarket cart, and instead of having sides, it is usually open and has two to three shelves. Carts are used in many different ways: for bussing dirty dishes, transporting food around the kitchen, delivering meals, serving food and beverages, and keeping janitorial supplies in one place. Carts may be made of stainless steel, aluminum, plastic, or other material, and some are enclosed.

SMALLWARES

Smallwares include pots, pans, knives and other hand tools, measuring tools, and utensils used for a variety of kitchen duties. Most pots and pans used in commercial kitchens are made of aluminum or stainless steel (sometimes with aluminum on the bottom). Aluminum is lightweight and an excellent heat conductor, but it reacts with some foods (especially acidic ones) and discolors light-colored foods such as eggs. Anodized aluminum removes many of these concerns, as it has a harder surface that does not react with acidic foods or discolor light foods. Heavy-duty aluminum pots work quite well in kitchens, and they last longer when they are washed by hand. While stainless steel is more durable than aluminum and does not react with any foods or cause discoloration, it is a poor conductor of heat. However, there are many stainless steel pots and pans available with aluminum-clad bottoms so they conduct heat better.

Cast iron and carbon steel are also used in pots and pans. **Cast iron** pans are heavy, durable, and when they get hot, they stay hot—which is helpful for browning foods. When properly seasoned, they can be used for nonstick cooking on the range or in the oven. Every time you use a cast-iron pan, it slowly develops a natural slick coating, called seasoning, which releases food easily. Seasoning also refers to the ongoing process of maintaining that finish so the cast iron does not rust. Before using a new cast iron pan, it will need to be seasoned by heating oil in it at a high temperature for an hour or so. To clean a cast-iron pan, scrub with a stiff brush and hot water, then wipe dry with a towel or set the pan over low heat until completely dry. No soap is needed. Then rub in a very thin layer of oil to maintain the seasoning.

Carbon steel pans weigh less than cast iron but perform very similarly. Carbon steel pans must be cleaned and seasoned like cast iron, and also cannot be used for prolonged cooking of acidic ingredients like tomato sauce. They are different from cast iron in that they heat fast and evenly and are a favorite for high temperature cooking. Carbon steel pans can also be used on induction heating equipment.

When looking at knives, **high carbon stainless steel** makes a knife blade with excellent durability and edge retention. High carbon stainless steel blades stay sharp longer than stainless steel blades and are easier to sharpen. Knives made from better quality stainless steel can hold a good edge. **Forged knives**, meaning they are created from one solid piece of metal and are higher quality and heavier than stamped knives created from a large sheet of metal. A **stamped knife** is thinner and less expensive.

Table 4-3 will help you identify and describe cookware, knives, hand tools, measuring tools, and serving utensils found in the commercial kitchen.

Table 4-3 Smallwares in Commercial Kitchens

Name	Description
a. Saucepan	With straight or slanted sides, the saucepan is the workhorse of rangetop cooking.
b. Saucepot	Saucepots have two handles and are deeper than saucepans. Used to make soups, sauces, stews, and more. Wide bottom for maximum heat conduction.
c. Stockpot	A large, straight-sided pot that is taller than a saucepot and is used to prepare stocks and soups. Thick base for a slow simmer.
d. Double boiler	The double boiler is used to cook foods that can't be cooked over direct heat (such as melting chocolate). The food is placed in the top part and water boils in the bottom.
e. Brazier	The broad and shallow brazier is designed for browning meats and long, slow cooking on the back of the range. Ideal to make stews and braised meats.
f. Sauté pan	The sauté pan is shallow and either straight-sided or slope-sided. Both are used for sautéing, frying, browning, and making egg dishes. The slope-sided pan lets the cook flip and toss the food during cooking.

g. Stir-fry pan 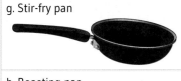	Stir-fry pans are used to stir-fry vegetables and other foods. They are from 11 to 14 inches in width and deeper than a sauté pan. Their deep curved sides allow movement of food during cooking. They may have a non-stick coating.
h. Roasting pan 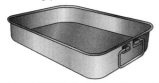	Roasting pans are shallow to allow heat to penetrate meats and poultry but deep enough to contain the juices. Heavy duty construction and large sizes.
i. Sheet pan 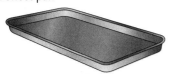	A shallow, rectangular pan (18 × 26 inches) used in the kitchen and bakery. Used to cook bacon, bake cookies and cakes, and roast and broil some proteins. Half pan is 18 × 13 inches.
j. Bake pan 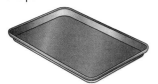	Rectangular pans like sheet pans, but deeper (about 2 inches deep). Used for baking.
k. Steam table pan, also called hotel pan, counter pan 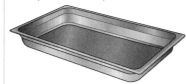	Stainless steel pans used to hold foods in steamtable, cook foods in oven or steamer, and also store foods. Standard size is 12 × 20 inches and standard depth is 2-1/2 inches. Fractions of this size (half pan, quarter pan, etc.) are available as well as deeper pans.
l. Bain-marie inserts 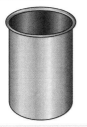	Round, tall, stainless steel containers used to hold foods in a bain-marie (water bath) or to store foods.
m. Chef's knife (French knife) 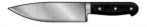	If you only had one knife, the Chef's knife would be the most useful. Designed for heavy-duty cutting, chopping, and other jobs. Length is often 10 inches and the blade tapers to a point.
n. Utility knife 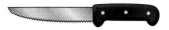	Narrow, pointed blade frequently used in fruit and vegetable preparation and slicing cooked poultry. Most range from 5 to 8 inches long and have a scalloped edge to make a cleaner cut.
o. Paring knife	A small knife, often with a 2- to 4-inch pointed blade, which is used to trim and cut fruits and vegetables.
p. Boning knife 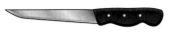	Boning knives are used to remove bones from raw meat, poultry, and fish. Stiff blades are used for removing bones from raw meat and poultry, while more flexible blades are used for lighter work including filleting fish. A boning knife used for filleting fish is often called a fillet knife.

(continues)

Table 4-3 Smallwares in Commercial Kitchens (continued)

Name	Description
q. Slicer	Slicers, with long slender blades, are used to slice cooked meats and poultry.
r. Serrated slicer	A serrated slicer looks like it has teeth. The teeth allow it to slice breads, cakes, and other foods you do not want to crush when slicing.
s. Steel	The steel is used to true and maintain knife blades.
t. Peeler	The peeler's swiveling blade is used for peeling fruits and vegetables.
u. Cook's fork	A heavy-duty fork used to lift and turn pieces of meat as well as hold them while carving.
v. Offset spatula	An offset spatula is used to turn food, such as hamburgers, during cooking. The blade is bent or offset so that it slides easily underneath food while your hand is kept away from the heat.
w. Straight spatula	With its long, flexible blade, the straight spatula is used for spreading frosting on baked goods and also for scraping bowls.
x. Sandwich spreader	A short spatula with a flexible blade used to spread butter, etc. on bread and fillings on sandwiches.
y. Rubber spatula	A flexible rubber or plastic blade is used in folding in procedures and scraping out bowls. Must use heat-resistant spatulas for hot foods.
z. Melon ball scoop	Also called a melon baller, it is used to scoop out balls of fruit from melons and other appropriate fruits and vegetables.
aa. Zester	With its tiny sharp-edge holes, a zester is used to remove the colored part of lemon, lime, or orange in thin strips.
bb. Colander and strainer	Stainless steel or aluminum bowl with small holes or mesh used to drain liquid from washed salad greens and other foods. A colander has handles and can sit in the bottom of a sink. A strainer is hand held.
cc. China cap (chinois)	A china cap is used to strain liquids, such as stock or soup, into another container.

dd. Sieve	The sieve is used for sifting flour and other dry ingredients.
ee. Grater	A metal box grater is used to shred or grate cheese, vegetables, or other foods. One side usually has smooth-edge holes for grating while two sides have rough-edge holes, and the fourth side has a diagonal slit.
ff. Skimmer	A perforated disk used by a cook to remove solid pieces or froth from stocks and other liquids.
gg. Wire whip	Whips are used to beat, whip, and blend liquid ingredients. Heavy whips are heavy duty and have fewer wires than balloon whips. Balloon whips have more flexible wires and are excellent for whipping eggs and mixing thin liquids.
hh. Pastry bag and tips	Using a cone-shaped cloth (sometimes made of plastic) fitted with a metal tip, you can decorate cakes or other foods. Tips vary in their size and produce different shapes such as a flower or simply written letters.
ii. Pastry brush	A pastry brush is used to brush egg wash on rolls about to go in the oven, brush on a glaze, and other uses.
jj. Tongs	A tool used to pick up foods, such as cooked spaghetti.
kk. Spoons: solid, perforated, and slotted	Large stainless steel spoons used to serve, stir, and mix. Perforated and slotted spoons are used when liquid must be drained. Perforated spoons have small holes while slotted spoons have slots.
ll. Measuring cups and spoons	Measuring cups for liquids have measuring lines well below the rims to prevent spilling. Measuring cups for solids allow you to fill them and then level off the top.

FOOD HOLDING AND SERVING EQUIPMENT

Once food is prepared, you want to hold it (keep it warm or cold in optimum conditions) so that you can maximize sales or service and minimize waste. This includes keeping French fries crispy and hot and keeping pizza from drying out or getting overcooked. At the same time, cold food can dry out or change color due to oxidation. Blowing (convected) air, and the drying effect of heat lamps or radiant warmers can ruin food quickly. Given that you need to keep your prepared food out of the danger zone: above 135°F (57°C) or hot foods and below 41°F (5°C) for cold, here are some options.

If not served immediately, hot foods that have already been cooked need to be held. Hot food may be put into a **steam table** (**Figure 4–17**) that keeps food above 135°F (57°C) to prevent bacterial growth. Steam tables are useful in cafeterias, hospital tray service, buffets, and other serving lines. Stainless steel pans, called hotel or counter pans, are used to hold foods in the steamtable.

Steam tables using gas heat up quicker and are less likely to malfunction than electric steam tables. Electric steam tables are more mobile, are more energy efficient and you can control the temperature better.

The space where a hotel pan fits into the steam table is called a well. Wells are either sealed or open. If you look into a **sealed well**, you will not see the heating element (if electric) or flame (if gas), because it is *under* the bottom of the metal well. This way, you can add water directly into the bottom of the well, and once the unit is heated up, some of the water turns to steam (moist heat) that will keep the food in the hotel pan warm. Moist heat is especially good to keep moist items like soups, vegetables, pasta, and rice warm. Be sure to keep the water below boiling and cover the foods or otherwise limit the air flow from above so foods stay warm and don't dry out. Sealed wells contain a built-in drain for removing the hot water.

Open wells have an exposed heat source at the bottom, and you can use dry or moist heat to keep foods warm. To use dry heat, you simply put the pan directly into the well over the heat source. Dry heat is especially good for holding crispy foods, such as fried foods, without losing quality. To use moist heat, first you have to fill a spillage pan with water and place that in the well. Then you place the food pan inside the spillage pan. Open wells are harder to clean than sealed wells.

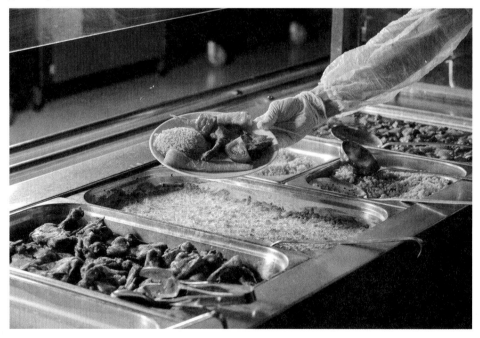

FIGURE 4-17 Steam Table

© Ercan senkaya/Shutterstock

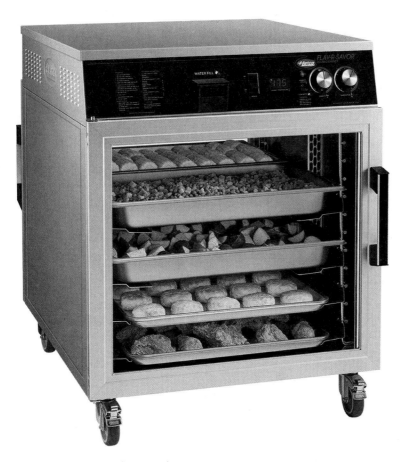

FIGURE 4-18 Holding Cabinet (Half-Size)

Courtesy of Hatco Corporation.

A **bain-marie** can also be used to keep hot foods hot. To use one, round stainless steel bain-marie pots are first filled with cooked foods and then placed directly into a hot water bath heated by electricity, gas, or steam. Whereas the steam table is more often used in the serving area, the bain-marie is used in the hot production area to hold soups, sauces, etc.

Another way to keep food warm is to use a **hot holding cabinet** (**Figure 4-18**) that keeps hot foods at appropriate temperatures without drying them out. They come in different heights and can accommodate sheet pans and steam table pans. Most have wheels and are, therefore, mobile. It is not unusual in some operations for foods to be prepared, placed in the holding cabinet, and then removed and put into a steam table for service.

Overhead **heat lamps** using infrared bulbs hanging about eight inches above a plate are often used to keep plated food warm before service. They are also used to keep meat warm at meat carving stations and maintain the heat and quality of French fries after coming out of the fryer. Infrared bulbs produce infrared radiation, which keeps the food hot. They are only meant to keep any item warm for a very short time, such as a few minutes, otherwise the food will start to dry out.

Most **electric heat strips** (also called strip warmers) also use infrared radiation and are more effective and less drying than heat lamps because they can radiate heat over a larger area. A typical strip warmer has one or more rows of heating elements inside a metal or ceramic cover that radiates the heat (Alley, 2017). A strip warmer is often about six inches wide and can be up to six feet in length. Whereas bulb-style lamps are designed more for warm individual plates, strip warmers can keep larger quantitites of food warm. They are used when you need more heat than a bulb can generate and work especially well in cafeterias and buffet lines.

SPOTLIGHT ON USING EQUIPMENT SAFELY

Working in a commercial kitchen has many hazards such as hot oil in a fryer, steam kettles with boiling liquids, sharp knives and slicer blades, electric equipment that can give you a shock, and mixers that might pull in your loose sleeve. Here are 15 tips to avoid accidents.

1. Only use equipment on which you have been trained.
2. Use equipment only for its intended purpose and follow directions.
3. Be sure safety devices are in place and use guards appropriately.
4. Pay attention to what you are doing when using any equipment (your cell phone should be put away).
5. When using electrical equipment, make sure the cord and plug are in good condition. Also, be sure your hands are dry and your feet are not in water.
6. Do not wear bulky clothes, dangling jewelry, or name badges hanging from lanyards near equipment as they might get caught up in a moving part.
7. Be sure gas pilot lights are on before turning on burners or ovens.
8. Be aware of correct temperatures for cooking on each piece of equipment.
9. Use the right size pots and pans to keep food from spilling over.
10. Keep an eye on foods as they are cooking.
11. Use dry potholders. Wet potholders conduct heat to your hands.
12. Turn a machine off before making adjustments or when walking away for a minute.
13. Open lids of pots and doors of steamers away from you, and do so slowly. When using a pressure steamer, make sure the pressure gauge returns to "0" before opening. Steam causes severe burns!
14. Don't turn your back on hot fat, and don't overfill fryer baskets.
15. Turn off and let equipment cool before cleaning. Also, unplug any electric machine before taking it apart and cleaning.

To hold cold foods, refrigerators are generally used. Refrigerated holding cabinets, which look just like their hot cabinet counterpart, are also available. Both hot and refrigerated holding cabinets are electric and on wheels so they are mobile.

REFRIGERATION EQUIPMENT

For any area of the kitchen, there are a number of choices for refrigeration. The major storage area for refrigerated goods are usually **walk-in refrigerators**. Once you open the door, you walk into a room where refrigerated goods are located on shelves. Walk-in refrigerators come in many different sizes and can store large quantities of food.

The food preparation and service areas generally use refrigerators such as the following.

- **Reach-in refrigerators**: These look a lot like your home refrigerator and have one or more solid or glass doors only on *one side* of the refrigerator. Reach-in refrigerators often have one or more glass doors that are used to merchandise bottles of soft drinks, water, sandwiches, etc. Smaller reach-in refrigerators are placed under counters when appropriate.
- **Pass-through refrigerators**: This refrigerator is basically the same as the reach-in model except pass-throughs have doors on *two opposite sides* so an employee can load finished salads on one side, and a server can grab the salads from the opposite side. Pass-through refrigerators help reduce congestion.
- **Roll-in refrigerators**: This refrigerator is basically the same as the reach-in except that it has no shelves. This allows an employee to roll a pan rack into the refrigerator for storage. A pan rack holds sheet pans (18 x 26-inches), which are used in cooking and storage.

Undercounter refrigerators are also useful to hold small quantities of food.

The NSF standards indicate that you need to hold cold foods from 33°–41°F (0–5°C) in open air display cases and food bar/salad bar environments. To do this, you need to have the foods chilled nearly to freezing before putting them out. But once the food is out, you will need to rely on clear plastic strip covers or a flow of cold air (such as an air curtain) to control temperature increases. Amtekco offers a "Flow Over" cooling system for its food and salad bars in which cold air cools foods from below and also circulates air over the top of the food (Amtekco, 2018). Food should be illuminated/displayed using cool light bulbs or LEDs.

WAREWASHING EQUIPMENT

Keeping your pots and pans, as well as your eating and serving utensils and your glassware and china clean, can use up to 20% of your labor hours in foodservice. It is also the most intensive use of your water resources. For example, a 44-inch rack conveyor dishwasher uses approximately 2,400 gallons of water per day and costs between $27,000/year for gas or $43,000/year for electric (Delagah, 2015). ENERGY STAR certified dishwashers save water, reduce run times, use sensors to keep the machine in idle, and also use heat exchangers to save energy. It is also important to use the proper size dishwasher. Sizes are constrained by the number of dishracks per hour and the wash cycle time.

Dishwashers are designed to clean and sanitize dishes. If hot sanitation is used, the final rinse of the dishmachine must reach 180°F. Low temperature machines must add a sanitizing solution to the final rinse. The sanitizer (such as chlorine or a quaternary sanitizer) must be strong enough (in ppm or parts per million) to register on an appropriate test strip.

There are several types of commercial dishwashers available depending on how many dishes need to be washed and how quickly.

1. The **door-type dishwasher** accommodates one rack full of dishes. A dishwashing rack is 19 inches by 19 inches. Once the rack is placed in the door-type dishwasher, the door is closed, and the cleaning cycle starts. In just minutes, you have cleaned and sanitized dishes.

2. For larger foodservices with more dishes, **conveyor-type dishwashers** are larger machines and they move full racks of dishes through regular wash, power rinse, and sanitizing rinse cycles. Some machines also feature prewash and/or airdry cycles.

3. For very high-volume operations, a **flight-type dishwasher** (**Figure 4-19**), also called a rackless conveyor or belt conveyor, is used. The flight-type dishwasher operates on the same principles as the conveyor-type dishwasher except

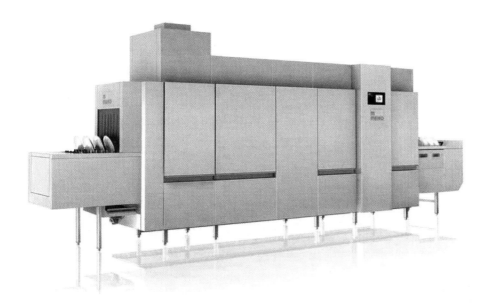

FIGURE 4-19 Flight Type Dishwasher (Dirty dishes enter on left side.)
Courtesy of MEIKO International.

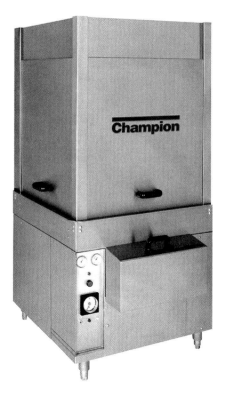

FIGURE 4-20 Front- or Side-Loading Pot Wash Machine

Courtesy of Champion Industries.

that the dishes and other items are hand-placed between rows of pegs on a conveyor belt. Flatware is placed in a rack. Two employees keep the dishes going through smoothly, one to load and one to empty. Specifying a high efficiency flight machine with an Energy Star rating can increase your efficiency by 40%, which could translate to $850/year savings in electricity and 52,000 gallons of water/year (Sherer, 2010)

Like dishwashers, **pot wash machines** save labor and make the kitchen a more pleasant environment. They come in many sizes from the ability to hold six sheet pans to 60. Pot washers have longer cycles than traditional dishwashers and more powerful pumps for higher pressure. They can be front or side loading. **Figure 4-20** shows a pot wash machine that can be loaded from the front or side.

4.4 DESCRIBE CONSIDERATIONS TO SELECT DINNERWARE, BEVERAGEWARE, AND FLATWARE

Unless you are only using disposable products, you will need to buy dinnerware (plates, bowls, and other dishes), glasses, and flatware or utensils. While pots and pans may last many years, glasses and dishes do break and have to be replaced regularly. Choosing these items should take some time. Here are some considerations.

1.   Dishes, glasses, and even utensils should work together on the table *and* reflect your concept or brand.
2.   Durability and price are major factors. Some higher-end flat dishes may offer a warranty against chips, while another line of dishes may simply state that they are resistant to scratches and chips.

3. Before buying any dishes, think about your menu items and how you intend to plate them for maximum presentation value. That will help you determine the shapes and sizes you will need.
4. Also consider the size of your tables.
5. To reduce breakage, consider if your staff will be able to easily handle the dishes and glasses. Do they fit well into the dishwashing racks? Will they present any storage issues?

Dinnerware refers to plates, bowls, and dishes. Ceramic dinnerware is made from clay, which is baked and then glazed to seal the surface. Depending on what is added to the clay, as well as the different firing procedures, the results will vary. Here are some popular choices for dinnerware made from clay, from less to more expensive.

1. **Stoneware** comes in a variety of styles. It is not only strong but also thick in appearance when compared with the next choices. Another concern is the weight of stoneware, which makes a server's tray a lot heavier.
2. **Porcelain china**, also just called **china**, refers to dinnerware made of a fine-particle clay that includes kaolin and is fired at a higher temperature than stoneware. This results in dinnerware that is very durable and nonporous. The process also allows the body to be thinner and yet quite strong. Along with its bright white color, porcelain is a natural on many tablecloths. For extra durability, look for porcelain that is vitrified. Vitrification is a process in which the clay is brought to its melting point and results in a stronger dish.
3. **Bone china** includes bone ash that is used as a refractory material and the firing temperature is lower. Bone ash gives the plate a lustrous appearance and makes it less likely to break. It is the strongest china you will find and also the most expensive. Bone china is lightweight with thin, delicate edges that add to its attractiveness and sense of refinement.

While stoneware, porcelain china, and bone china are all breakable, commercial **melamine**, made from plastic, is lightweight and doesn't break, so it is great for child-friendly foodservices and outdoor dining. Melamine is more attractive now than it was years ago and some melamine is made to imitate stoneware or china. Other plastic and glass dinnerware options are available, as well as wood. Wood dinnerware is made from woven wood that's been sealed, so it is nonabsorbent and dishwasher safe.

Beverageware includes everything that holds a beverage, from cocktail glasses to water goblets and coffee mugs. Most beverageware is made from glass or plastic. Some beverageware, such as bar glasses that are frosted in the freezer, are made from tempered glass (also known as safety glass) that will not break as easily as untempered glass. Plastic drinking glasses are obviously more durable than glass, and they are less expensive, but they are not as classy as glass. A popular plastic used in beverageware (because it is BPA free) is styrene acrylonitrile resin or SAN. Coffee cups may be purchased as part of the dinnerware, so they are often stoneware or china, but they can also be made of the plastic SAN or tempered glass.

Glassware, especially wine glasses, are often made from glass but higher-end foodservices may choose some crystal glasses. **Lead crystal** uses the normal ingredients of glass but substitutes lead for another ingredient. Because of this, lead crystal has a distinctive sparkle and becomes softer, so it can be worked into cut designs as well as give a wine glass a thin rim. Lead crystal is also heavier than glass. Because of concerns about lead safety, lead-free crystal, simply called crystal glass, is available. **Crystal glass** is not quite as sparkly as lead crystal but its appearance is favored over glass.

Flatware includes forks, knives, spoons, and any utensils to be used by the guest. There are a number of factors to consider for this big purchase.

1. **Style**. There are many styles available, some are quite simple or classic, while others are more modern.
2. **Pattern**. The unique design of each set of flatware you look at is referred to as the flatware pattern. For example, Regency is a simple but elegant pattern.

Several different flatware companies may produce a Regency pattern, but each one will be a little different.

3. **Material**. Most flatware is made from stainless steel. There are three types of stainless steel: 18/10, 18/8, and 18/0. Each of these types contain 18% chrome (the first number). The second number represents the amount of nickel. The more nickel there is, the stronger and shinier the steel is. So, 18/10 stainless steel is the highest grade and it also tends to be heavyweight and, of course, more expensive than the other grades. The next level, 18/8 stainless steel with its shiny appearance, is a good choice for many operations. Budget-minded operators may choose the 18/0 which is still relatively durable.

4. **Weight**. Flatware weights include medium- and heavy-weight (18/0), and extra heavy-weight (18/8 and 18/10). Heavier weight utensils have a sturdier feel and are often used in upscale operations.

5. **Finish**. The finish depends on the flatware you choose but may include mirror/polished, matte, satin, and silver- or gold-plated finishes.

4.5 WRITE EQUIPMENT SPECIFICATIONS

An equipment **specification** is a detailed description of the equipment. When you look at foodservice equipment, be sure to examine the specification sheet for any piece in which you are interested. **Figure 4–21** shows a sample specification sheet for a gas charbroiler that is available in several sizes. Note that each size has its own model number. **Table 4–4** also includes information on specifications, standard features, and accessories. This specification sheet has a second page (not provided here) that includes the dimensions of the different models and installation information.

Writing an equipment specification can help you determine exactly what you are looking for in a piece of equipment. In organizations that require you to request price quotations or more formal bids from *several vendors, you must write an equipment specification*. When writing a specification, be clear, exact, and make sure that several bidders could bid on the specification. Some general requirements to include in an equipment specification are as follows.

1. Name of the piece of equipment and how many are needed.
2. A brief statement about how the equipment will be used.
3. Utility and plumbing requirements (what you have available).
4. Specific features such as size/capacity, style or model, materials (including finishes and colors), description of controls, and performance characteristics. In some cases, drawings may be included.
5. Any accessories that are needed.
6. Any certifications desired such as NSF or UL, or Energy Star rating.
7. Desired conditions of the warranty, such as to include parts and labor. Warranties do not usually cover planned maintenance or repairs due to misuse or carelessness (Weber, 2015).
8. Delivery information including dates, how much you are willing to pay, and when you want the ownership of the equipment to switch to the buyer.
9. Installation requirements such as who will set the equipment in place, who will install the equipment, who will pay for installation, who will make the utility connections, who will start up the new equipment and assure it is working properly, who will clean up the area after installation, and who will apply for permits (if needed).
10. If there are changes or delays, which party will be responsible?
11. Payment terms and cancellation terms.

A bid for equipment may include one brand name, several brand names, or no brand names along with the criteria that must be met.

Garland

Item: _____

Quantity: _____

Project: _____

Approval: _____

Date: _____

Heavy Duty Gas Radiant Char-Broilers w/Adjustable or Non-Adjustable Grates

Heavy Duty Gas Radiant Char-Broilers

Models:

☐ GTBG24-AR24 ☐ GTBG36-AR36 ☐ GTBG48-AR48 ☐ GTBG60-AR60

☐ GTBG24-NR24 ☐ GTBG36-NR36 ☐ GTBG48-NR48 ☐ GTBG60-NR60 ☐ GTBG72-NR72

Model GTBG24-AR24

Standard Features:

- SS front, sides and back
- 4" SS adjustable legs
- 3/4" NPT gas regulator on all 24" to 60" wide models with "T" gas manifold connection for straight through rear or flush-mount gas connections.
- 1" NPT gas regulator for GTBG72-NR72 model only. Has "T" gas manifold connection for straight through or nearly flush-mount gas connections.

- SS front rail; 4" (102mm) deep overall with 3 1/2" (89mm) top work surface
- SS large capacity crumb tray
- Reversible cast iron broiler racks in 3" wide sections with 1/8" and 3/16" brand marks.
- 21-1/2" (546mm) broiling grid depth
- 2-position adjustable broiler grates or fixed-position non-adjustable grates
- One cast iron radiant over a 18,000 BTU stainless steel tube burner for every 6" of broiler width.
- One two position hi/lo valve control for each burner.

Optional Features:

☐ SS skirt for dais/counter surface mounting. The stainless steel skirt will reduce overall unit height by 1 3/4" (44.45mm).

☐ SS spatter-guard

☐ Removable wire holding shelf for spatter guards available for 24" and 36" models

☐ Broiler grate cleaning tool

☐ Fajita broiling grate: 9" wide, replaces 3 standard grate sections on the left or right end of the broiler. Limit one per broiler.

☐ Stainless stand with solid top and holding shelves, and adjustable feet

☐ Stainless stand with solid top and holding shelves, and casters, (locking front)

☐ Set of revisible cast iron broiler racks with 4 brand marks per 3" section. Brand 3/16" wide.

☐ Removable stainless steel attachment condiment rail with universal 1/9 or 1/3 food pan cut outs (pans supplied by others)

Specifications:

Garland gas radiant broilers are available with adjustable or non-adjustable cooking racks, in five nominal imperial widths from 24"(600mm) to 60"(1500mm), and with model GTBG72-NR72 only 72"(1800mm), 13" (330mm) high and 32" (814mm) deep. Reversible cast iron grates in 3" (76mm) wide sections overall cooking area depth 21 1/2" (546 mm). One 18,000 BTU burner with individual valve control per 6" of broiler width. Large stainless steel catch tray, stainless steel front, sides, and back.

Garland Commercial Ranges Ltd.
1177 Kamato Road,
Mississauga, Ontario
L4W 1X4 CANADA

General Inquiries 1-905-624-0260
USA Sales, Parts and Service 1-800-424-2411
Canadian Sales 1-888-442-7526
Canada or USA Parts/Service 1-800-427-6668

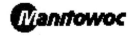

FIGURE 4-21 Sample Manufacturer Equipment Specification Sheet

Courtesy of Garland.

Table 4-4 Equipment Information Sheet

Equipment Name: _____

Manufacturer's Name and Phone Number: _____

Model Number: _____ Serial Number: _____

Date Installed: _____ Original Cost: _____ Life Expectancy (years): _____

Warranty Expires: _____ Type of Warranty: _____

Company for Repairs/Service Contract _____

Preventive Maintenance:

Interval (such as weekly)	Describe Work to Be Done.

Spare Parts Required:

Maintenance Records:

Date:	By:	Work Performed:	Cost:

Courtesy of Garland Commercial Ranges.

When writing a specification, the following words have specific meanings.

- "Shall" refers to a requirement.
- "Should" or "may" refers to a feature that is not a requirement.

Using past experience and manufacturers' literature, foodservice operators can write up specifications but may request the expertise of an engineer or foodservice consultant to get everything right. This helps prevent problems such as installing a new fryer and realizing the hood above it is too small. Salespeople can help too, but don't let them write the specification.

Also, make sure you know who will provide service for new equipment in the event that it breaks.

4.6 DEVELOP AN EQUIPMENT MAINTENANCE PROGRAM

To keep a foodservice running smoothly, you depend on both your employees and your equipment to do their jobs. On their days off, you hope your employees get plenty of time to relax, sleep, and eat so they return to work well rested and ready to go. Your equipment also needs attention to work well. To keep equipment operating smoothly and efficiently, it is important to do the following.

1. All employees who use a piece of equipment need to be trained on *how to operate* the equipment properly, stressing personal safety.
2. Employees also need to be trained on *how to clean* the equipment properly and safely as well as how often it should be cleaned. A master cleaning schedule details which employees are responsible for cleaning floors, equipment, etc., at given times, such as 9 PM daily or weekly on Tuesday mornings. For example, a grill cook may be responsible for daily cleaning of a griddle and a utility worker performs a more heavy-duty weekly cleaning after which the griddle is seasoned. Information on how to operate and clean equipment is discussed in the Installation and Operation Manual that comes with each piece of equipment.
3. Supervisors and managers need to check that employees are using and cleaning equipment properly every time they walk through the facility.
4. Employees also need to report any problems with equipment, such as a screw is missing or an electrical cord is looking frayed and worn, to their supervisors.
5. Develop a preventive maintenance program.

Just like you service a car with fresh oil, most of your equipment, along with the HVAC system, needs regular preventive maintenance. **Preventive maintenance** is service, such as inspection or calibration, that is regularly performed on a piece of equipment to increase its lifespan and lessen the chance of it failing to work. Recommendations for preventive maintenance are listed in the *Installation and Operation Manual*. For example, the manual for a convection oven recommends routine oven cleaning (including the inside, outside, and the blower wheel), as well as annual maintenance to check the venting system for possible deterioration from moisture and other substances that are vented out.

To set up a preventive maintenance program, first you need to have some basic information along with the *Installation and Operation Manuals* either in a binder or as digital copies on the computer. For each piece of equipment, an Equipment Information Sheet (Table 4-4) should be maintained that includes key information, such as the model number, when it was purchased, recommended preventive maintenance, and when it was serviced. Just as you can buy a service contract for Best Buy to repair the new computer you bought there, foodservices can purchase service contracts for new equipment. Service contracts vary widely in what they include—the contract may include just maintenance services or it may include maintenance and repair. Service providers who are members of Commercial Food Equipment Service Association (CFESA) get training and certification by the manufacturers themselves for all hot and cold foodservice equipment. A foodservice may, for example, have a service contract for their HVAC system including cleaning the exhaust hoods and ducts, but do much of the preventative maintenance themselves on basic equipment like convection ovens and griddles.

Once you have the Equipment Information Sheets prepared, you can make a **Master Maintenance Schedule** listing the preventive maintenance for each item that needs to be done, along with how often—weekly, monthly, bimonthly, quarterly, semi-annually, and annually. A Master Maintenance Schedule can then be put onto a calendar and managers then allot time to specific employees to perform the maintenance. Maintenance that is performed by an outside company should also be noted on the schedule. **Table 4-5** shows common maintenance issues that can be prevented by having a quality maintenance program.

Table 4-5 Common Equipment Maintenance Issues

- Failure to calibrate temperatures for cooking and refrigeration.
- Poor gasket seals or door latches on walk-in refrigerators, freezers, and steamers.
- Condenser coils and fans on refrigeration have dust, dirt, or ice buildup on them.
- Hoods are not clean and grease is building up in filters and on stainless steel.
- Ducts and grease traps are not cleaned regularly.
- Clogged filters in HVAC system or blocked fans in convection or refrigeration.
- Mixers and food processors are overloaded, which causes damage.
- Inspection and lubrication of all moving parts on slicers, mixers, and toasters.
- Failure to check temperatures and pressures of pumps and rinse arms in dishwasher.
- Hard water stains (lime scale) build up in dishwashers and ice makers.
- Lime scale buildup and solenoid failures in boilers, steam kettles, and coffee makers.

SUMMARY

4.1　Explain how to select foodservice equipment.

- When selecting equipment, consider the manufacturer's reputation; how energy efficient the equipment will be; what the equipment is made of; the appropriate size to pick, if the equipment will be easy to use, clean, and maintain; if the equipment is multifunctional and will save you labor; purchase price, freight charges, and installation costs; quality of the warranty; and if the equipment is certified by organizations such as NSF International.
- Stainless steel is used most often in kitchen equipment such as tables and steamers. Stainless steel is very durable, easy to clean, and does not react with foods. Because stainless steel is a poor conductor of heat, most pots and pans are made from aluminum, which is a good heat conductor. Small amounts of aluminum may be added to the bottom of pots and pans to help conduct heat.
- Whereas a manufacturer's salesperson or representative works directly for one manufacturer, an independent manufacturer's representative shows a number of product lines from more than one manufacturer. However, they can only represent noncompetitive product lines and their salaries are based on commission. You can also buy equipment online or from many full-service food distributors.

4.2　Choose an appropriate power source.

- Power for cooking will come from electricity, natural gas, propane, or steam.

- Each kitchen will be supplied with electricity through an electric panel that contains circuit breakers and fuses. Each panel has a limit as to how much power it can supply. The panel will be rated in Amps (amperes of electricity). Circuit breakers and fuses are also rated in Amps.
- Electric equipment can be wired directly to a power source or will require a cord and plug connection.
- Heat produced by gas is measured in BTUs. Gas cooking equipment is rated in BTUs and each piece of gas equipment is also given an efficiency rating. Because of the inefficiency of gas-fired burners and pilot lights, all natural gas and liquid propane cooking equipment must be placed under the ventilation hood so that unburned gases are drawn out of the kitchen.
- Many large buildings have steam available from heating to use in the kitchen for cooking. Steam needs to be consistently available year-round and at a consistent pressure in order for steam cooking equipment to perform.

4.3　Describe features of common kitchen equipment.

- A typical range has burners on top and oven(s) underneath. Some ranges also include a broiler, charbroiler, or griddle.
- Electric induction cooktops use a magnetic field to heat up pots and the cooktop stays cool.

- Heat distribution in range ovens can be uneven. Convection ovens use radiant heat and forced air to evenly distribute the heat and speed up cooking.
- Convection ovens cook food faster than standard ovens and are more energy efficient in part because you need to set the temperature at 25°–50°F (15°–30°C) lower than for a conventional oven for most foods.
- Other ovens include deck ovens (commonly used for pizza and baking), conveyor ovens, microwave ovens, and combination steamer ovens. Combination steamer ovens can be used in one of three ways: convected heat, pressureless steam, or a combination of both. They are perfect for cooking proteins (meat, poultry, etc.) because the dry heat will do the cooking while the moisture from the steam will prevent drying out and shrinkage.
- Rapid cook ovens easily fit on a countertop and often use microwaves combined with impinged convection to quickly heat up sandwiches and other foods.
- Cook-and-hold ovens are for slow or overnight cooking to tenderize meats and minimize moisture loss.
- Steam-jacketed kettles are ideal for blanching, boiling, simmering, rethermalizing, and stewing. They heat up faster and heat foods more evenly than pots on the range.
- Steamers are popular for cooking vegetables quickly and defrosting items. Most steamers use either convection or pressure to speed up the cooking process even more.
- All steamers hold steam table pans of various sizes.
- Tilt skillets are very versatile and can be used like a griddle and also to stir-fry, fry (by filling it with oil), and braise.
- Griddles are polished, flat cooking surfaces used to cook eggs, pancakes, burgers, and more. Clamshell griddles apply heat to both sides of the product to speed cooking.
- Thicker griddle plates, such as one inch, are more heavy duty and hold onto more heat.
- Griddles must be cleaned daily and seasoned according to the manufacturer's instructions.
- Most charbroilers (under-fired) are either radiant charbroilers (transmit radiant heat waves up into the food) or lava rock charbroilers (lava rocks above the burners heat up and radiate heat up).
- Broilers use heat from above. Cooks adjust the cooking temperature by raising or lowering the grate holding the food.

- A salamander is a small broiler than can melt cheese or cook a steak. It may be mounted on the wall or above the range. Cheese melters look like salamanders but they can only be used to melt cheese, toast bread, or brown the top of a casserole.
- Double-sided panini presses cook paninis faster than on a griddle.
- A fryer purposely has a "cold zone," an area designed to capture breading crumbs and food debris. This lower temperature zone keeps the crumbs from carbonizing, which gives the oil a burnt flavor and darkens the oil so that it needs to be replaced more often. Some fryers have built-in filters to remove debris.
- With manual slicers, the operator's right arm moves the carriage holding the meat past the rotating blade to slice. With automatic slicers, a separate motor moves the carriage holding the food being sliced, back and forth over the blade, which is useful when slicing large amounts of product. Automatic slicers can also be operated manually. Fully automatic slicers can be programmed to slice and are only used in high-volume operations.
- Employee safety is a major concern with slicers. Full-knife ring guards (Figure 4-12) are available for most models, and they protect the employee because the knife edge is not exposed. Employees also have to pay strict attention when the slicer is taken apart to be washed.
- A buffalo chopper uses an S-shaped blade and rotating bowl to turn large pieces of vegetables into small pieces and to finely chop meats.
- In a typical batch bowl food processor, the employee drops the food into a bowl. As the food drops down, it enters a pillar inside the bowl that contains an S blade or a disc that cuts the food into the desired shape and size. Bowl size varies from about one to six quarts. A wide variety of cutting discs allow you to accomplish grating, slicing, ripple cutting, brunoises, waffle-cut, shredding, sticks, Julianne, French fries, and strips. Continuous-feed food processors are excellent when you have large quantities of food to process.
- Most mixers are referred to as planetary mixers, meaning that the beater (also called the agitator) moves around the bowl (which is stationary) during operation.
- All mixers are electric and most models have three speeds. Most models come with a beater (called a paddle) for doing most

mixing, a wire whip for making whipped cream, and a dough hook for mixing doughs such as pizza dough. Safety guards look like a cage at the top of the bowl and they help make sure employees don't get near the moving beaters.

- Immersion blenders can be placed directly into a pot of food to blend, puree, or emulsify.
- Work tables are usually made of stainless steel to ensure durability, corrosion resistance, and cleanability. The typical work table is five to six feet long and 30 inches wide. It has a flat top with four legs and a storage shelf underneath the work surface.
- Racks and carts help with transporting food around the kitchen.
- Table 4-3 lists important smallwares, including pots, pans, knives, other hand tools, measuring tools, and utensils.
- Whereas the steam table is more often used in the serving area, the bain-maire is used in the hot production area to hold soups, sauces, etc. Hot holding cabinets, heat lamps, and electric heat strips are also used to keep hot food hot.
- Refrigerators may be walk-ins, reach-ins, pass-throughs, or roll-ins.
- Dishwashers may be door-type dishwashers that accommodate one rack, conveyor-type dishwashers that move full racks of dishes through the cycles, or flight-type dishwashers where dishes are placed directly between rows of pegs on a conveyor belt.
- Pot washers have longer cycles than traditional dishwashers and more powerful pumps for higher pressure. They can be front or side loading.

4.4 Describe considerations to select dinnerware, beverageware, and flatware.

- Dishes, glasses, and utensils should work together on the table and reflect your concept.
- Factors to consider include appearance, durability, price, and potential breakage. Also think about your menu items and how you intend to plate them for maximum presentation value. That will help you determine the shapes and sizes you will need.
- Foodservices often choose either stoneware or china for dishes. Stoneware is quite heavy. For extra durability, look for porcelain china that has been vitrified.
- Commercial melamine dishes, made from plastic, is lightweight and doesn't break.
- Beverageware is often made from glass or a BPA-free plastic called SAN.
- Flatware made from 18/8 stainless steel is a good choice for many operations.

4.5 Write equipment specifications.

- A specification should include the name of the equipment, how many are needed, how the equipment will be used, utility and plumbing requirements, specific features such as the size or material, accessories needed, any certifications, warranty features, delivery information, installation requirements, payment terms, and cancellation terms.
- In a specification, "shall" means required, and "should" refers to a feature that is not required.

4.6 Develop an equipment maintenance program.

- Preventive maintenance is service, such as inspection or calibration, which is regularly performed on a piece of equipment to increase its lifespan and lessen the chance of it failing to work. Recommendations for preventive maintenance are listed in the *Installation and Operation Manual*.
- A foodservice manager has the choice of doing the maintenance in-house or having a service contract with an outside company.
- For each piece of equipment, an Equipment Information Sheet (Table 4-5) should be maintained that includes key information, such as the model number, when it was purchased, recommended preventive maintenance, and when it was serviced. Using these sheets, you can make a Master Maintenance Schedule listing the preventive maintenance for each piece of equipment.

REVIEW AND DISCUSSION QUESTIONS

1. Why is stainless steel used for most large foodservice equipment such as ovens?

2. List six considerations when buying equipment.

3. What factors influence whether you buy equipment that uses electricity, gas, or steam?

4. When would you decide to buy a deck oven rather than a convection oven? A combi-oven rather than a rapid cook oven?

5. How do steam kettles maintain heat?

6. List five ways you can cook in a tilt skillet.

7. What is the different between a charbroiler and a broiler? A broiler and a salamander?

8. When would you use a buffalo chopper as opposed to a food processor?

9. Compare a commercial blender with an immersion blender.

10. Compare the materials used to make most commercial pots and pans and the materials used in knives.

11. Which type of pan is used to brown meats and make stews? Which type of pan is used in the bakery? Which type of pan is used in the steam table?

12. Which type of knife is used for heavy-duty cutting, chopping, and other jobs? What tool is used to true knife blades?

13. What is used to beat, whip, and blend liquid ingredients?

14. When might infrared radiation be used in a kitchen?

15. Which type of dishwasher would you find in a large hospital foodservice? What type of dinnerware might be used? Justify your answer.

16. What is an equipment specification and what is included in it?

17. Why is it important for a manager to set up an equipment maintenance program and how would he or she do that?

SMALL GROUP PROJECT

For the foodservice concept that you created in Chapter 1, do the following.

1. Recommend four pieces of equipment for purchase. Two should be for cooking equipment and two for food preparation equipment.

2. Develop a specification for each piece of equipment to be purchased (from #1) using the format given in the chapter. When developing a specification, be sure to consider the following.
   • The menu and the form in which food will be purchased.
   • Number of meals to be served.
   • If the equipment will save labor.
   • If the equipment can be operated by current employees.
   • Availability of utilities.
   • The budget.
   • Cost to run and maintain.
   • Space in the kitchen.

Explain how these considerations affected your choices.

3. Using a website such as www.WebstaurantStore.com, find each of the pieces of equipment you want to purchase that meets the specifications you set in #2. Submit a copy of the manufacturer's spec sheet for each of the four pieces of equipment.

REFERENCES

Alley, K.M. 2016. Hot stuff. *Foodservice Equipment Reports*. Retrieved from www.fermag.com/articles/7323-hot-stuff

Amtekco. (2018). Flow over food bar. Retrieved from http://www.amtekco.com/pdf/FlowOverFoodBar.pdf

Culliton, K. (2018). Planchas vs. griddles: What exactly is the difference? *Foodservice Equipment Reports*. Retrieved from https://www.fermag.com/articles/print/8549-planchas-vs-griddles-what-exactly-is-the-difference

Delagah, A. 2015. Conveyor dishwasher performance field evaluation report. *FSTC Report Number P20004-R0*. Los Angeles, CA: The Metropolitan Water District of Southern California. Retrieved from http://bewaterwise.com/

Environmental Protection Agency. (2016). *Energy saving tips for small businesses: Restaurants*. Retrieved from https://www.energystar.gov/buildings/tools-and-resources/energy_star_small_business_restaurants

Foodservice Equipment & Supplies. (2016). What to consider when specifying a steamer. *The Quarterly Product Knowledge Guide*. Retrieved from http://www.fesmag.com/products/thequarterly/cooking-equipment/13404-what-to-consider-when-specifying-a-steamer

Foodservice Equipment & Supplies. (2017). A guide to conveyor ovens. *The Quarterly Product Knowledge Guide*. Retrieved from https://fesmag.com/products/guide/cooking-equipment/14976-the-quarterly-product-knowledge-guide-conveyor-ovens

Foodservice Equipment & Supplies. (2018a). A guide to commercial slicers. *The Quarterly Product Knowledge Guide*. Retrieved from https://fesmag.com/products/guide/prep-equipment/slicers/16104-the-quarterly-product-knowledge-guide-slicers

Foodservice Equipment & Supplies. (2018b). Dough Mixers for Pizza Restaurants. *The Quarterly Product Knowledge Guide*. Retrieved from https://fesmag.com/products/guide/prep-equipment/15547-the-quarterly-product-knowledge-guide-dough-mixers

Food Service Technology Center. (2018). Steamers.

Gisslen, Wayne. (2015). *Professional cooking* (8th edition). Hoboken, NJ: John Wiley & Sons, Inc.

Katom Restaurant Supply. (2018a). Choosing your broiler: Cheese melter vs salamander. Retrieved from https://www.katom.com/learning-center/cheese-melters-salamanders.html

Katom Restaurant Supply. (2018b). Differences between porcelain, stoneware, and china dinnerware explained. Retrieved from https://www.katom.com/cat/dinnerware/porcelain-vs-stoneware-vs-china.html

Foodservice Consultants Society International and North American Association of Food Equipment Manufacturers Liaison Committee. (2015). *Recommended guidelines for foodservice equipment catalog specification sheets*. Retrieved from http://www.fcsi.org/wp-content/uploads/2015/11/Spec-Sheet_guidelines_revised-2015.pdf

Sherer, M. (2010). Warewashers welcome the 'Star.' *Foodservice Equipment Reports*. Retrieved from https://www.fermag.com/articles/245

Sherer. M. (2012). Mixing It Up. *Foodservice Equipment Reports*. Retrieved from https://www.fermag.com/articles/2032-special-report-mixing-it-up/

Sherer, M. (2015a). FER focus: The need for speed. *Foodservice Equipment Reports*. Retrieved from https://www.fermag.com/articles/5833-fer-focus-the-need-for-speed

Sherer, M. (2015b). FER focus: Griddle me this. *Foodservice Equipment Reports*. Retrieved from https://www.fermag.com/articles/4937

Sherer, M. (2018). By the slice. *Foodservice Equipment Reports*. Retrieved from https://www.fermag.com/articles/8115-by-the-slice

Thomas, C., Norman, E. J., & Katsigris, C. (2014). *Design and equipment for restaurants and foodservice* (4th ed.). Hoboken (NJ): John Wiley & Sons, Inc.

Weber, T. (2015). What to expect from a warranty. *Foodservice Equipment Reports*. Retrieved from http://fesmag.com/features/foodservice-issues/12987-what-to-expect-from-a-warranty

© Denis Val/Shutterstock

Design and Layout of Foodservices

LEARNING OUTCOMES

5.1 Develop a business plan and organize the planning team.

5.2 Design the environment.

5.3 Plan the flow of food and work.

5.4 Layout a foodservice.

5.5 Explain the process from blueprints to inspection.

INTRODUCTION

Design refers to developing a new foodservice including steps like selecting its location, creating the concept including menu and atmosphere, picking equipment and tables, laying out a kitchen and dining area, and then building. Design work is also needed for a renovation of an existing kitchen and/or dining room, which may include expansion. For example, a school may want to update its straight-line cafeteria into a larger cafeteria with scattered stations featuring varied cuisines and menu items. **Layout** is the process of arranging the actual physical facilities—such as where the walls will be, where the ovens will be, and how the tables and chairs will be arranged in the dining room.

There are many factors to consider in design and layout such as the following.

- Is there too much or too little space in certain areas? Does the layout allow for efficient use of the space?
- Will employees be able to do their jobs in an efficient manner? Will there be bottlenecks in the dining room or kitchen due to inadequate aisles or poor traffic patterns? Will employees have to walk too far to get to the storage areas?
- Will there be enough (but not too much) cooking equipment in the kitchen?
- Will employees be able to maintain appropriate sanitation standards, and will the design minimize the risk of injuries?
- Will the facility be energy efficient?
- Will the employees be comfortable and work in appropriate temperatures and humidity with clean air, adequate lighting, and noise control?
- Will the new design comply with all regulations?

- Can the project be completed within budget?
- Will the foodservice have to be closed (meaning lost sales) for renovations to be completed?

Although foodservice consultants and other specialists will help answer these questions, foodservice owners and managers need to be knowledgeable about the process of designing and laying out a new or renovated operation in order to make the right decisions.

5.1 DEVELOP A BUSINESS PLAN AND ORGANIZE THE PLANNING TEAM

Planning a new business or doing a renovation of an existing facility *begins* with formulating the details of the project into a written plan known as a **business plan** or **prospectus**. The business plan explains why the project is important (the rationale) and the goals of the project, such as serving new customers and being profitable. A business plan describes the business in detail and is used to seek and secure approvals and/or loans. It includes the following sections.

1. Business Overview. This section includes a description of the business including its mission and vision. For example, the mission of Aramark, a foodservice contractor, is to "enrich and nourish lives." While the overall intention of a company is depicted in the **mission statement**, the **vision statement** looks ahead at what the company wants to achieve. This section also includes information about the company's key products or services, major business goals and objectives, the legal structure of the business (such as corporation), the size of the company, and the company's history and profitability (if applicable). In the case of an existing business that is planning a renovation or expansion, the goal and objectives of the project should be explained. For example, if a foodservice plans to expand and update the dining area, the goal may be to increase sales. The objectives then state what to do to achieve the goal, so the objectives may be to increase the dining room by 150 square feet and update the dining room decor, both of which will help attract more customers.
2. Industry Analysis. The industry, such as fast casual restaurants, needs to be described, including whether this segment is growing, mature, or (hopefully not) declining. Barriers to entry are noted as well as the typical customer profile and an analysis of the competition.
3. Operating Plan. This section includes details about the location of the business; the menu; how much total space is needed and how the space will be allocated to each function; business operations including who will manage it, when it will be open, and how foods will be purchased, produced, and served; who the customers will be and how many will be served; the labor needed; how regulatory requirements will be met; and how the operation will be unique.
4. Marketing Analysis and Plan. The market analysis includes detailed information on target customers (including demographics such as age and level of education) and an analysis of what are the competing businesses in the area. The marketing plan starts with marketing goals and objectives and describing what is unique about your business. The marketing plan explains how you will attract and keep customers using your product or service as well as pricing information. The marketing plan also discusses how the company will promote and distribute the product/service to prospective customers (such as home delivery, etc.).
5. Financial Feasibility Study and Plan. The financial feasibility study examines the start-up costs for a new business or the renovation/expansion costs for an existing business. For a new business, you have to develop a **pro forma income statement** in which you project your sales and expenses (food, beverage, labor, lease, etc.) for a period of time, such as two years. By projecting sales and

expenses, you can estimate your net profit. A cash-flow statement is also useful as you need to forecast how money will flow in and out of your business so that you do not run out of money during the start-up phase. For a renovation, the costs of the project must be fully laid out and justified through, for example, increased sales or cost savings. The financial plan will need to show how the business can pay for building or renovation costs and succeed financially over time.

The emphasis for a business plan involving a renovation or expansion will be the financial justification. For example, will a kitchen renovation result in increased sales that will justify the expense, and how quickly will the renovation costs be paid off?

Anyone building a new business or renovating an existing business will certainly need help from his or her colleagues as well as specialists. The group of individuals who work together to plan a new facility or renovate an existing one are known as the **planning team**. Once you have a business plan, you can bring members onto your team. The planning team naturally includes the foodservice manager(s) and the owner or administrator. Depending on the needs, the planning team may also include any of the following.

1. Architect. The architect designs all kinds of buildings and spaces within buildings, while considering the function, safety, and economics of each project. The planning team should only hire an architect who is licensed and registered to practice in the state where the work will be done. Architects are licensed professionals who take the design of the foodservice through many steps until final drawings are produced. For example, the architect designs how space will be used, helps select materials, determines how utilities and plumbing will work (with assistance from engineers), and prepares drawings from which contractors will submit bids. Final drawings specify all aspects of the building or space—such as mechanical, electrical, plumbing, location of windows, doors, etc. They are used by the necessary authorities to approve the project and also by the architect to supervise construction.

2. Engineer. The term *engineer* is very broad and includes many specialized disciplines of people who are trained to use science and technology to develop solutions to technical problems. Mechanical engineers design systems such as heating, cooling, ventilation, and plumbing (includes water and steam). Electrical engineers work on lighting and power requirements. Structural engineers work on designing new buildings.

3. Interior designer. An interior designer develops floor plans for dining areas and other non-kitchen areas to make these spaces functional and to match the desired atmosphere. Interior designers recommend possible color schemes, textures, tables and other furniture, as well as wall and window coverings. They usually work with the architect to design the lighting. Architectural firms often employ an interior designer.

4. Foodservice consultant. **Foodservice consultants** provide expertise and experience when such expertise is not available in house. An excellent resource is the Foodservice Consultants Society International (FCSI). FCSI is a professional organization composed of consultants who specialize in many areas including space planning, kitchen design, kitchen equipment, operations, feasibility studies, and interior/dining room design. FSCI members work on a fee-for-service basis and do not try to sell you products from certain manufacturers. They are required to stay independent from the supply end and they must abide by a strict Code of Ethics and Professional Conduct.

5. Equipment representatives. Companies that manufacture foodservice equipment, such as Hobart, have sales representatives who are very knowledgeable about their products and can help you make appropriate equipment choices.

6. Builder/contractor. A builder/contractor would be hired to build the new building or renovate/expand an existing space using the plan and specifications of the architect.

Although foodservice consultants and equipment representatives are very helpful, always do your own analysis to be sure you are getting the best and most energy-efficient equipment for your money.

Not every member of the planning team will be involved in every decision. One person, usually the foodservice manager or owner, needs to be in charge of the team and ensure appropriate meetings and coordination.

The planning team knows that major factors influencing the design and layout are the menu and type of foodservice system (conventional, ready-prepared, assembly/serve, or commissary). For example, the amount of space and equipment needed for a conventional system are quite different from each of the other systems. The menu tells you which foods need to be purchased and the recipes will show the form in which each food needs to be purchased, such as fresh, frozen, or canned. By also considering the volume of meals to be produced each day, hours of service, and number of seats in the dining room, the planning team can now estimate the amount and kind of space needed to store foods (including freezers, refrigerators, and dry goods storage) as well as determine what equipment is needed and the space needed for the kitchen and dining area.

The planning team also considers who the customers and employees will be. It is especially important to consider the age and mobility of customers. For example, the space needed for a dining room in a family restaurant will be quite different from a dining room in a retirement facility. Older guests may not be as mobile and require walkers or wheelchairs, so these dining rooms often need space to store walkers and mobility scooters while guests eat and have taller tables for wheelchairs to fit under. Planners also look at the total number of employees, how many of each gender (for locker/rest room space), how many employees work on a shift, and what each position will be doing. This information will help ensure that enough space is allocated to each area so employees and guests are comfortable and can move around easily.

The planning team must be aware of various building codes and regulations that they need to meet. Regulations and requirements exist at federal, state, county, and local levels. For example, building permits are needed from local authorities before building a new structure, demolishing part or all of a structure, or altering or adding to an existing structure. Permits are also needed to install or modify fire suppression systems. Any demolition or building must be done in accordance with local building codes that ensure that all buildings meet minimum safety and structural standards. During the construction process, building inspectors will come in at certain points to ensure that everything is being done according to the building code.

The *Food Code* (2017), released every four years by the Food and Drug Administration, provides scientifically sound guidance on food safety and sanitation. It includes guidance in areas such as plumbing, sinks, lighting, floors and walls, ventilation, and trash disposal that are all pertinent to building or renovation. It is referred as a model code because it acts as a guide for local, state, and other jurisdictions when updating their own codes. The planning team will need to ensure compliance with the local food/health code.

Additional regulations include the Life Safety Code and Americans with Disabilities Act. The **Life Safety Code**, developed by the National Fire Protection Association's (NFPA), gives guidance on building construction, renovation, and operational features to minimize the effects of fires, smoke, and panic. Facilities participating in the Medicare and Medicaid programs (such as hospitals) must be compliant with the Life Safety Code as well as NFPA's Health Care Facilities Code.

The **Americans with Disabilities Act (ADA)** addresses making businesses accessible for disabled customers and employees, such as requiring handicapped parking spaces with extra space and aisles in the business that are at least three feet wide. The ADA protects the rights of people who have a physical or mental impairment that substantially limits their ability to perform one or more major life activities, such as walking or hearing. People with disabilities must not be treated in a different or inferior manner. New buildings have to be completely compliant with ADA; and if an existing building

Table 5-1 Some Requirements of the Americans with Disabilities Act
1. An adequate number of accessible parking spaces must be available and clearly identified with a sign including the International Symbol of Accessibility. Parking spaces must be a minimum eight feet wide with a five-foot wide striped aisle next to it.
2. The accessible route from the parking space to the building entrance must be firm, slip resistant, and at least three feet wide. If the accessible route crosses a curb, there must be a curb ramp, and other accommodations must be made if the route is too steep.
3. The opening width of the entrance must be at least 32 inches and the door handle must be operable with one hand. The closer must be on a time delay.
4. The accessible route *within* the building must also be at least three feet wide and cannot be blocked by items such as a drinking fountain.
5. At least 5% of seating (and standing) spaces in an eating place must be accessible to people in wheelchairs. The table should be between 28 to 34 inches above the floor with sufficient knee space.
6. In a counter service situation, there must be at least three feet of counter space that is not higher than 36 inches above the floor where someone with a wheelchair can order.
7. Accessible rest rooms must be available and meet a number of requirements (size, door pulls, sinks, etc.).

Data from "2010 ADA Standards for Accessible Design." U.S. Department of Justice, 2010. Retrieved from https://www.ada.gov/regs2010/2010ADA Standards/2010ADAstandards.htm

undergoes a renovation, the renovated space must be compliant with ADA. **Table 5-1** gives some of the ADA requirements. Employers are also asked to work with employees with disabilities to structure the way a job is performed so a disabled employee can successfully do the job.

When considering renovations or new construction, there are a number of resources to get ideas and information. In addition to talking to equipment companies directly and using their websites, attend trade shows such as the National Restaurant Association and the North American Association of Food Equipment Manufacturers (NAFEM). NAFEM represents over 500 foodservice equipment and supplies manufacturers. You can also talk to managers in similar foodservices and perhaps visit their operation to see their setup and equipment. Foodservice equipment trade magazines and journals are good sources of information. For example, *Foodservice Equipment & Supplies*, a monthly publication covering commercial and on-site foodservice, contains up-to-date articles on the industry, how operators are using new equipment, and actual layouts of new or renovated facilities.

5.2 DESIGN THE ENVIRONMENT

Before discussing how to design and lay out kitchen and dining areas, we need to look at the environment in which employees work and customers eat. The heating and air conditioning, ventilation, lighting, noise control, as well as the materials and colors used in floors, walls, and ceilings affect the work environment as well as the atmosphere in the dining area. A foodservice manager does not need to know all the details about each of these but does need to know some basics including terminology.

HEATING, VENTILATION, AND AIR CONDITIONING

A well-designed heating, ventilation, and air conditioning (HVAC) system is crucial to maintaining appropriate air quality, temperature, and humidity within the foodservice. The right combination of temperature and humidity keeps everyone comfortable. HVAC isn't just about heating and cooling; it is also about air quality. Air quality is maintained by removing contaminated air (called exhaust air) and bringing in outside air (called **makeup air**), as well as proper air movement within the building. Depending on the climate and other factors, HVAC systems may include filters (or other air cleaner) and dehumidifiers to maintain air quality.

Facilities may use a split HVAC system with a furnace or heat pump, an air conditioning system, and ductwork for the air to flow. Heat is produced using sources such as steam, fuel oil, natural gas, or electricity. Air conditioning usually requires electricity. Fans and air ducts located in ceilings and walls allow conditioned air to move from area to area or room to room to maintain comfort. Air going into the kitchen or dining room from the HVAC system is called **supply air**, while the air returning to the HVAC system from the kitchen or dining room is called the **return air**.

Air conditioners use the scientific principle that when a liquid converts to a gas, it absorbs heat. The major components of the air conditioning system are the evaporator, compressor, and condenser. When hot air flows over the cold evaporator coils, the refrigerant inside absorbs heat as it changes from a liquid to a gas, so the air becomes cooler and also less humid. To continue cooling, the air conditioner must convert the refrigerant gas back to a liquid. To do that, a pump, called the compressor, moves the hot gas *outdoors* into the condenser coils where the gas reverts back to a liquid, giving up its heat to the outside air flowing over the condenser's coils. The condenser coil is what gets rid of the heat in the system, and it may be water cooled or air cooled. Think of air conditioning as a cycle: liquid refrigerant changing to gas, compression, and then conversion to a liquid again.

Nearly all air conditioning systems once used halogenated chlorofluorocarbons (HCFCs) as the refrigerant, but these are being gradually phased out, with most production and importing stopped by 2020 and all production and importing stopped by 2030, according to the U.S. Environmental Protection Agency. As these refrigerants are phased out, ozone-safe hydrofluorocarbons (HFCs) are expected to dominate the market.

The size of the air conditioning system is based primarily on the size of the space and the amount of heat generated. A specialist is required to do a heating and cooling load calculation to determine the size air conditioning system you will need. An economizer may be added to the outdoor unit to allow the use of outdoor air for cooling when the outside air is below a certain temperature and humidity. This way you can cool a building without running the compressor.

Instead of using a split system, most businesses use a packaged HVAC unit that sits on the roof. With a package unit, all the components are housed in one cabinet stored on the top of the building. Both heating and air conditioning are in the cabinet along with the compressors and the fans. The unit connects directly into the building's ventilation system to circulate the air. With installation of a humidistat on a rooftop unit, it can also control humidity. One disadvantage of this system it that it is not always as energy efficient as a split system.

Keeping the temperature and humidity at comfortable levels is important, particularly in hot kitchens. It is also important to maintain air quality. Cooking produces smells, smoke, and grease that must be ventilated to the outside. This is where kitchen hoods come in. They are built over kitchen equipment to capture grease, heat, moisture, odors, smoke, and other cooking products (**Figure 5-1**). Filters in the hood help to capture grease as the air is exhausted to the outside. Otherwise the grease would build up in the ducts and cause a fire.

When air is removed through an exhaust hood, it must be replaced with an equal volume of air—called makeup air—that often comes from the outside. Keep in mind that fans are used to pull air out of the building and also pull outside air into the building. When pulling outside air in, the air intake vents should not be placed in locations close to odors such as trash dumpsters or automotive exhaust. In kitchens with large exhaust requirements, it may not be practical to supply all the makeup air through the building HVAC system, so an independent makeup air supply may be needed. Standards for proper ventilation to ensure acceptable air quality have been set by the American Society

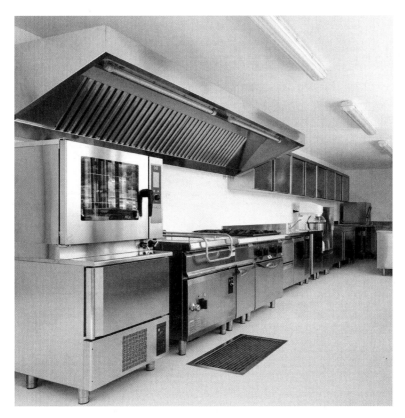

FIGURE 5-1 A Kitchen Hood Over Cooking Equipment

© Alexandre zveiger/Shutterstock

of Heating, Refrigeration, and Air Conditioning Engineers (ASHRAE). For example, the ventilation rate (in cubic feet of air per minute (cfm)) for a commercial kitchen is 14 cfm per person based on 20 people working in a 1,000-square feet (ASHRAE, 2016).

Clogged hood filters are a fire hazard and also hamper the ability for smoke, odors, etc., to be pulled out of the kitchen. Hood filters must be cleaned frequently either by hand or by running through the dishwasher. The ducts must also be cleaned and maintained. Many health codes specify exactly how often kitchen exhaust systems must be cleaned and may even specify which companies you can use to clean the ducts.

In some cases, such as space limitations or when venting is not feasible, a **ventless hood** may be used. This type of hood is a compact, portable unit that doesn't require fans or ductwork because it uses two or more levels of filters to remove grease and other contaminants from the air. Some ventless hoods use electronic filtration along with charcoal filters to help remove odors, etc. You can buy equipment with its own ventless hood, such as a combi-oven, or buy a ventless hood to install over an existing piece of equipment. However, gas-fired equipment can't be used with ventless hoods— only electric equipment. Also, any high-volume kitchen would need traditional hoods. While ventless hoods are often cheaper, they require frequent cleaning and maintenance and don't always remove all the odors.

The air system also has to be balanced. Air transfer between the kitchen and dining room must flow towards the kitchen. This ensures that grease, smoke, fumes, heat, steam, and odors do not enter the dining area. For a new or renovated facility, an engineer will draw a diagram showing airflow. All airflow has a direction—either positive or negative. The kitchen should have negative air pressure (meaning more air is removed than supplied to it) as this ensures that odors etc., do not leave the kitchen and go into surrounding areas such as the dining room. The dining area generally has positive

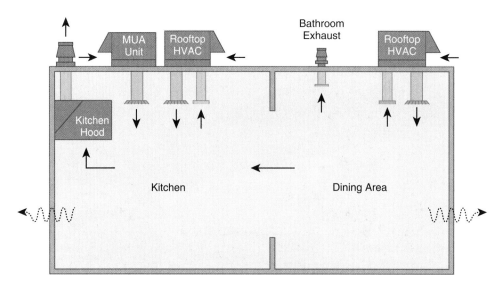

FIGURE 5-2 How Air Flows in a Quick-Service Restaurant

"Guidance on Demand-Controlled Kitchen Ventilation." U.S. Department of Energy, 2015. Retrieved from https://betterbuildingssolutioncenter.energy.gov/sites/default/files/attachments/Guidance-on-Demand-Controlled-Kitchen-Ventilation.pdf

pressure (meaning more air is brought in than removed). Air flows from areas with positive pressure to areas with negative pressure.

Figure 5–2 is a schematic representation of how air flows in a quick-service restaurant. Rooftop HVAC units pull in air from the kitchen and dining areas and also return conditioned air to those areas. In addition, air from the kitchen hood and bathrooms is exhausted out of the building, and a separate makeup air unit helps supply fresh air that has been heated or cooled back into the kitchen. The arrow from the dining area into the kitchen shows how air flows.

Demand-controlled kitchen ventilation (DCKV) saves energy by adjusting the quantity of kitchen hood exhaust and incoming outdoor air to reflect the amount of cooking taking place under the hood. Periods of reduced cooking activity are opportunities for ramping down the air flow to the exhaust hood (U.S. Department of Energy, 2015). A tempered DCKV system can heat or cool the replacement air as needed.

Hoods, conventional or ventless, also incorporate fire suppression systems to extinguish fires quickly and efficiently. Fire suppression systems use chemicals, not water because water does not extinguish grease fires and just makes them worse. When a fire starts, it is automatically detected by sensors in the hood or ductwork, and chemical is released from nozzles located throughout the hood onto the appliances. A manual pull station can also be used to release the chemical. As the system is discharged, gas and/or electric cooking power will be shut down to the appliances. Inspections of kitchen fire suppression systems must be conducted at least every six months by qualified people in accordance with the National Fire Protection Association's and the manufacturer's requirements.

LIGHTING

The interior designer or lighting consultant is involved with determining appropriate lighting requirements and making purchasing recommendations. Lighting in the dining area is quite different from kitchen lighting. Whereas lighting in the dining room should add to the desired ambiance, lighting in the kitchen must be bright to improve employee accuracy and productivity as well as reduce eyestrain. Other areas, such as the host area or the rest rooms have different lighting needs. Keep in mind that natural light is usually quite desirable, and that the colors and surfaces of walls, ceilings, and floors reflect light to varying degrees so they will affect the lighting chosen.

Designers use several types of light. **Indirect lighting** (sometimes called ambient lighting) is pointed upward and mostly washes the ceiling and upper walls with light instead of aiming at a certain spot. Indirect lighting, such as recessed lights or natural sunlight, often provide the main light source in a room and are complemented by direct and accent lighting. **Direct lighting** is used to put light in a specific area—such over a table in the dining room or over a grill in the kitchen. **Accent lighting**, a form of direct lighting, is used to add interest by, for example, highlighting artwork or architectural features or simply using colorful backlighting behind the bar. In **Figure 5-3**, the large pendant lights close to the ceiling, and the two sconces on the left wall, act as indirect lighting for this restaurant. The glass shades of the pendants help throw off lots of ambient light. Direct lighting over each table and the station on the right is provided by smaller pendants with solid shades. In the food preparation area, bright recessed ceiling lights help employees prepare foods.

In addition to considering where light fixtures need to be placed, designers also consider the intensity of the light. The light intensity for a dining room varies. If you consider a typical limited-service restaurant, it is brightly lit (including a lot of natural light from big windows) to speed up service and get customers out the door faster. Many other operations use dimmer lighting to communicate to guests that they can stay longer and enjoy themselves. Dining room lighting needs to be adjustable (using a dimmer) to different occasions or times of day. More light is usually desirable for breakfast meals and business lunches and less light for leisurely dinners. At the end of the day, the lights can be turned on full for the staff to clean up the dining room. In the kitchen, bright lighting is needed to allow employees to do their work and for their safety.

The most common measure of light output from a lightbulb is the **lumen**. While lumens measure the amount of visible light emitted by the lightbulb, **foot-candles** measure the amount of light falling on a given surface. A foot-candle (or lux) is defined as the illuminance on a one square foot surface from a uniform source of light. Foot-candles are useful when you need to quantify the amount of light present in a given area.

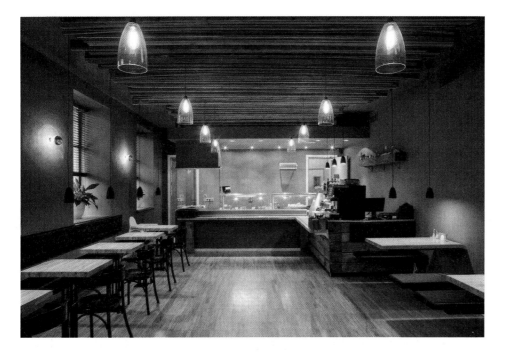

FIGURE 5-3 Indirect and Direct Lighting in a Restaurant

© Aleks Kend/Shutterstock

Table 5-2 Minimum Lighting Intensity for Foodservices	
Minimum Lighting Intensity	**Area**
10 foot candles (108 lux)	• Walk-in refrigerators and freezers • Dry food storage areas • In other areas when being cleaned
20 foot candles (215 lux)	• In areas used for handwashing, dishwashing, and potwashing • In areas used to store equipment and/or utensils • Inside equipment such as reach-in refrigerators • Buffets and salad bars • Displays of produce or packaged foods • Restrooms
50 foot candles (540 lux)	• Food preparation areas including working with knives, slicers, or other equipment

Data from *2017 Food Code*, p 186, by the U.S. Public Health Service and Food & Drug Administration, 2017. Retrieved from https://www.fda.gov/Food /GuidanceRegulation/Retail Food Protection/FoodCode/ucm595139.htm

Guidelines for light intensity (measured in foot-candles) are available from the Illuminating Engineering Society, the federal *Food Code* (see **Table 5-2**), building codes, and some local food/health codes.

Another way to look at light is the **color rendering index (CRI)**. The color rendering index (CRI) is a measure of how well an artificial light shows natural colors compared with daylight or incandescent light. The higher the CRI, the better the artificial light source is at rendering colors accurately. A CRI of 80 to 100 is considered very good/excellent while lower numbers do not render colors as accurately.

CRI is independent of color temperature. A bulb's color temperature (measured in degrees Kelvin) ranges from warmer light (think yellow to red) to cooler light (think blue or white), and lets you know what the look and feel of the light produced will be. For example, warm white bulbs give off some orange and yellow colors, and work well in calm, cozy settings such as some dining rooms. Cool white emits a more neutral white light and is better for task lighting. Daylight bulbs give off a blue–white light that mimics daylight, and these bulbs are excellent for lighting foods and task lighting.

There are several types of light bulbs used in foodservices, each with its own special characteristics.

1. The traditional light bulb is the **incandescent**. While it is inexpensive and makes food look natural, the incandescent bulb gives off heat, does not last very long, and uses more energy than many other bulbs. Incandescent bulbs tend to capture color better than fluorescent lighting, but fewer are being manufactured because they are not energy efficient.

2. **Fluorescent tubes** are often used in foodservice kitchens as they are bright and more energy efficient than incandescent bulbs. They are also durable and spread light over a large area. They are slightly more expensive than incandescent bulbs but last a lot longer. Daylight fluorescent tubes are usually recessed into the ceiling of cooking and food preparation areas.

3. **Compact fluorescent lamps (CFLs)** are ideal to save energy and money as they are about three times more efficient than incandescent bulbs, they last for years, and they don't emit heat. CFLs contain a small amount of mercury and old bulbs should be given to qualified recyclers or Home Depot. Because CFLs often need time to warm up and they also do not last as long if they are frequently turned on and off; they work best in offices and walk-in coolers where the lights are mostly kept on. Warm white CFLs can be used in dining areas.

4. **LED (light-emitting diode) bulbs** produce light approximately 90% more efficiently than incandescent light bulbs (Energy Star, 2018), and the bulbs have

a very long life. Although their initial cost is higher than for many other bulbs, they can last up to 10 times longer. In addition, they only give off tiny amounts of heat and put out much brighter light than incandescents. In restaurants, they are used, for example, outdoors, in menu boards, and also for some uses in the dining room.

No matter which type of bulb you use, you can save energy by using **occupancy sensors**, which detect motion and then turn the light on in rooms such as storage rooms, break rooms, and restrooms.

When designing kitchen lighting, also keep these points in mind.

- According to the federal *Food Code*, light fixtures must be easy to clean. Grease and dust do accumulate on fixtures, so they must be cleaned regularly.
- The *Food Code* also requires that light bulbs are shielded, coated, or otherwise shatter-resistant in areas where food is being handled; food packages are open; or over clean equipment, utensils, or linens. Fluorescent tubes often have shields that protect food and employees from falling glass if the bulb breaks. Local food/health codes often have specific requirements.
- Because of the humidity in dishrooms and walk-in refrigerators, lighting used in these areas should be labeled as "Vapor Proof" or "Suitable for Damp Locations." Vapor-proof light fixtures use rugged housings that protect the socket and wiring from moisture, dirt, and grease so they are also used in exhaust hoods.
- When using bright fluorescent lights in a kitchen, you have to make sure they don't cause glare. To reduce glare, metal work tables and countertops should have a matte or satin finish.

The color and surfaces of the ceiling, walls, floors, tables, etc., as well as the height of the ceiling, all impact lighting.

The Life Safety Code, developed by the National Fire Protection Association's (NFPA), gives guidance on emergency lighting—basically lighting to help people get out of a building in the event of a fire or other event. Emergency lighting must work for at least 90 minutes and have its own power source (in case of a power failure). Local building codes and the National Electrical Code also have guidelines for emergency lighting.

Noise Control

The intensity of sound is measured in **decibels**. Whispering to someone is about 30 decibels whereas normal conversation is 60 decibels (National Institute for Occupational Safety and Health, 2018). Depending on the desired atmosphere, the dining room may be relatively quiet or a bit louder. Noise can harm employees and bother guests when they occur at high levels and/or continue for a long time. The National Institute for Occupational Safety and Health (2018) recommends that employees should be not exposed to noises of 85 decibels or louder for eight hours (a work shift) to minimize chances of hearing loss.

Kitchens are full of noise, from commercial dishwashers to conversation to the fans in the exhaust hoods. The designer works on reducing kitchen noise as well as keeping that noise from filtering into the dining room through a number of means.

1. <u>Kitchen</u>. Since much foodservice equipment, such as a dishwasher, is noisy, the designer will compare the decibels produced by different models. The designer also considers where to place equipment to minimize noise. Large operations often put dishwashing functions into its own room because of the noise and also the humidity. Insulation and soundproof doors can also be used to keep noise from getting into other areas.

2. <u>Dining Room Materials</u>. Many of the materials used today in dining rooms create noise: guests walk on hard floors (such as wood) and sounds bounce off hard

tabletops, bars, and glass windows. Tall ceilings and open kitchens just create more sound. To offset noise in a dining room, designers can use sound-absorbing ceiling tiles and fabric-covered wall panels. The use of movable partitions made of sound-reduction materials can also decrease unwanted noise and, at the same time, create smaller spaces. Carpeting in adjacent areas, such as the lobby and by restrooms, can help decrease noise. Even window coverings, tablecloths, and padding in chairs can dampen noise.

3. <u>HVAC System</u>. HVAC systems can create and transmit unwanted noise so selection of an appropriate system along with well-designed ductwork and proper installation are vital to decrease noise. ASHRAE recommendations, such as keeping air flow below 1,500 feet per minute as it exits diffuser and grills, can help reduce noise. If air ducts are too small, it forces air to travel too fast and that creates background noise in the kitchen or dining room. Lined ducts significantly reduce noise and improves thermal performance. Lastly, HVAC systems need to be maintained regularly to keep quiet.

4. <u>Music</u>. A quality sound system with excellent speakers can add to a guest's experience, whereas an inexpensive system with poor audio speakers may just create more noise. In the dining room, the sound in different sections of the room should not vary by more than 10 decibels.

FLOORS, WALLS, AND CEILINGS

When choosing floors for a foodservice, there are a number of considerations.

1. <u>Safety</u>. Slip resistance is important to meet code requirements for the Americans with Disabilities Act as well as decrease the likelihood of falls by employees.
2. <u>Durability</u>. Floors have to be able to endure lots of foot traffic, as well as a knife falling on the ground or a glass jar falling and breaking, without damage.
3. <u>Cleanability</u>. Because foodservice floors are often subject to moisture, spilled foods, and splattered grease, they must be easy to clean and able to withstand frequent cleaning.
4. <u>Nonporous</u>. The last thing you want is for the floor to absorb moisture, acids, or grease.
5. <u>Comfort</u>. Floors need to be comfortable for employees who stand on them for hours at a time. For floors that are still rather hard, such as concrete, anti-fatigue mats can be used. Anti-fatigue mats are usually made of rubber and provide cushioning for employees working at the potwashing station or cash register, for example. Anti-fatigue mats are also made for use in wet areas or areas where grease is an issue, where they also help reduce slips and falls.
6. <u>Appearance/beauty</u>. Floors can add to the atmosphere in the dining room as well as the quality of the work environment in the kitchen.
7. <u>Building code/health code requirements</u>. Codes usually give guidance about flooring, wall, and ceiling choices, as it is preferable to have durable surfaces that are easy to keep clean, as well as fire-resistant surfaces for ceilings.

For foodservices, designers specify commercial grade flooring instead of residential grade flooring. Commercial grade flooring is designed to be more durable and slip-resistant than residential flooring.

Table 5-3 describes several possible flooring options for kitchens. The most popular options are quarry tile and epoxy-coated concrete. While epoxy-coated concrete and composite sheet vinyl are much less expensive than quarry tile; quarry tile is the most long-lasting of all the choices. Neither wood flooring nor carpeting would be appropriate in kitchens—water and moisture would ruin them in short order.

Whichever flooring is chosen, coving will be required by code. For example, if a foodservice is laying a sheet of composite vinyl, where the sheet hits the wall, it will be

Table 5-3 Types of Non-Wood Flooring for Kitchen Areas			
Description	**Advantages**	**Disadvantages**	**Best Uses**
Quarry tile (unglazed red clay tile)	Very durable, slip-resistant, easy to clean, nonporous, long lasting	Keeping grout clean can be difficult, grout may deteriorate, high initial cost	Anywhere in kitchen, excellent in moist areas, offices, restrooms
Epoxy-coated concrete (coating is about ¼" thick)	Durable, slip-resistant, easy to clean, nonporous, no seams or grout, withstands high temperatures, variety of colors, low cost	Not as durable as quarry tile	Anywhere in kitchen
Composite sheet vinyl (with slip-resistant coating)	Durable, slip-resistant, easy to clean, resists moisture, comes in many different colors/patterns, softer and more comfortable than concrete or tile, low cost	Not as durable as quarry tile, less resistant to grease, may dent or stain, requires routine maintenance	Best for moderate traffic areas away from fryers
Glazed ceramic tile	Durable, easy to clean, nonporous, decorative, available in many colors/patterns	Keeping grout clean, very hard surface that may require rubber mats for employees, slippery, high initial cost	On walls behind equipment, in display kitchens, in rest rooms

turned up the wall from 4 to 6 inches (depending on the code) and then cut. **Coving** then is basically a curved edge that links the floor with the wall so there are no gaps (that would be hard to clean) or sharp edges. Floors will also be sloped toward floor drains. Floor drains are usually required in areas such as sinks and dishwashers.

Carpet and solid hardwood floors are frequently used outside of the kitchen. Carpet is popular for the dining room, but is not a good choice for high traffic areas such as where servers are picking up plates or in front of beverage stations. While carpet is cheaper, has a warmer appearance, and keeps noise down, solid hardwood floors are more popular in dining rooms because, besides their timeless appeal, they are more durable and easier to clean. Because solid hardwood floors can be sanded and refinished many times, they last for decades. In recent years, alternatives to solid hardwood floors (which are expensive) have emerged that cost less. Here's a list that starts with the least expensive option to the most expensive.

1. *Commercial vinyl sheet flooring* is 100% plastic and is very resistant to water. It can mimic the appearance of wood quite well. Vinyl flooring ranges from inexpensive to moderately expensive.

2. *Luxury vinyl planks* are also 100% plastic. Plank vinyl flooring is installed plank by plank to create a natural wood look. The planks look distinct and have a textured surface so the floor looks very authentic. They resist moisture unless moisture gets in between the planks. Textured surfaces can be slip resistant and a good choice for high traffic areas.

3. *Laminate flooring* is made of pressed wood with an image of wood on the top that is covered with a thin layer of plastic for protection. Laminate flooring installs much like real hardwood. If water gets between the boards, it will cause the floor to swell. Also, it resists dents better than solid hardwood, but is not indestructible.

4. *Engineered hardwood* is more expensive than vinyl or laminate flooring but not usually as expensive as solid hardwood flooring. Engineered wood has a plywood base topped with a thin layer of wood that can be sanded and refinished a few times, perhaps more depending on the quality. Engineered wood deals with moisture better than solid hardwood because plywood is more stable than solid wood. It can get scratched or dented just like regular hardwood floors.

Although wood floors are not as warm as carpet, you can soften up the appearance of a wood floor by covering part of it with an area rug as long as the rug is not a tripping hazard.

Like flooring, walls need to be nonporous, easy to clean, and durable. Many walls in the kitchen are made of wallboard and covered in a paint with an enamel or semi-gloss finish to allow cleaning. However, painted walls are not durable in areas where they are likely to be splattered frequently with water or food and require cleaning. A wall made with ceramic tile (such as found in bathrooms) or stainless steel can be easily cleaned day after day. Although they are much more expensive to install (especially the stainless steel), ceramic tile is frequently found in wet areas and stainless steel in cooking areas. Attention needs to be paid to keep grout between the ceramic tiles clean and in good repair. Both materials are reflective and may cause glare from light fixtures. To keep costs down, ceramic tile or stainless steel may be used to a height of perhaps six feet (or wherever the protection is no longer needed) and then wallboard is used above that height.

Fiberglass-reinforced plastic (FRP) panels look like wall paneling and are economical to install in kitchens, restrooms, and service areas. In addition to being tough and nonporous, they are easy to keep clean and maintain. FRP panels are available in many colors and finishes, including panels that look like ceramic tile or wood.

Common ceiling materials include acoustic tile, painted wallboard, and painted plaster. Acoustic tiles are individual units that fit into a grid running across the ceiling. Ceiling tiles vary in terms of several characteristics:

1. How much sound it blocks and absorbs.
2. How much light it reflects.
3. How resistant it is to water and humidity.
4. How resistant it is to fire.
5. How resistant it is to soil.
6. How washable it is.

Dining room and kitchen ceilings are normally lighter than the wall color. Ceilings often help add light and remove some noise from the room.

PLUMBING

Although the engineer and architect plan the plumbing, it is important for foodservice managers to know some basics.

- Handwashing sinks must be available in food preparation, food dispensing, warewashing areas, and rest rooms. The number of sinks is often based on the total square footage.
- Plumbing lines carrying water and waste are usually located in the concrete floor. This makes it hard and expensive to make changes because you have to tear up concrete.
- Floor drains must be provided where water may gather and need to drain, such as by the dishwasher or steam equipment.
- Air gaps are used to prevent backflow. Once clean water leaves the faucet, it is either used or sent down the drain. In the event of a drain back up or flood, the contents of the drain line (which could include sewage) should never be able to back up into a sink or touch the clean water supply. An **air gap** is an interruption in the drain pipe from a sink to prevent sewage from flowing into the sink. **Figure 5-4** shows how the drains under a kitchen sink empty just above a trough that collects the dirty water. The air gap prevents any dirty water from going back into the sink. An air gap is also required for ice machines.
- When buying equipment using water or steam, it is important to consider the water and steam pressure needs for installation, including where to locate the water and steam inlets.

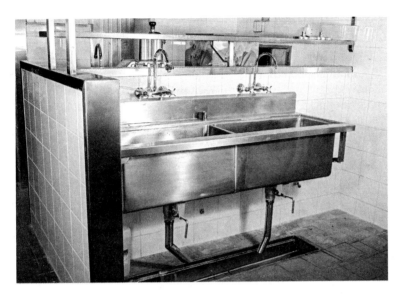

FIGURE 5-4 Example of an Air Gap Under the Sink

© Suprun Vitaly/Shutterstock

SPOTLIGHT ON SUSTAINABLE FOODSERVICE DESIGN

Today, both the government and parts of the construction industry are working with businesses to help design, construct, and operate efficient green buildings that save valuable resources such as water and cost less money to operate. The U.S. Green Building Council's trademarked LEED certification process (LEED stands for "Leadership in Energy and Environmental Design") is the national benchmark for green construction. LEED certification is available for different situations, such as new retail construction or existing interior spaces. The Green Restaurant Association (GRA) also has its own certification program.

To earn LEED certification, a building must meet certain prerequisites in each of the following categories, as well as accumulate 40 additional LEED points.

- Sustainable Sites
- Location and Transportation
- Water Efficiency
- Material and Resources
- Energy and Atmosphere
- Indoor Environmental Quality

If a building gets more than 40 points, higher levels of certification, such as LEED Silver for 50 points or LEED Gold with 60 points, are possible. A LEED Accredited Professional can help a foodservice owner examine and pursue certification goals.

Here are some examples of what a hotel restaurant did to get LEED certification

- Sustainable Sites: At least half of the space outside of the building was restored with native planting. Reflective roofing materials were put on over three-quarters of the roof surface.
- Location and Transportation: The location is within ¼ mile of local bus lines so employees and customers can use the bus.
- Water Efficiency: Water use was reduced by ⅓ through the use of low-flow fixtures. Water for landscaping was minimized and supplied by a nonpotable source.
- Energy and Atmosphere: No CFC-based refrigerants were used. One-third of the electricity is from renewable sources (solar panels).
- Materials and Resources: Over 20% of the build materials were made from recycled materials. Almost half of the building materials were extracted and/or made within 500 miles of the site.
- Indoor Environmental Quality: Adhesives, sealants, paints, stains, and carpeting comply with the Volatile Organic Compounds (VOC) limits. Lots of daylight is available.
- Innovation and Design Process: Over 40% of building materials were sourced locally.

5.3 PLAN THE FLOW OF FOOD AND WORK

Employees move through kitchens and dining rooms every day, as they transport food to storage, work areas, and customers, and simply go about their jobs. The flow of food from receiving to plated meals is referred to as **product flow**, and the flow of employees doing their jobs is referred to as **work flow**. The actual flow of food and work depend a lot on the menu (what foods are produced), the volume of customers served within a specific time period, and the style of service (how food is delivered to customers). For example, a restaurant may offer wait service whereas a hospital offers self-service in the employee/visitor café and room service for patients during specific hours.

The major work areas to consider when planning the flow of food and work are

- Receiving
- Storage and issuing
- Cold and hot food preparation
- Service and dining areas
- Warewashing (meaning washing dishes, glasses, flatware, and also pots and pans)
- Support services (such as restrooms, employee lockers, offices, janitors' closets).

The flow of food starts when foods are received and then stored (see **Figure 5-5**). The receiving area includes the loading dock where trucks pull up to get unloaded. The floor of the loading dock should be at the standard height of the bed of a delivery truck (about 48 inches). Adjustable height loading docks are available to accommodate varied truck heights.

Foods are stored in one of three areas: refrigerators, freezers, or at room temperature. Kitchens need a storage room dedicated to holding foods such as canned tomatoes and dry cereals that don't require any refrigeration. This type of storage area is referred to as **dry stores**. When baked goods (such as fresh bread) arrive, they are often left on a rack closest to the area where employees will use them. But staples such as canned tomatoes and crackers, that are stored for a longer period of time, will go into dry stores.

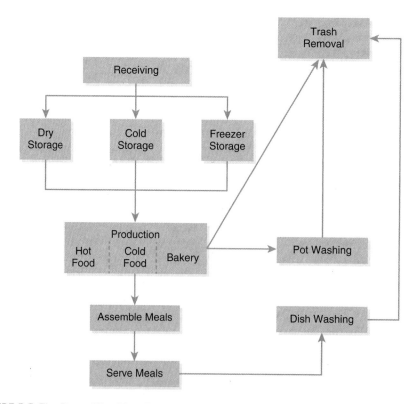

FIGURE 5-5 The Flow of Food in a Typical Kitchen

Refrigerated storage normally includes one or more walk-in refrigerators. Three walk-in refrigerators (one for meat and poultry, one for dairy and eggs, and one for produce) are ideal, and they should be close to the receiving area as well as production areas. Each walk-in refrigerator or freezer should have an interior safety release (so no one gets stuck inside) and an interior thermometer linked to an exterior thermometer so the temperature can be monitored without opening the door.

In addition to food storage, cleaning supplies must be stored, and they must be stored separately from food. Space is also needed for paper goods, dishes, glasses, uniforms, aprons, towels, and table linens.

Whereas many operations allow employees to enter the storage areas and get what they need (sometimes that requires documentation of supplies being withdrawn), some operations have a centralized ingredient room. In a **centralized ingredient room**, employees measure and weigh the ingredients for each recipe to be prepared that day. Employees do some preparation of ingredients as needed, such as slicing celery, and then assemble all the ingredients for a recipe together on a cart to be picked up or delivered to the cooks. This provides quality control, less chance for theft, and allows a lower-paid employee to do what the cook would normally do. If a central ingredient room is used, it should be close to the storage areas and have enough tables and aisle space to prepare and assemble ingredients and place onto carts.

Food preparation is normally separated into separate areas for hot food and cold food preparation, which are also called **production areas**. The production areas are the heart of the kitchen. Hot food preparation includes tasks such as battering up fish, making a casserole, or roasting meat. Typical equipment includes ovens, ranges, steam equipment, grills, and cook's tables. Cold food preparation, also referred to as the **pantry** or **garde manger**, includes cutting vegetables as well as making salads, appetizers, and any other cold dishes on the menu, including some desserts. This area needs lots of table space, sinks for washing vegetables and fruits, and refrigeration.

Once foods are prepared, some may be held at hot or cold temperatures until served while other foods are cooked to order. The last production step is to assemble the meals, then it is time for service. **Service** is the presentation of food to the customer. Sit-down restaurants often have a window from the kitchen into the dining area (called a **pass window**) where finished plates are passed to servers to serve to customers in the dining room. The reason why a pass window works so well is that it gives the cooks and servers each their own space so they stay out of each other's way. After preparing and cooking foods, cooks deliver the dirty pots, pans, and utensils to the potwashing area to be cleaned and sanitized before their next use.

Whereas sit-down restaurants use **wait service**, quick-service restaurants use **counter service** in which customers order at the counter, get their meals, and then sit down in the dining room or take the food elsewhere to eat. Cafeterias serving college students often use both counter- and **self-service**, and need lots of space for customers to choose what to eat and pay. Hospitals use **tray service** in which patient meals are assembled on trays and the trays are transported to the patient's bedside.

For employees to work efficiently, they need to be able to do their work with the least number of motions and a minimum of walking. In an ideal kitchen, employees travel the shortest distances possible (usually a straight line) without getting in someone's way. So a server should be able to quickly pick up a cold dessert for a customer or a cook drop off dirty pots to the pot washer without interrupting anyone. To plan for smooth product flow and work flow, keep these considerations in mind.

1. Storage areas should be between the loading dock and the productions areas. More frequently used items should be stored in the most convenient locations—such as near the storeroom entrance and about waist height.

2. It's best to keep the production area close to the service/dining areas to reduce distance traveled and help maintain food temperatures.

3. To reduce congestion and improve traffic flow, main traffic aisles should be at least five feet wide and most other aisles at least four feet wide. Much consideration needs to be paid to developing good traffic flow patterns.

4. Each work area should have adequate storage space for tools used in that area. For example, a baker needs space for baking pans, mixing bowls, spatulas, scales, and flour sifters. The receiving area should have enough room for a receiver's desk, scales, hand trucks and carts, pallet jacks, and deliveries.

5. In production areas, adequate space is also needed for raw materials and finished products so refrigeration and/or freezer space must be available.

6. Since most dirty pots and pans are generated by the production areas, pot and pan washing should be close by. Likewise, dishwashing should be as close as possible to the dining area.

These considerations are examples of how good design keeps workers and materials moving efficiently.

The field of **materials handling** examines how efficiently products can be stored and move through a facility. Some basic principles of materials handling include storing materials close to the point of use, minimizing the distance that products are moved, reducing the number of times a product is moved or handled, and using gravity to move products or assist in their movement.

Figure 5-6 shows the work areas in a university dining hall. Trace the product flow from delivery to the dining area as well as the flow of dirty dishes and pots and pans to the dishwashing/potwashing areas. How would you rate product flow and overall work flow?

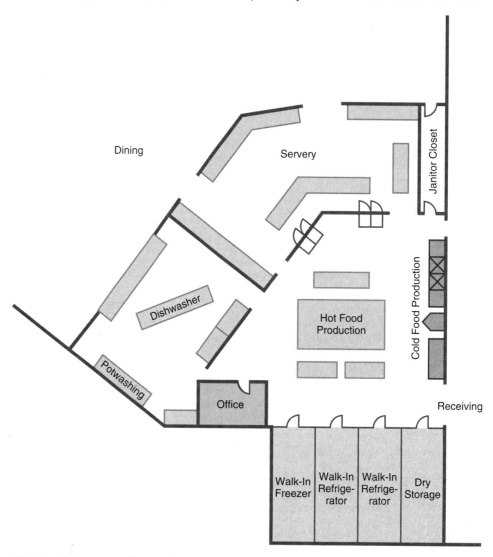

FIGURE 5-6 University Dining Hall and Kitchen

5.4 LAYOUT A FOODSERVICE

To lay out a foodservice, first the amount of square feet for kitchen and the dining room needs to be determined. For a typical foodservice, the kitchen area (including storage, cooking, warewashing, offices, etc.) is about 40 to 50% of the total space. The dining area then is about 50 to 60% (Thomas, Norman, & Katsigris, 2014). One way to calculate dining room space is to use general seating guidelines for the number of square feet needed for each seat, such as the following.

K–12 school cafeteria	10–15 square feet per seat
Banquet service	10–15 square feet per seat
Counter service	11–15 square feet per seat
Full service restaurant	12–18 square feet per seat
Fine dining restaurant	16–20 square feet per seat

This breakdown of space for kitchen versus the dining room is only an estimate and is influenced by factors such as the menu, whether foods are cooked from scratch or not, style of service, volume of meals produced, and the local fire code. Within the kitchen area, at least 50% of that space is generally used for food preparation and cooking, while storage is about 20%, and the remaining space is used for warewashing, aisles, offices, lockers/rest rooms, etc.

Aisle space is very important in any kitchen or dining room. Aisles are not just for people (and some people may be in wheelchairs) but also for employees to open oven doors and refrigerator doors as well as roll carts and trucks. Main traffic aisles should be about five feet wide, and most other aisles should be at least four feet wide.

LAYOUT GUIDELINES

When deciding where to place equipment, think about how an employee can get his or her job done with the smallest number of motions and steps. For example, **Figure 5-7** shows workflow for a potwashing area. Dirty pots and pans are delivered to the prescrape area, and then the potwasher works from left to right to scrape, wash, rinse, sanitize, and place each piece to air dry. A shelf with hooks is often located above the pot sink for additional drying and/or storage space. This work flow design is called the **straight line arrangement**, and it is often put against a wall. The potwashing area may have its own room or it may be against a wall in the dishroom. Instead of a three-compartment sink, some foodservices use a mechanical pot/pan washer. It is similar to a one-compartment dishwasher but is made to handle the grime found in pots and pans and also to accommodate their bulky sizes. **Figure 5-8** show a U-shaped layout for potwashing using a pot/pan washing machine.

Now let's start at the beginning when food enters the facility. The receiving area needs to be large enough to accommodate a loading dock (if available), room for deliveries, and space for a receiver's desk, scales, hand trucks, and carts. The receiving clerk

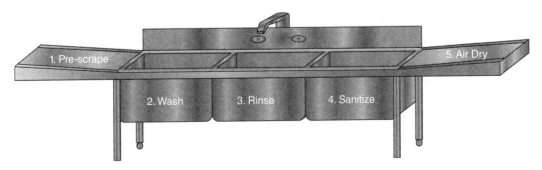

FIGURE 5-7 Straight Line Arrangement for Potwashing Area

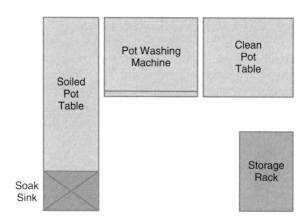

FIGURE 5-8 U-Shaped Arrangement for Potwashing Area

needs enough room to check in deliveries properly, so the planning team needs to consider how often deliveries will come in and the volume of goods that will be received at any one point in time. Keep in mind that in some operations, such as a hospital foodservice, the receiving clerk will be using a loading dock that is often not in the foodservice itself. Instead, many departments use the same hospital loading dock and the clerk will need some extra time and proper equipment (such as platform trucks and hand trucks) to transport items to the storage areas.

In storage areas, the objective is to store as much as possible within the space allotted while making all items accessible and giving employees enough room to add fresh stock. For an average foodservice, *per meal served*, you will need *approximately* 0.25 to 0.50 cubic feet of space in dry stores and 1 to 1.5 cubic feet of space in refrigerated storage (Thomas, Norman, & Katsigris, 2014). Note that the cubic space required does not include aisle space; it is strictly the space for the food itself.

To lay out a storage area, you need to be familiar with some basics about shelving. Storage shelving can be purchased as stationary or mobile. Mobile shelving has small wheels (called casters) at the bottom, which allow you to move the unit, making it more versatile. When storeroom space is limited, high-density shelving units may be useful as the shelving units are mounted at the top onto a track system so that several shelving units are right next to each other and can be easily rolled apart to get access.

Shelving used in storage areas is purchased in standard depths, such as 24 inches or 30 inches. The length of each unit is usually in whole feet from two foot to six foot. If a storage room is eight feet wide, you can place 30-inch deep shelving unit on the walls and have a three-foot aisle between the shelving units. For a walk-in refrigerator whose interior is seven feet wide, you can place a 24-inch deep shelving unit on the walls and again have a three-foot aisle in the middle. Keep in mind that all food items must be stored at least six inches off the ground. Also, shelving in humid areas, such as refrigerators, freezers, or warewashing areas, must be corrosion resistant, so shelving made of stainless steel or epoxy-coated chrome are good choices.

Walk-in refrigerators and freezers come in standard sizes although a custom unit can be ordered and built (expect it to cost a lot more money). When considering how much food you can put into a walk-in, it is important to look at the *interior* dimensions so you can determine how much shelving you will need.

Next let's look at how to lay out a cold food preparation area. Typical equipment for this area includes stainless steel work tables, sinks, a food chopper or processor (which sits on a work table), and refrigeration. If the cold food employees also make sandwiches, a table, slicer, and sandwich station will be needed. **Figure 5-9** shows a straight-line arrangement for a cold food preparation area where work starts at the left (washing vegetables in the sink) and progresses to the right until salads or other items are ready to go into the refrigerator. A larger cold food area may use a **parallel arrangement** in which you have two or more straight lines that are parallel. In Figure 5-9b, an employee

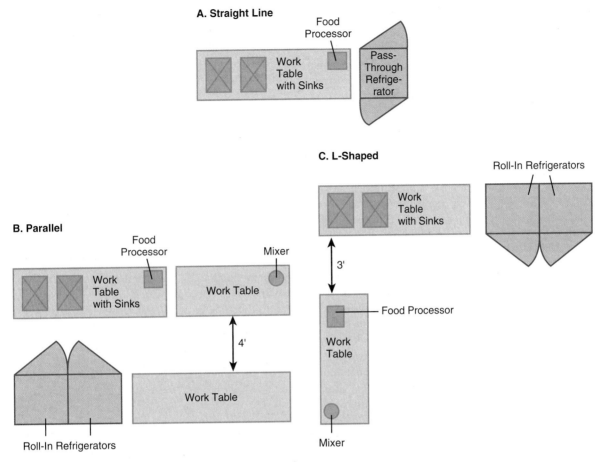

FIGURE 5-9 Possible Layouts for Cold Food Preparation Area

has a work table next to the double sinks to prepare foods, and can then turn around and plate foods on the other table and place them into the refrigerators. Finally, you could also arrange the equipment in an **L-shape arrangement** (Figure 5-9c).

Whereas the cold food preparation area is often located at the sides of the kitchen, the hot food preparation area is often in the center of the kitchen and adjacent to the serving area. The equipment for preparing hot food is dependent on the menu and whether the operation is conventional, ready-prepared, assembly/serve, or commissary. In a conventional kitchen, the hot foods area may include equipment such as a range, oven, grill, fryer, steam equipment, refrigeration, and preparation tables with under-counter drawers and shelves and overhead racks to hold pots, pans, and utensils. If the foodservice also does some baking, a separate room or corner of the kitchen is set up with baking ovens, a mixer, tables, and other tools.

How the equipment is laid out will depend to some degree on the shape and size of the kitchen as well as the stations that are needed. A **station** is a designated area in the kitchen where a certain part of production takes place. Examples include a grill station, sauté station, or vegetable/soup station. Having an area in the kitchen devoted to the equipment and tables for a cook to make vegetables and soups, as an example, is helpful for work flow. The following are additional factors to be aware of when arranging the hot food production area for optimal work flow.

1. Before placing any equipment in a kitchen, you have to consider whether it requires electric, gas, or steam as well as where the utility connections are in the kitchen. Some equipment also requires a water connection. Getting the right utility and/or water connections to a piece of equipment can be quite expensive.

2. Some steam cooking equipment can generate their own steam and, therefore, don't need a steam connection. When steam equipment is used that does need a steam connection, you will see all the steam equipment placed together. Also, floor-mounted steam-jacketed kettles that tilt (to let cooks pour the contents into a container) require a floor drain in front of the kettle (in case something spills).

3. Foodservices are required to put a vent hood over cooking equipment (see Figure 5-1) so cooking equipment is placed together. The vent hood is equipped with fans to pull smoke, heat, grease, moisture, and odors to the outside.

4. Equipment used to cook items to order (such as steak on a grill) should be placed closer to the dining area, but still under the ventilation hood.

5. When equipment is placed against a wall, or back to back, there must be some space (at least one foot) at the back of the equipment so that the area can be cleaned. Equipment on casters using flexible gas lines makes cleaning and maintenance easier as well.

Figure 5-10 gives ideas on how a hot food preparation area may be laid out using parallel, back-to-back, and L-shape arrangements. In the parallel arrangement, the cooking equipment is in a line with work tables opposite, so a cook can, for example, pull a pan out of the oven and place it on the table or perhaps in a rack (**Figure 5-11**). There is a hood (designated by the dashed line) above the cooking equipment to help keep the air fresh and clean. In the **back-to-back arrangement**, which is a variation of the parallel plan, two rows of equipment are back-to-back with a hood overhead. Tables are opposite each row of equipment. The **L-shaped arrangement** would work well in a corner. In any kitchen, you also need room for holding foods and assembling meals.

Once meals are assembled, they need to be served. Nowadays, many servers only use the service area to pick up meals because they put in their orders electronically on tablets or POS (point-of-sale) terminals. Counter-service restaurants need a larger

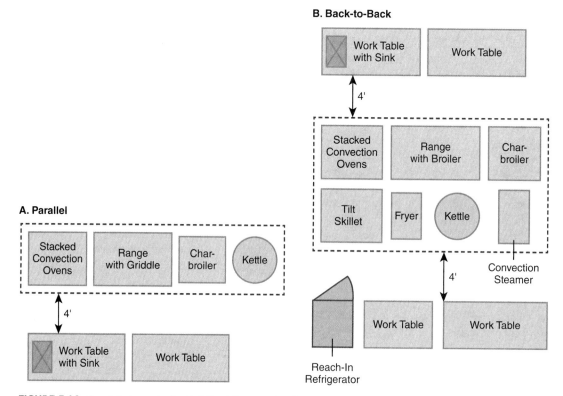

FIGURE 5-10 Possible Layouts for Hot Food Preparation Area

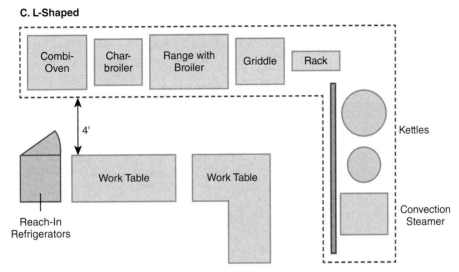

C. L-Shaped

Dashed line indicates exhaust hood.

FIGURE 5-10 Possible Layouts for Hot Food Preparation Area

service area because in-house customers will order and pick up at the counter. Well-designed counters are needed to serve customers in a timely manner and the service area also needs room for stations where customers pick up napkins, condiments, and sometimes pour their own beverages. Drive-through service or take-out also need additional room to be provided.

In a cafeteria, the amount of square feet devoted to serving customers is quite large. The cafeteria not only includes stations to pick up food but also cashiers. Flatware, napkins, and condiments are often placed just outside the cashiers in the dining area. You may remember lining up to enter a school cafeteria that used a straight-line pattern and you had to stay in line as you moved along (usually slowly) and picked up your beverage

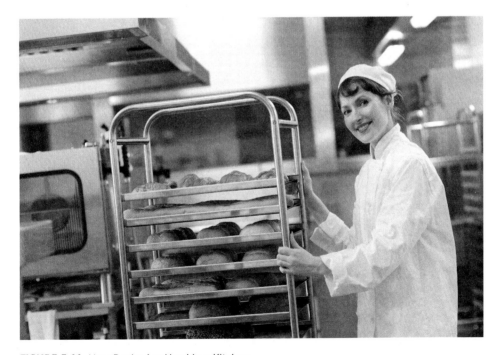

FIGURE 5-11 How Racks Are Used in a Kitchen

© Wavebreakmedia/Shutterstock

and other meal items. A slight improvement on the straight-line cafeteria is a **bypass line** in which sections of the line are indented, such as separating hot foods from sandwiches, so a customer could bypass hot foods and go directly to sandwiches.

Many cafeterias in business and industry, colleges and universities, and healthcare use a system that requires more space and is known as a **scramble (scatter) system** or **hollow square cafeteria** (**Figure 5-12**). In a hollow square cafeteria, customers pick up a tray and then walk around and look at the foods offered at each station before deciding on what to eat. Some stations, such as a salad bar, may be self-service, while other stations have an employee who will make a sandwich to order, grill a hamburger, or stir fry a custom dish. While scramble systems require more space, service is generally faster, the variety of food is better, each station can be as big or small as needed, and there may be room for exhibition cooking.

Major factors in designing dining areas are the number of seats and the style of tables and chairs to be used. For example, round tables encourage conversation but square or rectangular tables save more space. A mix of fixed seating, such as booths, which customers enjoy for their comfort and privacy, and regular tables, which can be moved around as needed, works well in many operations. Depending on the size of the dining room, you may want one open space or you may want to create smaller rooms. Movable wall partitions or screens can help create smaller spaces and they also absorb some noise.

Dining rooms must include space for aisles and wait stations that are stocked with everything the waitstaff needs to set tables, etc., and also a terminal if a point-of-sale software system is used. Many dining rooms have about 18 inches between tables and chairs, but the ADA requires at least a 36-inch aisle from the entrance of the dining room to any wheelchair-accessible table.

The dishroom is usually a separate room because it is noisy, hot, and steamy, and it is located close to dining areas. In the case of cafeterias, customers will often place their trays on a conveyor belt that brings their dishes right into the dishroom. A well-designed dishroom has a sound-absorbing ceiling, lots of light, and excellent ventilation.

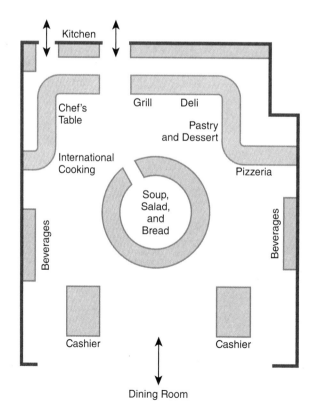

FIGURE 5-12 Hollow Square (Scramble System) Cafeteria

A dishroom should have a clear flow from incoming soiled dishes, glasses, and flatware to the dishwasher and then to clean items. Soiled and clean wares must be kept separate to prevent cross-contamination. Soiled wares are collected on tables on one side of the dishwasher, and you need more table space for soiled dishes than for clean dishes. Because flatware can be hard to get clean, dirty flatware is usually placed into a tub of water with presoaking solution in it. Dishroom employees first scrape the dishes and then prerinse them using a water spray. Next, dishes are put into dishwasher racks (19 × 19 inches) or directly on the dishwasher's belt to go through the dishwasher's cycles. When the dishwasher has finished, clean dishes are removed and organized. Space is needed to store clean dishes until they are transported out in dish carts, etc.

There are several types of commercial dishwashers available depending on how many dishes need to be washed and how quickly. The **door-type dishwasher** accommodates one rack full of dishes. A dishwashing rack is 19 inches by 19 inches. Once the rack is placed in the door-type dishwasher, the door is closed, and the cleaning cycle starts. In just minutes, you have cleaned and sanitized dishes. For larger foodservices with more dishes, **conveyor-type dishwashers** are larger machines and they move full racks of dishes through regular wash, power rinse, and sanitizing rinse cycles. Some machines also feature prewash cycles. For very high-volume operations, a **flight-type dishwasher**, also called rackless conveyors or belt conveyors, is used. The flight-type dishwasher (**Figure 5-13**) operates on the same principles as the conveyor-type dishwasher except that the dishes and other items are hand-placed between rows of pegs on a conveyor belt. Flatware is placed in a rack. Two employees keep the dishes going through smoothly, one to load and one to empty.

Dishrooms in smaller operations may be set up in a straight-line similar to the potwashing area, with the door-type dishwasher replacing the three-compartment sink and table space on each side to collect dirty dishes and organize clean dishes. **Figure 5-14** shows how an L-shaped dishroom would be set up in a corner using a door-type dishwasher and also how a dishroom might be organized in a larger operation using a flight-type dishwasher. The size of the room will depend largely on volume of dishes, which determines the size of the dishwasher.

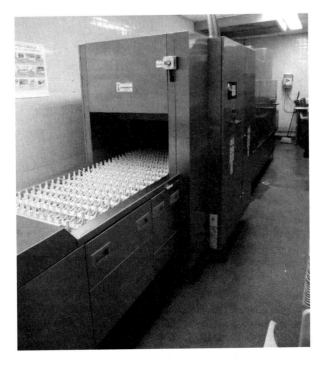

FIGURE 5-13 Flight-Type Dishmachine

Courtesy of MEIKO International.

A. L-Shaped Dishroom with Door-Type Dishwasher

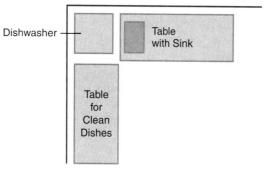

B. Dishroom with Flight-Type Dishwasher

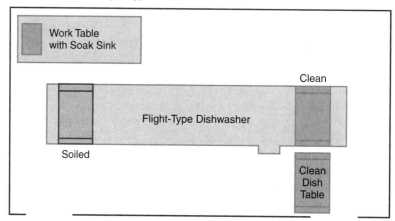

FIGURE 5-14 Dishroom Arrangements

Finally, space needs to be designed for support services.

1. <u>Janitor's closet(s)</u>. This room must have a low sink for washing mops and space where mops are hung for airing. Cleaning chemicals and tools, such as brooms, are also stored here.

2. <u>Washing area for trash cans and food trucks/carts</u>. A separate room may be needed to wash and sanitize (using a steam hose) food trucks/carts that carry trays to patients in a healthcare facility. Trash pails can also be washed in this area. The walls and floor in this area need to be tiled and constructed for easy, thorough cleaning. Excellent floor drainage is also needed.

3. <u>Rest rooms and employee lockers</u>. Restrooms will be needed for guests and separate restrooms for employees. Employees will also need lockers. The local health department code, along with ADA regulations, will determine how many toilets are required.

4. <u>Offices</u>. Offices for managers are normally placed adjacent to the areas, such as the production area, which they oversee. A large window in an office overlooking the kitchen is not unusual so a production manager can keep an eye on what is going on.

PREPARE A SCHEMATIC DRAWING

A **schematic drawing** (**Figure 5–15**) is a floor plan showing where walls, doors, windows, equipment, and tables will be placed in the foodservice. Usually, the architect prepares two or three schematic drawings, along with a cost estimate for each one, after reviewing the business plan and discussing what is needed with the planning team members.

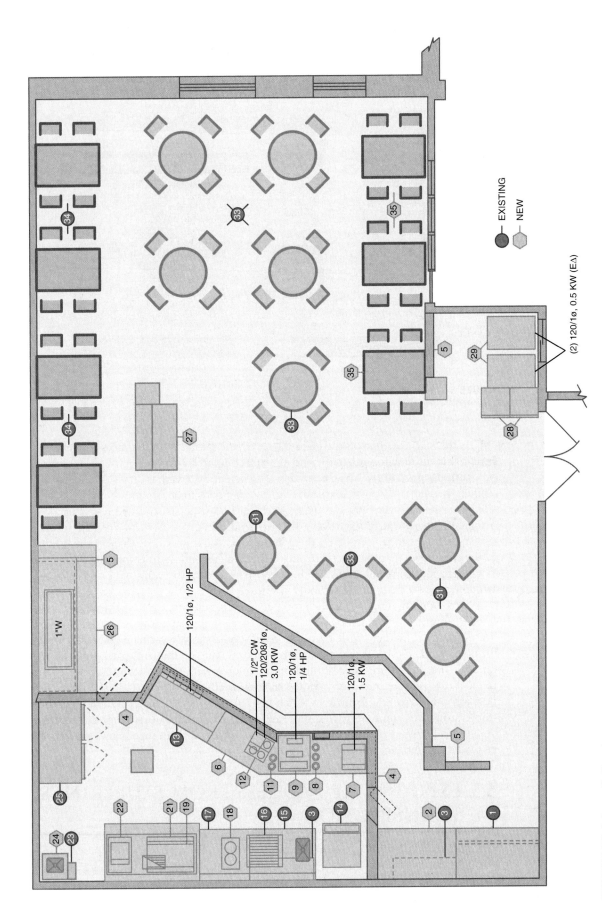

FIGURE 5-15 Schematic Drawing

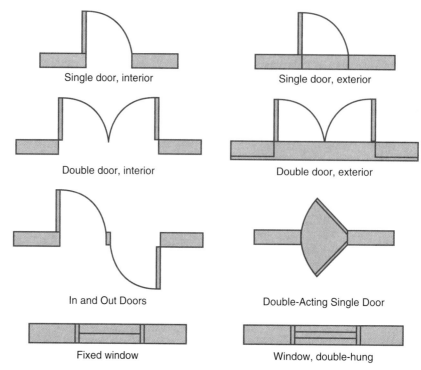

Single door, interior

Single door, exterior

Double door, interior

Double door, exterior

In and Out Doors

Double-Acting Single Door

Fixed window

Window, double-hung

FIGURE 5-16 Architectural Symbols

At this stage, anyone on the planning team can go through the process of developing a schematic drawing either by hand or using computer-aided design (CAD) software programs designed to lay out an operation. A schematic drawing is drawn to scale, so if a ¼-inch scale is used, ¼-inch on the drawing corresponds to one foot in the actual operation. For ¼-inch scale, you can use ¼-inch squared paper (also called graph paper—4 squares per inch) if you are doing this by hand. First, you need to draw the proper size and shape of the operation on the graph paper. You may choose to draw the outline of the entire operation or just the front- or back-of-the-house (this includes receiving, storage, production, and service). Once you have drawn the walls, you can draw the windows and doors using the symbols in **Figure 5-16**.

Next, you can move around equipment and table/chair templates (**Figure 5-17**) to test out a number of layouts. Be sure the templates use the same scale as the graph paper. Templates for equipment with doors that open should show how much space is required for opening. You can cut out the templates for cooking equipment, place them in the kitchen, and then move them around until a good arrangement is found. Then check to see if the aisles are sufficiently wide. Once the arrangement seems to work, trace the flow of food and work to evaluate whether your plan is efficient. Don't be afraid to move things around to come up with a more efficient layout, but always keep in mind the guidelines discussed earlier such as keeping cooking equipment together so a hood can be placed above them.

5.5 EXPLAIN THE PROCESS FROM BLUEPRINTS TO INSPECTION

Once the planning team agrees on a layout and design, the architect creates a set of precise construction drawings *and* detailed specifications. Specifications are prepared ahead of construction to describe exactly how the construction should proceed. As such, specifications describe in detail the materials to be used, methods of installation, quality

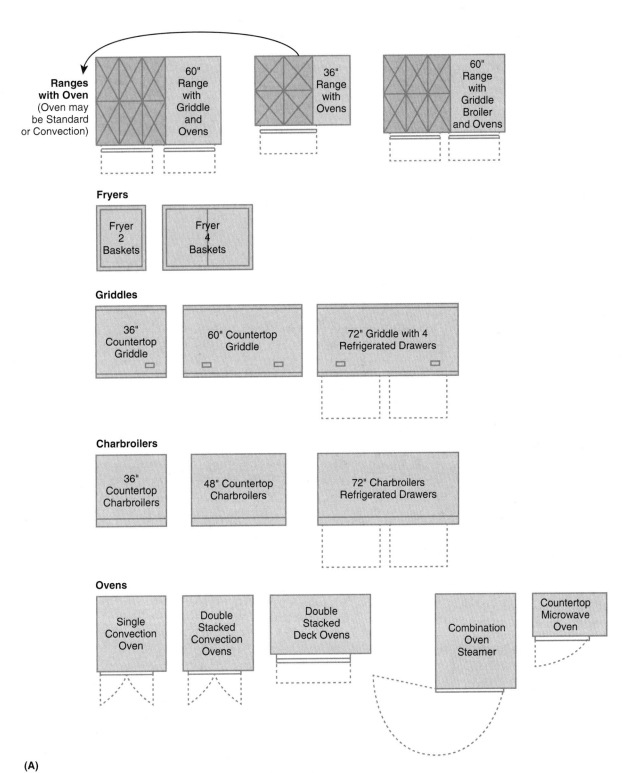

(A)

FIGURE 5-17 Templates of Selected Kitchen Equipment Drawn to ¼-Inch Scale (*continues*)

standards to which to adhere, and specifications for all equipment. The construction plans and specifications must, of course, meet all applicable building and health codes. If you are renovating an existing foodservice and plan to remain open during construction, the local health department must approve your plan to provide meals in a safe and sanitary manner during construction.

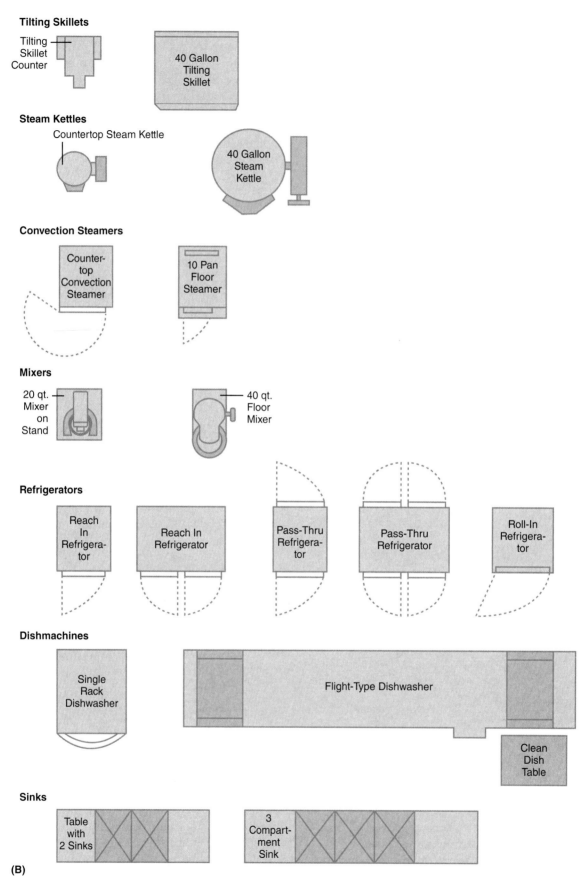

(B)

FIGURE 5-17 (continued) Templates of Selected Kitchen Equipment Drawn to ¼-Inch Scale

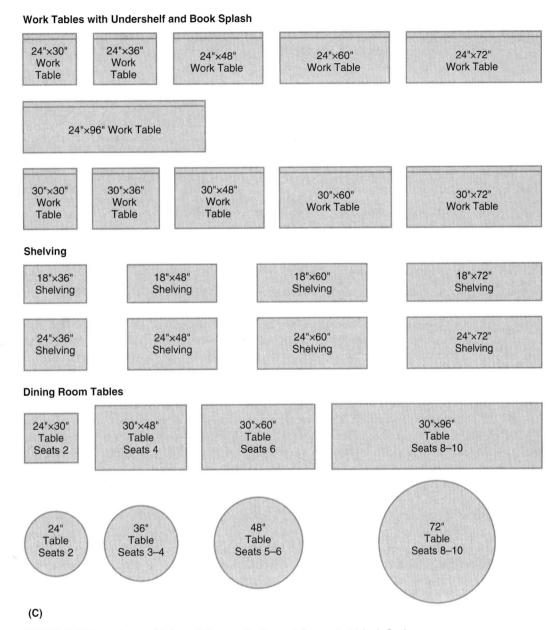

(C)

FIGURE 5-17 Templates of Selected Kitchen Equipment Drawn to ¼-Inch Scale

Working with the engineers and interior designer, the architect completes the final set of drawings, also called **blueprints**. In addition to drawings that show placement of equipment and walls, the architect makes separate drawings for utilities including plumbing, electrical, and gas. Some basic guidelines on reading blueprints are as follows.

1. Each blueprint includes a title block that includes the name and address of the operation, the scale used, and the date the drawing was prepared. In addition, each room is labeled.
2. Each blueprint is marked as a plan, elevation, or section. A floor **plan** shows a space from above. An **elevation** is a view looking sideways at the object, such as a drawing of how the front of a restaurant will look including windows and doors. A **section** is a cut-through view of the object.
3. The thickest lines on a blueprint represent the sides of an object, such as a table, that are visible to the eye. Dashed lines are often hidden lines—meaning they show the sides of an object that would not be visible.

Because renovations and new construction are so expensive, a Request for Proposal (commonly called a bid) is usually sent out to a number of companies that are asked to submit prices on a project. To send out a **Request for Proposal (RFP)**, you need the following contract documents at a minimum.

1. General Conditions and Scope of Work (Includes obligations and rights of both parties and the amount of work needed to complete the project)
2. Drawings (Blueprints)
3. Specifications
4. Construction schedule (usually a timeline or Gantt chart)

Everything in these documents must be clearly stated to avoid misinterpretations and problems.

The goal of sending out bids is to ensure open competition and hopefully get better prices by asking companies to bid against each other. The Request for Proposal document outlines the bidding process and contract terms, and explains how the bid should be formatted and presented. The bid document is a legally binding contract and includes bidder qualifications and the payment schedule. The RFP also includes criteria that will be used to choose which vendor will get the contract. The planning team should evaluate proposals once they are returned.

If the only criterion is price, an Invitation for Sealed Bid (IFB) is normally sent out. An IFB is more often used when clearly specified equipment is being purchased. In the case of a sealed bid, the award is given to the responsible vendor with the lowest price who meets the terms and conditions.

Once a bid is awarded, construction can start. Construction is usually the longest phase of any project. General contractors, subcontractors, and tradesmen work to bring the architect's plans to life. During construction, the architect inspects and oversees the progress to ensure that procedures and materials comply with plans and specifications. Members of the planning team should be involved as well and communication with the architect is important. Planning team members can help check in new equipment and make sure it is installed as described in the Installation and Operation Manual.

Toward the end of construction, the architect and planning team need to develop a punch list (although some organizations will use an outside professional to do this). A **punch list** is a list of items and tasks that need to be completed or fixed before a construction project can be considered finished. During the inspection, all equipment should be turned on and undergo a performance test. Often, someone who works for the manufacturer of the equipment will do the performance test to be sure it works properly and will make adjustments as needed. This person should also demonstrate to employees how to operate, clean, care for, and maintain the equipment. It is imperative to go through the punch list and performance check before you allow the construction company to leave. Once they begin another project, it is hard to get them to come back for repairs or adjustments.

SUMMARY

5.1 Develop a business plan and organize the planning team.

- A business plan explains why a project, such as a new or renovated foodservice, is important and the goals of the project. It includes these sections: business overview, industry analysis, operating plan, marketing analysis and

plan, and financial feasibility study and plan (including a pro forma income statement).

- The emphasis for a business plan involving a renovation or expansion will be the financial justification.
- The group of individuals who work together to plan a new facility or renovate an existing

one are known as the planning team. Once you have a business plan, you can bring members onto your team that may include an architect, engineer, interior designer, food-service consultant, equipment representative, and builder/contractor.

- The planning team knows that major factors influencing the design and layout are the menu and type of foodservice system. They also consider who the customers and employees will be, and which building codes and regulations must be met, such as the Americans with Disabilities Act.

5.2 Design the environment.

- The heating and air conditioning, ventilation, lighting, noise control, as well as the materials and colors used in floors, walls, and ceilings affect the work environment as well as the atmosphere in the dining area.
- Most businesses use a packaged HVAC unit that provides heating and air conditioning and sits on the roof. It connects directly into the building's ventilation system.
- Exhaust hoods are built over kitchen equipment to capture grease, heat, moisture, odors, smoke, and other cooking products. Filters in the hood help to capture grease as the air is exhausted to the outside. When air is removed through an exhaust hood, it is replaced with an equal volume of air called makeup air. Figure 5-2 shows how air flows in a quick-service restaurant. Air should flow from the dining area into the kitchen to keep kitchen odors out of the dining room.
- Designers use indirect, direct, and accent lighting in foodservices. In the kitchen, bright lighting is needed to allow employees to do their work and for their safety, so fluorescent tubes are frequently used.
- Light bulbs are shielded, coated, or otherwise shatter-resistant in areas where food is being handled, food packages are open, or over clean equipment, utensils, or linens.
- Designers use various ways, such as using sound-absorbing ceiling panels, to decrease noise in a foodservice.
- In a foodservice, floors are rated on their slip resistance, durability, cleanability, porosity, comfort, and appearance. The most popular options are quarry tile and epoxy-coated concrete. While epoxy-coated concrete is quite a bit less expensive than quarry tile, quarry tile is the most long-lasting of all the

choices. Neither wood flooring nor carpeting would be appropriate in kitchens.
- Plumbing pipes carrying waste and water are usually located in the concrete floor, which makes it expensive to make changes. Air gaps are used (Figure 5-4) to prevent backflow.

5.3 Plan the flow of food and work.

- The flow of food from receiving to plated meals is referred to as product flow, and the flow of employees doing their jobs is referred to as work flow. The actual flow of food and work depend a lot on the menu (what foods are produced), the volume of customers served within a specific time period, and the style of service (how food is delivered to customers). Food flows from receiving and storage through cooking, serving, and washing of dishes and pots and pans (Figure 5-5).
- Whereas many operations allow employees to enter the storage areas and get what they need, some operations have a centralized ingredient room where employees measure and weigh the ingredients for each recipe to be prepared that day so the cook doesn't have to do that.
- Production areas are normally separated into hot and cold production.
- Meals may be served using waitstaff, counter servers, self-service, or tray service.
- Tips are given to help plan for smooth product flow and work flow, such as having storage areas between the loading dock and the production areas, having production areas close to the service area, and making sure main traffic aisles are at least five feet wide (and most other aisles at least four feet wide).
- Some basic principles of material handling include storing materials close to the point of use, minimizing the distance products are moved, reducing the number of times a product is moved or handled, and using gravity to move products or assist in their movement.

5.4 Lay out a foodservice.

- To lay out a foodservice, first the amount of square feet for the kitchen and the dining room need to be determined. For a typical foodservice, the kitchen area (including storage, cooking, warewashing, offices, etc.) is about 40 to 50% of the total space. The remainder is dining.

- Within the kitchen area, at least 50% of that space is generally used for food preparation and cooking, while storage is about 20%, and the remaining space is used for warewashing, aisles, offices, lockers/rest rooms, etc.
- Figures 5-8 through 5-10 show how equipment may be laid out in different parts of the kitchen using straight line, L-shaped, U-shaped, and back-to-back arrangements.
- When laying out equipment, keep in mind the utility connections that are needed and also if a hood is necessary.
- Cafeterias may use a straight line (possibly with bypass lines too) or more commonly a scramble or hollow square system.
- A dishroom should have a clear flow from incoming soiled dishes, glasses, and flatware to the dishwasher and then to clean items. Soiled and clean wares must be kept separate to prevent cross-contamination (Figure 5-14).
- Spaces must also be laid out for a janitor's closet, washing area for trash cans/food trucks, rest rooms, employee lockers, and offices.
- A schematic drawing is drawn to scale, so if a ¼-inch scale is used, then ¼-inch on the drawing corresponds to one foot in the actual operation. Figure 5-15 gives an example.

5.5 Explain the process from blueprints to inspection.

- Once the planning team agrees on a layout and design, the architect creates a set of precise construction drawings (blueprints) *and* detailed specifications. Specifications describe in detail the materials to be used, methods of installation, quality standards to which to be adhered, and specifications for all equipment.
- Because renovations and new construction are so expensive, a Request for Proposal (a bid) is usually sent out to a number of companies who are asked to submit prices on a project. The RFP includes the General Conditions and Scope of Work, blueprints, specifications, and construction schedule.
- Once a bid is awarded, construction can start. The architect inspects and oversees the construction and the planning team is also involved.
- Toward the end of construction, the architect and planning team need to develop a punch list (although some organizations will use an outside professional to do this).

REVIEW AND DISCUSSION QUESTIONS

1. Compare and contrast design and layout.
2. Describe what each member of the planning team is responsible for.
3. Name three sets of regulations that influence building construction and renovations and explain the overall purpose of each one.
4. What is NAFEM and why is it important?
5. Where are exhaust hoods placed and what do they do? Why are exhaust hoods a potential fire hazard?
6. Explain how air should flow between the kitchen and dining area. What is make-up air?
7. Explain when each of the following is used: direct lighting, indirect lighting, and accent lighting.
8. Explain how foot candles are used in choosing lighting.
9. Where is there a lot of humidity in a foodservice and how does it affect your choice of lighting?
10. Name five considerations when choosing flooring. Why is quarry tile a good choice anywhere in a kitchen?
11. What is an air gap?
12. Explain LEED certification.
13. Describe different ways that sanitation, safety, noise control, and sustainability can be built into a new or renovated space.
14. Name four considerations to ensure smooth product flow and work flow.
15. How does a layout for cold food preparation differ from one for hot food production?
16. What is an RFP and a punch list?
17. How does a foodservice manager keep up with new developments in design and layout?

SMALL GROUP PROJECT

For the foodservice concept that you created in Chapter 1, do the following.

1. Using guidelines in this chapter, estimate how many square feet will be needed for the storage areas (dry food storage room, walk-in refrigerators, freezer) *and* hot and cold food production areas.
2. Using ¼-inch graph paper, draw the size needed for the storage and production areas (a rectangular space usually works well).
3. Next, draw all walls needed and show where there are doors going to a loading dock and also going into a dining area/cafeteria.
4. Using the templates, lay out the hot production area, cold production area, and put shelving in the storage areas.

REFERENCES

ASHRAE. (2016). *Ventilation for acceptable indoor air quality*. Retrieved from https://ashrae.iwrapper.com/ViewOnline/Standard_62.1-2016

Energy Star (Environmental Protection Agency). (2018). *Learn about LED lighting*. Retrieved from https://www.energystar.gov/products/lighting_fans/light_bulbs/learn_about_led_bulbs

Environmental Protection Agency. (2020). *Energy saving tips for small businesses: Restaurants*. Retrieved from https://www.energystar.gov/buildings/tools-and-resources/energy_star_small_business_restaurants

Levin, A. (2017). Ventilation: Now and for the future. *Foodservice Equipment Reports*. Retrieved from http://www.fesmag.com/features/foodservice-news/14485-ventilation-now-and-for-the-future

Lewis, S. A. (2013). How to make smart flooring choices. *Restaurant Development + Design*. Retrieved from http://rddmag.com/design/67-make-smart-flooring-choices

National Institute for Occupational Safety and Health. (2018). *Noise levels by decibels*. Retrieved from https://www.cdc.gov/niosh/topics/noise/infographic-noiselevels.html

Thomas, C., Norman, E. J., & Katsigris, C. (2014). *Design and equipment for restaurants and foodservice* (4th ed.). Hoboken (NJ): John Wiley & Sons, Inc.

U.S. Department of Energy. (2015). *Guidance on demand-controlled kitchen ventilation*. Retrieved from https://betterbuildingssolutioncenter.energy.gov/sites/default/files/attachments/Guidance-on-Demand-Controlled-Kitchen-Ventilation.pdf

U.S. Public Health Service and U.S. Food and Drug Administration. (2019). *2017 Food Code*. Retrieved from https://www.fda.gov/food/fda-food-code/food-code-2017

Standardized Recipes and Food Cost

LEARNING OUTCOMES

6.1 Measure ingredients accurately.

6.2 Convert units of measure.

6.3 Use yield percent.

6.4 Develop a standardized recipe and adjust recipe yield.

6.5 Calculate cost of a recipe and portion.

6.6 Calculate food cost percentage.

INTRODUCTION

To use recipes to produce a quality product and keep food costs under control, you need to know everything possible about accurate measuring and converting measurements and recipe yields. How you apply math in the kitchen will affect your success. This chapter covers the basics of measuring ingredients and converting measurements, as well as using yield percent to determine how much to purchase for certain ingredients. The importance of standardized recipes is explained along with instructions on how to calculate the cost of a recipe. Finally, food cost percentage is discussed.

6.1 MEASURE INGREDIENTS ACCURATELY

In a recipe, ingredients are measured in one of three ways.

1. <u>Count:</u> Some ingredients are measured simply by counting. A recipe may call for 10 eggs or three large apples.
2. <u>Weight:</u> Weight is frequently used for solids and is measured in pounds and ounces such as 4 ounces of meat or 1 ounce of cheese in a sandwich. *Weight is more precise than volume, especially for solid ingredients.* Scales for weighing are either mechanical or digital. Metric units for weight are grams and kilograms.
3. <u>Volume:</u> Volume, such as 1 quart of soup, measures the amount of space occupied by the soup. Units of volume measurement are teaspoons, tablespoons, fluid ounces (often incorrectly called ounces), cups, pints, quarts, and gallons.

© Denis Val/Shutterstock

179

Common metric measures of volume are milliliters and liters. Volume is measured using measuring spoons and measuring cups, and sometimes ladles or scoops. There are two types of measuring cups, depending on whether they are used for dry or wet ingredients.

To measure the volume of a liquid, use a measuring cup designed to measure liquids. Liquid measuring cups are usually made of glass and have a handle. Place the measuring cup on a flat surface and check that the liquid goes up to the proper line on the measuring cup while looking directly at it *at eye level*.

Measuring cups for dry ingredients, such as flour, are often made of metal or plastic. They are designed to be filled to the top and then leveled off. To measure the volume of a dry ingredient, such as flour, spoon it into the measuring cup and level it off with a table knife. Do not pack the cup with the dry ingredient—that is, don't press down on it to make room for more—unless the recipe says to. You can pack the cup when you are measuring brown sugar, butter, or margarine.

Liquid measuring cups indicate that 1 cup = 8 ounces, but what they really mean is 1 cup = 8 *fluid ounces*. **Fluid ounces** is a measure of volume, not weight. Even 8 fluid ounces of water doesn't weigh exactly 8 ounces—it weighs 8.3 ounces. Eight fluid ounces of honey weighs 12 ounces. Dry ingredients are even more variable. For instance, 1 cup of all-purpose flour weighs 4.5 ounces and 1 cup of chocolate chips weighs a little over 6 ounces. **Table 6-1** gives kitchen measurement equivalents that are important to know.

In the metric system, there is only one basic unit for each type of measurement.

- The **gram** is the basic unit of weight. A **kilogram** contains 1,000 grams.
- The **liter** is the basic unit of volume. A liter contains 1,000 **milliliters**.

A kilogram is a little more than two pounds. A liter is a little more than one quart.

Recipes use abbreviations such as Tbsp for tablespoon. Common abbreviations are listed in **Table 6-2**. **Table 6-3** shows decimal equivalents for ounces (weight) and

Table 6-1 Equivalents of Common Units of Measurement		
Unit	**Equivalents**	
1 tablespoon	3 teaspoons	1/2 fluid ounce
¼ cup	4 tablespoons	2 fluid ounces
⅓ cup	5 tablespoons + 1 teaspoon	2¾ fluid ounces
½ cup	8 tablespoons	4 fluid ounces
1 cup	16 tablespoons OR 48 teaspoons	8 fluid ounces
1 pint	2 cups	16 fluid ounces
1 quart	2 pints	32 fluid ounces
1 gallon	4 quarts OR 8 pints	128 fluid ounces
1 liter (1000 ml)*		33.8 fluid ounces
30 milliliters (ml)*		1 fluid ounce
½ pound	8 ounces	
1 pound	16 ounces	
1 ounce	28 grams	
1 pound	454 grams	
1 kilogram (1000 g)*	2.2 pounds	

*Quantities are metric measurements.

Table 6-2 Common Abbreviations in Recipes	
Abbreviation	**Meaning**
AP	as purchased
EP	edible portion
approx.	approximately
lb or #	pound
oz	ounce
kg	kilogram
g	gram
fl oz	fluid ounce (volume, not weight)
tsp or t	teaspoon
Tbsp or T	tablespoon
c or C	cup
pt	pint
qt	quart
gal	gallon
ml	milliliter
L	liter

Table 6-3 Decimal Equivalents for 1–16 Ounces	
Ounces	**Pounds**
1 oz	0.06 lb
2 oz	0.12 lb
3 oz	0.19 lb
4 oz	0.25 lb
5 oz	0.31 lb
6 oz	0.38 lb
7 oz	0.44 lb
8 oz	0.50 lb
9 oz	0.56 lb
10 oz	0.62 lb
11 oz	0.69 lb
12 oz	0.75 lb
13 oz	0.81 lb
14 oz	0.88 lb
15 oz	0.94 lb
16 oz	1 lb

Table 6-4 Decimal Equivalents 1–8 Fluid Ounces	
Fluid Ounces	**Cups**
1 fl oz	0.125 cups
2 fl oz	0.25 cups
3 fl oz	0.375 cups
4 fl oz	0.50 cups
5 fl oz	0.625 cups
6 fl oz	0.75 cups
7 fl oz	0.875 cups
8 fl oz	1 cup

Table 6-4 shows decimal equivalents for fluid ounces (volume). For example, 8 ounces is half a pound so it is 0.5 pounds.

6.2 CONVERT UNITS OF MEASURE

In a quantity foods kitchen, you must be able to convert cups to tablespoons, ounces to pounds, and lots more. When converting cups to teaspoons, you are just changing one volume measurement to another volume. When converting ounces to pounds, both are weight measurements. At times, you will also need to convert a volume to a weight measurement (or the reverse) such as when a recipe calls for cups but you have to order it in pounds. Whichever type of conversion you need to make, you can use what is called the bridge method. You can even use the bridge method to convert metric measures to U.S. standard measures (as shown in Example 6.2.2 D).

The **bridge method** is a series of steps to use when you need to convert from one type of measurement to another. To use the bridge method, you will need the information in Table 6-1. To explain the steps, let's convert 7 pints to quarts.

Step 1. First, identify what type of conversion you need to do. In this case, it is volume to volume. Also identify the units you will use to get to the final conversion. In this example, you can go from pints to quarts directly, or you can go from

$$Pints \rightarrow cups \rightarrow quarts.$$

Step 2. If the number you need to convert is a fraction or contains a fraction such as 1¾, first convert it to a decimal. (In the case of 1¾, convert to 1.75). Since "7" is a whole number, place "7 pints" over 1 as follows and place a multiplication sign next to it.

$$\frac{7 \text{ pints}}{1} \times$$

Step 3. Next, we are going to multiply "7 pints/1" by another fraction. The *bottom* of the new fraction will always have the unit found in the first fraction. This way, you can cross them out when you do the multiplication.

$$\frac{7 \text{ pints}}{1} \times \frac{}{\text{pint}}$$

Step 4. Now you have to insert the appropriate relationship between cups and pints: one pint contains 2 cups.

$$\frac{7 \text{ pints}}{1} \times \frac{2 \text{ cups}}{1 \text{ pint}}$$

Step 5. Now you repeat Steps 3 and 4, putting cups at the bottom of the last fraction. The next and final unit is quarts so you insert the right relationship (1 quart = 4 cups).

$$\frac{7 \text{ pints}}{1} \times \frac{2 \text{ cups}}{1 \text{ pint}} \times \frac{1 \text{ quart}}{4 \text{ cups}} =$$

Step 6. Calculate the answer by crossing out the pints and cups, then multiplying across the top and then the bottom.

$$\frac{7 \text{ \sout{pints}}}{1} \times \frac{2 \text{ \sout{cups}}}{1 \text{ \sout{pint}}} \times \frac{1 \text{ quart}}{4 \text{ \sout{cups}}} = \frac{14}{4} \text{ quarts} = 3.5 \text{ quarts}$$

Whenever using this method, remember that the first fraction is the amount you need to convert over "1." The other fractions must show the correct relationship between two measurements, and you must be able to cancel out the measurement units.

An alternative (quicker) way to solve this is shown next. You can go directly from pints to quarts as long as you remember that 1 quart has 2 pints.

$$\frac{7 \text{ \sout{pints}}}{1} \times \frac{1 \text{ quart}}{2 \text{ \sout{pints}}} = 3.5 \text{ quarts}$$

More examples are shown in Example 6.2.1. To convert ounces to pounds or pounds to ounces, when you have less than 16 ounces, you can often use Table 6-3.

Besides converting cups to tablespoons, an example of within-volume conversions, or ounces to pounds, an example of within-weight conversions, you can also convert three

EXAMPLE 6.2.1. HOW TO USE THE BRIDGE METHOD TO CONVERT WITHIN VOLUME OR WEIGHT

Problem A: A recipe calls for ⅔ cup of flour. How many tablespoons are in ⅔ cup?

This problem requires converting cups to tablespoons, both volume measurements. First you need to convert ⅔ into a decimal (0.66).

$$\frac{0.66 \text{ cups}}{1} \times \frac{16 \text{ Tablespoons}}{1 \text{ cups}} = 10.5 \text{ tablespoons}$$

Problem B: You need 60 ounces of crushed pumpkin to make muffins. How many pounds will you need?

This problem requires converting ounces to pounds, both weights.

$$\frac{60 \text{ ounces}}{1} \times \frac{1 \text{ pound}}{16 \text{ ounces}} = \frac{60}{16} \text{ pounds} = 3.75 \text{ pounds} = 3 \text{ lb } 12 \text{ oz}$$

You should convert 0.75 pounds to ounces (use Table 6-3) to get 12 ounces. If you don't have the table, just multiply 0.75 × 16 oz in a pound.

Problem C: Convert 26 tablespoons to cups.

This problem requires converting tablespoons to cups, both volume measurements.

$$\frac{26\ T}{1} \times \frac{1\ cup}{16\ Tablespoons} = \frac{26}{16} = 1.625\ cups = 1^5/_8\ cups$$

Using Table 6-3, 0.625 cups equal 5 fluid ounces. If you don't have the table, just multiply 0.625 × 8 fluid ounces in a cup.

Problem D: For an upcoming event, you need to make 200 servings of soup (portion size is 6 fl oz). How many gallons of soup will you need to make?

This problem requires converting fluid ounces to gallons, both volume measurements. We will go from fluid ounces to quarts to gallons. But first, multiply 200 servings by 6 fl oz to get how many total fluid ounces of soup are needed.

$$200\ servings \times 6\ fl\ oz/serving = 1200\ fluid\ ounces$$

$$\frac{1200\ fl\ Oz}{1} \times \frac{1\ quart}{32\ fl\ oz} \times \frac{1\ gallon}{4\ quarts} = \frac{1200}{128}\ gallons = 9.375\ gallons$$

You can also convert 0.375 pounds to fluid ounces. Just multiply 0.375 by 128 fluid ounces in a gallon to get 48 fluid ounces (1½ quarts).

EXAMPLE 6.2.2 HOW TO USE THE BRIDGE METHOD TO CONVERT BETWEEN VOLUME AND WEIGHT

Problem A: A recipe calls for 1¾ cups of flour and you need to know how many ounces that represents.

This problem requires converting volume to weight. In Appendix D, you will find that 1 cup of flour weighs 4.3 oz. So, you will convert from cups to ounces. First, convert 1¾ to a decimal.

$$\frac{1.75\ cups}{1} \times \frac{4.3\ oz}{1\ cup} = 7.5\ ounces$$

Problem B: You have extended a home recipe to make 100 servings. You now need 50 tablespoons of chopped bell peppers and you would like to convert that amount to pounds.

This problem requires converting volume to weight. In Appendix D, you will find that 1 cup of chopped bell peppers weighs 5.3 oz/cup. So, you will convert from tablespoons to cups to ounces to pounds.

$$\frac{50\ T}{1} \times \frac{1\ cup}{16\ T} \times \frac{5.3\ oz}{1\ cup} \times \frac{1\ pound}{16\ oz} = \frac{265}{256}\ pounds = 1.04\ pounds\ (1\ pound\ 1\ ounce)$$

Problem C: A salad recipe calls for 8½ pounds of fresh, cherry tomatoes. How many pints of tomatoes do you need?

This problem requires converting pounds (weight) to pints (volume). In Appendix D, you will find that 1 pound of cherry tomatoes equal 3 cups. So, you will convert from pounds to cups to pints.

$$\frac{8.5\ lb}{1} \times \frac{3\ cups}{1\ lb} \times \frac{1\ pint}{2\ cups} = \frac{25.5}{2} = 12.75\ pints\ or\ 12\ pints + 1\frac{1}{2}\ cups$$

Problem D: You have 10 bottles of wine and each contains 750 milliliters. How many 4-fluid-ounce servings will the 10 bottles provide?

This problem involves converting a metric measurement of volume (milliliters) to the U.S. system of volume (fluid ounces). *You can use the bridge method to convert metric measurements* as long as you know the conversion factor, which in this case is 30 milliliters equals 1 fluid ounce. First, you need to calculate how many total milliliters of wine you have.

(continues)

EXAMPLE 6.2.2 HOW TO USE THE BRIDGE METHOD TO CONVERT BETWEEN VOLUME AND WEIGHT (continued)

$$10 \text{ bottles} \times 750 \text{ mL/bottle} = 7{,}500 \text{ mL total wine}$$

$$\frac{7500 \text{ ml}}{1} \times \frac{1 \text{ fl oz}}{30 \text{ mL}} = 250 \text{ fl oz}$$

If you divide 250 fluid ounces by 4 fluid ounces/glass, you get 62.5 servings of wine.

cups of flour (volume) to ounces (weight). As you know, almost every ingredient, such as flour, that a baker uses is weighed. Also, weight is more accurate. And yes, you can convert cups of flour to pounds of flour as long as you know how much one cup of flour weighs in ounces. Part D of Appendix D includes a chart "Weight and Measure Equivalents for Common Foods" with that information. To convert volume to weight or weight to volume, we will continue to use the bridge method, as seen in Example 6.2.2.

6.3 USE YIELD PERCENT

In a kitchen, two recipes need to be prepared. One recipe calls for five pounds of russett potatoes that must be washed and forked before going into the oven. The other recipe calls for 10 pounds of trimmed green beans. When trimming green beans, the ends of each bean are cut off and any discolored or damaged sections removed. In the baked potato recipe, the cook can simply grab 5 pounds of potatoes from the storeroom. For the green beans, the cook will need more than 10 pounds because there will be some waste. This shows the difference between AP and EP quantities.

- **AP (as purchased) quantity** is the weight or volume of an item exactly as it was purchased. The recipe calling for 5 pounds of washed potatoes gives an example of an AP weight.
- **EP (edible portion) quantity** is the weight or volume of an item after all inedible or nonservable parts are trimmed off (Gisslen, 2018). Ten pounds of trimmed green beans is an example of EP weight. If you take about 11⅓ pounds of whole green beans from the refrigerator and clean and trim them, you will have 10 pounds of trimmed product. The weight (or volume) of product that wasn't used is called the **trim**. Not all trim is wasted. Some vegetable trim, for example, is used to make stock or soup.

Basically, the AP quantity minus the trim equals the EP quantity.

Yield percent is the percent of a food that is edible. For instance, whole green beans have an 88% yield. That means that if you have 10 pounds of whole green beans, you will have 8.8 pounds left after cleaning and trimming (just multiply 10×0.88). Of course, many ingredients, such as flour, are 100% edible. Other ingredients, such as a top round roast or fresh head of broccoli, are not 100% edible. The top round will shrink in size and weight during cooking and the broccoli needs to be trimmed. **Table 6–5** gives yield percents for fruits, vegetables, and fresh herbs. Appendix D gives yield percents for additional foods, including meat, poultry, and seafood.

In the commercial kitchen, we use yield percent in two ways. First, in purchasing, if a recipe lists the EP quantity needed, we will need to use the yield percent to calculate what to purchase (the AP quantity). Second, sometimes a production employee just needs to figure out how many servings can be obtained from a purchased amount. We will look at each of these situations now.

Table 6-5 Yield Percent for Fruits and Vegetables

Fruits	Yield Percent	Vegetables	Yield Percent
Apples, cored, unpeeled cored, peeled	91% 78%	Artichokes (edible leaves and base)	40%
Apricots	93%	Asparagus	53%
Avocado	67%	Beans, green or wax	88%
Bananas	64%	Beans, lima, in pods	44%
Blackberries	96%	Beets, whole, with full tops	40%
Blueberries	98%	Beets, whole, with no tops	70%
Cantaloupe	51%	Broccoli, spears	61%
Cherries (flesh)	62%	Brussels sprouts	80%
Coconut	48%	Cabbage, green, red, or white (trimmed without core)	80%
Figs (no stems)	97%	Cabbage, Chinese	59%
Grapefruit (segments without membranes)	52%	Carrots, with full tops	59%
Grapes (no stems)	93%	Carrots, without tops	82%
Honeydew, chunk	67%	Cauliflower, florets	60%
Lemon, juice	43%	Celeriac	86%
Lime, juice	47%	Celery	83%
Mango	69%	Chard	77%
Orange, sections with membrane	71%	Collards	57%
Orange, sections without membrane	50%	Cucumber (peeled, sliced)	84%
Papayas	65%	Eggplant (peeled, sliced)	81%
Peaches, peeled and pitted	76%	Endive (trimmed, cored)	86%
Pears, peeled and pitted	78%	Fennel (trimmed, cored)	86%
Pineapple, chunks	56%	Garlic (peeled, chopped)	87%
Plums, flesh	94%	Jicama, peeled and cubed	92%
Pomegranates	44%	Kale (leaves without stems)	64%
Raspberries	96%	Leeks (bulb and lower leaf)	44%
Strawberries	88%	Lettuce, butter/bibb	72%
Tomatoes (cored and trimmed)	88%	Lettuce, Romaine (trimmed, cored)	75%
Tomatoes (peeled, cored, seeded, chopped)	78%	Lettuce, iceberg (chopped)	65%
Watermelon (rind and seeds removed)	52%		
		Lettuce, leaf green or red	77%
		Mushrooms, trimmed and sliced	89%
		Okra	86%
		Onions, sliced or rings	84%
		Onions, diced	91%

(continues)

Table 6-5 Yield Percent for Fruits and Vegetables (continued)			
Fruits	**Yield Percent**	**Vegetables**	**Yield Percent**
		Peas, shelled	38%
		Peppers, sweet, diced	81%
		Potatoes, peeled and quartered	81%
		Radishes	63%
		Rutabagas, peeled	93%
		Shallots	88%
		Spinach	70%
		Squash, summer (not peeled)	95%
		Squash, winter - acorn	74%
		Squash - butternut	84%
		Squash - Hubbard	68%
		Squash - spaghetti	69%
		Sweet potatoes, hand peeled	88%
		Fresh Herbs	**Yield Percent**
		Basil	56%
		Cilantro	46%
		Oregano	78%
		Parsley, Italian	40%
		Rosemary	80%
		Tarragon	80%

Data from U.S. Department of Agriculture. (1975.) *Food yields: Summarized by different stages of preparation (Agriculture Handbook No. 102)*. Agricultural Research Service.
U.S. Department of Agriculture. (2019/2020). *Food Buying Guide for Child Nutrition Programs*. https://foodbuyingguide. fns.usda.gov/Appendix/DownLoadFBG Produce Marketing Association.
Lynch, F. T. (2010). *The Book of Yields: Accuracy in Food Costing and Purchasing* (8th edition). Hoboken: John Wiley & Sons, Inc. (fresh herb data)

When purchasing foods, use the following formula to determine what to purchase for a recipe that lists an ingredient in an EP format. An example is given in Example 6.3.1.

$$\text{As purchased quantity (AP)} = \frac{\text{Edible portion (EP) quantity}}{\text{Yield percent (in decimal form)}}$$

Remember that the yield percent does not take into account any mistakes made in the kitchen such as dropping foods on the floor or excessive spoilage or trimming.

In the next situation, you have the AP quantity and want to calculate the EP quantity.

EXAMPLE 6.3.1 HOW TO CALCULATE AP QUANTITY FROM EP QUANTITY

A recipe calls for 4 pounds of chopped celery. How much do you need to purchase?

$$\frac{\text{EP quantity}}{\text{Yield percent}} = \text{AP quantity}$$

$$\frac{4 \text{ pounds}}{0.75} = 5.3 \text{ pounds}$$

When calculating the purchase quantity, always round up. So you will want to make sure you get 6 pounds of celery.

EXAMPLE 6.3.2 HOW TO CALCULATE EP QUANTITY FROM AP QUANTITY

A cook wants to cut up 10 pounds of whole cantaloupes as cubes to use in fruit salad, but first she wants to know how much it will yield.

Edible portion quantity (EP) = As purchased quantity (AP)
× Yield percent (in decimal form)

5 lbs EP = 10 lbs AP (cantaloupe) × 0.50 (yield percent)

Using the formula, 10 pounds of whole cantaloupes will yield 5 pounds of cantaloupe when cut up for fruit salad.

6.4 DEVELOP A STANDARDIZED RECIPE AND ADJUST RECIPE YIELD

A recipe contains both the amount of ingredients and the instructions for a cook to use to make a certain product. A written recipe is a communication tool and is vital to producing good dishes, but it cannot tell you everything. Judgment is still needed.

Recipes have the following limitations.

1. Ingredient quality varies.
2. Equipment and how it is used varies from kitchen to kitchen.
3. The person cooking the food may make a wonderful, or terrible, product.
4. Even the same cook may not prepare a recipe the same way every time.
5. The weather and the kitchen's temperature and humidity also vary and will affect some ingredients and how some products come out.
6. Instructions are not always totally precise.

These limitations can be mostly overcome by using a standardized recipe.

A **standardized recipe** is a recipe that has been tested and adapted for use in a specific kitchen location so any cook in that kitchen can follow the written instructions to produce the same quantity and quality of food every time. Many people have the mistaken idea that a standardized recipe contains a foolproof set of ingredients, amounts, and instructions that will work every time in every kitchen for every cook. If you transplant a recipe standardized for one kitchen to another kitchen that has different ingredients, equipment, and cooks, the recipe may or may not work. If it doesn't work, that kitchen may make adjustments in the recipe to fit its equipment and cooks and to achieve the precise yield, flavor profile, and quality standards needed.

The standardized recipe is useful in many ways. Standardized recipes provide:

- Consistent flavor, appearance, and texture.
- Consistent yield and reduced risk of overproduction.
- Accurate nutritional information.
- Food cost control. (Food cost/serving is more accurate.)
- Labor cost control. (Food production staff can use their time more efficiently.)
- Easier for food purchasing and inventory.

Using standardized recipes also removes some stress for cooking staff as they are less likely to make mistakes.

All standardized recipes (see **Table 6-6** for an example of one) should include the following information.

1. Recipe name or title.
2. Recipe category (The corn muffin recipe is placed in "Quickbreads"—this category is given the code "QB" and then each recipe is numbered.)
3. Recipe yield (total number of servings).
4. Portion size.
5. Ingredient names and weight and/or volume needed. (Keep in mind that weight is used most often in quantity recipes and is more accurate than volume, especially for solid ingredients).
6. Preparation instructions/directions including cooking time and temperatures.
7. Panning or portioning information.
8. Serving suggestions such as garnishes to be used.

Recipes may also include food safety (HACCP) information; nutrient information; optional ingredients, recipe variations, and food costs. Recipes should be printed in large print so a cook can read the recipe from a short distance.

To develop a standardized recipe in a foodservice, the recipe should first be thoroughly reviewed for issues such as the following.

1. Are the ingredients listed in the order they are used?
2. Is each ingredient described appropriately and in enough detail? Is each ingredient available in your kitchen or do you need to write in a substitute?

Table 6-6 Standardized Recipe Example

Corn Muffin
Yield: 100
Portion: 1 muffin

Ingredients	Weight
Flour, white, general purpose	2⅞ lbs
Cornmeal	2¾ lbs
Milk, nonfat dry	4½ oz
Sugar, granulated	5¼ oz
Baking powder	4⅜ oz
Salt	1 oz
Eggs, whole frozen	1¼ lbs
Water	6 pounds (2 qts, 3½ cup)
Oil, soybean	1⅛ lbs
Cooking spray, nonstick	2 oz

Directions:
1. Blend flour, cornmeal, milk, sugar, baking powder, and salt in mixer bowl.
2. Combine eggs and water, add to ingredients in mixer bowl. Blend at low speed about 1 minute. Scrape down bowl.
3. Add oil, mix at medium speed until blended.
4. Lightly spray 9-12 cup muffin pans with nonstick cooking spray. Fill each cup ⅔ full.
5. Bake for 15 to 20 minutes at 425°F OR at 375°F in a convection oven for 15 minutes.

Nutrition: 160 cal, 22 g carbohydrate, 4 g protein, 6 g fat, 24 mg cholesterol, 252 mg sodium, 95 mg calcium.

3.   Are AP and EP used correctly in the ingredient list?
4.   Is it clear how much of each ingredient should be used?
5.   Are the proportions of ingredients similar to other recipes?
6.   Are the directions clear? Will the cooking staff understand all directions and cooking terms? Do the cooking staff possess the skills needed?
7.   Are the procedures correct?
8.   Do the cooking time and temperature seem to be right?
9.   Do the directions refer to equipment and tools that should be used? Are the equipment and tools the best ones for the job? Are they available?
10.   Does the yield look realistic?
11.   Is the portion size appropriate? Does the portion size need to be increased or decreased?
12.   Is the recipe too costly for your operation? Is it too labor intensive?
13.   Does the recipe meet your requirements for nutrition? For example, is it too high in calories or sodium?

At this stage, the written recipe should be customized to your kitchen.

The next step is to prepare the recipe. It is easier at this stage to test a smaller recipe rather than one that makes 200 servings. If your recipe is for 20 servings and you know you will increase the yield later, just make the smaller recipe now and see if you have any success before increasing the yield. When preparing the recipe, make notes if you change anything. For instance, you may find that the cooking time is too short; note the time it really took for the item to be prepared.

Once the recipe is made, it is time to evaluate it from a number of perspectives.

- First, measure the total yield and then verify the number of portions it produces. Is the total yield accurate? Does it make the correct number of portions in the portion size given? Yields can vary depending on a number of factors such as cooking times and temperatures as well as ingredients. Note the actual yield information on the recipe.
- Second, pull together a variety of people (employees, customers, etc.) to taste test and evaluate the product. Don't let the size of the group get too big—10 people is enough so you can have a good discussion among the participants. Ahead of time, set up a table for the food testing. Be sure to have plates, utensils, napkins, water for drinking, pencils, and evaluation forms (**Table 6-7**).

With these results and feedback, you can determine if the results were good enough to use the recipe as is or whether it is worthwhile to make some changes to the recipe and test it again. The final decision may be that the recipe was not very good and should be rejected with no further testing.

If you decide to continue testing, you will need to adjust the recipe as needed, such as for taste or yield. Here are some general guidelines.

- Involve the production staff in the process.
- Change one ingredient/procedure at a time, being sure to record all changes on the recipe.
- Evaluate each product for quality and quantity produced.
- Repeat the process as needed.
- Once you have the quality and quantity you want, if you need to, you can increase the overall yield.

Once the recipe seems to be just right in quality and quantity, make it one more time to do a final check for consistency.

Sometimes, you need to increase or decrease the yield of a recipe. For instance, your recipe produces 25 portions but you need 50. That's an easy one to do, since you just double the ingredients, as shown here.

Table 6-7 Food Evaluation Form					
Food Evaluation Form Recipe Name: _____ Please rate the following traits of this product using the scale provided.					
	Very Undesirable	**Moderately Undesirable**	**Neither Desirable nor Undesirable**	**Moderately Desirable**	**Very Desirable**
The **appearance** of the food	1	2	3	4	5
The **taste** of the food	1	2	3	4	5
The **temperature** of the food	1	2	3	4	5
The **texture** of the food (moist, firm)	1	2	3	4	5
The **overall acceptability** of the food	1	2	3	4	5
Total Score: _____ Mean Score: _____ Comments:					

"Measuring Success with Standardized Recipes," by U. S. Department of Agriculture, Food and Nutrition Service, with the National Food Service Management Institute, 2002, p. 53. University, MS: National Food Service Management Institute.

$$
\begin{array}{llll}
\text{Flour} & 12 \text{ lbs} \times 2 & = 24 \text{ lbs} \\
\text{Water} & 8 \text{ lb} \times 2 & = 16 \text{ lbs} \\
\text{Yeast} & 6 \text{ oz} \times 2 & = 12 \text{ oz.} \\
\text{Sugar} & 12 \text{ oz} \times 2 & = 24 \text{ oz} = 1\frac{1}{2} \text{ lbs}
\end{array}
$$

Of course, you can easily change the yield of a recipe using the computer or find a free program on the Internet (such as https://www.webstaurantstore.com/recipe_resizer .html), but you should know how it is done. Let's say you need to adjust a recipe yield from 50 portions to 175 portions. What you need is a multiplier (also called a conversion factor or just factor), such as "2" in the previous example.

1. To determine the multiplier, divide the desired yield by the current yield.

$$
\frac{Desired\ Yield}{Current\ Yield} = Multiplier
$$

$$
\frac{175}{50} = 3.5
$$

2. Then you multiply each ingredient in the recipe by 3.5.

$$
\begin{array}{lll}
\text{Flour} & 12 \text{ lbs} \times 3.5 = 42 \text{ lbs} \\
\text{Water} & 8 \text{ lb} \times 3.5 = 28 \text{ lbs} \\
\text{Yeast} & 6 \text{ oz} \times 3.5 = 21 \text{ oz.} \\
\text{Sugar} & 12 \text{ oz} \times 3.5 = 42 \text{ oz}
\end{array}
$$

3. Change the amounts into more common measurements, such as 42 ounces of sugar can be written as 2 lb, 10 oz.

SPOTLIGHT ON BAKER'S PERCENTAGES

Baker's percentages is a useful concept for bakers. Compared with making an item such as meatballs, where the meatballs will probably come out fine even if you don't measure every ingredient precisely, baking is not as forgiving. Maintaining the correct proportions of ingredients in a baking recipe are essential to get desirable results, such as a tender brownie or crusty loaf of bread. To get quality baked products, baking ingredients are almost always weighed.

When using baker's percentages, 100% represents the amount of *flour* in the recipe (*not* the total of all the ingredients). Other ingredients are then expressed as percentages of the flour. For example, if a recipe (often called a formula in baking) calls for 10 pounds of flour and 4 pounds of shortening, the flour is 100% and the shortening is 40%. If a formula specifies 130% sugar for 10 pounds of flour, then you will need 13 pounds of sugar. Baker's percentages express ingredient proportions, not total percentages. They are useful to create new formulas or change the yield. The following is an example.

White Bread		
Ingredient	**Weight**	**Percentage**
Flour, white, enriched	50 lb	100%
Water	33 lb	33%
Salt	1 lb	2%
Yeast	0.6 lb	1.2%

To calculate the percentage of salt, for example, do the following calculation.

$$\frac{1\ lb\ salt}{50\ lb\ flour} \times 100 = 2\%$$

6.5 CALCULATE COST OF A RECIPE AND PORTION

Once a recipe is standardized, you can calculate how much it costs to produce that recipe and how much one portion costs. Knowing the cost/portion will help you set prices for each menu item and control food costs. Before you learn how to calculate cost of a recipe, you need to calculate AP Cost/Unit.

CALCULATE AP COST/UNIT

As discussed earlier in the chapter, AP quantities refer to foods as they are purchased—such as 20 pounds of raw ribeye roast, 5 pounds of butter, 1 case of apples, or 5 pounds of elbow macaroni. The price paid for these foods is the AP (as purchased) cost. Food-services buy products in a wide variety of units, from cases to pounds to dozens.

In a quantity kitchen, you may need to determine the cost of 2 pounds of butter, 6 ounces of cooked ribeye roast or 6 apples being used to make apple pie. In the case of the butter, you purchase it by the pound and your recipe calls for 2 pounds, so you can simply double the price to find your cost. But sometimes, a product is purchased in a unit different from the unit used in the recipe. For example, the ribeye roast was purchased by the pound, but now you want to find the cost per ounce. Another issue with the ribeye roast is that you purchased it raw, and you need the cost per ounce after it has been cooked, so you will also need to consider yield. For the apples, you purchased them by the case, but now you want the cost per apple. (Luckily, the size of the apple, such as 125, tells you how many apples are in the case.)

To calculate the AP cost per unit, use the following formula. Note that the "unit" on each side of this equation must be the same unit—such as pounds or cups.

$$\frac{AP\ cost}{Number\ of\ Units\ Purchased} = AP\ cost\ per\ unit$$

Now you can review several examples of calculations.

EXAMPLE 6.5.1 HOW TO CALCULATE AP COST/UNIT—SUGAR

The restaurant buys 25-pound bags of granulated sugar. Each bag costs $15.50. Calculate the AP cost per pound and per cup.

Cost Per Pound:

$$\frac{AP\ cost}{Number\ of\ Units\ Purchased} = \frac{\$15.50}{25\ pounds} = \$0.62/pound$$

Cost Per Cup:

Because the unit is now cups, you need to convert a 25-pound bag of sugar into cups. Appendix D shows that 1 pound of sugar contains 2.25 cups. Now use the bridge method to make this conversion.

Bridge Method:

$$\frac{25\ pounds}{1} \times \frac{2.25\ cups}{1\ pound} = 56.25\ cups$$

$$\frac{AP\ cost}{Number\ of\ Units\ Purchased} = \frac{\$15.50}{56.25\ cups} = \$0.275/cup$$

EXAMPLE 6.5.2 HOW TO CALCULATE AP COST/UNIT—MILK

The restaurant buys gallons of whole milk for $3.09 each. Calculate the AP cost per cup and per fluid ounce.

Cost Per Cup:

Since the unit is cups, convert 1 gallon into cups.

Bridge Method:

$$\frac{1\ gallon}{1} \times \frac{4\ quarts}{1\ gallon} \times \frac{4\ cups}{1\ quart} = 16\ cups$$

$$\frac{AP\ cost}{Number\ of\ Units\ Purchased} = \frac{\$3.09}{16\ cups} = \$0.193/cup$$

Cost Per Fluid Ounce:

The unit is now fluid ounces, so convert 1 gallon into fluid ounces (or use Table 6-1).

Bridge Method:

$$\frac{1\ gallon}{1} \times \frac{4\ quarts}{1\ gallon} \times \frac{4\ cups}{1\ quart} \times \frac{8\ fluid\ ounces}{1\ cup} = 128\ fluid\ ounces$$

$$\frac{AP\ cost}{Number\ of\ Units\ Purchased} = \frac{\$3.09}{128\ fluid\ ounces} = \$0.024/fluid\ ounce$$

EXAMPLE 6.5.3 HOW TO CALCULATE AP COST/UNIT—ROMAINE LETTUCE

The restaurant buys a case of romaine lettuce for $30. Each case contains 24 heads and each head weighs 22 ounces. Calculate the AP cost per head and AP cost per ounce.

Cost Per Head:

$$\frac{AP\ cost}{Number\ of\ Units\ Purchased} = \frac{\$30.00}{24\ heads} = \$0.125/head$$

Cost Per Ounce:

To calculate cost per ounce, you need to calculate the number of ounces in a case.

$$24 \text{ heads} \times 22 \text{ ounces/head} = 528 \text{ ounces}$$

$$\frac{AP\ cost}{Number\ of\ Units\ Purchased} = \frac{\$30.00}{528\ ounces} = \$0.057/ounce$$

CALCULATE INGREDIENT COST

To calculate the cost of a recipe, you will be going through these steps to determine the cost of each ingredient.

1. When an AP quantity is given for an ingredient, check the unit of the AP quantity and the unit on which the cost is based. If the unit is the same, such as when the recipe calls for 2.5 pounds of butter and butter costs $4.00/pound, you are all set to go to Step 2. However, if the units are not the same, you will need to do a calculation so that the recipe unit matches the purchasing unit. For example, if the purchasing unit is gallon and the recipe says quarts, you can divide the number of quarts by four to convert to gallons.

2. Next, determine if any ingredients are given in an EP quantity. For example, if the recipe calls for 2 pounds of peeled and quartered potatoes, there is trimming loss and you will need more than 2 pounds of potatoes for this recipe.

   a. As shown earlier, use the following formula to calculate the AP quantity from the EP quantity. The following shows the AP quantity needed for a recipe that calls for 2 pounds of peeled and quartered potatoes.

$$\frac{EP\ quantity}{Yield\ \%} = AP\ quantity$$

$$\frac{2\ pounds}{0.81} = 2.47\ pounds\ (round\ to\ 2.5\ lbs)$$

3. Calculate the cost of each ingredient using the following formula. The unit for the AP quantity and the cost unit must be the same.

$$AP\ quantity \times AP\ cost\ per\ unit = Ingredient\ Cost$$

$$5\ pounds \times \$10.50/pound = \$52.50$$

4. Add up the cost of all the ingredients to get the total recipe cost.

Example 6.5.4 shows how to calculate ingredient cost for a recipe when none of the ingredients have to be fabricated. In other words, there is no waste for any of the

EXAMPLE 6.5.4 HOW TO CALCULATE INGREDIENT COST (NO WASTE)

Baked Apples—Cost for each Ingredient	
Ingredients	**Cost**
12 apples, Red Delicious	$41.00/case (80 count)
¾ pound butter	$4.00/pound
¾ cup brown sugar	$1.35/pound
2 teaspoons cinnamon	$4.48/pound

(continues)

EXAMPLE 6.5.4 HOW TO CALCULATE INGREDIENT COST (NO WASTE) (continued)

12 apples: *The unit in the recipe is one apple (or sometimes we just say "each"), and the cost is given for a case that contains 80 apples. So, we can simply divide the case cost by 80 apples to get the cost/apple. Then we multiply the cost/apple by 12 apples to get the ingredient cost.*

$$\frac{AP\ cost}{Number\ of\ Units\ Purchased} = \frac{\$41.00}{80\ apples} = \$0.512/apple$$

AP quantity $\times$ AP cost per unit = Ingredient Cost
12 apples $\times$ \$0.512/apple = \$6.14

¾ pound butter: *The ingredient unit and cost unit are the same: pound.*
AP quantity $\times$ AP cost per unit = Ingredient Cost
0.75 pound butter $\times$ \$4.00/pound = \$3.00

¾ cup brown sugar: The cost is given in cost/pound, so you need to convert ¾ cup of brown sugar to pounds. Appendix D shows that one cup of brown sugar weighs 7 ounces.

Bridge Method:

$$\frac{0.75\ cup}{1} \times \frac{7\ ounces}{1\ cup} \times \frac{1\ pound}{16\ ounces} = 0.33\ pound$$

AP quantity $\times$ AP cost per unit = Ingredient Cost
0.33 pound brown sugar $\times$ \$1.35/pound = \$0.45

2 teaspoons cinnamon: Since the cost is in pounds, you need to convert 2 teaspoons to pounds. One tablespoon of cinnamon weighs 0.250 ounces.

Bridge Method:

$$\frac{2\ teaspoons}{1} \times \frac{1\ tablespoon}{3\ teaspoons} \times \frac{0.250\ ounces}{1\ tablespoon} \times \frac{1\ pound}{16\ ounces} = 0.01\ pound$$

AP quantity $\times$ AP cost per unit = Ingredient Cost
0.01 pound cinnamon $\times$ \$4.48/pound = \$0.04

EXAMPLE 6.5.5 HOW TO CALCULATE INGREDIENT COST (WITH TRIMMING LOSS)

Spaghetti Squash Italian Style—Cost for each Ingredient	
Ingredients	**Cost**
1 cup shallots, minced	\$6.89/pound
1 quart canned diced tomatoes, drained	\$7.15/#10 can
6 pounds spaghetti squash, peeled	\$0.99/pound

1 cup shallots, minced: *First, 1 cup needs to be converted to pounds. One cup minced weighs 5.5 ounces.*
Bridge Method:

$$\frac{1\ cup}{1} \times \frac{5.5\ ounces}{1\ cup} \times \frac{1\ pound}{16\ ounces} = 0.34\ pounds$$

Next, calculate the AP quantity. The yield percent for shallots is 88%.

$$\frac{EP\ Quantity}{Yield\ \%} \times \frac{0.34\#}{.88} = 0.39\ pounds\ (AP\ quantity)$$

Last, calculate the cost.
AP quantity $\times$ AP cost per unit = Ingredient Cost
0.39 pounds shallots $\times$ \$6.89/pound = \$2.69

1 quart canned diced tomatoes, drained: First, you need to calculate the AP cost per quart. A #10 can holds 3 quarts.

$$\frac{AP\ cost}{Number\ of\ Units\ Purchased} = \frac{\$7.15}{3\ quarts} = \$2.38/quart$$

Next, calculate the AP quantity. The drained weight yield percent is 66%.

$$\frac{EP\ Quantity}{Yield\ \%} \times \frac{1\ quart}{.66} = 1.52\ quarts\ (AP\ quantity)$$

Last, calculate the cost.
AP quantity × AP cost per unit = Ingredient Cost
1.52 quarts × $2.38/quart = $3.62

6 pounds spaghetti squash, peeled: First, calculate the AP quantity. The yield percent is 69%.

$$\frac{EP\ Quantity}{Yield\ \%} = \frac{6\ pounds}{.69} = 8.7\ pounds\ (AP\ quantity)$$

Because the AP quantity and price are in pounds, you can move right to calculating the cost.
AP quantity × AP cost per unit = Ingredient Cost
8.7 pounds × $0.99/pound = $8.61

ingredients. Example 6.5.5 shows how to calculate ingredient costs for ingredients when there is waste. For example, shallots have to be trimmed and minced, and canned tomatoes have to be drained. For each of the ingredients in 6.5.5, you need to determine the AP quantity using the appropriate yield percent.

CALCULATE RECIPE COST AND PORTION COST

To calculate the cost of a recipe, simply add up the cost of all of the ingredients. Once you have the recipe cost, you can divide that cost by the number of portions the recipe makes. Now you have the cost per portion.

$$\frac{Total\ recipe\ cost}{Number\ of\ portions} = Cost\ per\ portion$$

So, if a recipe costs $80 to make, and it yield 20 portions, then you do the following.

$$\frac{\$80.00}{20\ portions} = \$4.00/portion$$

The cost per portion is important to know, especially for setting menu prices.

Example 6.5.6 shows the ingredient costs for Chicken Marsala with Mushrooms and Tomatoes. The recipe cost and portion cost are shown at the bottom. Here's an explanation of each column.

- Each ingredient and the recipe quantity are listed in the first two columns on the left.
- The third column shows the recipe quantity in the same unit as the purchasing unit. For example, the recipe calls for 50 boneless chicken breasts that are 6 ounces each. The purchasing unit is pounds, so you will have to convert the recipe quantity. If you multiply 50 chicken breasts × 6 ounces, you get 300 ounces, which can then be divided by 16 ounces/pound to give you 18.75 pounds.
- The fourth column, Quantity to Purchase, includes Yield Percent and AP Quantity. The Yield Percent column includes yield percents for typical ingredients, such as onions and tomatoes, that need to be fabricated. It also includes

EXAMPLE 6.5.6 RECIPE: CHICKEN MARSALA WITH MUSHROOMS AND TOMATOES

Recipe Yield: 50 servings
Portion Size: 1 piece chicken + 1 cup sauce

Ingredient	Recipe Quantity	Recipe Quantity in Purchasing Unit	Quantity to Purchase Yield Percent	AP Quantity	AP Cost	Ingredient Cost
Chicken breast (boneless) 6 oz. (AP)	50 ea	18.75#	—	18.75#	$3.85/#	$72.19
Flour	2.5 cups	0.67#	100%	0.67#	$0.89/#	$ 0.60
Olive oil	1 cup	0.24 L	100%	0.24 L	8.51/L	$ 2.04
Butter	1#	1#	100%	1#	$4.00/#	$ 4.00
Onion, minced (EP)	1#	1#	90%	1.11#	$0.50/#	$ 0.56
Tomatoes, peeled, seeded, chopped (EP)	3 qt	4.8#	78%	6.15#	$1.75/#	$10.76
Mushrooms, sliced (EP)	5#	5#	89%	5.62#	$2.59/#	$14.56
Marsala, dry	2 qt	2 qt	—	2 qt	$14.55/qt	$29.10
Stock, chicken	2 qt	2 qt	—	2 qt	$0.50/qt	$ 1.00
Basil, fresh, chopped (EP)	1 cup	0.06#	56%	0.11#	$8.88/#	$ 0.98
Recipe Cost						$135.79
Portion Cost						$ 2.72
(# means pound)						

100% when, for example, you are using oil or butter. Three of the ingredients do not show a yield percent—chicken, marsala, and chicken stock. As these items cook, there will be some loss in cooking—but that does not affect what you will purchase because that has already been taken into account.

- To get the AP Quantity, simply multiply the third column by the Yield Percent.
- The AP Cost is obtained from personnel involved in Purchasing.
- The Ingredient Cost in the final column is obtained by multiplying the AP Quantity by the AP Cost. For example, multiply 18.75 pounds of chicken by the cost of $3.85/pound to get $72.19.

Sometimes, you may not know the number of portions in a recipe or other item such as a 3-gallon bulk container of ice cream. Use this formula to calculate the number of portions.

$$\frac{Total\ EP\ Quantity}{Portion\ Size} = Number\ of\ Portions$$

If you need to know how many ½- cup servings of ice cream are in a 3-gallon container, first you need to calculate how many cups are in 3 gallons.

$$3\ gallons \times 16\ cups/gallon = 48\ cups$$

$$\frac{48\ cups}{0.5\ cups} = 96\ 1/2\ cup\ servings$$

Example 6.5.7 gives additional examples for calculating the number of portions.

EXAMPLE 6.5.7 HOW TO CALCULATE NUMBER OF PORTIONS

$$\frac{Total\ EP\ Quantity}{Portion\ Size} = Number\ of\ Portions$$

Example: 7.5 cups of cubed honeydew will be portioned into ½ cup servings. How many servings will it make?

$$\frac{7.5\ cups}{0.5\ cups} = 15\ portions\ or\ servings$$

Example: You have cleaned and chopped romaine lettuce and have 54 ounces of product. If each Caesar salad contains 4 ounces of romaine, how many servings will it make?

$$\frac{54\ ounces}{4\ ounces} = 13.5\ portions\ or\ servings$$

6.6 CALCULATE FOOD COST PERCENTAGE

An important number for any foodservice operation is its food cost percentage. **Food cost percentage** is the proportion of food sales spent on food. The formula for food cost percentage is to divide food cost by food sales as shown here. The food cost and food sales must come from the same period of time, such as the month of October. The example here shows the food cost percentage for the period January 1, 2021 to March 31, 2021.

$$\frac{Food\ cost}{Food\ sales} \times 100 = Food\ cost\ percentage\ \frac{\$83.492}{\$238,183} \times 100 = 35.1\ \%$$

To calculate the food cost for this period, use the following formula.
Beginning Inventory + Food Purchased − Ending Inventory = Cost of Food Sold
Here's an example.

Beginning Inventory – 1/1/2021	$24,000
Purchases for January – March	+ $87,000
Food Available for Sale	$111,000
Ending Inventory – 3/31/2021	− $27,508
Cost of Food Sold	$ 83,492

In restaurants, food cost percentage is usually close to 33% and labor cost percentage close to 35% (Reynolds & McClusky, 2013), although some restaurants keep food cost and/or labor cost percentages down a bit lower, such as 25%. Food and labor costs run a wide range due to different foodservice concepts, customers, menus, and other considerations.

SUMMARY

6.1 Measure Ingredients Accurately

- Ingredients are measured by count, weight (pounds and ounces), or volume (such as cups, fluid ounces, tablespoons, and teaspoons).
- Liquid measuring cups are usually made of glass and have a handle. Place the measuring cup on a flat surface and check that the liquid goes up to the proper line on the measuring cup while looking directly at it at eye level. Measuring cups for dry ingredients, such as flour, are often made of metal or plastic.
- Table 6-1 is list of measurement equivalents that you must know. Table 6-2 lists common abbreviations used in recipes.

- Gram (and kilogram) is the basic unit of weight in the metric system. Milliliters (and liter) are the basic unit of volume.

6.2   Convert Units of Measures

- The following is an example of how to use the bridge method to convert 60 ounces to pounds.

$$\frac{60 \ \cancel{ounces}}{1} \times \frac{1 \ pound}{16 \ \cancel{ounces}} = \frac{60}{16} \ pounds$$
$$= 3.75 \ pounds = 3lb \ 12oz$$

6.3   Use Yield Percent

- In a recipe, a quantity may be expressed in AP or EP format.
  - AP (as purchased) quantity is the weight or volume of an item exactly as it was purchased. A recipe calling for 5 pounds of washed potatoes is an example of an AP weight.
  - EP (edible portion) quantity is the weight or volume of an item after all inedible or nonservable parts are trimmed off (Gisslen, 2018).
- Yield percent is the percent of a food that is edible. For instance, whole green beans have an 88% yield (see Table 6-5). That means that if you have 10 pounds of whole green beans, you will have 8.8 pounds left after cleaning and trimming (just multiply 10 × 0.88).
- When purchasing foods, use the following formula to determine what to purchase for a recipe that lists an ingredient in an EP format. An example is given in Example 6.3.1.

$$\text{As purchased quantity (AP)} = \frac{Edible \ portion \ (EP) \ quantity}{Yield \ percent \ (in \ decimal \ form)}$$

- To calculate the EP quantity from the AP quantity, use this formula.

Edible portion quantity (EP) = As purchased quantity (AP) × Yield percent (in decimal form)

6.4   Develop a Standardized Recipe and Adjust Recipe Yield

- A standardized recipe is a recipe that has been tested and adapted for use in a specific kitchen location so any cook in that kitchen can follow the written instructions to produce the same quantity and quality of food every time.
- Standardized recipes have many benefits: consistent quality and yield, accurate nutrition information, improved food cost and labor cost control, and they are easier for food purchasing and inventory.

- All standardized recipes (see Table 6-6) should include recipe name, category, yield, portion size, ingredient names and quantity needed, directions, panning or portioning information, and serving suggestions/garnishes.
- To develop a standardized recipe from a recipe, first the recipe needs to be thoroughly reviewed and analyzed, and appropriate changes made. Next, the recipe should be prepared. Then you can verify the total yield/number of portions as well as get a group of people to evaluate the product (see evaluation form in Table 6-7).
- If you decide to continue testing, you will need to adjust the recipe as needed, such as for taste or yield. Here are some general guidelines.
  - Involve the production staff in the process.
  - Change one ingredient/procedure at a time, being sure to record all changes on the recipe.
  - Evaluate each product for quality and quantity.
  - Repeat the process as needed.
  - Once you have the quality and quantity you want, if you need to, you can increase the overall yield.
- To adjust a recipe yield, determine the conversion factor or multiplier as follows—then multiply each ingredient by the factor.

$$\frac{Desired \ Yield}{Current \ Yield} = Multiplier/Factor$$

6.5   Calculate Cost of a Recipe and Portion

- To calculate the AP cost per unit, use the following formula. Note that the "unit" on each side of this equation must be the same unit—such as pounds or cups. See Examples 6.5.1 and 6.5.2.

$$\frac{AP \ Cost}{Number \ of \ Units \ Purchased} = AP \ cost \ per \ unit$$

- To calculate the cost of a recipe, use these steps.
  - If an AP quantity is given for an ingredient, the unit of the AP quantity needs to match the unit it is purchased in. If the units are not the same, you must do a calculation so the AP unit matches the cost unit—such as you need 2 pounds of butter for a recipe and you buy it by the pound.
  - For ingredients given in an EP quantity, you will have to calculate the AP quantity using yield percent.

- Calculate the cost of each ingredient using this formula.

AP quantity $\times$ AP cost per unit = Ingredient Cost

- Add up the cost of all ingredients to get the total recipe cost.
- Divide the total recipe cost by the number of portions to obtain the cost/portion.
- When you do not know the number of portions in a recipe, use this formula to calculate the number of portions.

$$\frac{Total\ EP\ quantity}{Portion\ Size} = Number\ of\ Portions$$

6.6 Calculate Food Cost Percentage

- Food cost percentage is the proportion of food sales spent on food. The formula for food cost percentage is to divide food cost by food sales as shown here.

$$\frac{Food\ cost}{Food\ sale} \times 100 = Food\ cost\ percentage$$

$$\frac{\$83,492}{\$238,183} \times 100 = 35.1\%$$

- To calculate the food cost for this period, use the following formula.

Beginning Inventory + Food Purchased − Ending Inventory = Cost of Food Sold

REVIEW AND DISCUSSION QUESTIONS

1. List the ways ingredients may be measured.
2. List the equivalents of: 1 gallon, 1 quart, 1 cup, and 1 tablespoon.
3. Explain how you would convert 15 cups of seedless grapes into pounds using the bridge method.
4. Explain what AP and EP are.
5. Carrots have an 82% yield. What does that mean? If you have 5 pounds of carrots (without tops), what will they yield? If you need 5 pounds of sliced carrots for a recipe, how many pounds do you need to purchase?
6. What are the advantages of having cooks use standardized recipes?
7. Describe the process to standardize a recipe.
8. To change the yield of a recipe, how do you get a multiplier?
9. Use the AP cost/unit formula to calculate the cost of one apple when a case of apples (80/case) costs $26.00.
10. Use the Ingredient Cost formula to calculate the cost of 3 cups of vegetable when the cost per quart is $5.50.
11. How do you calculate food cost percentage and why is it important?

SMALL GROUP PROJECT

When you created the menu for your foodservice concept, you included recipes for all items on the menu for one day (for cycle menus) OR recipes for at least 25% of the menu items (for restaurant-style menus). For this part of the project, you will need two recipes. Make sure the recipes you pick are not all from one category of the menu, such as soups or salads. Vary the recipes.

1. Convert two of your recipes so each yield 140 portions.
2. Determine the total cost to make one of your recipes and include the cost per portion as well.

REFERENCES

Blocker, L., & Hill, J. (2016). *Culinary Math* (4th ed.). Hoboken (NJ): John Wiley & Sons, Inc.

Dopson, L. R., & Hayes, D. K. (2017). *Food & Beverage Cost Control* (6th ed.). Hoboken, NJ: John Wiley & Sons, Inc.

Dressen, L., Nothnagel, M., & Wysocki, S. (2011). *Math for the Professional Kitchen*. Hoboken (NJ): John Wiley & Sons, Inc.

Gisslen, W. (2018). *Professional Cooking* (9th edition). Hoboken (NJ): John Wiley & Sons, Inc.

King Arthur Flour. (2020). Ingredient weight chart. https://www.kingarthurbaking.com/learn/ingredient-weight-chart

Lynch, F.T. (2010). *The Book of Yields: Accuracy in Food Costing and Purchasing* (8th ed.). Hoboken: John Wiley & Sons, Inc.

Reynolds, D., & McClusky, K. W. (2013). *Foodservice Management Fundamentals*. Hoboken (NJ): John Wiley & Sons, Inc.

U. S. Department of Agriculture, Food and Nutrition Service, with the National Food Service Management Institute. (2002). *Measuring success with standardized recipes*. University, MS: National Food Service Management Institute.

U.S. Department of Agriculture. (2019/2020). *Food Buying Guide for Child Nutrition Programs*. https://foodbuyingguide.fns.usda.gov/Appendix/DownLoadFBG

U.S. Department of Agriculture. (1975.) *Food yields: Summarized by different stages of preparation (Agriculture Handbook No. 102)*. Agricultural Research Service.

© Denis Val/Shutterstock

Food Purchasing

LEARNING OUTCOMES

7.1 Outline the distribution system for food and supplies.

7.2 Describe the organization and objectives of a purchasing department.

7.3 Explain how prepurchasing activities are accomplished.

7.4 Summarize federal food safety laws and agencies involved.

7.5 Outline how varied buying methods work.

INTRODUCTION

To many people, purchasing is the simple act of buying something at a store or ordering an item online and having it delivered. For a foodservice system, **purchasing** involves studying your menu and recipes, specifying the ingredients you will use, comparing quality and prices, then choosing which producers, manufacturers, and/or distributors (also called **suppliers** or **vendors**) you will order from, and then finally receiving and paying for the goods. In reality, the person in charge of purchasing does more than just order and receive goods and make sure the bills get paid. For example, purchasing agents have to find, evaluate, and pick which suppliers they want to work with as well as maintain an ethical and professional relationship with them. Because purchasing is more complex, some professionals prefer to use the term **procurement** because it is more comprehensive and includes purchasing as well as the other processes essential to securing goods and services. Within the foodservice industry, the terms purchasing and procurement are generally interchangeable. This chapter will use the term purchasing.

Working as a purchasing agent or buyer involves a lot of planning, information gathering, decision making, and activities including the following.

1. Review the menu and recipes (preferably costed out) and talk to the Chef and Production staff to see which products to buy to produce the menu while meeting quality standards.

2. Find and evaluate suppliers in your region who carry the products you need.

3. Select suppliers and/or create a list of approved suppliers. Make sure any supplier you pick is ethical, current in health inspections, and has no conflicts with your business, such as lawsuits, ownership, or conflicting union contracts.
4. Determine how much to buy.
5. Request and evaluate price quotations from suppliers.
6. Negotiate with suppliers.
7. Place orders and administer purchasing contracts.
8. Receive and inspect products when delivered (often completed by a receiving clerk)
9. Process invoices and payments to suppliers.
10. Store products in a safe manner and manage the inventory.

While performing these activities, the buyer is always trying to get good value for the money spent and to have adequate food supplies on hand to serve meals.

In the foodservice systems model, food and labor are the two major inputs and also the biggest expenses in a foodservice. When purchasing food is done well, money is saved and meals are served that meet customer expectations. On the other hand, when purchasing is accomplished in a haphazard fashion, food costs can be higher than budget and unhappy customers may not return, thus decreasing sales.

Technology has made purchasing less time consuming and helped communications between the supplier and the foodservice. According to Dale Wilkinson, National Account Manager for US Foods, "Online ordering from your desk or from your phone cuts ordering time in half. You can also get updated information on vendor inventory online and know exactly where your delivery truck is." US Foods is a foodservice **distributor**, meaning they provide food and supplies to restaurants and other foodservices. Not only has technology saved time but it has also allowed distributors to better communicate with customers. For example, they will let you know immediately when an item you order is out of stock so you can substitute with a different item. You can also receive emails or texts immediately when a food is recalled or a shortage is predicted, or when a price changes dramatically.

Sourcing and sustainability have become important purchasing issues, especially for foodservices leading the fight against pollution and climate change. Distributors can switch you to "locally sourced" produce when available, or they can help if your goals are to purchase from minority or women-owned businesses. Many suppliers can now provide information for farm-to-table operations, and let you know which products are organic, vegan, halal, free range, wild caught (for seafood), or non-GMO. GMO, the abbreviation for **Genetically Modified Organisms**, refers to products that are bioengineered. When a gene from one organism is purposely moved to improve or change another organism in a laboratory, the result is a GMO. Many genetically modified crops, such as corn, have been modified to resist insects or herbicides.

This chapter will examine many of the tasks buyers perform as part of their jobs, such as how to evaluate potential suppliers and develop food specifications (a detailed description of a food). Federal food safety laws and agencies and common purchasing methods are also discussed. A detailed discussion on how to develop food specifications for specific foods is included at the back of this chapter. Food receiving and inventory management are covered in the next chapter.

7.1 OUTLINE THE DISTRIBUTION SYSTEM FOR FOOD AND SUPPLIES

Any physical good that can be purchased has to go through a **supply chain**, such as from a farm to a food processor and then to a distributor who sells the item to a foodservice. **Supply chain management** is a common business term that refers to conscious efforts to ensure the supply chain runs efficiently and effectively.

So, let's take a look at the supply chain for foods served in a restaurant or foodservice. Many of the vegetables eaten in foodservices across the country come from farms in California such as those found in the Central Valley. Some vegetables will go directly from the field to area restaurants in what is known as farm-to-table operations, while most of the vegetables will be shipped somewhere to be processed (such as frozen) or used as ingredients by a manufacturer to make products like salsas or soups.

The supply chain, also called the **distribution channel**, is; therefore, the pipeline foods travel from their point of origin through various businesses to arrive at a foodservice for preparation and service to customers. **Figure 7-1** shows the typical distribution channel for foods. The source of foods could be growers such as farmers who grow crops, or ranchers who raise livestock such as cattle. Dairy, poultry, and hog producers are also called farmers. Most foods produced by farmers and ranchers will move on to a processor and/or manufacturer. For example, a processor washes fresh salad greens, cuts them into smaller pieces, and packages them for sale to foodservices. Food processing typically involves activities such as washing, slicing, dicing, freezing, canning, or pasteurizing (for milk). A manufacturer, such as a bread company, buys raw materials like wheat flour, which a processor has produced by milling wheat. A manufacturer like Arnold Bread use a series of processes with varying numbers of steps to make their breads and rolls.

The next participant in the distribution channel is the **distributor**. Distributors act as intermediaries or links between the processors/manufacturers and foodservices. Each foodservice depends on a variety of distributors for the right products for their operation. Distributors do more than just deliver food, as many help with menu planning and provide ingredient and nutritional information as well as promotional materials. Distributors are also referred to as wholesalers, vendors, and suppliers. Distributors may fall into one of several categories.

1. **Specialty distributors** handle only one category or niche of goods—such as dairy, coffee, baked goods, ice cream, or fountain beverages (soft drinks).
2. **Full-line distributors** and **broadline distributors** sell a wide variety of food and nonfood supplies. What makes the two different is that broadline distributors also sell foodservice equipment such as sheet pans or mixers. Examples of national broadline distributors include Sysco, US Foods, Performance Food Group, and Gordon Food Service. Large national distributors often ask their suppliers to produce some private label foods for them, which are called **packers' brands**. For example, Sysco has its own line of Italian staples known as Arrezzio. In fact, some large distributors actually operate their own processing facilities to produce quality meats, seafood, fruits, and vegetables.
3. **Cash-and-carry distributors** are used by smaller restaurants and foodservices that may not have large enough orders for delivery by a full-line or broadline

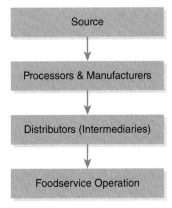

FIGURE 7-1 Distribution Channel for Foods

distributor. The cash-and-carry distributor could be Restaurant Depot (an outstanding outlet for small operations) or a wholesale club such as Costco, BJ's, or Sam's Club or a store run by a distributor, such as a Gordon Food Service Store.

Although most full-line and broadline distributors carry milk and bread, many foodservices buy these very perishable items directly from a dairy or bakery. Whereas a distributor may make one or two deliveries (also called "drops") a week to a foodservice, bread and milk are delivered more often.

In addition to distributors, another intermediary who works with foodservices is the **broker**. A broker represents food processors or manufacturers and brings product samples to foodservices to promote their use. If the foodservice decides to order a product from a broker, the broker will earn a sales commission and place the order with a distributor. The broker never maintains an inventory or fills orders and they are not technically employees of the companies they represent. They do help the foodservice use and market their product. Brokers often represent several companies with different product lines. Examples of brokers include Acosta Foodservice and Waypoint.

The distribution channel for foods can change depending on the buying power of the foodservices. As mentioned, smaller foodservices that don't meet the minimum order requirements of a distributor are often forced to shop at a cash-and-carry distributor. On the other hand, large companies that buy a lot of food (and, therefore, have increased buying power) can go directly to processors and manufacturers to buy products and save money by removing the distributor. Some products may be made to the custom specifications of the large foodservice. This is how franchise restaurants (such as Burger King) and foodservice contractors (such as Sodexo) do much of their purchasing. Multi-unit operations often have products delivered to their own **central distribution centers**, from which trucks deliver to the individual foodservice units.

In addition, some multi-unit foodservices may own a commissary. A **commissary** adds value by processing food from a bulk state and reducing labor at each operation. For example, commissary workers may take large cuts of beef and cut unique steaks, fajita strips or cubes, or make specialty burger patties. They may also make proprietary recipe items such as sauces, soups, salad dressings, or pies to ensure consistency, or they can chop and blend all the fresh vegetables needed for salads. They can even make individual salads, sandwiches, wraps, and snacks for convenience stores like 7-11, Wawa, and Sheetz (Smith, 2016). The foods are made to exact specifications and shipped directly to the foodservices, sometimes with labels, prices, and bar codes already on them. Large college campuses sometimes use a "central commissary dining hall" with a larger-than-average kitchen to produce all of the grab-and-go items (like a sandwich or salad) for their vending machines, coffee shops, and convenience stores. Commissaries help save time and labor at the point of service and will become more important as a way to reduce costs.

7.2 DESCRIBE THE ORGANIZATION AND OBJECTIVES OF A PURCHASING DEPARTMENT

How the purchasing function is organized depends a lot on the size of the foodservice and whether it is an independent or multiunit operation. The person responsible for purchasing is generally in charge of organizing, staffing, directing, and controlling the purchasing activities, as well as coordinating with other departments such as accounting to pay the invoices.

In small independent foodservices, the owner/manager and/or chef are usually in charge of purchasing along with their other duties. In medium independent foodservices, a full-time purchasing agent is not normally needed, so the owner/manager often supervises ordering completed by the kitchen manager (chef), head bartender, and

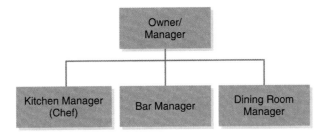

FIGURE 7-2 Example of Medium Foodservice Organization in Which Owner/Manager Supervises Purchasing by Managers

dining room manager (**Figure 7–2**). A clear policy should always spell out exactly who has the authority to place orders.

In larger independent foodservices, an assistant manager may be responsible for purchasing. Even larger foodservices may employ a full-time purchasing director who supervises buyer(s) as well as a receiving clerk and/or storeroom manager (**Figure 7-3**).

In a multiunit restaurant chain or a foodservice contractor, a corporate purchasing director and staff (e.g., food buyer, beverage buyer, supply buyer) select and purchase the items needed as well as oversee the central distribution center or commissary when used. If there is no central distribution center or commissary, the corporate purchasing director still negotiates regional or national contracts with processors and manufacturers. By guaranteeing to buy a certain amount of product, the corporate purchasing director can get lower prices. The corporate purchasing department does not usually procure all of the items needed by every foodservice unit as that would be impossible.

At the local foodservice unit level, the unit manager orders many needed items from the central distribution center and/or commissary (**Figure 7-4**). Foods that are not available from them are often purchased from suppliers approved by the corporate purchasing department or the unit manager may be allowed to purchase some items from other suppliers. If neither a central distribution center nor commissary is used, the unit manager orders foods using the regional/national contracts, as well as orders from other approved suppliers and some local suppliers. This is important to businesses that want to support the local community.

Regardless of how the purchasing function is organized in a foodservice, the objectives of purchasing remain similar. The following is a discussion of common purchasing objectives.

1. <u>Buy the correct products and services</u>. Many factors affect which is the right product or service to purchase. When purchasing food, a buyer considers factors such as the quality desired, the budget, the kitchen equipment available, the skills of the food preparation/cooking staff, service style, and customer satisfaction. For example, you may choose whole frying chickens for a fried chicken dish. But first you will need to decide whether the chickens will be fresh or frozen (frozen chicken is less expensive but it will take time to thaw out, and once it is cooked,

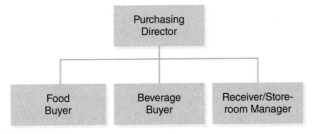

FIGURE 7-3 Example of Purchasing Department in Large Foodservice Organization

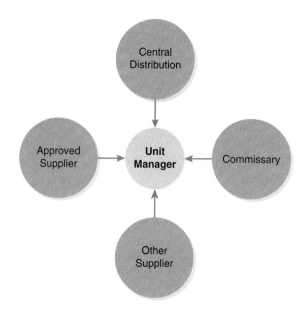

FIGURE 7-4 Where a Unit Manager May Purchase Food

it will be slightly drier). You also need to consider whether the cooks have the time and skills to cut up the chicken properly.

2. <u>Obtain maximum value from purchases</u>. Buyers analyze prices and products from different vendors to determine whether price and product quality give maximum value for their operation. Good value means less waste. One supplier might trim their meats more closely, give you shorter stems on your heads of broccoli, or remove the dark and torn outer leaves from lettuce that would be discarded anyway.

3. <u>Evaluate and select appropriate suppliers</u>. Excellent suppliers are those who are committed to quality standards, give value, and make timely deliveries. More on this topic is discussed shortly.

4. <u>Establish and build good relations with suppliers</u>. When the relationship involves friendliness and trust, conflicts will be easier to resolve and buyers can gain better value for their business.

5. <u>Maintain the foodservice's competitive position in the marketplace</u>. A good purchasing department makes sure the prices paid are as good as or better than your competition so the foodservice can compete with other operations in your region or marketplace.

6. <u>Buy appropriate quantities of products for delivery at the right time to minimize **stockouts** (running out of an item) and investment in inventory</u>. Inventory takes up space and also requires money, so it is best to keep just enough inventory to prevent running out of items (which isn't always easy to do).

7. <u>Monitor supply markets and trends and strive to find new and better products and sources of supply</u>. New foodservice products are constantly being introduced. Some may be great to add new flavors, add variety, or help save a cook's time. New sources of supply may provide more consistent ingredients or reduced recipe cost.

8. <u>Select and implement appropriate technology</u>. Technology can save time and improve ordering, receiving, and inventory management.

9. <u>Develop and use policies and procedures</u>. Policies and procedures help guide the purchasing function. For example, it is important to make clear who has the power to spend the organization's money and how much money they are

Table 7-1 Common Guidelines for Ethics in Purchasing
1. <u>Follow applicable laws and regulations governing the purchasing function</u>. The **Uniform Commercial Code (UCC)**, passed and overseen by all states, governs commercial transactions including purchasing and the obligations of a buyer to its employer. The UCC also covers warranties and the law of warranty recognizes three types of warranties. In general, a supplier must uphold any warranties that a product will perform in a certain manner. The UCC also contains rules about contracts, including when a contract must be written, what it must contain, and how to handle offering and acceptance of contracts.
2. <u>Avoid activities that would compromise or give the perception of compromising the best interests of your employer</u>.
3. <u>Refrain from purchasing when there is a conflict of interest</u>. A conflict of interest is "a conflict between the private interests and the official or professional responsibilities of a person in a position of trust" (Merriam Webster, 2016). This can occur, for example, if you place an order with a company that part of your family owns.
4. <u>Do not accept or solicit money, discounts, gifts, meals, entertainment, or services from present or future suppliers that could influence your purchasing decisions</u>. Most organizations have specific guidelines on what you can and can't accept from a supplier.
5. <u>Refrain from publicly endorsing products</u>.
6. <u>Purchase without prejudice to get the maximum value for each dollar spent</u>.
7. <u>Promote positive relationships with your suppliers by being professional, competent, courteous, and impartial</u>.
8. <u>Do not disclose confidential or proprietary information</u>.

authorized to spend (weekly or per order). Also, employees doing online ordering need to keep their passwords secret as any place where money is changing hands can lead to problems such as embezzlement. To prevent problems such as unauthorized purchases or goods purchased for personal use, it is best to assign related buying functions to different people (at least two different people). This way, no single person has complete control over all buying activities. In addition, you don't want the same person who approves purchases to receive the orders and it is best to have yet another person who reviews the invoices and reconciles the financial records.

10. <u>Abide by ethical standards</u>. Ethics is often defined as norms for conduct that describe acceptable and unacceptable behavior. Many organizations and professions have their own code of ethics to guide their members and establish trust. For example, the Code of Ethics developed by the Academy of Nutrition and Dietetics includes guidance relevant to purchasing when it discusses conflicts of interest (Peregrin, 2018). **Table 7-1** lists some common ethics guidelines, such as not accepting or soliciting money, discounts, gifts, meals, entertainment, or services from present or future suppliers that could influence purchasing decisions.

7.3 EXPLAIN HOW PREPURCHASING ACTIVITIES ARE ACCOMPLISHED

Before buyers can place an order, they need to know what to order, how much to order, when to order, and who to order from. This section will look at these important prepurchasing activities.

Using the menu and recipes, along with input from the chef and other personnel, the buyer can start the process of selecting what to buy. For example, if the menu calls for whole green beans and baby carrots as side dishes, you could buy them in a variety of grades and package sizes, and also fresh, frozen, or canned, so decisions will need to be made. It is best to take the time to develop a food specification for each item you purchase. A **food specification** is a written detailed description including size, color, quality requirements, packaging information, and any other relevant information. Specifications typically include the following information.

1. Name of product. This is the common name for the food, such as boneless chicken breast or canned kidney beans.

2. Intended use of the product. This is very important because it affects what type of product you should buy. For example, if you are buying eating apples, they need to be a different variety and higher quality than apples for pie filling.

3. Description: The description includes the market form of the food and other pertinent information. **Market form** includes the temperature of the food (refrigerated, frozen, room temperature, or dry), its shape (whole or cut up in some way such as sliced cheese), and whether it is raw or cooked. The description section also includes information related to size, such as the weight for portion-controlled items (10-ounce steaks or 6- to 6.5-ounce chicken breasts) or count per container (size 150 Gala apples). Size 150 tells you that one case contains 150 apples and also indicates size. The size 150 apple is a small apple and weighs about 4.5 ounces. (To compare, a size 48 apple weighs 14 ounces.) The description may include point of origin for certain foods, such as Vermont cheddar or Washington State apples, or requirements such as certified grass-fed beef or organic.

4. Quality indicators. Two indicators of quality include inspection and grading. For example, the inspection and grading of meat and poultry are two separate programs within the U.S. Department of Agriculture (USDA). **Inspection** for safe and wholesome meat, poultry, and processed egg products is mandatory while **grading** for quality is voluntary. The USDA currently grades meats, poultry, shell eggs, butter, cheeses, and fresh and processed fruits and vegetables. In some cases, purchasing agents prefer to use a brand, such as Heinz ketchup, instead of a grade to designate quality. Purchasing agents may also state "U.S. Grade A or equivalent" so that suppliers with equivalent quality products can participate in the price quotation or bid.

5. Unit on which price is quoted/packaging information. The unit on which the price is quoted will vary and could be per case, pound, can, bunch, or other package size. For example, meats are normally priced per pound, gallons of milk per gallon, many fresh herbs per bunch, and canned goods per case. A common can size is the #10 can and they are packed six to a case, but there are other can sizes as well (see **Table 7-2**). Packaging information for fresh produce varies from product to product, and at least two different size packages are available for most

Table 7-2 Common Can Sizes for Foodservices

Case Size Number and Number/Case	Approximate Volume of Food	Approximate Weight of Food	Principal Products
No. 1 (Picnic) (48/case)	1¼ cups	10½ to 12 oz.	Condensed soups, some fruits and vegetables
No. 300 (24/case)	1¾ cups	14 to 16 oz.	Some fruits and meat products
No. 2 (24/case)	2½ cups	18 or 20 oz.	Juices, ready-to-serve soups, some fruits
No. 2½ (24/case)	3½ cups	26 or 30 oz.	Fruits, some vegetables
No. 5 (12/case)	5¾ cups	46 or 51 oz.	Institutional size: Condensed soups, some vegetables, meat and poultry products, fruit, vegetable juices
No. 10 (6/case)	12 cups (3 quarts) to 13⅔ cups	6 pounds to 7 pounds 5 oz.	Institutional size: Fruits, vegetables, some other foods.

Data from *Food Buying Guide for Child Nutrition Programs*, p. I-15 - I-16, by U.S. Department of Agriculture, 2017.

produce. For example, California avocadoes come in single layer boxes called **flats** that weigh 12.5 pounds, as well as boxes called **lugs** that contain two layers of avocadoes and weigh about 25 pounds.

6. <u>Other requirements</u>. Depending on what you are buying, there will likely be additional requirements to state.
    - A buyer may include the maximum amount of waste allowed (for produce) or **drained weight** (for canned fruits), specific ingredient or nutrient requirements, and delivery requirements such as the temperature you want the product to be when delivered.
    - To ensure fresh products, some buyers may add a reference to expiration dates, such as on a specification for milk or bread.
    - A buyer may also stipulate that a product is **Kosher** (for the Jewish religion) or **Halal** certified (for the Muslim religion). Kosher food is divided into meat (no pork, shellfish, or birds of prey allowed), dairy, and pareve (a neutral food that contains no meat or dairy). Meat and dairy are not eaten together. Pareve foods such as fruits, vegetables, grains, and water in their natural state are considered Kosher. Kosher meat must be slaughtered in a special way. For Muslims, all foods are considered Halal (permitted) except animals not properly slaughtered using Islamic rules, pork, carnivorous animals and birds of prey, and blood (Islamic Food and Nutrition Council of America, 2019). Halal meat and poultry must be slaughtered and processed according to Islamic requirements.
7. <u>Acceptable substitutions</u>. In some cases where appropriate, a buyer may allow substitutions, hopefully previously agreed upon by both buyer and vendor. In this case, at the end of the specification, it will state "or equal." Vendors do experience shortages, or "outs" as they are called, so establishing acceptable substitutions in advance is helpful.

Specifications should be written and given to suppliers before orders are placed so that price quotations consider the desired quality of the products needed. When writing specifications, buyers do the following.

- State requirements in clear and appropriate terms so that several suppliers will be able to quote prices. If a buyer writes a product specification that only one supplier can provide, that supplier has little incentive to give a good price. Getting quotes from several suppliers helps to keep prices down because the suppliers know they have to compete against each other. Buyers can review a distributor's database to see the specifics about any of the items they sell.
- It is also important to rely on more than just U.S. grades to ensure quality. First, there can be quite a bit of variation within a grade, such as in USDA Choice beef or U.S. No. 1 fresh produce. Second, fresh meat or produce do lose quality after grading depending on how it is packed and transported and how long it takes to get to the foodservice. Third, many imported fruits and vegetables are not graded and grading is voluntary.

Nowadays with more preprepared ingredients and menu items available, a chef has more options to consider. For example, when a successful sandwich shop uses shredded lettuce for many of its menu items, the buyer may develop a specification for heads of lettuce (that will be washed and shredded in-house) or prewashed shredded lettuce. Of course, it is more cost-effective (less expensive) to buy heads of lettuce than lettuce that has been washed and shredded, but then the cost of washing and shredding the lettuce in the foodservice has to be added to the cost of the heads of lettuce to really compare the costs accurately. A manager may do a **make-or-buy analysis** not only to compare the costs of the two options (including food and labor costs) but also the quality of each product as well as the labor/skills/equipment required for in-house preparation (see **Table 7-3**). If buying prewashed, shredded lettuce provides the quality needed, while also freeing up labor time that could be put to another use, the choice may be to buy shredded lettuce.

Table 7-3 Make-or-Buy Analysis for Italian Beef Lasagna				
Italian Beef Lasagna		**Stouffers**	**Whole Foods**	**Modified**
	<u>Scratch</u>	<u>Frozen RTB</u>	<u>Heat and Eat</u>	<u>Frozen RTB</u>
Servings	24	24	24	24
Time to Prep (minutes)	40	5	2	6
Cooking time (minutes)	55	70	25	70
Total Food Cost	$29.00	$15.40	$82.00	$16.00
Labor Cost @ $18/hr	$12.00	$1.50	$0.60	$1.80
Gas/Electric Cost	$4.75	$3.75	$1.35	$3.80
Total/Prime Cost	$45.75	$20.65	$83.95	$21.60
Cost per Serving	$1.91	$0.86	$3.50	$0.90
Average Customer	5	3.5	4.5	4
Rating out of 5 Stars	★★★★★	★★★ ½	★★★★ ½	★★★★

Before you place an order, you have to figure out how much to order and when to order it. Order dates are based on when deliveries are made. Delivery dates depend on when the supplier is in your area. Buyers don't usually have a lot of choice in terms of when deliveries will be made. Full-line and broadline distributors often deliver twice a week, such as Monday and Thursday, or whenever they are doing deliveries in your area. Vendors who supply more perishable products, such as milk and baked goods, often deliver more frequently. If the distributor delivers on a Thursday morning, for example, the buyer may need to place the order by Wednesday morning. **Lead time** is the time between when an order is placed and when it is delivered. Lead time must be considered to avoid running out of something.

When deliveries are made, most items go right into storage. Every foodservice stores foods, beverages, and supplies for use when needed. The amount of foods, beverages, and supplies that are on hand are referred to as the **inventory**. It's important to have a large enough inventory so you are not running out of items between deliveries, but you also need to avoid having excess items sitting in storage for these reasons.

1. When the inventory is larger than it needs to be, the foodservice is tying up money in the inventory instead of investing the money somewhere else, such as making improvements or hiring a new employee.
2. The space for the inventory costs money. The less inventory space needed, the less expensive the storage costs.
3. It takes longer to count up the stock when the inventory is larger than it need be.
4. If food is stored too long, the greater the chance it will spoil.
5. Excess food may also encourage theft by employees.

By ordering the ideal amount of products to be delivered and then used close to delivery, a buyer can maintain a lean inventory. **Just-in-time purchasing** is when a buyer purchases goods so that they're delivered just as they're needed to meet customer demand.

The buyer determines the optimal amount to order using the menu and/or par values. For example, if a foodservice has a two-week cycle menu and sirloin steak is on the menu once in the cycle, the buyer will use the menu to order that item in just before it is needed. The amount of steak ordered will be based on the number of servings that are forecast and then subtracting any steak that may be in inventory. A **forecast** is a prediction of how much of each menu item will be needed for a specific time period or meal. Using the menu and forecast to determine order quantities works best with foods that are not used on a daily or almost daily basis, and foods (such as meats and poultry) that are quite expensive (so you don't want to over order).

For foods and ingredients that are used frequently in the kitchen, such as pancake mix, salad greens, or gallons of milk, a par value may be used. A **par value** is the amount of a product that is needed to meet production requirements for one order period plus a small amount of safety stock. Par values represent the maximum amount of a food to keep on hand, and they work best for foods where consistent amounts are used between orders. For example, in a foodservice that uses 4-ounce hamburgers every day, it would be best to set a par value for hamburgers. So, if the par for 10-pound boxes of hamburgers is set at six and there are two boxes in stock plus one box will be used before the new order comes in, the buyer will order five boxes to get back up to six boxes. Par values need to be constantly evaluated and adjusted to keep them as accurate as possible.

Most large purveyors (such as Sysco or US Foods) with online ordering systems allow you to create a personal order guide for your foodservice operation, which includes the items you normally order. This guide is usually printable so you can take it to your storage areas to see what you have "on hand" prior to placing an order. If you have the order guide on a tablet, you can enter your inventory right into the ordering system.

The final prepurchasing activity to be discussed is finding suppliers. Names of potential suppliers can be collected by using national and local trade magazines and directories, attending trade shows and conventions (such as the National Restaurant Association Show), speaking with managers of nearby foodservices, and conducting Internet searches.

Buyers can use the criteria listed in **Table 7-4** to compare suppliers and then develop a list of approved suppliers. The most important criteria revolve around price, quality, timely deliveries, and sanitation practices. Every time a supplier makes a delivery, the delivery costs money. Whenever a supplier can make one large drop shipment to a foodservice instead of shipping it in batches, the buyer should be able to get a better price. Buyers also have a responsibility to ascertain that the sanitation practices of their vendors meet their standards. To do so, buyers should inspect each vendor's facility as well as ask questions such as how many employees are HACCP certified or if all their meat/poultry suppliers operate under a HACCP plan.

Table 7-4 Qualities of a Good Supplier
• Has helpful and responsive sales personnel who are knowledgeable about the products, the market, and the needs of the individual foodservice.
• Has planned and productive sales calls.
• Offers products that meet quality and quantity needs (in stock).
• Delivers on a timely basis with few back orders, substitutions, or rejections (when an item in a delivery arrives in poor condition and is sent back).
• Has fair, reasonable, and competitive prices.
• Uses current technology such as computerized ordering with out-of-stock notices.
• Invoices correctly and issues prompt credits.
• Maintains clean facility and trucks.
• Is honest and fair.
• Has a financially sound business.

SPOTLIGHT ON SUSTAINABLE PURCHASING

Sustainable purchasing is better for the environment. Here are some ways foodservices try to implement sustainable purchasing. For specific information for each food group, look at the *Sustainable Food Purchasing Guide* by the Yale Sustainable Food Project (available online).

1. *Source local foods especially when fresh and in season.* By sourcing local foods, you are supporting local farms and communities. An excellent resource for purchasing local foods is *Procuring Local Foods for Child Nutrition Programs* by the USDA (available online).
2. *Buy organic foods.* **Organic** food is produced by farmers who emphasize the use of renewable resources and the conservation of soil and water to enhance environmental quality for future generations. Before a product can be labeled organic, a government-approved certifier inspects the farm where the food is grown to make sure the farmer is following all the rules necessary to meet US Department of Agriculture organic standards. Organic is really important for fruits and vegetables with the most pesticide residues, especially when the skin is eaten. Examples include strawberries, spinach, apples, grapes, peaches, pears, tomatoes, potatoes, and bell peppers.
3. *Serve meals that are plant-based.* An animal-based diet requires more fertilizer, water, energy, and pesticides than a vegetarian diet. Studies show that changing from beef to chicken, fish, eggs, or vegetable-based entrées has less harmful effects on the environment and can reduce greenhouse gases. Beef is also more expensive to produce than any other meat or poultry. Chefs have been adding more plant-based recipes to the menu and using more plant ingredients such as beans and nuts. A diet higher in plant-based foods and lower in animal foods not only has less environmental impact but is also healthier.
4. *Buy sustainable fish.* For information on specific seafood to purchase, visit the websites of the Monterey Bay Aquarium Seafood Watch (United States) or SeaChoice (Canada). Green Chefs, Blue Ocean is a comprehensive, interactive online sustainable seafood training program and resource center.
5. *Start a garden to grow herbs, vegetables, and other foods.* More chefs are growing some of their own produce and herbs. When growing your own foods and serving them, the chef needs to consult with the local health department to get the necessary permission (may require a variance) to do so.
6. *Buy coffee and tea from sustainable operations.* Some conventional growers use mass production methods involving excessive chemicals and pesticides. To avoid those problems, there are several certification programs, such as Fair Trade or Rainforest Alliance Certified, where coffee is grown more sustainably. You can also buy certified organic coffee.
7. *Reduce bottled beverages.* Encourage the use of reusable cups and "bottleless" beverage options, and source bottles from companies that use less plastic or glass in their bottles.

7.4 SUMMARIZE FEDERAL FOOD SAFETY LAWS AND AGENCIES INVOLVED

Many federal agencies, along with state and local agencies, are responsible for making sure that the foods Americans eat are safe and labeled accurately. The following are several federal agencies and how each is involved. The U.S. Department of Agriculture (USDA) and Food and Drug Administration (FDA) oversee much of the food supply, but other agencies also play roles in specific areas.

- The U.S. Department of Agriculture's *Agricultural Marketing Service* (AMS) sets grade standards and currently grades fruits and vegetables (fresh and processed), meat, poultry, shell eggs, butter, and some cheeses. Grading is *voluntary*. Grading is often done cooperatively between the USDA and the state department of agriculture. The Agricultural Marketing Service is also responsible for setting standards for organic foods.
- The U.S. Department of Agriculture's *Food Safety and Inspection Service* (FSIS) inspects meat, poultry, and processed egg products for safety and wholesomeness. Inspection of these foods is *mandatory*. FSIS enforces the Federal Meat Inspection Act, the Poultry Products Inspection Act, and the Egg Products Inspection Act.

- The <u>Food and Drug Administration</u> (FDA), an agency within the Department of Health and Human Services, is responsible for ensuring the safety of the food supply (including imported foods) and it also regulates food labeling. The FDA is responsible for enforcing the Food, Drug, and Cosmetic Act, Fair Packaging and Labeling Act, and Nutrition Labeling and Education Act. To enforce various regulations, the FDA performs inspections of businesses that manufacture, process, or pack foods (except for meat, poultry, and processed eggs where the FSIS is responsible). In 2016, the FDA published final rules on a new Nutrition Facts label for packaged foods (**Figure 7-5**), which are currently in use. The label better reflects new scientific information on the link between diet and chronic disease.
- The <u>U.S. Department of Commerce's *National Oceanic and Atmospheric Administration (NOAA) Fisheries*</u> section oversees the Seafood Inspection Program, a voluntary program that inspects and grades seafood (fresh and frozen).
- The <u>U.S. Public Health Service</u> (part of the U.S. Department of Health and Human Services) along with the FDA have set the standards for Grade A fresh milk. The U.S. Public Health Service also works with states to ensure safe, wholesome milk.
- The <u>Alcohol and Tobacco Tax and Trade Bureau</u> (part of the U.S. Department of the Treasury) enforces laws covering the production and labeling of alcoholic beverages with at least 7% alcohol. The FDA monitors alcoholic beverages that are under 7% alcohol.

This is not a comprehensive list of federal agencies. It is meant to show the agencies that are most involved.

Table 7-5 explains components of the major food laws, starting with the Pure Food and Drug Act of 1906, which defines **misbranded foods** (if the food label contains false or misleading information or omits required information) and adulterated foods. **Adulterated foods** are those that are harmful to health; prepared, packed, or held under unsanitary conditions; or contain filth or part of a diseased animal. In 1938, The Food, Drug, and Cosmetic Act defined the following terms.

- **Standards of identity** define the nature of a specific food in terms of types of ingredients the food must contain and/or how it is made. For example, one of the requirements for an item to be labeled *fruit jam* is that it is made from crushed fruit. If made from fruit juice instead of crushed fruit, it must be labeled *fruit jelly*.
- **Standards of fill** for a container set out requirements as to how much food must be in the container so the container appears well-filled and the buyer is not deceived. For example, some standards for canned fruit specify minimum weights of solid food that must be present after being drained of liquid.
- **Standards of quality** set minimum requirements for the quality of a product. For example, canned fruits are often graded on color, appearance, flavor, odor, uniformity in size, and the presence of defects or blemishes.

7.5 OUTLINE HOW VARIED BUYING METHODS WORK

Once the specifications are written and other prepurchasing activities are completed, the buyer is ready to get prices and give orders to suppliers. Depending on the circumstances, the buyer will use informal purchasing or formal purchasing.

The buyer basically goes through these steps in the **informal purchasing** process to order foods.

1. First, determine exactly how much to purchase using various tools such as the menu and par values.

Nutrition Facts

8 servings per container

Serving size   2/3 cup (55g)

Amount per serving

Calories   230

% Daily Value*

Total Fat 8g	**10%**
Saturated Fat 1g	**5%**
Trans Fat 0g	
Cholesterol 0mg	**0%**
Sodium 160mg	**7%**
Total Carbohydrate 37g	**13%**
Dietary Fiber 4g	**14%**
Total Sugars 12g	
Includes 10g Added Sugars	**20%**
Protein 3g	
Vitamin D 2mcg	10%
Calcium 260mg	20%
Iron 8mg	45%
Potassium 235mg	6%

* The % Daily Value (DV) tells you how much a nutrient in a serving of food contributes to a daily diet. 2,000 calories a day is used for general nutrition advice.

FIGURE 7-5 Nutrition Facts Label

Food and Drug Administration (https://www.fda.gov/food/new-nutrition-facts-label/whats-new-nutrition-facts-label)

Table 7-5 Major Food Laws

Pure Food and Drug Act (1906)
- Defined "misbranding" and "adulteration."
- Made it a federal crime to sell misbranded or adulterated foods, beverages, or drugs in interstate commerce.

Federal Food, Drug, and Cosmetic Act (1938)
- Replaced and expanded on the Pure Food and Drug Act (1906).
- FDA was given authority to oversee the safety of food and inspect where foods were made.
- Required that food labels contain the common name of the food and prohibited false or misleading statements on food label.
- Provided Standards of Identity, Standards of Quality, and Standards of Fill.
- Required color additives to be subject to rigorous standards of safety before being used in food and artificial colors had to be declared on the label.

Miller Pesticide Amendment (1954)
- Set safety limits for pesticide residues on domestic and imported agricultural products such as fruits.

Food Additives Amendment (1958)
- Required manufacturers of new food additives to establish their safety.
- Established a list of additives that are generally recognized as safe (GRAS).
- Prohibited approval of any food additive shown to induce cancer in humans or animals.
- Required all additives to be declared on food label.

Color Additive Amendment (1960)
- Defined "color additive" and "unsafe color additive" and required that only color additives listed as "suitable and safe" for a given use could be used in foods.
- Required manufacturers to establish color additive's safety *before* marketing.
- Specific factors to be used by FDA to determine if a color additive was safe, such as cumulative effect in the diet.

Fair Packaging and Labeling Act (1966)
- Required the food label to state name of product, name and address of manufacturer/packer/distributor, net quantity of contents, and list of ingredients (from highest in weight or volume to lowest).

Nutrition Labeling Regulations (1973)
- Called for voluntary nutrition labeling and required nutrition information on foods fortified with vitamins, minerals, or protein, or any food making a nutritional claim.

Nutrition Labeling and Education Act (1990)
- Required uniform nutrition labeling on packaged food based on serving size (except fresh meat and poultry).
- Required more detailed declaration of some ingredients.
- Regulated nutrition content claims and health claims and made them consistent.

Food Safety Modernization Act (2010)
- Requires food facilities to implement a written HACCP plan.
- Mandates regular inspections, based on risk, for food facilities (including some foreign facilities).
- Requires certain food testing to be carried out by accredited laboratories.
- Gives FDA more tools to respond quickly when problems emerge, such as detaining products, mandatory recalls, and suspension of a facility's registration.
- Gives FDA more authority to ensure that imported products are safe and meet U.S. standards.

2. Request price quotations from suppliers, often by phone, on the items you need to order.
3. Evaluate prices and possibly negotiate some prices with suppliers.
4. Select the supplier(s) and place the order(s). This is often completed on the same day that the buyer gets the price quotations.
5. Receive shipment according to the delivery schedule. Keep in mind the lead time (or lag time) between when an order is placed and when it is received and the fact that your inventory continues to be used up between when you place the order and when you receive the order.
6. Review and approve the invoice.

Informal purchasing works well for items with prices that change frequently (such as fresh meat and produce) and smaller orders.

To start the process, the buyer goes through the menu and walks through the storage areas to determine how much to order for each item. Next, the buyer calls several suppliers and records the prices (and date) on a form so there is a formal record. In some cases, a supplier may fax in prices. After evaluating the prices and possibly negotiating with a supplier, the buyer is ready to place the order by computer, phone, or fax.

The buyer has to prepare a **purchase order** (**Table 7-6**), which is a sales agreement stating the items to be purchased, pricing, credit terms, and delivery date. The purchase order is often completed online and it functions as a written sales contract. The purchase order includes the name and address of the supplier and the buyer. The term F.O.B. (Free on Board) identifies who pays to ship the goods and who owns them while they're in transit. If the purchase order says F.O.B. the supplier's address, the buyer must arrange and pay for shipment from the supplier. From the time the goods leave the supplier, the buyer owns the goods. On the other hand, if the purchase order says F.O.B. the buyer's address, the supplier is responsible for shipping to the buyer and assumes responsibility if the goods are damaged on route to the buyer.

Informal purchasing works differently in a foodservice that is part of a larger organization (such as a hospital) with **centralized purchasing**. A centralized purchasing department oversees all of the purchasing within the organization, and the foodservice department has to work with this department to get the ordering done. When a school district's foodservice office makes purchasing decisions and consolidates purchases for all schools, that is centralized purchasing. The foodservice buyer will still determine what and how much needs to be ordered, which is written up as a **purchase requisition** and given to central purchasing. Central purchasing will then use the purchase requisition to get prices, decide which suppliers to use, and place the purchase orders.

Whereas informal purchasing involves getting price quotes quickly, there are times when **formal purchasing**, which takes more time, is desirable or required. Formal purchasing is especially useful for staples, such as canned tomatoes, that have a relatively stable price and are used frequently. A foodservice can usually get a better price for canned tomatoes (and other similar items) if they commit to one distributor for a period of time, such as six months. In tax-supported institutions, such as many schools and hospitals, foodservices must use formal purchasing when the purchase goes above a certain amount of money to make sure the money is well spent.

Table 7-6 Purchase Order Form

Purchase Order

Emily's Deli
16 North Main St.
Anytown, CO
Vendor: Sysco, Pocomoke City, MD
F.O.B. Emily's Deli, Anytown, CO

Purchase Order No.: _____
Order Date: _____

Line	Item Description/Specification	Pack Size	Quantity	Price/ Unit	Extended Price
1					
2					
3					
4					
5					
6					

Formal purchasing uses a procurement process known as competitive proposals or bids. The most common are **Requests for Proposal (RFP)** or an **Invitation for Bid (IFB)**. Since the bidding cycle has a number of steps, and each step takes time, the timing of each step must be carefully considered so the process starts early enough to be completed properly. It is not unusual for the process to start six or more months ahead of when the items will be purchased. The steps in the bidding cycle are described here.

1. If the only criterion for the award is price, an IFB is normally developed, which includes product needs, specifications, and amounts that almost any vendor could provide. The bid may request prices for a one-time purchase or prices over a given period of time. Each vendor is asked to hand in a **sealed bid** by a given date and time. A sealed bid means each vendor must submit their price offer in a sealed envelope that won't be opened until the given time.

2. If a foodservice doesn't have generic specifications for a product, or wants additional services provided, they should develop a RFP that outlines the goods and/or services needed. Like the IFB, the RFP outlines the bidding process and contract terms. The bid document is a legally binding contract and includes bidder qualifications and the date the bid is due. The RFP also includes criteria that will be used to pick the winning vendor. The winning vendor will not necessarily have the lowest overall price but will best meet the criteria. If a school foodservice, for example, wants a foodservice contractor to run the school cafeterias within a district, the school district will write up a RFP for meals and services.

3. The RFP or IFB is sent to qualified distributors/vendors. In some cases, a public announcement to solicit vendors to respond is required.

4. Sometimes, a Prebid Meeting is held with interested vendors to review what is needed and answer questions.

5. At the deadline, the RFP bids are evaluated using the pre-established criteria. The successful bidder(s) is determined and receives the award.

6. Sealed bids sent in response to an IFB are generally opened at a stated time and place and the awardee is the one with the lowest overall bid.

Formal purchasing is designed to provide open competition and make sure that the money spent results in the best product at the lowest possible price.

The following are some variations on informal and formal purchasing.

1. **Group purchasing.** Certain foodservices purchase some products through a **group purchasing organization (GPO)**. For example, a group of hospital foodservices in a region may work jointly with a GPO to put their orders together (such as for milk). The GPO then uses the greater buying volume to get better prices for the foodservices involved.

2. **Standing orders.** With a standing order, a driver pulls up at a foodservice and takes inventory of certain items such as packages of fresh bread and rolls. Using par levels, the driver writes up a delivery ticket of what needs to be stocked. Then the driver grabs the items from the truck and stocks up the bread racks in the foodservice. Once the driver has finished stocking, the delivery slip is handed in so that it gets paid at a later date. Standing orders may be used for breads and rolls, milk, ice cream, beer kegs, and tablecloths/napkins.

3. **Prime vendor contract.** The prime vendor contract is based on the idea that a distributor will generally give better prices to a foodservice when the foodservice purchases large volumes of food and beverages over a period of time from them. (The same thing happens when a consumer goes to Costco or Sam's Club—because they are buying larger size packages than at a supermarket, the prices are lower.) A prime vendor contract is special pricing that a distributor offers to foodservices for the items they frequently buy over a specific period of time. The pricing is often based on **cost-plus pricing** (cost of the product plus a fixed markup) for items with stable prices such as canned goods. With cost-plus

pricing, the cost of an item can go up or go down. The foodservice should have the right to audit the distributor periodically to make sure the correct cost was charged. Sometimes, pricing may be based on **cost plus percentage** (cost of the product plus an additional percentage) or market pricing. **Market pricing** is simply the current price on the market and it is used for items with prices that fluctuate frequently, such as produce and seafood. With cost plus percentage pricing, prices increase in proportion to cost.

In today's world, the quantities you purchase can have a dramatic effect on the price you pay. So, if you are a small, independent business, it may help you to leverage purchasing power with other small businesses by joining a Group Purchasing Organization. The GPO combines the purchasing power of its members to negotiate pricing with both suppliers (such as US Foods or Sysco) and manufacturers (such as Dole, Heinz, Kraft, or Tyson). As a GPO member, you could serve on the committee that chooses which foods, small equipment, or cleaning chemicals on which to negotiate pricing. The overall spending power of the group gives you leverage and increases your importance as a customer.

The main job of the GPO is to promote competition and innovation in the procurement and purchasing process. Businesses that use the services of a GPO, on average, save about 15% versus individual purchasing or "street pricing" (Hale Group, 2012). In healthcare foodservice, some of the major GPOs include Vizient ($100 billion annually and includes more than 50% of acute-care hospitals) and Premier ($50 billion annually and includes 76% of all community hospitals) (Gooch, 2017). Foodbuy is an example of a GPO that restaurants may use. Because each group is trying to increase its market share and purchasing power, they often recruit new foodservices that pay a fee to join a GPO. However, if you work with your national distributor or prime vendor, they may be able to add you to existing contracts free of charge.

Whichever buying method is used, buyers always want optimal prices. But what is an optimal price? **Table 7-7** shows an example of meat prices (as purchased—AP—before trimming and cooking) that a foodservice obtained from two suppliers. Some buyers will take this meat order and award each item to the supplier who bid the lowest price (shown in Table 7-7 with an underline), so the order will be split between the two suppliers. This is known as **line–item purchasing** (or **cherry picking**) because buyers examine the prices on each line item and then award each item to the lowest bidder. Other buyers will look at the cost of the total order for Supplier A and Supplier B

Table 7-7 Line-Item Purchasing vs. Bottom-Line Purchasing

Product	Amount	Supplier A Price	Supplier B Price
Beef Rib Steak, IMPS 1103, USDA Choice (high), 10 oz.	45 pounds	$9.39/pound	$9.69/pound
Lamb, boneless shoulder, rolled and tied, IMPS 208, 2.5 to 3 pounds each, USDA Choice (high)	20 pounds	$8.79/pound	$9.10/pound
Pork tenderloin (IMPS 415), US No. 2, 1.5–2 pounds each	30 pounds	$3.99/pound	$3.89/pound
Hamburger patties from USDA Choice ground sirloin, 4 oz. each	70 pounds	$4.55/pound	$4.59/pound
Top round roast, IMPS 169, USDA Choice, 17–20 lb. ea.	60 pounds	$3.03/pound	$2.99/pound
TOTAL	By line item: $1,212.95	$ 1218.35 Supplier A	$ 1235.45 Supplier B

and award the entire order to whoever has the lowest bottom line (known as **bottom-line purchasing**). As shown in Table 7-7, Supplier A is less expensive overall than Supplier B, but a buyer could save even more money by using line-item purchasing ($1,212.95). One advantage of line-item purchasing is that each supplier gets some business so that they feel it is worth the time to bid prices. If the buyer continually gives the entire order to Supplier A because they are less expensive, at some point, Supplier B is not going to want to spend time giving prices for no benefit.

Optimal AP prices are easy to point out. However, the optimal price to pay should be based on edible-portion (EP) costs for items such as meats that shrink in cooking, fresh vegetables that are trimmed, or canned fruits that have different drained weights. In these situations, the buyer can easily calculate EP cost by using this formula (discussed more in Chapter 6).

EP cost = AP price divided by yield percentage

As an example, let's use the top round roast in Table 7-7. A cooking yield test on a 20-pound top round roast from Supplier A and Supplier B gave these yield percentages: 0.80 for Supplier A and 0.72 for Supplier B. Now we can calculate the EP cost/pound

Supplier A: $3.03 divided by 0.80 = $3.79 EP cost/pound
Supplier B: $2.99 divided by 0.72 = $4.15 EP cost/pound

So, even though Supplier B has a lower AP price, its EP price is 36 cents higher/pound than Supplier A.

SUMMARY

7.1 Outline the distribution system for food and supplies.

- The distribution channel (or supply chain) for foodservices starts at the source (such as a farm or ranch) and continues to processors and manufacturers, distributors, and finally to foodservice operations. Distributors, also called wholesalers, may be cash-and-carry distributors, specialty distributors, full-line distributors, or broadline distributors such as Sysco that sell food and equipment.
- A broker represents food processors or manufacturers and calls on foodservices to promote their products. If a foodservice buyer orders the product, the broker places the order with a distributor and earns a sales commission. Brokers are not employees of the companies they represent.
- Large and multi-unit foodservices that buy a lot of food have increased buying power and can go directly to processors and manufacturers to buy products and save money. Multiunit operations often have products delivered to their own central distribution centers, from which trucks deliver to the individual foodservice units. Some multiunit operators also own a commissary to process and prepare foods to ensure consistency at each unit.

7.2 Describe the organization and objectives of a purchasing department.

- How the purchasing function is organized depends a lot on the size of the foodservice and whether it is an independent or multiunit operation. In small independent foodservices, the owner/manager and/or chef usually do the purchasing. In medium independent foodservices, a full-time purchasing agent is not normally needed, so the owner/manager often supervises ordering completed by the kitchen manager (chef), head bartender, and dining room manager. In larger, multiunit foodservices, one or more people are devoted to purchasing (Figure 7-3).
- In a multiunit operation, a unit manager may order from the central distribution center or commissary (if used) as well as approved and other suppliers.
- The objectives of a purchasing department are to buy the right products and services, obtain maximum value from purchasers, evaluate and select appropriate suppliers, establish and build good relations with suppliers, maintain

the foodservice's competitive position in the marketplace, buy appropriate quantities of products for delivery at the right time to minimize stockouts and inventory investment, monitor supply markets and trends, strive to find better products and sources of supply, select and implement appropriate technology, develop and use policies and procedures, and abide by ethics standards (see Table 7-1).

7.3 Explain how prepurchasing activities are accomplished.

- Before buyers can place an order, they need to know what to order, how much to order, when to order, and who to order from.
- To determine what to order, a buyer must develop a food specification. A specification includes the following information: Name of product, intended use of product, description (such as market form and size), quality indicators (such as inspection or grading required and/or a brand name), unit on which price is quoted and packaging information (such as flat or lug for produce), and any other requirements (such as maximum amount of waste allowed).
- It is important to rely on more than just U.S. grades to ensure quality. First, there can be quite a bit of variation within a grade, such as in USDA Choice beef or U.S. No. 1 fresh produce. Second, fresh meat or produce do lose quality after grading depending on how it is packed and transported and how long it takes to get to the foodservice. Third, many imported fruits and vegetables are not graded and grading is voluntary.
- With more preprepared ingredients and menu items available, such as lettuce that has already been washed and cut, a buyer has more options to consider. A manager may do a make-or-buy analysis to compare the food and labor costs of buying washed and cut lettuce versus doing that work in the kitchen. The analysis should also examine the quality of each product as well as the labor/skills/equipment required for in-house preparation.
- Full-line and broadline distributors often deliver twice a week or whenever they are doing deliveries in your area. Vendors who supply more perishable products, such as milk, deliver more frequently. If the distributor delivers on a Thursday morning, for example, the buyer may need to place the order by Wednesday morning.

- When the inventory is larger than it needs to be, the foodservice is tying up money in the inventory instead of investing the money somewhere else. The space for inventory also costs money. Excess food can spoil and may encourage employee theft.
- For menu items that are only on the menu once a week, the buyer may order those items in just before they are needed. For foods and ingredients that are used frequently in the kitchen, such as gallons of milk, a par value (the amount of a product that is needed to meet production requirements for one order period plus a small amount of safety stock) is often used. Par values represent the maximum amount of a food to keep on hand, and they work best for foods where consistent amounts are used from order period to order period.
- Table 7-4 lists qualities of a good supplier.

7.4 Summarize federal food safety laws and agencies.

- The U.S. Department of Agriculture's *Agricultural Marketing Service* sets grade standards and grades fruits and vegetables (fresh and processed), meat, poultry, shell eggs, butter, and some cheeses. Grading is *voluntary*. The Agricultural Marketing Service also sets standards for organic foods.
- The U.S. Department of Agriculture's *Food Safety and Inspection Service* inspects meat, poultry, and processed egg products for safety and wholesomeness. Inspection of these foods is *mandatory*.
- The Food and Drug Administration is responsible for ensuring the safety of the food supply, including imported foods, and it also regulates food labeling. To enforce various regulations, the FDA performs inspections of businesses that manufacture, process, or pack foods (except for meat, poultry, and processed eggs where the FSIS is responsible).
- The U.S. Department of Commerce's National Oceanic and Atmospheric Administration (NOAA) Fisheries section oversees the Seafood Inspection Program. The U.S. Public Health Service along with the FDA set standards for Grade A fresh milk.
- Table 7-5 explains components of major food laws, such as how the Food, Drug, and Cosmetic Act defined standards of identity, standards of fill, and standards of quality.

7.5 Outline how varied buying methods work.

- Buyers use various methods to purchase goods: Informal purchasing (asking suppliers for price quotations on a regular basis mostly for items with prices that change frequently like fresh meat and produce), formal purchasing (bid buying involving a Request for Proposal or Invitation for Sealed Bid) group purchasing, and prime vendor contracts (committing to buy a number of items over a period of time using cost-plus, cost plus percentage, or marketing pricing.)
- Foodservices that are part of a larger organization may need to hand purchase requisitions to a centralized purchasing department that does the buying.

- A purchase order is a sales agreement stating the items to be purchased, pricing, credit terms, and delivery date.
- Once buyers have prices from several suppliers, some buyers will use line-item purchasing while others use bottom-line purchasing to decide who gets the order(s).
- Optimal AP prices are easy to point out. However, the optimal price to pay should be based on edible-portion (EP) costs for items such as fresh vegetables that are trimmed, meats that shrink in cooking, or canned fruit that have different drained weights. Sometimes, a supplier has a lower AP price than others but a higher EP price.

REVIEW AND DISCUSSION QUESTIONS

1. Describe the distribution channel for foods. What is another term for distribution channel?
2. What types of distributors do food purchasers buy from?
3. As a purchasing manager, what would you want to achieve in addition to getting competitive prices?
4. What is a conflict of interest?
5. Why do buyers develop food specifications? Describe the components of a food specification.
6. Why would a manager do a make-or-buy analysis?
7. Why is it important for the purchasing agent to not maintain too large of an inventory?
8. How is a par value set?
9. As a purchasing agent, what are you looking for in your suppliers?
10. Which federal agencies are involved in making sure that foods are safe to eat and labeled accurately?
11. How do inspection and grading differ?
12. Distinguish between standards of identity, standards of fill, and standards of quality.
13. Compare and contrast informal and formal purchasing, including their advantages and disadvantages.
14. Explain how group purchasing and also prime vendor contracts work. What are their advantages and disadvantages?
15. What's the difference between line-item purchasing and bottom-line purchasing?
16. What events in the environment—such as anything related to the economy or climate—could have an effect on prices?

SMALL GROUP PROJECT

For this part of the project, you will need the two recipes that you converted to 140 portions in Chapter 6.

1. For each recipe, you will complete **Table 7–8**, Quantities to Purchase for Recipes, which is also posted on the Companion Website in

Word format. Fill in the ingredient names in the first column and how much of each ingredient is needed in the second column.
2. If the recipe quantity is in cups (such as flour), and you need to order flour by the pound, convert from cups to pounds in the third column. At this point, you can use the *Distributor*

Table 7-8 Quantities to Purchase for Recipes

RECIPE NAME: _____

Recipe Yield: 100 servings

Portion Size: _____

Ingredient	Amount Needed	Amount Needed in Purchasing Unit	Quantity to Purchase	
			Yield %	AP Quantity

Catalog on the Companion Website to preview purchasing units.

3. If an item in a recipe still needs to be trimmed (such as fresh broccoli) or cooked (such as a raw beef roast), use the yield percentage as discussed in Chapter 6 to determine the quantity to purchase. You don't need to do this for items such as portion cut meats or chicken.

4. Calculate the Quantity to Purchase—the final column.

5. Next, develop a specification for each item you need to order and enter it on the *Purchase Order* in the second column.

6. Now you can use the *Distributor Catalog* on the Companion Website to find the exact items you will purchase along with the packaging information. Enter the pack size and quantity needed on the Purchase Order (on the Companion Website in Word format). Make sure the quantity entered will cover your needs. If an ingredient, such as eggs, is used in more than one recipe, add up how many total eggs you need before you fill in the Purchase Order.

7. In addition to ordering for the recipes, you also need to order the following (enough for 200 servings).
    - Fluid low-fat milk (½ pints) *plus* one other beverage.
    - Two condiments: portion-controlled packaging or bulk.
    - One fresh fruit to be eaten whole.
    - One ready-to-serve dessert.
    - Dinner rolls (prepared).

8. You will be handing in the completed *Quantities to Purchase for Recipes* for *each* recipe *and* the Purchase Order.

REFERENCES

Code of Federal Regulations. (2020). *Subchapter B - Food for human consumption, Part 135, Frozen desserts*. Retrieved from https://www.ecfr.gov/cgi-bin/text-idx?SID=8bc97923842340f4a315557acf5b4592&mc=true&node=sp21.2.135.b&rgn=div6

Feinstein, A. H., Hertzman, J. L., & Stefanelli, J. M. (2017). *Purchasing: Selection and Procurement for the Hospitality Industry*. Hoboken (NJ): John Wiley & Sons, Inc.

Gooch, K. (2017). 4 of the largest GPOs/2017. *Becker's Hospital CFO Report*. Retrieved from https://www

.beckershospitalreview.com/finance/4-of-the-largest-gpos-2017.html

The Hale Group. (2012). GPOs in foodservice — landscape & growth opportunities. Retrieved from http://www.halegroup.com/~halegrou/wp-content/uploads/2012/05/GPOs-in-Foodservice.pdf

Islamic Food and Nutrition Council of America. (2019). What Is Halal certification? Retrieved from https://www.ifanca.org/Pages/Faq.aspx

National Oceanic and Atmospheric Administration. (2018a). What is aquaculture? Retrieved from https://oceanservice.noaa.gov/facts/aquaculture.html

National Oceanic and Atmospheric Administration. (2018b). Seafood commerce & certification. Retrieved from https://www.fisheries.noaa.gov/topic/seafood-commerce-certification

National Oceanic and Atmospheric Administration. (2019). U.S. aquaculture. Retrieved from https://www.fisheries.noaa.gov/national/aquaculture/us-aquaculture

NOAA Fisheries. (N.D.). *Seafood Inspection Manual*. Retrieved from https://www.fisheries.noaa.gov/national/seafood-commerce-certification/seafood-inspection-manual

North American Meat Processors Association. (2010). *The Meat Buyer's Guide*. Reston (VA): NAMP.

Peregrin, T. (2018). Revisions to the Code of Ethics for the nutrition and dietetics profession. *Journal of the Academy of Nutrition and Dietetics, 118*(9), 1764–1767.

Produce Marketing Association. (2003). *Fresh produce manual*. Retrieved from http://www.americanfruitandproduce.com/uploads/data/pm.pdf

Smith, D. P. (2016). The convenience store threat. *FSR Magazine*. Retrieved from https://www.foodnewsfeed.com/fsr/convenience-stores/convenience-store-threat

U.S. Department of Agriculture. (2014). *Institutional Meat Purchase Specifications, Fresh beef, Series 100*. Retrieved from https://www.ams.usda.gov/sites/default/files/media/IMPS_100_Fresh_Beef%5B1%5D.pdf

U.S. Department of Agriculture, Food and Nutrition Service. (2015). *Procuring local foods for child nutrition programs* (FNS-465). Retrieved from https://theicn.org/icn-resources-a-z/procuring-local-foods-for-child-nutrition-programs/

U.S. Public Health Service. (2017). Grade "A" Pasteurized Milk Ordinance. Retrieved from https://www.fda.gov/downloads/Food/GuidanceRegulation/GuidanceDocumentsRegulatoryInformation/Milk/UCM612027.pdf

Yale Sustainable Food Project. (2008). *Sustainable food purchasing guide*. Retrieved from https://www.sare.org/Learning-Center/SARE-Project-Products/Northeast-SARE-Project-Products/Sustainable-Food-Purchasing-Guide

© Denis Val/Shutterstock

Resource Guide to Writing Specifications for Specific Foods

This section will give guidelines for developing specifications for these food groups: Fresh fruits and vegetables, processed produce and grocery items, meat, poultry and eggs, seafood, and milk and dairy products.

FRESH FRUITS AND VEGETABLES

Buying fresh fruits and vegetables can be challenging for a number of reasons.

- For many fruits and vegetables, the buyer must choose a **variety**. For example, apples come in varieties such as Fuji, Honeycrisp, Granny Smith, or Jonathan. Each variety has its own flavor, texture, and sometimes color. Also, some varieties, such as Jonathan, are better for baking, whereas Honeycrisps are excellent for baking or eating.
- Produce prices change frequently, in part because the supply of produce varies depending on when a fruit or vegetable is in season and also how the weather has affected the quality of the harvest. Some fruits and vegetables are mainly available during the months they are in season, which is also the time when prices are (usually) lowest. For example, California sweet peppers are available from May through November, but imported sweet peppers are available any time during the year.
- Produce is packed in many different ways. For example, onions come in bags in several sizes including 50 pounds, or onions may be packed in 40- or 50-pound cartons. Strawberries are often packed in a 12-pound flat, each holding 12 pints.
- Although much produce is graded using the USDA grades names of U.S. Fancy, U.S. No. 1, and U.S. No. 2, the grade names and number of grades can vary from item to item. For example, the grades for apples are U.S. Extra Fancy, U.S. Fancy, U.S. No 1, and U.S. Utility. The grades for peaches are U.S. Fancy, U.S. Extra No. 1, U.S. No. 1, and U.S. No. 2.

To develop specifications for fresh fruits and vegetables, resources such as those listed in **Table 7-9** are needed to find information about varieties, availability during the year, packaging, and grades.

Table 7-9 Resources for Writing Produce Specifications
• Especially useful for grading and availability: • USDA Produce Information Sheets (https://www.fns.usda.gov/ofs/produce-information -sheets)
• Especially useful for grading, availability, varieties, and packaging: • Produce Marketing Association's *Fresh Produce Manual* (2003, available online).

• Especially useful for the grades used for a specific fruit or vegetable:
  • USDA Agricultural Marketing Service
    • Vegetable Grade Standards (https://www.ams.usda.gov/grades-standards /vegetables)
    • Fruit Grade Standards (https://www.ams.usda.gov/grades-standards/fruits)

Grading of produce is voluntary and the USDA Agricultural Marketing Service sets the grading standards and performs grading for a fee. State departments of agriculture offer fruit and vegetable grading services under cooperative agreements with the USDA Agricultural Marketing Service (AMS). The grader considers the following factors, with appearance generally being the most important.

- Appearance: Such as appropriate color and shape, well-formed, and proper trimming.
- Defects: Such as blemishes, broken skin, decay/spoilage, foreign material, or damage due to insects, bruising, freezing, or disease.
- Maturity: Mature enough to ensure proper ripening if not ripe.
- Size: Appropriate size, uniform sizes.
- Texture: Appropriate texture such as a firm apple.

Inspection and grading are usually performed at the same time. All imported produce is subject to random inspection as it enters the country, but only a small percentage actually gets inspected.

Here are guidelines for developing a specification for fresh fruits or vegetables. **Table 7–10** includes sample specifications.

1. Name of product: For most fresh produce, you need to include the variety. For example, state navel orange instead of orange, and russet potatoes instead of potatoes. If buying precut fresh produce, such as chopped onions, buyers should state if they want the items prewashed and exactly how they are to be precut. (*Note that there is no grading available for precut produce.*)
2. Intended use: The intended use could vary from making fresh fruit cups, cooking broccoli for a side dish, to having eating apples available.

Table 7-10 Sample Produce Specifications
Fresh seedless whole watermelon
Cut up for fruit dishes and sliced for dessert.
U.S. No. 1 (high end). Elongated seedless. 15 to 25 pounds each. Firm and symmetrical. Fully ripened.
85-pound fiberboard case. Slab-packed.
Fresh whole potatoes
For baked potatoes.
Russet potatoes. U.S. No. 1 (high end). 110 count. Washed.
50-pound carton

3. Description:
    - Buyers indicate the size of an item in different ways such as by specifying "jumbo" onions or the count per box for potatoes. For example, using **Figure 7-6**, you can see that a 100-count carton of potatoes contains 100 potatoes that are mostly between 7 to 9 ounces each. Potatoes in a 120-count carton are smaller in size. Size may also be indicated in the packaging, such as a lug of tomatoes that contains two layers of tomatoes. The tomatoes in the lug may be packed 6 × 6 (36 tomatoes/layer), which are considered "large" tomatoes.
    - For certain items, such as sweet peppers (which can be green, orange, red, or yellow), the color needs to be given.
    - For other items, such as bananas, the degree of ripeness needs to be stated—such as green, turning yellow, or ripe.
    - If certified organic produce is desired, it must also be stated. Organic fruits and vegetables are produced without using most conventional pesticides; fertilizers made with synthetic ingredients or sewage sludge; bioengineering; or ionizing radiation.

4. Quality:
    - Foodservices use the higher grades, such as U.S. Fancy or U.S. No. 1. Since there is a lot of variation within U.S. No. 1, buyers often request the high end of U.S. No. 1. Produce with lower grades are often sent to food processing plants to make juices, soups, jams, and canned fruits and vegetables.
    - There are not many brand names in fresh produce, and if "Chiquita®" bananas are specified, it is a good idea to still include the desired grade, such as high U.S. No. 1.
    - In terms of quality, a buyer knows that once an item is cleaned and trimmed, there will be some waste (see yield table in Appendix D), so the buyer may include the maximum amount of waste allowed.

5. Unit on which price is quoted/packaging information. The unit on which the price is quoted is often the carton but could also be based on per bag, per pound, or per bunch. Buyers should also include the minimum acceptable weight of one carton or bag, as well as how the fruit or vegetable is packed in a carton. **Slab-packed** items, such as potatoes, are placed into a carton without any packaging materials. An item that is more fragile, such as apples, may be layered in a case with cardboard in between the layers. Some produce may be layered in a **cell pack** in which each item sits in its own spot and is protected from touching any other fruit or vegetable in the case.

6. Other requirements. Precut fresh produce must be refrigerated and, therefore, delivered on a refrigerated truck.

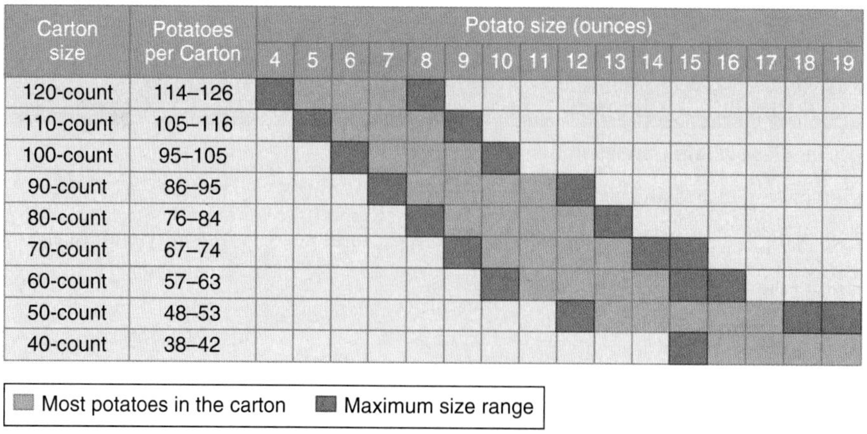

Carton size	Potatoes per Carton	Potato size (ounces) 4–19
120-count	114–126	
110-count	105–116	
100-count	95–105	
90-count	86–95	
80-count	76–84	
70-count	67–74	
60-count	57–63	
50-count	48–53	
40-count	38–42	

☐ Most potatoes in the carton   ■ Maximum size range

FIGURE 7-6 Size Range of Most Popular Idaho Russet Potatoes

Courtesy of Idaho Potato Commission.

PROCESSED PRODUCE AND SELECT GROCERY ITEMS

This section will look at processed fruits and vegetables (such as canned and frozen) as well as some grocery items to include pasta, noodles, rice, and vegetable oils. The FDA has established over 280 standards of identity largely for staple grocery items.

USDA Agricultural and Marketing Services grade canned or frozen fruits and vegetables as a voluntary service. Canned fruits and vegetables are graded on qualities such as color, appearance, flavor, odor, uniformity in size, defects/blemishes, and the quality of the packing medium. Buyers may use the U.S. grades when purchasing these items. Because the exact grades for each canned fruit or vegetable vary, it's useful to check the USDA AMS website (under "Grades and Standards") for the correct grades.

The top quality for many canned or frozen fruits and vegetables is U.S. Grade A (which may also be called "U.S. Fancy") and then U.S. Grade B (which may also be called "U.S. Choice"). For example, the grades for canned peas or canned freestone peaches are U.S. Grade A, U.S. Grade B, U.S. Grade C, and Substandard. The grades for frozen berries are U.S. Grade A or U.S. Fancy, U.S. Grade B or U.S. Choice, and U.S. Grade D or Substandard. A number of processed fruits and vegetables come in different cuts and/or sizes as shown in **Table 7–11**.

Two considerations for canned fruits or vegetables are drained weight and the style of packing medium. **Drained weight** refers to the weight of the can's content once the liquid is completely drained. Of course, the higher the drained weight, the more product you have to serve. The standards for each USDA-graded canned fruit and vegetable include a minimum drained weight, but the buyer can include this on a specification.

For canned fruit, the buyer must specify the packing medium—if the fruit is to be packed in water, its own juice, pear juice, light syrup, or heavy syrup. **Brix** is the measurement of the sugar content of a watery solution such as the packing medium

---

Table 7-11 Cuts and Sizes for Selected Processed Fruits and Vegetables

Canned Fruits

Apricots: halves: sized by count in #10 can: 66–86 (large), 86–108 (medium), 108–130 (small)

Apples: applesauce, diced, sliced, rings

Peaches: diced, slices, quarters, halves
    Peach halves: sized by count in #10 can: 40/50 count (small), 35/40 count (medium), 30/35 count (large), 25/30 count (extra large)

Pears: diced, slices, halves
    Pear halves: sized by count in #10 can: 50/60 count (small), 40/50 count (medium), 30/40 count (large), 25/30 count (extra large)

Pineapple - crushed, tidbits, chunks, slices
    Pineapple slices: sized by count in #10 can: 110 count (small), 66 count (medium), 52 count (large)

Frozen Fruits

Cranberries: halves, whole

Mango: chunks, halves

Peaches: slices, halves

Pineapple: tidbits, chunks

Canned Vegetables

Corn: whole kernel, cream corn

Potatoes: diced, sliced, whole

Tomatoes: sauce, puree, ground, crushed, diced, chopped, whole peeled, stewed

(continues)

Table 7-11 Cuts and Sizes for Selected Processed Fruits and Vegetables (continued)
Frozen Vegetables
Asparagus: cuts and tips, spears
Green beans: cut, French cut (cut lengthwise), whole
Broccoli: chopped, floret, spears
Carrots: diced, sliced, whole baby
Corn: whole kernel, cobette, cob
Okra: cut, whole
Onions: diced, chopped, pearl onions
Potatoes for French fries: crinkle cut, curly, shoestring, straight-cut, steak/wedge, waffle (skin-on is an option for many of these)
Peppers (green, red): diced, strips
Spinach: chopped, leaf

in canned fruit. Therefore, it is expected that heavy syrup (which is sweeter than light syrup) has a higher Brix than light syrup. Canned fruit graded by the USDA includes requirements for minimum Brix levels for different packing mediums. Buyers can specify a Brix level for canned fruits along with the type of packing medium desired. One benefit of a higher Brix is that fruits packed in heavy syrup do not break as easily as fruits packed in less sugar. One disadvantage of a higher Brix is that the product contains more added sugar, which is not nutritious.

To evaluate the quality of a canned product, a **can-cutting test** can be useful. In a can-cutting test, a buyer picks one product, such as fruit cocktail in light syrup, and gets different brands for a testing panel to compare and evaluate. A distributor like Sysco has its own brand of canned fruit with different quality levels, so a buyer may want to compare those too. Ahead of time, it is important to decide which characteristics will be examined and how they will be evaluated. In many cases, the testing will be done blind—meaning that the brand name is blinded to those evaluating the products. **Table 7-12** is an example of an evaluation form for a can-cutting test.

Pasta is made from flour and water that is rolled and cut into a wide variety of pasta shapes (**Figure 7-7**). Pasta may be dried or fresh. The best dried pasta is made from

Table 7-12 Score Card for Can-Cutting Test			
Sample	**A**	**B**	**C**
Overall Appearance			
Color			
Texture			
Taste			
Size			
Clearness of Liquid			
Uniformity of Size			
Lack of Defects			
Rate above characteristics from 1 to 5 (5 = best quality) **Team to fill in below after completion of top section**			
Vendor/Brand			
Drained Weight			
Number of Svg./can			
EP Cost/Svg.			

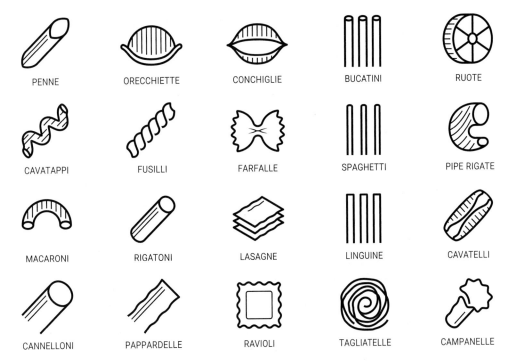

FIGURE 7-7 Pasta Shapes

© Alexandr III/Shutterstock

semolina, a high–protein flour made from durum wheat. Because this flour is so high in protein, it helps the pasta maintain its shape during cooking. High-quality pasta should be yellow in color (due to the semolina), brittle, and able to hold its shape well during cooking.

Pasta may also be made with whole wheat flour (or semolina with whole wheat flour) or gluten-free flours (such as those made from rice, corn, lentils, or chickpeas). Some pastas include additional ingredients—such as egg solids (to make egg pasta) or vegetable purees (such as spinach pasta).

Asian cuisine uses a wide variety of noodles (**Figure 7–8**), some made from wheat and others made with different starches, such as rice noodles and bean thread noodles. Chinese noodles use flour and water and some add egg as well. Soba noodles are an example of Japanese wheat noodles that are thin and include some buckwheat. Udon noodles are long, white thick noodles that are also Japanese.

When choosing rice, buyers need to consider the variety of rice and also the shape and length of the kernel. Long-grain rice is three to five times as long as it is wide. The cooked grains are separate and fluffy and work well in dishes such as pilaf and rice salads. Medium grain rice is a little shorter and plumper than long-grain rice after cooking and has a greater tendency to cling together, so it works well in paella and risotto. Short-grain rice is very sticky and is used in rice puddings and Japanese cooking.

Milled white rice has been milled to remove the outer bran covering. Brown rice has the bran layer left on so it requires more time to cook than white rice. Brown rice is also chewier and nuttier in flavor than white rice. Other examples of rice varieties (**Figure 7–9**) include the following.

- *Arborio rice* is an Italian, short-grain rice that is used to make risotto, a creamy rice dish.
- *Basmati rice* is an aromatic, long-grain rice with a nutty flavor that is widely used in India and works well in stir-fries and curries.
- Originally from Thailand, *jasmine rice* is a long-grain white rice that is more floral in flavor than basmati. Steaming it works well and it is excellent in Mediterranean dishes.

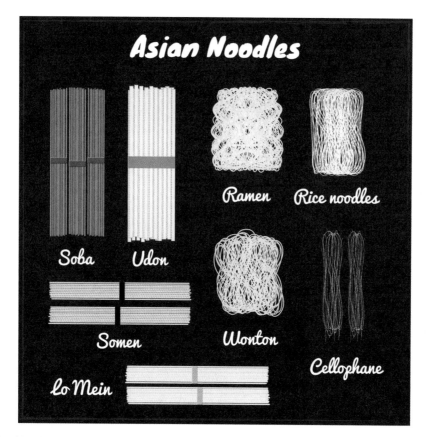

FIGURE 7-8 Asian Noodles

© Minur/Shutterstock

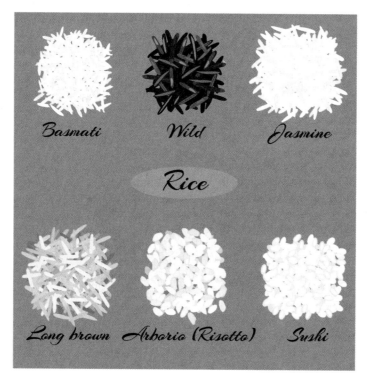

FIGURE 7-9 Rice Varieties

© Everilda/Shutterstock

- *Wild rice* is not a true rice but actually a grain. Its long dark kernels have a unique, nutty flavor.
- *Moolgiri rice* is a low glycemic index rice that is popular on low carbohydrate and diabetic diets.

Table 7–13 gives information on selected vegetable oils. There are USDA standards for olive oil. U.S. Extra Virgin Olive Oil has excellent flavor and odor while U.S. Virgin Olive Oil has good flavor and odor. Both of these oils are made from olives that are

Table 7-13 Characteristics and Uses of Oils

Oil	Characteristics	Uses
Almond oil	Light golden color. Clean flavor.	Sautéing, frying.
Avocado oil	Buttery, nutty flavor with green color.	Sautéing. Flavoring finished dishes and in salad dressings.
Canola oil	Light yellow color. Neutral flavor.	Sautéing, stir-frying, salad dressings, baked goods.
Corn oil	Golden color. Bland flavor.	Sautéing, stir-frying, baked goods. Too heavy for salad dressings
Hazelnut oil	Dark amber color. Nutty and smoky flavor.	Good for flavoring finished dishes such as pasta, potatoes, and beans. Used in salad dressings. Sautéing.
Olive oil	Color and flavor depend on olive variety, level of ripeness, and how oil was processed.	Extra virgin or virgin—good for flavoring finished dishes and in salad dressings, strong olive taste. Pure olive oil—can be used for sautéing and in salad dressings. Light olive oil—the least flavorful, good for sautéing and stir-frying.
Peanut oil	Pale yellow color. Mild nutty flavor.	Sautéing and stir-frying. Good for salad dressings.
Pecan oil	Flavorful.	Works well in salad dressings. Sautéing and stir-frying.
Pine nut oil	Subtle and mild.	For flavoring finished dishes such as pesto, sauces, and soups.
Safflower oil	Golden color. Bland flavor.	Sautéing and in baked goods. Used in salad dressings
Sesame oil	Sweet nutty flavor. Toasted sesame seed oil has a more intense flavor.	Good for sautéing, flavoring dishes, and in salad dressings.
Soybean oil	Light color. Bland flavor.	Good for sautéing, frying, and in baked goods. Good oil for salad dressings.
Sunflower oil	Somewhat neutral flavor.	Good for sautéing, frying, and in baked goods, if refined. Good oil for salad dressings.
Walnut oil	Medium yellow to brown color. Rich, nutty flavor.	For flavoring finished dishes and in salad dressings. Heating produces some bitterness.

Reproduced from Drummond, K. E., & Brefere, L. M. (2016). *Nutrition for foodservice and culinary professionals.* John Wiley & Sons.

ground into a paste and then pressed to extract oil. No heat or processing is involved. U.S. Olive Oil consists of a blend of refined olive oil and virgin olive oils without further processing.

The following are guidelines for writing specifications. Sample specifications appear in **Table 7–14**.

1. <u>Name of product</u>: State the exact name including canned, frozen, etc., as appropriate. Use the names from the Standards of Identity when appropriate. For example, canned fruit cocktail is not the same as canned fruit salad.

2. <u>Intended use</u>: The intended use should include the menu item(s).

3. <u>Description</u>:
   - For canned fruit, the buyer must specify the packing medium—if the fruit is to be packed in water, in its own juice, or in pear juice. Most fruits also come packed in light or heavy syrup. Heavy syrup has more sugar than light syrup. Some canned fruits are also available in extra light syrup or extra heavy syrup.
   - For many processed fruits and vegetables, the buyer must specify the cut and/or size (see Table 7–11).
   - Buyers may also specify minimum drained weight for canned fruit and vegetables.
   - Buyers specify the type and shape of the pasta or noodles. Some pasta brands have a number on their container for long pasta such as spaghetti. As the number increases, the pasta is thicker.
   - For pasta, buyers often specify the type of grain used, such as semolina and/or whole wheat. For noodles, specify the width, such as ¼-inch or ½-inch.
   - Buyers specify the variety of rice along with whether it is long-grain, medium-grain, or short-grain.
   - When a buyer wants a blended oil, the percentage of each oil should be given. For example, a buyer may order a blend of 90% soybean oil and 10% olive oil or 50% canola oil and 50% olive oil.

4. <u>Quality</u>:
   - When buying processed fruits or vegetables, buyers usually specify a federal grade or equivalent, *and/or* a specific brand name. Even when using a brand name such as Dole for pineapple slices, there may be two or more levels of quality for that product so the name must be complete. When appearance is important, U.S. Grade A (U.S. Fancy) is the most appropriate choice. A lower grade could be used when appearance is not important, as in baking.
   - A buyer may specify minimum drained weight for canned goods.

Table 7-14 Sample Processed Produce Specifications
Canned yellow clingstone peach slices.
Used as dessert for patients.
U.S. Grade A or equivalent yellow clingstone peach slices. Packed in juice. Must be peeled. Minimum drained weight: 68.5 oz.
6/#10 cans.
Frozen whole kernel sweet corn.
Used as side dish.
Yellow/golden in color. Non GMO. U.S. Fancy or equivalent.
12/2.5# per fiberboard case. Net weight: 30 pounds per case.
Shipment of frozen vegetable must be at or below 2°F (−17°C).

- Pasta and rice are often purchased by name brand. There are USDA grades for milled rice from U.S. No. 1 to U.S. No 6.
- For olive oil, buyers specify a brand, quality level (extra virgin, virgin, or olive oil), dark colored glass bottles, and appropriate freshness dates.

5. <u>Unit on which price is quoted/packaging information</u>:
    - Prices are normally per case.
    - Canned fruits and vegetables are packed most often in a case of six #10 cans. Some are packed in other can sizes shown in Table 7-2.
    - Pasta is often packaged in a bulk 20-pound case or as 20 one-pound boxes in a case. Rice is often packaged in a bulk 25-pound bag or in a case of smaller packages.
    - Oil is usually available in a case containing six one-gallon bottles. Smaller size bottles are available.
    - Two other important grocery items are cold cereals and portion-controlled packets of condiments. Cold cereals are sold in individual boxes of 72/case or in cases containing four bags (about 30 oz. each) for bulk dispensers. Portion-controlled salad dressings are often 60/case. Other portion-controlled condiments are often 200/case, but mustard is often 500/case and ketchup 1,000/case.

6. <u>Other requirements</u>:
    - For some items, requirements for freshness dating may be used.

MEAT

Foodservices spend a large proportion of their purchasing dollars on meat, poultry, and seafood. This section will look at meats including beef, veal, pork, lamb, bison, and game meats such as venison. We will start by looking at beef.

The beef carcass is cut lengthwise into two sides of beef. Each side is then cut into the **primal cuts** seen in **Figure 7-10**. Primal cuts, such as the rib, are further divided

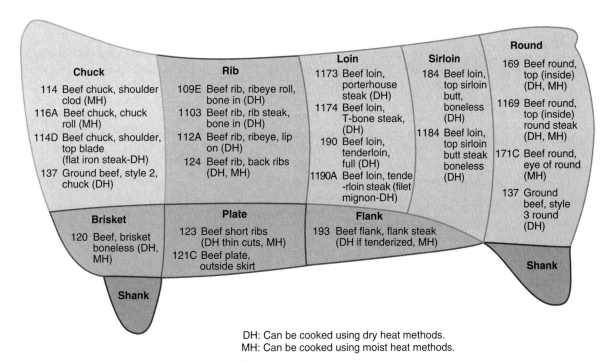

DH: Can be cooked using dry heat methods.
MH: Can be cooked using moist heat methods.

FIGURE 7-10 Examples of Beef Cuts Using IMPS

Data from "Institutional Meat Purchase Specifications" by USDA Agricultural Marketing Service, 2014.

into cuts of meat for cooking. Generally speaking, meat that touches the backbone is tender and can be cooked using dry-heat methods. The most tender cuts include those from the loin, sirloin, and ribs, which have ample fat distributed throughout the meat (called **marbling**). Marbling is associated with tenderness. The round (rear of animal) and chuck (shoulder) contain some cuts that are moderately tender and others that are less tender. Less tender cuts need to be cooked using moist-heat cooking methods such as braising. Less tender cuts also come from the shank, brisket, plate, and flank. Any muscles that get a lot of exercise, such as the legs and neck, will be firmer and tougher than the muscles along the spine of the animal.

Figure 7-10 shows popular cuts of beef used in foodservice. Each cut includes the Institutional Meat Purchase Specifications (IMPS) numbers. The Institutional Meat Purchase Specifications are a series of meat product specifications maintained by the USDA Agricultural Marketing Service. They were developed as voluntary specifications and are widely used in foodservice. Purchasers such as restaurants, hotels, schools, and other foodservices reference the IMPS when buying meats. For example, here is the full IMPS for the porterhouse steak found under "Loin" in Figure 7-10.

"Item No. 1173 - Beef Loin, Porterhouse Steak - The steaks shall be prepared from any IMPS short loin item. The maximum width of the tenderloin shall be at least 1.25 inches (3.2 cm) when measured parallel to the length of the back bone." (USDA, 2014, p. 68)

In addition to the IMPS number, you may include the quality grade, thickness of surface fat, and/or the weight of each item (such as a roast or steak). **Table 7-15** shows the categories of IMPS for meats. Using the website noted at the bottom of Table 7-15, you can access all of the IMPS.

All beef cattle start their lives eating grass, but conventional cattle then spend their last months in a feedlot being fattened up with grains such as corn. The grains put weight on cattle quickly, and results in beef that has more fat than grass-fed animals. **Grass-fed cattle** only feed on grass, forage, hay, or silage so they grow at a slower pace and are not normally slaughtered until up to 12 months later than grain-fed cattle. This helps explain why, compared with grain-fed beef, the flavor of grass-fed beef is more robust. As for **organic beef**, regulations require that cattle are raised in living conditions accommodating their natural behaviors (like the ability to graze on pasture), are fed 100% organic feed and forage, and do not receive antibiotics or hormones.

Veal is the meat from a calf or young beef animal. A veal calf is raised until about six to seven months when they weigh about 500 pounds. Male dairy calves are frequently used to produce veal. Veal meat has a light color, fine texture, and is naturally tender.

Pork from domestic pigs is another popular meat. There are four primal cuts into which pork is separated. From the (rear) leg comes fresh ham roasts while the belly/spareribs provide bacon and spareribs. The loin (which is tender) offers pork chops, loin roasts, and country style ribs; while the shoulder (which is tough) provides ground pork for sausage as well as roasts and other cuts. Some pork cuts, such as ham and bacon, are often cured—meaning they are exposed to a combination of salt, sugar, nitrite

---

Table 7-15 Institutional Meat Purchase Specifications Numbering System

- 100 Fresh Beef
- 200 Fresh Lamb and Mutton
- 300 Fresh Veal and Calf
- 400 Fresh Pork
- 500 Cured, Cured and Smoked, Cooked Pork Products
- 600 Cured, Dried and Smoked Beef Products
- 700 Variety Meats and Edible By-Products
- 800 Sausage Products

"Institutional Meat Purchase Specifications" by USDA Agricultural Marketing Service, 2014. Retrieved from https://www.ams.usda.gov/grades-standards/imps

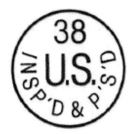

FIGURE 7-11 Inspection Mark on Meat

Courtesy of USDA Agricultural Marketing Service.

and/or nitrate to prevent spoilage and add flavor. Some pork products are both cured and smoked, meaning they were exposed to a wood fire to add a distinct flavor.

The Federal Meat Inspection Act requires that all meat sold commercially must be inspected and passed to ensure that it is safe and wholesome. Federal inspection personnel from the USDA's Food Safety and Inspection Service must be present during livestock slaughter operations and their inspection both before and after slaughtering ensures that the meat is fit for human consumption. Inspected facilities must maintain and follow written Sanitation Standard Operating Procedures and Hazard Analysis and Critical Control Point (HACCP) plans. In addition to inspecting the meat products, federal personnel (or equivalent state personnel) inspect the facilities and equipment to confirm sanitary conditions are maintained. **Figure 7-11** shows the inspection mark used on raw meat.

Meat grading is voluntary. Beef, veal, and lamb are often graded, a service that is purchased by the meat company. Higher grades are more tender and juicier and come from younger animals. Lower grades are tougher and require moist-heat cooking methods or they are mechanically tenderized or ground up for hamburger.

The following is a guide to writing up meat specifications. **Table 7-16** contains sample specifications.

1. <u>Name of product</u>. The buyer must state the type and cut of meat, preferably with the IMPS number.
2. <u>Intended use</u>. The name of the menu item and how the meat will be cooked should be included here.
3. <u>Description</u>.
   - State chilled or frozen. Some fresh meats, such as ground beef, are vacuum sealed in a plastic-type film to reduce the oxygen and keep the meat fresh for a longer period of time.

Table 7-16 Sample Beef Specifications
Strip Loin Steak, Center-Cut, Boneless, IMPS #1180A
Entrée—grilled
10 oz. portion ± 0.5 oz., U.S. Choice (High), cut from USDA Yield Grade 2 carcass. Surface fat shall not exceed 1/4″ at any point. Refrigerated.
16/10 lb. case, individually wrapped, layered.
Fresh hamburger patties.
Used for burgers.
8 oz. homestyle patties made from U.S.D.A. Choice (high) ground chuck. No more than two days from packaging to delivery.
20 patties/10-pound box. Stack packed in moisture-proof box.

- State special requirements such as USDA certified organic meat or grass-fed beef.
- State the weight range for roasts (such as 16–19 pounds for a rib roast) and portion cuts (such as 6 oz. ± 0.5 oz). Appendix E contains information about weight ranges for roasts and portioned meats.
- State the thickness of portion cuts. If a piece of meat is over 1-inch thick, it is generally allowed that the thickness range from ¼-inch thicker to ¼-inch thinner than the desired thickness. For portion cut meat, you can also state a portion weight tolerance. For example, a 10-ounce steak has a portion weight tolerance of plus or minus 0.5 ounces so each steak should be between 9.5 and 10.5 ounces. See Appendix E for more information.
- State the maximum fat thickness (either average or at any one point) such as ¾ inch for roasts or ¼-inch for portion cuts. See Appendix E for more information.
- For roasts, state if they must be netted (using stretchable netting) to make them firm and compact or tied with string.
- When ordering hamburgers, buyers must specify the size (such as 2 oz., 3.2 oz., 4 oz., 5 oz., etc.), seasoned or unseasoned, the lean-to-fat ratio, and whether to use ground beef, angus beef, ground turkey, or other product. A lean-to-fat ratio of 75/25 means that the meat contains 25% fat. A leaner product will be 80/20 or 87/13 or 90/10.
- State if the item is to be cured, smoked, or **dry aged**. Beef can be dry aged to increase its flavor and tenderness. The process involves storing beef in the refrigerator at a controlled temperature and humidity for several weeks, during which time the natural aging processes (including evaporation) result in improved tenderness and a concentrated meat flavor. Dry aging increases the price.

4. <u>Quality</u>.
    - <u>Grades for beef</u> are determined by the age, flavor, and extent of marbling, which tells you how tender and juicy the beef will be. The highest grade is USDA Prime, which is produced from young, well-fed cattle. USDA Prime meat has lots of fat and flavor and is used mostly in top restaurants and foodservices. Next is USDA Choice grade with less marbling. Buyers often choose USDA Choice to meet almost all needs. Within USDA Choice beef, there are three levels: High Choice, Average Choice, and Choice. The USDA Select grade is very lean and lacks the tenderness and flavor of higher grades (**Figure 7-12**). There are several more grades below USDA Select: USDA Standard, Commercial, Utility, Cutter, and Canner, but they are not suitable for foodservices. Figure 7-12 shows the grade shields for USDA Prime, Choice, and Select.
    - <u>Grades for veal</u> are USDA Prime, Choice, Good, Standard, and Utility. USDA Prime and Choice qualities are normally chosen as they are juicier, more tender, and tastier than lower grades.
    - <u>Pork is not graded like the other meats</u> because the quality of pork is very consistent. Pork is only graded on yield, meaning the amount of usable lean meat from a carcass. The grades are U.S. No. 1, U.S. No. 2, U.S. No. 3, U.S. No. 4, and U.S. Utility. Yield grade U.S. No. 1 is the highest grade with the most muscle and the lowest amount of fat while U.S. No. 4 has more fat and less muscle. Buyers usually specify U.S. No. 1 or U.S. No. 2.
    - <u>Grades for lamb</u> are USDA Prime, Choice, Good, and Utility. USDA Prime and Choice qualities are normally chosen as, again, they are juicier, more tender, and tastier than lower grades.

5. <u>Unit on which the price is quoted/packaging information</u>. Meat pricing is usually per pound or per case. For example, if you are buying 50 pounds of beef roasts that range from 15 to 18 pounds each, the supplier can't always send you exactly 50 pounds. In that situation, the price is set by the pound, not the case. However,

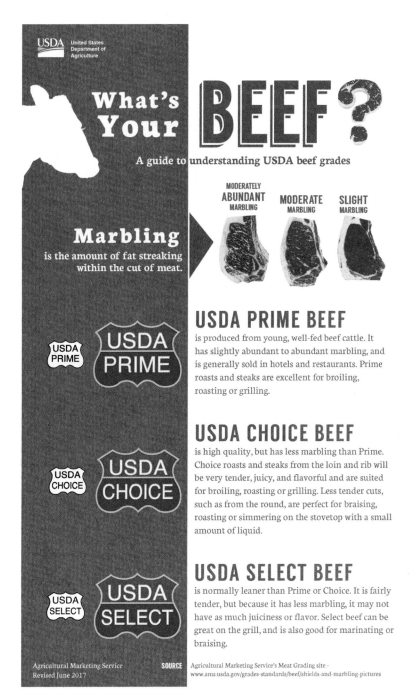

FIGURE 7-12 USDA Beef Grades

Courtesy of USDA Agricultural Marketing Service.

if you are buying hamburgers (4 ounces each) or other portion-controlled meats, they are usually packed in layers in a 10-pound box with patty paper between each layer. A buyer can also specify that each portion be wrapped individually before layering in a case. In either case, the price will be per box. Bacon comes mainly in a bulk pack, **shingle pack** (where it is layered like shingles on a roof), or a **layout pack** (where it is laid out on oven paper so the cook just has to place the paper on a sheet pan to cook). Bacon is available in different sizes or thicknesses. A size of 9/11 means that there are 9 to 11 slices per pound. Bacon is often packed in 15-pound boxes.

6.   Other requirements.
   • A buyer may state the minimum yield after cooking or use U.S. yield grade numbers 1 through 5 (available for beef and lamb only). U.S. Yield Grades range from 1 (lean and heavily muscled) to 5 (plenty of fat and less muscled). Yield grades work differently from quality grades. For example, Prime beef can never have a Yield Grade of 1 or 2 because Prime beef is quite fatty and has less muscle than lower grades such as Choice or Select. Also, the Choice grade can't get a Yield Grade of 1.

POULTRY AND EGGS

The term poultry refers to edible birds domestically raised for human consumption, such as chicken, turkey, and duck. Each kind of poultry is divided into classes (**Table 7–17**) that are based on age and tenderness. Younger birds are naturally tender and can be cooked using almost any method. Older birds have good flavor but will need moist–heat cooking to make the meat tender. Most foodservices use younger, tender poultry such as broiler/fryer chickens, roasting chickens, or young turkeys.

Table 7-17 Poultry Classes

Chicken

A. **Rock Cornish game hen or Cornish game hen**. A Rock Cornish game hen or Cornish game hen is a young, immature chicken (under 5–6 weeks old), weighing not more than two pounds ready-to-cook weight, which was prepared from a Cornish chicken or the progeny of a Cornish chicken crossed with another breed of chicken.

B. **Rock Cornish fryer, roaster, or hen**. A Rock Cornish fryer, roaster, or hen is the progeny of a cross between a purebred Cornish and a purebred Rock chicken, without regard to the weight of the carcass involved; however, the term "fryer," "roaster," or "hen," shall apply only if the carcasses are from birds with ages and characteristics that qualify them for such designation under paragraphs (c) and (d) of this section.

C. **Broiler or fryer**. A broiler or fryer is a young chicken (usually under 10 weeks of age), of either sex, that is tender-meated with soft, pliable, smooth-textured skin and flexible breastbone cartilage.

D. **Roaster or roasting chicken**. A bird of this class is a young chicken less than 12 weeks of age, of either sex, with a ready-to-cook carcass weight of 5.5 pounds or more, that is tender-meated with soft, pliable, smooth-textured skin and breastbone cartilage that is somewhat less flexible than that of a broiler or fryer.

E. **Capon**. A capon is a surgically unsexed male chicken younger than 4 months old that is tender-meated with soft, pliable, smooth-textured skin.

F. **Hen, fowl, or baking or stewing chicken**. A bird of this class is a mature female chicken (usually more than 10 months of age) with meat less tender than that of a roaster or roasting chicken and nonflexible breastbone tip.

G. **Cock or rooster**. A cock or rooster is a mature male chicken with coarse skin, toughened and darkened meat, and hardened breastbone tip.

Turkey

A. **Fryer-roaster turkey**. An immature turkey younger than 12 weeks old of either sex, that is tender-meated with soft, pliable, smooth-textured skin, and flexible breastbone cartilage.

B. **Young turkey**: A young female or male turkey from 5 to 8 months old, that is tender-meated.

C. **Yearling turkey**: A fully-mature female or male turkey under 15 months old, that is reasonably tender-meated.

D. **Mature turkey or old turkey**: A mature or old turkey of either sex in excess of 15 months old with toughened flesh.

United States Classes, Standards, and Grades for Poultry p. 3-4, by U.S. Department of Agriculture Agricultural Marketing Service, 2018.

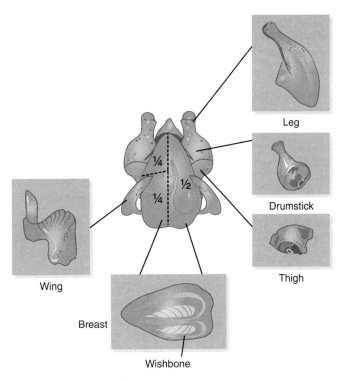

FIGURE 7-13 Whole Chicken and Its Parts

Reproduced from D. Mizer, M. Porter, B. Sonnier, and K. Drummond (2000). Food Preparation for the Professional, p. 340, Hoboken (NJ): John Wiley & Sons, Inc.

Whole birds or parts may be ordered, such as breast, thigh, or wings. **Figure 7-13** shows a whole chicken and how it is cut up to make half chicken, quarter chicken, breasts, wings, and legs (which can be cut to provide drumsticks and thighs). Fresh whole birds usually have the lowest price per pound. When ordering fresh poultry, keep in mind that it is very perishable with a short shelf life. Buyers also purchase processed poultry, such as breaded chicken tenders, which is almost always purchased frozen.

Inspection for safe and wholesome poultry by the USDA Food Safety and Inspection Service is mandatory according to the Poultry Products Inspection Act. Poultry grading by the USDA is voluntary and is paid for by the poultry producers. The grading shield and inspection stamp for poultry are shown in **Figure 7-14**.

Following is guidance on writing up a specification for poultry. **Table 7–18** gives a sample specification.

1. <u>Name of product</u>. The buyer must state the type of poultry, the cut (such as whole or wings), and whether raw or cooked, fresh or frozen.

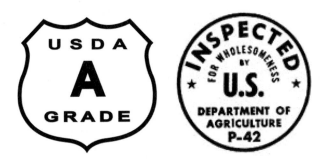

FIGURE 7-14 Grading Shield and Inspection Stamp for Poultry

Courtesy of USDA Agricultural Marketing Service.

Table 7-18 Sample Poultry Specification
Frozen boneless skin-on chicken breasts.
Main dish.
8-ounce split boneless skin-on chicken breasts. USDA Grade A.
24/8 oz. per case. Net weight 12.0 lbs. Product layered in cell packs or equivalent.

2. <u>Intended use</u>. The name of the menu item and how the poultry will be cooked should be included here.
3. <u>Description</u>.
   - Unless specified otherwise, fresh poultry will be delivered skin-on and bone-in. If you want, for example, chicken breasts without the bone or skin, state "boneless and skinless chicken breasts."
   - The buyer must state the weight range for whole birds (such as three pounds) and parts like chicken breasts (such as 4, 6, 8, 10, or 12 oz. each).
   - *The Meat Buyer's Guide* (North American Meat Processors Association) includes IMPS for poultry, which may be used.
   - If desired, state certified organic. Organic poultry means the animal was fed organic feed, did not receive antibiotics, and had access to the outdoors. Free-range chicken must have access to the outdoors.
4. <u>Quality</u>. There are three grades of raw poultry: USDA Grade A, B, or C. The factors that determine the grade are conformation (shape), amount of flesh, fat coverage, and defects such as presence of feathers, bruising, discoloration, and skin tears. USDA Grade A is most commonly purchased, but USDA Grade B poultry can be used when appearance is not as important, such as in soups, casseroles, or chicken salad. (The lowest poultry grades are mostly used for processed chicken products.) A brand of fresh poultry, such as Perdue or Tyson, may be used, but brands are more commonly used when ordering processed poultry products.
5. <u>Unit on which the price is quoted/packaging information</u>. The price is often per pound but can also be based on case price, especially for frozen products. Fresh poultry may be delivered packed in crushed ice, cello packs (a transparent film), or gas-flushed pack in which air is removed from the bag and replaced with carbon dioxide (to extend shelf life). Most processed poultry products, such as breaded chicken patties, are **individually quick frozen (IQF)**, and then layered in a case. IQF foods are frozen separately so that they are less likely to stick together when placed in a case. The case size varies for processed poultry products, but they are usually 10 pounds. For example, a 10-pound box may hold 54 three-oz. portions of cooked grilled breast strips or 40 four-oz. portions of uncooked breaded spicy breast filets.
6. <u>Other requirements</u>. If buying whole birds, specify if you want or don't want the organ meats (liver, heart). If buying processed poultry products, the buyer can use a brand name but should also state the proportion of white to dark meat, the amount of breading allowed, etc., in case the desired brand is not available.

When buying eggs, a buyer can purchase fresh shell eggs or processed eggs, which are also called **egg products**. Egg products refer to eggs that are removed from their shells and processed to produce whole eggs, egg yolks, or egg whites in refrigerated, frozen, or dried forms. All egg products must be pasteurized for safety reasons and as egg products are made, they are under continuous inspection by the USDA Food Safety and Inspection Service. A foodservice may purchase liquid whole eggs to make large batches of scrambled eggs, thereby saving the labor of cracking eggs. Liquid or dried eggs may also be used in the bakery, and they keep longer than shell eggs. Many *precooked* egg products are also available, including patties, omelets, scrambled eggs, and hard-cooked eggs.

Table 7-19 Sample Egg Specifications

Fresh shell eggs
Used mostly in breakfast dishes and in some baking recipes.
U.S. Grade A, Brown or White, Large.
Eggs shall be packaged in one dozen cartons and packed in fiberboard cases with 15 dozen per case. Price is per case.
Code date not to be less than 14 days from the date of delivery.
Frozen, fully cooked, round scrambled egg patty
Used to make breakfast sandwich.
Processed from pasteurized whole eggs. Each patty shall be 3.25 to 3.5 inches wide and weigh 1.5 ounces. Patties should be IQF. Patties should have egg flavor, texture, and appearance. Glenview Farms brand or equivalent.
Packaging to include plastic-film bags within fiberboard case. 120 per case.
The product should be delivered at or below 2°F (−16°C).

The shell of the egg permits exchange of moisture and gases from the egg. The shell is brown or white depending on the hen's breed. The Food and Drug Administration periodically inspects shell egg producers for clean facilities and adherence to practices to prevent egg-associated illness caused by Salmonella.

Free-range eggs must be produced by hens that are able to roam up and down in indoor houses with continuous access to the outdoors and food and water. **Cage-free eggs** are laid by hens that are able to roam up and down in indoor houses, and have access to fresh food and water. They are not required to have access to the outdoors. **Organic eggs** were laid by hens raised on organic feed and with access to the outdoors.

The following is guidance on writing up a specification for eggs. Examples of specifications are in **Table 7–19**.

1. Name of product. The buyer must state either fresh shell eggs or a specific egg product. Buyers often choose a specific brand for egg products.
2. Intended use. State the menu item the eggs will be used in. Shell eggs are best when appearance is important.
3. Description.
   - Graded eggs must meet size standards. Eggs range from jumbo to peewee in size (see **Table 7–20**). The most popular size is large. A large egg is 2 oz. and works well for most egg dishes such as scrambled eggs. Baking recipes also normally require large eggs.
   - Buyers describe the type of processed eggs.

Table 7-20 Minimum Weights for Different Sizes of Shell Eggs

Size	Weight of a Dozen Eggs
Jumbo	30 ounces
Extra Large	27 ounces
Large	24 ounces
Medium	21 ounces
Small	18 ounces
Peewee	15 ounces

Specifications for Shell Eggs, p. 4, by U.S.D.A. Agricultural Marketing Service, 2017. Retrieved from https://www.ams.usda.gov/sites/default/files/media/ S01ShellEggSpecGuideforVolumeBuyers.pdf

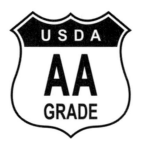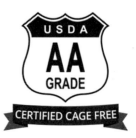

FIGURE 7-15 Grade Shield for Fresh Eggs

Courtesy of USDA Agricultural Marketing Service.

4. <u>Quality</u>.
   - The USDA Agricultural Marketing Service provides voluntary grading of shell eggs using three grades: US AA, A, B. The grades are based on the shape and condition of the shell as well as the firmness of the egg yolk and white. If you crack an AA egg into a pan, the yolk is high and round and the white is thick. As an egg ages, the yolk and whites become thinner, so the egg spreads more when cracked in a pan. Interior egg quality is, therefore, determined largely by freshness, whereas the shell's shape, texture and strength are determined largely by the age of the hen and quality of its feed. Buyers often purchase grade A eggs because grade AA eggs can be hard to find. Even if a buyer gets grade AA eggs, unless they are used quickly, the eggs will deteriorate to grade A. Grade A eggs are excellent for any purpose, especially where appearance is important as in fried or poached eggs. Grade B eggs can be used when appearance is not important, as in scrambled eggs, meatballs, or bakery items. The grade shield for eggs is shown in **Figure 7-15**.
   - Although processed eggs (egg products) are made under continuous USDA inspection, there are no grades for processed eggs and buyers usually choose a brand, such as Papetti's, that gives consistent quality and results.
5. <u>Unit on which the price is quoted/packaging information</u>.
   - Shell eggs are normally ordered in a 15-dozen or 30-dozen case. Buyers can also order a 2½ dozen box called a flat. Prices are per case.
   - Liquid egg products are often packed in two-pound cartons (15 to a case) or 20- or 30-pound bags. Frozen items are often packed in 30-pound plastic containers. The packaging varies depending on the manufacturer.
6. <u>Other requirements</u>.
   - Buyers may state that fresh shell eggs be held in refrigeration, including when delivered, at a temperature of no greater than 45°F.

SEAFOOD

Seafood includes fin fish and shellfish. Whereas fin fish, such as salmon, have fins and internal skeletons, **shellfish**, such as lobsters, have external shells and no internal bone structure. Fish and shellfish are naturally tender and cook quickly.

Seafood suppliers offer locally available seafood as well as seafood imported from Canada, Argentina, and many other countries. In 2016, over 80% of the seafood that Americans ate was imported from outside of the United States (NOAA, 2019). Foodservices in highly populated areas, especially those close to bodies of water, generally have more fresh seafood choices than foodservices in rural areas. The availability of certain seafood items and their prices can vary a lot during the year. If a buyer has only a few seafood suppliers, and if their seafood selection and/or quality do not match the needs of the buyer, a foodservice may decide they are better served by purchasing frozen seafood. Fresh seafood is highly perishable, like poultry, so buying frozen can be a safer choice. Today, much fish is frozen right on the boat to help maintain quality.

Suppliers sell seafood that is either **wild-caught seafood**, meaning it is caught from a lake, ocean, river or other natural habitat; or **farm-raised seafood**, meaning the seafood is raised using aquaculture. **Aquaculture** refers to breeding, raising, and harvesting fish and shellfish (NOAA, 2018a). Similar to the word agriculture, aquaculture basically is farming in water. There are two types of aquaculture: marine (farming in the ocean to produce oysters, shrimps, salmon, etc.) and freshwater (farming in ponds or other fresh water to produce catfish, trout, etc.). Marine aquaculture often occurs in net pens in the water or in tanks on land, while freshwater aquaculture occurs in ponds and other locations. Farm-raised fish can be more consistently supplied to foodservices and the quality is more stable.

Fishing practices worldwide along with warming oceans depleting fish populations are of concern to many foodservice buyers. Sustainable seafood comes from species of fish that are managed in a way that provides for today's needs without damaging the ability of the species to be available for future generations. The Seafood Watch or Fish-Choice website helps seafood buyers source sustainable seafood.

Managers and chefs have many considerations when deciding on a specific species for the menu. Salmon is an example of a family of fish. Families are large groups of fish and within each family, there are different species, such as Coho and King salmon. The wide variety of fish and categories of fish make purchasing a challenge. Here are some fish categories.

1. Fish that live all or most of their lives in the ocean are **saltwater fish**. **Freshwater fish** live all or most of their lives in streams, rivers, ponds, lakes, and reservoirs. Saltwater fish have a different flavor because of the salt in their flesh.
2. Fish also have different body shapes. Flounder is considered a flatfish whereas salmon is a round fish.
3. Some fish, such as salmon, are considered fatty fish while flounder is a lean fish (low in fat). Lean fish are still tender but may need some oil or butter during cooking to keep them moist. Moist-heating cooking methods, such as poaching, can also be used to keep a lean fish moist as well as provide variety in cooking methods.

When choosing finfish or shellfish, use the buying guide available at FishChoice (www.fishchoice.com/seafood-buying-guides), Fish Watch (www.fishwatch.gov), or SeafoodSource (www.seafoodsource.com). In addition to sustainability information, these websites explain what product forms are available and tell you about its availability, flavor, and texture. The market forms of fresh finfish are shown in **Figure 7-16**. Two popular forms are fillets, which are boneless sides of fish; and steaks, which are cross-section slices of fish.

Salmon and tuna are often described as "sushi grade." Although there are no actual regulations for "sushi grade," the fish is normally flash frozen while still on the boat and kept frozen for at least seven days at or below -4°F (-20°C), according to the federal 2017 *Food Code*, in order to kill any parasites in the flesh. So, fish used for sushi is often raw, but not "fresh" relative to when it was caught.

The safety of the seafood supply is overseen by the Food and Drug Administration and the U.S. Department of Commerce's National Oceanic and Atmospheric Administration (NOAA) Fisheries section. The FDA is responsible for the safety of fish that are imported into the United States. All seafood imports must comply with standards for safety and wholesomeness and the FDA monitors imported fish shipments. The FDA performs periodic inspections of plants (domestic and foreign) that process seafood.

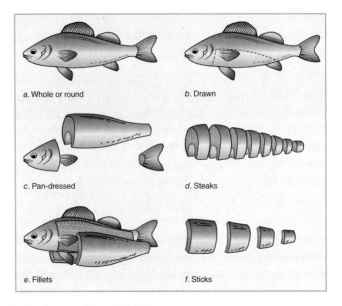

FIGURE 7-16 Market Forms of Fresh Finfish

Reproduced from D. Mizer, M. Porter, B. Sonnier, and K. Drummond (2000). Food Preparation for the Professional, p. 340, Hoboken (NJ): John Wiley & Sons, Inc.

The FDA also runs a mandatory program for all seafood processors within and outside of the United States (who ship food to the United States) in which processors are required to implement and maintain a Hazard Analysis Critical Control Point (HACCP) system. Using HACCP, the processors monitor critical points along the supply chain to prevent food safety problems. All HACCP programs require Current Good Manufacturing Practices (cGMP) to be in place first, such as personal hygiene and clean water requirements. Some U.S. companies that import seafood visit fish farms and processors overseas to ensure that their trading partners are following U.S. food regulations.

The NOAA Fisheries section oversees the **Seafood Inspection Program**. The Seafood Inspection Program is a voluntary, fee-for-service program that inspects and grades seafood (fresh and frozen). NOAA Fisheries certifies more than one-third of the seafood sold in the United States (NOAA Fisheries, 2018b). Grading standards are published for certain fish and shellfish (**Table 7–21**) as well as some processed fish such as breaded fish sticks. Grading standards for breaded products include a limitation on the breading, such as lightly breaded shrimp must contain 65% shrimp. Graded seafood has also been inspected. The Seafood Inspection Program also provides inspection services in foreign countries.

Finally, the **National Shellfish Sanitation Program (NSSP)** is a federal and state cooperative program recognized by the FDA to oversee shellfish safety from the quality of the water in the areas they grow to their processing and shipping. Shellfish (including oysters, mussels, scallops, and clams) must be delivered to a foodservice with a shellfish identification tag on the container that identifies where the shellfish were harvested and when. Once the shellfish are used up, the date should be put on the tag and the tag must be removed and held for 90 days.

The following is additional information to help write up specifications. **Table 7–22** contains sample specifications.

1. <u>Name of product</u>. The buyer must state the precise name, market form, and fresh or frozen.
2. <u>Intended use</u>. The name of the menu item should be included here as well as how it will be cooked. A fish that will be grilled and served needs to be more attractive than fish that will be used in a fish stew or fish taco.

Table 7-21 Fish and Shellfish with U.S. Grading Standards	
By Name	**By Market Form**
Catfish	Fish Fillet Blocks
Cod Fillets	Frozen Fried Fish Portions
Flounder Fillets	Frozen Fried Fish Sticks
Frozen Raw Breaded Scallops	General Fillets
Frozen Fried Scallops	Minced Fish Blocks
Frozen Raw Breaded Shrimp	Raw Breaded Fish Portions
Frozen Raw Scallops	Raw Breaded Fish Sticks
Haddock Fillets	Raw Fish Portions
Halibut Steaks	Whole and Dressed Fish
Headless Dressed Whiting	
Ocean Perch and Rockfish	
Salmon Steaks	
Shrimp Fresh and Frozen	

Seafood Inspection Manual (Part 5 Chapter 1), p. 1, by NOAA Fisheries, ND. Retrieved from https://www.fisheries.noaa .gov/national/seafood-commerce-certification/seafood-inspection-manual

3. <u>Description</u>.
   - The buyer may specify wild-caught or farm-raised.
   - There is no U.S.D.A. certified organic fish in the U.S. There are fish certified abroad as organic, but they are not recognized as organic in the United States.
   - When ordering fresh fish, such as whole fish or fillets, the buyer usually states a weight range or average weight because suppliers can't supply an exact weight, such as 6-oz. fillets.
   - Some shellfish items are sized by count. Lobster tails and crab legs are sized based on how many are in 10 pounds. For example, if lobster tails are marked as 10/12, it means there are 10 to 12 tails in a 10-pound box. Shrimp are sold

Table 7-22 Sample Seafood Specifications
Fresh boneless salmon fillets.
Main dish.
Wild-caught Coho salmon or Sockeye salmon produced in the U.S. 7–8 oz. fillet. Consistent in thickness and size. Must carry "Packed Under Federal Inspection" seal. Good flavor and odor.
Packed on crushed ice.
Frozen, Oven-Ready Breaded Fish Sticks
Used as main dish.
U.S. Grade A. 1.0 oz. each. Contents: 72% by weight Alaskan pollock, remainder is crispy style breading. IQF. Must be rectangular shaped and at least 3/8" thick. Uniform in size and weight. Must be processed in USDC/NOAA Seafood Inspection Approved facility.
10 lb. case. Moisture-proof packaging. Must be packed to prevent any more than 2% breakage/case.

U.S. Grade A/PUFI Mark

PUFI Mark

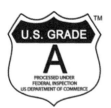 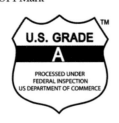 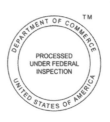 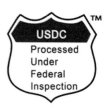

FIGURE 7-17 Grade Shields and Inspection Labels for Seafood

Courtesy of NOAA Fisheries. Retrieved from https://www.fisheries.noaa.gov/policy-advertising-services-and-use-marks-us-department-commerce

by count per pound, which is indicated on the label. For example, 51/60 are small shrimp, 31/35 are large shrimp, and 21/25 are jumbo shrimp.
- Include the **point of origin** if the menu includes a description such as Maine lobster.
- Processed fish, such as breaded fillets, are available in different sizes and each piece is uniform. The buyer must state the number of portions per case and size of each portion.

4. Quality.
- Grading generally looks at appearance, odor, flavor, size, and defects. For most items, grades are U.S. Grade A, U.S. Grade B, and Substandard. Grade A fish has good flavor, a uniform appearance, and usually no defects or blemishes. If a buyer wants to specify a grade, the U.S. Grade A designation is normally used (Figure 7-16) but Grade B may be acceptable for fish incorporated into casseroles, soups, and the like.
- Instead of grading, a buyer may specify that the seafood must be federally inspected. The "Packed Under Federal Inspection" label (**Figure 7-17**) certifies that the items were produced under continuous government inspection.
- For processed fish, such as frozen breaded fish sticks or battered shrimp, a brand name (such as Tampa Maid Foods) is often used to designate a certain level of quality.

5. Unit on which the price is quoted/packaging information.
- Fresh seafood is usually priced per pound. Frozen processed fish is priced per case or per bag.
- Fresh fish is often delivered slab-packed in plastic tubs in crushed ice. Some fresh fish may be packed in plastic in modified-atmosphere packaging so that it stays fresh longer. Shellfish that are still alive are *not* packed in ice or fresh water but are kept cold in moisture-proof containers.
- Frozen fish are usually individually quick frozen and wrapped in some way such as cello wrapped before being layer packed. Boxes for frozen products should be moisture-proof.

6. Other requirements.
- Buyers may specify minimum product yield.

MILK AND DAIRY PRODUCTS

Dairy products are unique in that many have a standard of identity established by the federal government. For example, following is part of the standard of identity for ice cream.

Ice cream contains not less than 1.6 pounds of total solids to the gallon, and weighs not less than 4.5 pounds to the gallon. Ice cream contains not less than 10% milkfat, nor less than 10% nonfat milk solids, except that when it contains milkfat in 1% increments above the 10% minimum. (CDR, 2018)

Table 7-23 Minimum Fat Content for Selected Dairy Products	
Milk, whole	3.25%
Milk, nonfat	0.0 – 0.5%
Yogurt, whole	3.25%
Yogurt, lowfat	0.5 – 2.0%
Yogurt, nonfat	0.0 – 0.5%
Heavy cream	36%
Light cream	18–30%
Half and Half	10.5–18%
Light whipping cream	30–36%
Sour cream	18%
Cottage cheese, creamed	4%
Ice Cream	10%
Cheddar cheese	31%
Cream cheese	33%
Mozzarella cheese	18–21%
Part-skim mozzarella cheese	12–18%
American cheese (Pasteurized processed cheese)	27%
Butter	80%

Data from *Code of Federal Regulations, Part 131 Milk and Cream and Part 133 Cheeses and Related Cheese Products*, by Food and Drug Administration, 2017. Retrieved from https://www.govinfo.gov/content/pkg/CFR-2018-title21-vol2/xml/CFR-2018-title21-vol2-part131.xml#seqnum131.110 and https://www.govinfo.gov/content/pkg/CFR-2018-title21-vol2/xml/CFR-2018-title21-vol2-part133.xml

Without 10% milkfat, the product cannot be labeled as ice cream. **Table 7-23** gives the minimum fat content for selected dairy products, such as butter which must contain at least 80% milkfat to be labeled "butter."

Milk is a highly perishable food because bacteria can grow well in it. Keeping it fresh and safe to drink is very important. All 50 states, the District of Columbia, and U.S. Territories participate in the Grade A Pasteurized Milk Ordinance program that safeguards milk by, for example, inspecting farms and milk plants, pasteurizing milk (heating it to destroy pathogenic bacteria), monitoring milk quality, and overseeing safe milk transport. It applies to farms, dairy plants, processors, and shippers that produce or transport Grade A products, including fluid milk, yogurt, and some other dairy products. This program was developed by the U.S. Public Health Service, which is part of the U.S. Department of Health and Human Services (U.S. Public Health Service, 2017). Milk plants also have to have HACCP programs in place and FDA inspectors visit to see how the HACCP plan is being implemented.

Outside of milk and butter, not many dairy products are graded. This occurs because graded milk is usually used to make yogurts, cheeses, etc., and most dairy products are also produced in inspected plants.

Cheese is made using milk from cows, goats, or sheep. Many cheeses are ripened, meaning that humidity, temperature, and oxygen are controlled to develop the cheese to maturity. During ripening, the cheese takes on its own unique flavor, texture, and aroma. Here are some categories of cheese.

1. Unripened cheeses include freshly made cheeses that are soft and white such as cottage cheese, ricotta cheese, or mozzarella.
2. Semisoft cheeses include Muenster cheese as well as fontina cheese from Italy.

3. Soft-ripened cheeses ripen from the outside in and are soft or runny when ready to eat. Examples include Brie and Camembert from France.
4. Hard cheeses are cured and range from mild to sharp in flavor, such as Cheddar, Monterey Jack, or Provolone.
5. Blue-veined cheeses contain mold cultures that gives cheeses, such as Roquefort, their appearance and flavor.
6. Goat cheeses are made from goat's milk and when these cheeses are not aged, they are white in color and mild in flavor.
7. Hard grating cheeses include Parmigiano-Reggiano from Italy.
8. Processed cheeses include **American cheese**. American cheese is a product made by blending one or more natural cheeses (often cheddar is included) with texture—and flavor-altering ingredients. Processed cheese does not ripen like natural cheese, has a mild flavor, melts well, and is less expensive (more cost-effective) than a natural cheese such as Cheddar.

The following are guidelines to write dairy specifications. **Table 7-24** contains sample specifications.

1. Name of product. The buyer must state the precise name of the product, which may include terms such as "low-fat" to designate the fat content.
2. Intended use. The name of the menu item(s) should be included as well as if it will be used in cooking.
3. Description.
    - A buyer usually requires fortification of fluid milk with vitamins A and D, as well as homogenization. Almost all of the U.S. milk supply is fortified with vitamin D because few foods in nature contain it. Dairies are required by law to add vitamin A to nonfat milk, lowfat (1%) milk, and reduced-fat (2%) milk. This is because vitamin A is "fat soluble," so there is less vitamin A in the milks with less fat. When milk is **homogenized**, its milkfat is divided into tiny pieces that are evenly dispersed throughout the milk. Otherwise, the fat would separate from the liquid and clump together.
    - A buyer may specify organic milk. **Organic milk** comes from cows that must have outdoor access year-round. In addition, they must graze for at least 120 to 200 days per year (depending on the region and weather), during which they get at least 30% of their calories from grass. They can be given

---

Table 7-24 Sample Milk and Cheese Specifications

Fluid milk, whole.

For drinking and cooking.

Grade A, pasteurized and homogenized. Vitamin A minimum 2,000 I.U./quart. Vitamin D minimum 400 I.U./quart. Milk fat not less than 3.25%. Milk solids (not fat) no less than 8.25%. Must be produced and sold in compliance with all federal and state health laws and regulations.

50 ½-pint cartons or plastic bottles/case. Easy-to-open, leak-proof cartons/bottles. Cases and cartons must be clean and free of unpleasant odors.

Code date not to be less than 8 days from date of delivery.

Sharp yellow cheddar cheese.

To slice for sandwiches.

Cabot brand sharp yellow cheddar cheese. Block. Aged minimum 5 months or to meet flavor profile.

10-lb. loaf in moisture-proof packaging. Random weight. One/case.

organic feed when grass is not available. Hormones to stimulate milk production or the use of antibiotics are not allowed.

- For yogurt, buyers must specify regular, low-fat, or nonfat. Buyers should also be sure to include the variety of the yogurt, such as traditional yogurt, Greek yogurt (thicker and higher in protein than traditional), Icelandic yogurt (less tart and creamier than Greek), Australian yogurt (richer and creamier than traditional), or nondairy yogurt using almond milk or soy milk. A brand name is often used.
- For some cheeses, such as Swiss cheese, the buyer should state whether domestic Swiss is acceptable or if it must be Emmentaler cheese, a medium-hard cheese that comes from the Emmental region in Switzerland.
- For cheese, the buyer must specify whether is it to be sliced, whole, grated, shredded, or crumbled.
- Buyers may specify a size when ordering sliced cheese. For example, sliced American cheese (yellow or white) comes in 5-pound loaves with 120 slices (0.66 oz. each) or 160 slices (0.5 oz. each) per loaf.
- Buyers must specify whether butter is to be salted or unsalted (sometimes called sweet butter). Some buyers will specify butter made with milk from grass-fed cows, such as Kerrygold butter made in Ireland. Some buyers may also specify a butter blend (usually by brand name) that uses butter and vegetable oils.
- The buyer must specify which size/form of butter to buy: a 50 to 55-pound block, one-pound blocks (called a print), a 1-pound box with 4 sticks, or a whipped tub. Butter is also available in individual portions as chips. A **butter chip** is a slice of butter on a small square of moisture-proof material and a paper on top of the butter. Butter chips come in different counts, such as 47, 50, 60, 72, or 90 per pound. The higher the count, the smaller the piece of butter. **Continental butter chips** are completely covered in foil. Butter is also available in portion control cups in counts such as 90 count. (Margarine is also available in one-pound prints and in portion-control cups or chips.)

4. Quality.
   - Grade A is specified for fluid milk. Most milk is graded and the grade is either Grade A or Manufacturing Grade. The difference is that Manufacturing Grade milk is allowed to contain more bacteria. Manufacturing grade milk is used to produce ice cream, cheese, butter, or other milk product.
   - Yogurt is not graded. Brand names are often used.
   - Some cheeses have federal grades and standards, including Cheddar, Colby, Monterey Jack, Swiss and Emmentaler, and bulk American cheese. For example, Cheddar cheese has the grades U.S. Grade AA, U.S. Grade A, U.S. Grade B, and U.S. Grade C. In general, cheeses are graded on flavor, body and texture, color, and appearance. The exact grades for each cheese may vary but they are available on the USDA AMS website under "Grades and Standards." Buyers often specify a brand name or equivalent or may specify U.S. Grade A or comparable quality for cheese.
   - Butter often carries a federal grade of U.S. Grade AA, U.S. Grade A, or U.S. Grade B (**Figure 7-18**). The grade is based on flavor, body, color, and salt. Some states, such as Wisconsin, use their own grading system for butter and cheese. Therefore, in Wisconsin, a container of butter will have "Grade A" on its label instead of "USDA Grade A." Buyers usually specify either USDA Grade AA, USDA Grade A, or a specific brand.
   - The quality of ice cream depends on the fat content (more is better), the amount of air worked into it (called **overrun**—less is better), and the quality of the flavorings. Premium ice cream has about 15 to 18% butterfat, high-quality flavorings (such as vanilla bean instead of imitation vanilla), and under

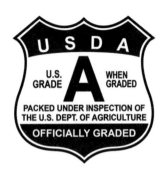

FIGURE 7-18 Federal Grade with Inspection Stamp Used for Butter and Cheeses

Courtesy of USDA.

50% overrun. Standard overrun for ice cream is 100%, which means that every pint of ice cream mix will mix with an equal amount of air to provide two pints of ice cream. Premium ice cream, at only 50% overrun, is heavier by volume than less expensive ice creams that contain more air. Many buyers taste test ice cream to determine which brand and flavors are most appropriate for their operation.

5. Unit on which the price is quoted/packaging information.
    *   Fluid cow's milk is priced per case. One case holds four 1-gallon containers, nine half gallons, 16 quarts, 50 half-pint paper cartons, or 75 4-fluid ounce cartons. If a milk dispenser is used, it requires a 5-gallon poly bag for each type of milk available.
    *   Yogurt is priced per case. Most cups (5–6 ounces) are packed 12/case. Yogurt is also packed in 2-pound tubs (6/case) and 5-pound tubs (4/case).
    *   Cheese is priced per case. Sliced American cheese comes in a case containing four or six 5-lb. loaves. Shredded cheese often comes in a 20-lb. case containing four 5-lb. bags. Blocks of cheese come in varying sizes, such as a 10-pound loaf of cheddar cheese.
    *   One-pound blocks of butter are packed 36 to a case. Butter chips are often packed in 17- or 30-pound boxes, and individual cups of butter are often in 8-lb. boxes.
    *   Ice cream is sold in bulk in 3-gallon round containers (tubs) or in individual portions packed in cases of 24 or sometimes 12.

6. Other requirements. Buyers may also state the maximum freshness date allowed at time of delivery.

© Denis Val/Shutterstock

Food Receiving, Storage, Inventory, and Issuing

LEARNING OUTCOMES

8.1 Receive products.

8.2 Store products safely.

8.3 Manage inventory including calculating food/beverage cost.

8.4 Issue products.

INTRODUCTION

Trucks filled with food and beverage deliveries arrive at foodservices across the country every day, starting early in the morning. **Receiving** these deliveries is an important job where the receiving clerk makes sure that the delivered items are exactly what was ordered and the quality of the items meet specifications. For example, the receiving clerk is responsible for making sure that moldy strawberries are neither accepted nor paid for, and the fresh chicken wings are really fresh and the correct weight. In other words, by inspecting incoming food, the receiving clerk is the front line for food safety in the foodservice.

Once an order is received, the receiving clerk stores the items until they are needed. Food, beverages, and supplies that are received but not yet used are referred to as **inventory**. Until the items are removed from inventory to be used in meal preparation, management is responsible for safeguarding what was received to prevent shrinkage. **Shrinkage** is the loss of product due to damage, waste, spoilage, and theft. This chapter will discuss in more detail receiving and storing foods, along with how to manage inventory appropriately to control costs.

8.1 RECEIVE PRODUCTS

The receiving clerk works in an area that includes the loading dock and receiving bay where trucks pull up to get unloaded (**Figure 8-1**). It also includes space for deliveries to sit while each order is checked in. The floor of the loading dock should be at the standard height of the bed of a delivery truck (approximately 48 inches). Adjustable height loading docks are available to accommodate varied truck heights.

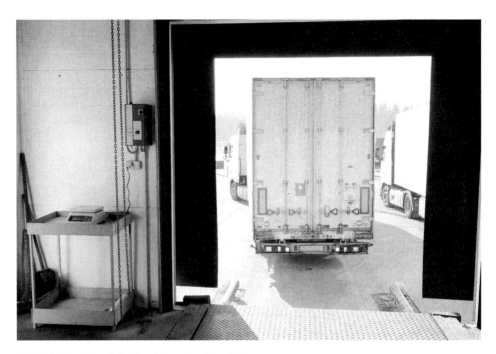

FIGURE 8-1 A Truck Pulling into a Loading Dock

© Vereshchagin Dmitry/Shutterstock

A receiving clerk needs the following equipment to complete the job satisfactorily.

1. A desk/table for completing paperwork and inspecting items.
2. A receiving or platform scale (**Figure 8-2**) for weighing items such as cases of meat, and a tabletop or counter scale for weighing smaller items. Scales must be checked regularly for accuracy.

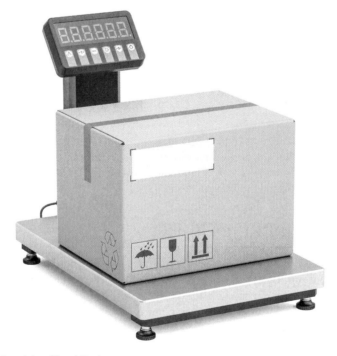

FIGURE 8-2 Receiving (floor) Scale

© AlexLMX/Shutterstock

3. Equipment for moving deliveries includes hand trucks (**Figure 8-3**), platform trucks (**Figure 8-4**), and U-boat platform trucks that are narrower and able to maneuver in tight aisles and doorways. You also need a hand or powered pallet truck, also called a pallet jack (**Figure 8-5**). A pallet truck is used to lift and transport a pallet—an open wooden or plastic platform (about 48" x 40") on which boxes are placed and either strapped to or shrink wrapped to keep boxes together. A pallet truck has two forks that fit into the pallet so the pallet can be lifted and moved around. A powered pallet truck has a motor to lift and move the load.

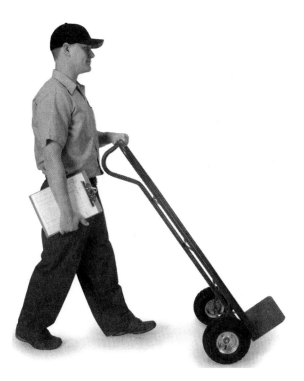

FIGURE 8-3 Hand Truck

© James Steidl/Shutterstock

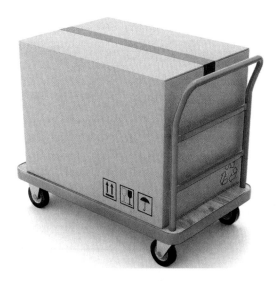

FIGURE 8-4 Platform Truck

© Mipan/Shutterstock

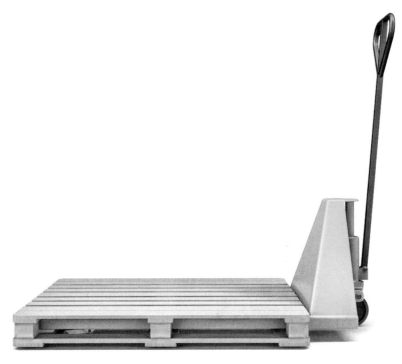

FIGURE 8-5 Pallet Truck

© Cherezoff/Shutterstock

4. Miscellaneous tools include a computer or similar device to access purchasing and inventory records, pencils, markers, clipboards, thermometers for taking food temperatures (an infrared thermometer can measure surface temperatures from up to four feet away and quickly checks food temperatures at receiving), barcode scanner (if used), date stamp, and tools for opening boxes and containers such as a box cutter, wire snips, and hammer.

STEPS TO RECEIVE PRODUCTS

Before a delivery comes in, the receiving area must be clean and tidy, and the scales, hand trucks, and other equipment also need to be clean and ready for use. The receiving clerk needs plenty of room to count, weigh, and check the quality of incoming products. In addition, the storage areas should be clean with everything on the appropriate shelves so that new merchandise can be put away safely and quickly.

When a delivery truck pulls up at the loading dock, and the driver opens the door at the rear of the truck, the receiving clerk should note both the timeliness of the delivery and assess the trailer temperature and cleanliness. Many receiving departments only allow deliveries within certain time frames, such as from 7:00 AM to 11:00 PM and from 1:00 to 3:00 to allow for lunch service and employee breaks. Once a truck arrives, the receiving clerk should look inside the truck to check for problems, such as the refrigeration is not on, the truck is filthy, or items have moved around a lot causing possible damage.

After the preliminary inspection, the receiving clerk goes through these steps.

1. The delivery person hands the receiving clerk an **invoice** or pick list that includes everything on the order and often, but not always, includes prices. At this point, the clerk may compare this to the purchase order.
2. Using **invoice receiving**, the receiving clerk will use the invoice to check the name/description and quantity of each item delivered. In some kitchens, the receiving clerk will have a receiving notebook with information about the

products commonly purchased. For example, it may include photos of tomatoes with scars and decay that should not be accepted or a copy of the label for frozen chicken breasts that can help identify the correct product. Checking the quantity will require counting the number of items or weighing items. When weighing items packed in ice, such as chicken, remove the chicken from the ice onto a sanitary surface to get the correct weight. Receiving clerks may also weigh portion-control items, such as hamburgers, to check for the proper weight.

Many foodservices are investing in labeling and scanning technology so they can scan **barcodes** on incoming boxes to keep track of what they have received (and their inventory). Distributors normally tag each case with a label and barcode. Some distributors provide foodservices with handheld scanners for barcode scanning (**Figure 8-6**) or apps that allow scanning with a tablet or smartphone. The barcode includes vertical lines and spaces, and the number beneath them is called the Global Trade Item Number (GTIN). The GTIN tells you the specific brand, pack unit, and product code. Larger foodservices may print barcode labels for items that don't arrive with barcodes, such as fresh produce, because barcode labels make it easier to track inventory. Use of the GTIN is helpful in tracing where the food originated, which is helpful in the event of a food recall.

3. When checking quantities, the clerk also checks for food quality and safety. **Table 8-1** shows temperature requirements for safe food and what fresh foods should look like.

    a. Temperatures must be taken on TCS (Time and Temperature Control for Safety) foods such as meats, poultry, seafood, and dairy. TCS foods require time and temperature controls to prevent the growth of bacteria. In many foodservices, the receiving clerk will be required to record those temperatures on a receiving log or other form. When taking temperatures, insert the thermometer into the thickest part of the food and make sure the stem does not touch the package. Sanitize the thermometer between uses. To test the temperature of reduced-oxygen packaging food, place the thermometer stem between two packages—do not puncture the packaging. Do the same for bags of pre-cut or pre-washed produce. For eggs, check the air temperature of the truck.

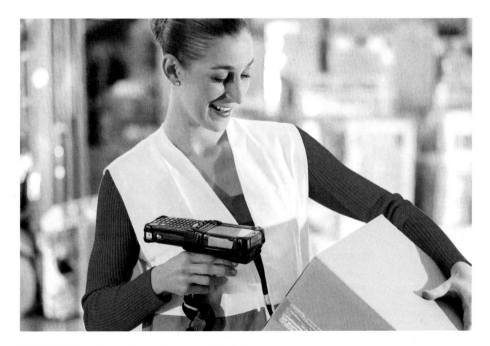

FIGURE 8-6 Employee Scans Barcode of Package

© Kzenon/Shutterstock

Table 8-1 Indicators of Good and Poor Quality Used When Receiving Foods

Food	Temperature*	Indicators of Good Quality	Indicators of Poor Quality
Meat	41°F (5°C) or lower.	Beef: Bright red color with creamy white fat. Aged beef is dark in color and vacuum-packed beef is purplish. Firm texture and no odor. Pork: Pinkish-red with white fat. Firm texture and no odor.	Beef: Green, brown, or gray coloring. Slimy/sticky feel. Strong unpleasant odor. Pork: Dark/greenish color. Slimy feel. Sour, unpleasant odor.
Poultry	41°F (5°C) or lower.	Yellowish skin. Light meat is pale pink with little fat. Dark meat is dark pink with some white fat. Firm texture. No odors. Glossy surface. Packed under ice.	Meat is grayish in color. Sticky surface. Foul, sour odor.
Fresh fish	41°F (5°C) or lower.	Whole fish: Bright, clear eyes and skin that shines. Bright red or pink moist gills. Cleaned with all traces of guts and organs removed. Cut fish: Firm flesh that springs back when pressed. Mild scent with no unpleasant odors. Both packed in ice.	Whole fish: Dull, cloudy, sunken eyes and skin with discolored patches. Faded red gills. Slimy touch. Strong fishy smell. Cut fish: Milky liquid on flesh. Soft texture that doesn't bounce back after pressing. Browning around the edges. Pungent odor.
Shellfish (After receiving, must be cooled to 41°F (5°C) or below within four hours.)	Live: Air temperature of 45°F (7°C) or lower and internal temperature no higher than 50°F (10°C). Shucked: 45°F (7°C) or lower.	Live: Closed, clean shells. Smell like the ocean (unless freshwater sourced). Must have an identification tag attached. Shucked: Plump meat free of shell or grit. Clear or slightly milky fluid (liquor). Mild odor.	Live: Slightly open or open shells that don't close when tapped. Broken shells or shells full of mud. Unpleasant odor. Shucked: Meat is dry and sticky or slimy. Unpleasant odor.
Shell eggs	Air temperature of 45°F (7°C) or lower.	Shells are clean and intact. No odors.	Shells are cracked and/or not clean. Sulfur-like smell.
Dairy products	45°F (7°C) or lower, then cool to 41°F (5°C) or lower.	Milk: Clean white color. Pleasant taste and odor. Butter: Yellow color. Smooth texture. Pleasant taste and odor. Cheese: Appropriate color, texture, and taste.	Milk: Off-white or yellow color. Sour taste. Thicker consistency, possibly with lumps. Unpleasant odor. Butter: Discolored. Sour taste and odor. Moldy. Cheese: Smells or tastes sour. Green, red, or black mold on packaging. Mold on rind is acceptable.
Fresh produce	41°F (5°C) or lower for cut melons, cut tomatoes, & cut leafy greens.	Bright color with few or no bruises and blemishes. Most should have firm texture. Pleasant, fragrant aroma.	Soft texture or limp. Unusual smell. Fuzzy growth (mold) or spots. Avoid greens with wilt, browning, rust, slime, or liquid in the bag or plastic box.
Canned, bottled, and pouched goods.		Cardboard boxes are intact and clean. Cans, bottles, or pouches are in good condition and clean.	Cans with deep dents, rust, or swollen ends are not acceptable. Broken bottles or pouches with holes. Missing labels.
Frozen goods	0°F (−18°C) or lower	Frozen solid in clean, intact packages.	Water or dampness inside case. Water stains on cardboard box indicate item thawed at some point.

*Data from *2017 Food Code*, p. 62, by the U.S. Public Health Service and Food & Drug Administration, 2017. *National Shellfish Sanitation Program Guide for the Control of Molluscan Shellfish*, p. 111, by the Interstate Shellfish Sanitation Conference, 2017.

    b. The receiving clerk should randomly open boxes and check for quality, looking at the oranges in the bottom of a case as well as in the top layer. Vacuum-packed products, such as meat, should not show signs of leaking or bloating. Fresh produce or canned goods that traveled in a freezer truck under an insulated blanket (so they didn't freeze) may have frozen anyway. If precut salads are frozen, they are ruined and canned goods may split or explode because of the cold. Rejected items should be set aside and reasons for rejection should be noted on the invoice.

    c. Even when receiving canned foods or dry goods such as flour or crackers, the cases should be visually inspected and some opened. Canned goods with deep dents, missing labels, rust, or swollen ends are not acceptable. A case of crackers can be opened to make sure the crackers are not broken. If a bag of flour is dirty or has holes in it, it needs to be returned. Any foods with signs of pests or pest damage should also be rejected.

    d. The receiving clerk has to keep an eye on any dates on the products, such as "Sell-By" Dates on milk or "Best If Used By" date on olive oil. Any outdated product should be rejected. Even items such as diet soft drinks should be rejected if out of date because sweeteners lose or change flavor over time.

    e. When examining quality of fresh produce, check the bottom of some of the boxes for moisture, dirt, or mold. This is an immediate clue that the contents need to be thoroughly inspected. Also, handle fresh produce with care! Most items are fragile and even dropping a box of apples just a few inches drastically shortens their shelf life.

4. Fresh shellfish (including oysters, mussels, scallops, and clams) must be delivered with a shellfish identification tag on the container that identifies where the shellfish were harvested and on what date. Once the shellfish are used up, the date should be put on the tag and the tag must be removed and held for 90 days. This is done in case a foodborne illness related to these shellfish occurs so that the source of the problem can be identified. This is especially critical if you serve raw oysters.

5. If the foodservice does not accept an item on the invoice, that item is returned to the supplier. The return is normally noted on the invoice itself with the signature or initials of the delivery person and receiving clerk. Quite often, the delivery person will submit a request for credit for the returned items using a handheld device (so the supplier will then send the foodservice a credit memo) or will print out a credit memo. The **credit memo** indicates the amount of money that does not need to be paid on the invoice and reduces the amount the foodservice owes to the supplier.

6. In some operations, the receiving clerk now checks the foodservice's purchase order against the supplier's invoice to make sure the right items were delivered along with the correct quantity and price. (Note that some foodservices ask the receiving clerk to use both the invoice and the purchase order together when checking in an order.) A credit memo will also be needed if pricing on the invoice is higher than on the purchase order.

7. After making adjustments (as needed) on the invoice for returns or for corrected prices, the final step is for the receiving clerk to sign the invoice. By signing the invoice, the foodservice is acknowledging receipt of the items.

8. The receiving clerk may be required to maintain a **receiving log** with the date and time of each delivery, along with name of the supplier, invoice number, purchase order number, and description of goods received. This log can be used to list items that were temperature-checked on delivery. Many health departments require this, but even if they do not, it is considered a "best practice" for receiving TCS foods.

9. At the end of the day, all supplier invoices (along with any credit memos) and receiving log (if used) are sent to accounting to be reviewed and paid. In some

cases, someone in the foodservice may check/sign off on the invoices before they go to accounting.

Once the paperwork is completed, cold and frozen foods should be put away as soon as possible. A standard should be set for how long foods remain in the receiving area before they are put away. For example, a foodservice may require that *foods be moved from receiving to storage within 30 minutes of delivery* with ice cream and frozen desserts put in the freezer immediately to maintain quality.

Receiving clerks should follow these guidelines when putting foods away.

1. *Most operations make sure all incoming food has receiving dates marked on it.* Distributors normally tag each case with a label and barcode, and this tag has the receiving date on it. For cases without these tags, the receiving clerk can use a **date label gun** designed to print a date on a sticker that is then put on the product. When employees take cans and products out of the cases, most foodservices will use the label gun to mark each can or item.

2. *When receiving clerks put foods into storage, they must use the first-in, first-out (FIFO) method* of stock rotation. Using the FIFO system, foods are shelved based on use-by or expiration dates, so older foods are used first. For example, if the boxes of cereal you just received in April have a use-by date of 7/18 of the current year, and the cereal in stock has a use-by date of 6/1 of the current year, the employee should put the cereals with the 6/1 date *in front of* the cereals with the 7/18 date. When putting foods away, employees must regularly check use-by and expiration dates and discard food that is beyond either date. For foods without use-by dates, the date the food was received can be used.

3. *When placed into storage, the box label or can label should be face out so employees can find what they need quickly.* Foods are often organized in storage areas by food group with frequently used foods closer to the storage area entrance so they can be picked up quickly. Heavier items also tend to be on lower shelves.

4. *Store raw meat, poultry, and seafood separately or away from ready-to-eat foods,* because you don't want poultry juices, for example, to accidentally contaminate a food that won't get any further cooking. If you must store these raw foods on the same shelving with ready-to-eat foods, always store the ready-to-eat foods *above* raw meat, poultry, or seafood. When storing raw protein foods in the same rack, they should be stored in the following top-to-bottom order: seafood, whole cuts of beef and pork, ground meats and ground fish, and whole or ground poultry on the very bottom shelf. This order is based on the fact that the minimum internal temperature of each food (once cooked) increases as you move down the rack from seafood to poultry. The food requiring the highest internal cooked temperature (whole or ground poultry) is at the bottom.

Some received items do not go directly into storage. Instead, they go directly from receiving to production. These items are referred to as **direct issues** and are expected to be used within a day. For example, every morning, a bakery delivers fresh breads, rolls, and other baked goods to a university dining hall. The breads and rolls go directly to the deli and grill stations in the dining hall, and the baked goods are rolled over to the dessert station to be sliced. Milk may also be considered a direct issue in some foodservices.

As you can imagine, being a receiving clerk is a demanding job, both physically and mentally. Some incoming orders can be quite large, or several orders arrive about the same time, and the receiving clerk needs to check in each order accurately and get foods put away as quickly as possible. In addition, drivers put pressure on the receiving clerk to sign off on the invoice as quickly as possible so they can get to their next stop. Besides working well under pressure, the receiving clerk needs to be very detail-oriented and attentive to food safety and cost issues.

SPOTLIGHT ON RADIO FREQUENCY IDENTIFICATION

Radio Frequency Identification (RFID) is now being used extensively by the supermarket industry, and you can expect to see more of it in foodservice operations. This new technology involves the use of radio waves to read and write information onto a tag attached to a box or pallet. What makes it different from barcodes is that the tag can carry a lot more information and does not have to be directly in front of a reader to be read. Multiple tags can be read from several feet away or more, depending on the type of tag used. RFID tags are being used to track food through the supply chain process from farm to manufacturer to consumer, which makes them extremely useful for recalls.

RFID tags come in passive and active types. A passive tag has no internal power source and instead responds to the electromagnetic field generated by an RFID reader. They help to improve food safety and lessen risk by tracking the temperature exposure and "use-by" dates. Active RFID tags have batteries, *cost a lot more*, but increase the range for reading them to over 300 feet.

According to the Grocery Manufacturers Association, the average cost of a food recall is about $10 million, so the use of RFID is growing and this has pushed the cost of the tags down. RFID tracking is becoming a central piece of the food industry compliance with the Food Safety Modernization Act (O'Boyle, 2016). It is being used by Gordon Food Service (working with Markon) in their 5-Star Food Safety Program.

8.2 STORE PRODUCTS SAFELY

Foods are stored in refrigerators, freezers, or at room temperature in dry storage areas. Guidelines to keep food safe in storage include the following.

1. *All foods need to be labeled with their product name and also dated.* Any food not in its original container, such as flour that has been put in a bin, must be labeled with the name of the food. Any ready-to-eat TCS food that will be held for more than 24 hours must be marked with a use-by date that is no more than seven days beyond when it was received. The same rule applies to TCS foods, such as egg salad, that are prepared in the foodservice. Once prepared, many foodservices label them with both the date the food was made and the use-by or discard date (**Figure 8–7**). If an employee combines two TCS foods with different discard dates, the new discard date should be the earliest of the two.

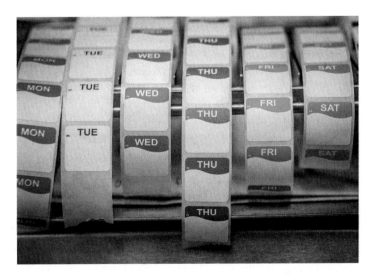

FIGURE 8-7 Example of Food Label Showing Use-By Date

© Pav-Pro Photography Ltd/Shutterstock

2. *All foods need to be stored at appropriate temperatures and humidity levels.* It is especially important to keep the doors of refrigerators and freezers closed. Poor gasket seals or door latches on walk-in refrigerators and freezers can also contribute to warm temperatures.

    a. Dry storage areas should be maintained between 50°F (10°C) and 70°F (21°C). Cold pipes and air conditioning ducts should be wrapped with insulation so that liquid condensate is not dripping on food or floors. Hot water and steam pipes should also be insulated to prevent the room from heating up. Higher temperatures shorten the shelf life of dry goods. High humidity in dry storage areas (over 60%) can cause cans to rust and grains (such as crackers) to get moldy. Good ventilation is important.

    b. TCS foods must be kept under refrigeration and at an internal temperature below 41°F (5°C). It is best to store meat, poultry, seafood, and dairy in the coldest part of the refrigerator (also called the cooler). Cut melons, cut tomatoes, and cut leafy greens are stored at 41°F (5°C) or lower, as they are also TCS foods. Shelving should be open to allow for air circulation, which helps maintain proper refrigeration temperatures, and all foods should be covered. Moisture forming on the refrigerator ceiling and black mold indicate poor air circulation and temperature inconsistencies. Condensation drainage systems in walk-in refrigerators should be checked regularly to make sure they are clean and working properly.

    c. Freezers must be able to keep frozen food solid, meaning a temperature at or below 0° F (−18° C). To keep frozen goods at proper temperatures, it is important to use open shelving, not overload the shelves, and watch for frost buildup. Some freezers go into a defrost cycle each day to reduce the chances of frost buildup. Other freezers, usually older ones, have a manual defrost cycle. Manual defrost cycles can be lengthy so it is usually best to move food to another freezer while it defrosts. All food items in the freezer need to be thoroughly wrapped and sealed to prevent freezer burn. Freezer burn is when the surface of a food loses moisture and dries out, and this affects the food's color, flavor, and texture once cooked. Freezer burn is more likely if the freezer temperature fluctuates above 0° F (−18° C) and if foods are stored too long. Individually quick frozen (IQF) foods, because of their large, exposed surface areas, are also more prone to freezer burn. IQF foods, such as fruits and vegetables, are frozen individually to maintain their quality once thawed.

    d. Storage areas must have at least one thermometer that measures air temperature and it must be accurate to within ± 3°F (± 1.5°C). Thermometers are placed in the warmest part of refrigerators and freezers (generally by the door). Many refrigerators and freezers have a remote thermometer placed by the door on the outside of the unit so an employee can do a temperature check without opening the door. Temperatures in all storage areas are checked often (at least twice a day) and documented. With a computerized temperature system, temperatures in refrigerators and/or freezers are constantly recorded, and managers are alerted when a unit has become too warm. Higher humidity helps fruits and vegetables stay fresh, so keep the relative humidity at 85 to 95 percent if you have a cooler containing just fruits and vegetables.

3. *Food storage areas must be kept clean and dry and allow for air circulation.* To keep floors clean and reduce cross contamination and pests, food is always stored at least 6 inches above the ground and 6 inches away from the wall. Any spills should be mopped up quickly, and regular cleaning (such as daily mopping) must be on a schedule. Upper shelving should be wire mesh or slotted to allow air circulation, but bottom shelves can be solid to prevent food being exposed to mop spray when floors are cleaned. Don't overload refrigerators or freezer.

4. *Food has to be stored properly to avoid cross-contamination.* Never store food near dirty linens, cleaning chemicals or pesticides, exposed waste or sewer lines, or under anything that could drip moisture. Also, never store food in a room such as a locker room, restroom, or garbage room. If food is put into a container, the container should be NSF approved for food use, leakproof, sanitized, covered, and labeled. Live shellfish should always be stored in their original container with the identification tag attached.

5. *For quality and safety reasons, food can be stored for limited periods of time in refrigerators or freezers.* **Table 8-2** shows recommended storage times and temperatures for many foods.

Food	Length of Time in Refrigerator at <41°F	Length of Time in Freezer at <0°F	Additional Notes
Table 8-2 Recommended Storage Times and Temperatures			
Fresh chicken and turkey	1–2 days	9–12 months	Iced-packed poultry can be stored in the refrigerator as is. Change the ice often and sanitize the container.
Cooked poultry dishes	3–4 days	4–6 months	
Fresh lean fish	1–2 days	6–8 months	Ice-packed whole fish can be stored in the refrigerator as is. Change the ice often and sanitize the container.
Fresh fatty fish	1–2 days	2–3 months	Ice-packed whole fish can be stored in the refrigerator as is. Change the ice often and sanitize the container.
Fresh shrimp, scallops, crawfish, squid	1–2 days	3–6 months	
Fresh meat: chops, steaks, roasts	3–5 days	4–12 months	Store in coldest part of refrigerator.
Ground meat, stew meat	1–2 days	3–4 months	Store in coldest part of refrigerator.
Cooked meat dishes	3–4 days	2–3 months	
Bacon	7 days	1 month	Once opened, keep the package tightly wrapped in foil.
Milk	7 days	3 months	Milk must be chilled to 41°F (5°C) or lower within four hours of being received.
Cheese, sliced	2 weeks	Not recommended	Rewrap cheese in fresh wrapping, such as plastic wrap, after it has been opened.
Eggs (shell)	3–5 weeks	Not recommended	Shell eggs should be kept in a refrigerator with an air temperature of 45°F (7°C) or lower.
Fresh apples	3 weeks	8–10 months	Apples can be stored at room temperature for one week. Apples produce ethylene so store them away from ethylene-sensitive fruits such as carrots, leafy greens, and broccoli.
Fresh bananas	2–5 days	2 months	Green bananas stored around 60–70°F (16–21°C) will ripen in 4–7 days.

(continues)

Table 8-2 Recommended Storage Times and Temperatures (continued)

Food	Length of Time in Refrigerator at <41°F	Length of Time in Freezer at <0°F	Additional Notes
Fresh citrus	10–14 days	Not recommended	Oranges may be held at room temperature for up to five days, grapefruit up to seven days. Store fresh citrus in a well-ventilated area. High humidity is helpful as long as there is sufficient air circulation.
Fresh berries and cherries	2–4 days	8–12 months	Blueberries last longer than other berries—up to seven days. If strawberries are stored closer to 32 °F with a relative humidity of 95%, they will stay fresh up to two weeks.
Most other fruits	2–7 days	8–12 months	Fruits can dry out so keep the relative humidity in the refrigerator at 85 to 95%. Bananas, peaches, and pears should only be frozen for 2–3 months.
Beets and carrots	10–14 days	8–12 months	Remove green tops to carrots prior to storage to increase shelf life because the tops need water.
Potatoes, White Sweet	Don't refrigerate! 1–2 weeks 2–3 weeks	8–12 months	Potatoes should be stored in a well-ventilated container, away from sunlight, and ideally at 45–55°F (7–13°C).
Corn in husks	1–2 days	8–12 months (if corn is cut off)	Corn in husks should be used quickly as the sugar turns to starch.
Most other vegetables	2–7 days	8–12 months	Vegetables can dry out so keep the relative humidity in the refrigerator at 85 to 95%. Don't freeze lettuces, greens, radishes, cucumbers, or artichokes

Data from Food and Drug Administration and U.S. Department of Agriculture.

6. *Use the first-in, first-out (FIFO) method of stock rotation to prevent food spoilage* (as discussed in the previous section).
7. *The following are notes for certain foods.*
   a. Certain fruits and vegetables do *not* need to be refrigerated and should be stored at room temperature, such as potatoes, sweet potatoes, onions, garlic, winter squash, beets, pineapple, and bananas.
   b. Keep onions away from other foods that may absorb odors such as butter, cheese, milk, and cake frosting.
   c. Because fruits produce ethylene gas (which enhances ripening) during refrigeration, they can cause most vegetables and a few non–ethylene-producing fruits to deteriorate quicker. Ideally, ethylene-producing fruits should be stored in the refrigerator as far from ethylene-sensitive fruits and vegetables as possible (**Figure 8-8**).
   d. Fresh greens and lettuces, herbs, berries, corn, sprouts, and ripe peaches are the most perishable so they should be stored in the back of the refrigerator where it is coldest.
   e. Fresh whole fish or poultry that is packed in ice should be stored with the ice in a self-draining container and kept in the refrigerator. The ice should

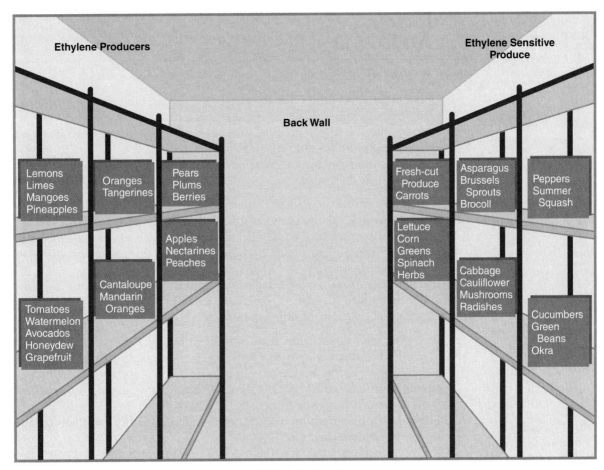

Ethylene Producers

Ethylene Sensitive Produce

Back Wall

Lemons
Limes
Mangoes
Pineapples

Oranges
Tangerines

Pears
Plums
Berries

Apples
Nectarines
Peaches

Cantaloupe
Mandarin
Oranges

Tomatoes
Watermelon
Avocados
Honeydew
Grapefruit

Fresh-cut
Produce
Carrots

Asparagus
Brussels
Sprouts
Brocoll

Peppers
Summer
Squash

Lettuce
Corn
Greens
Spinach
Herbs

Cabbage
Cauliflower
Mushrooms
Radishes

Cucumbers
Green
Beans
Okra

Walk-in Refrigerator

FIGURE 8-8 Ethylene-producing Fruits Should Be Stored in the Refrigerator as Far from Vegetables and Ethylene-sensitive Fruits as Possible.

U.S. Department of Agriculture. Retrieved from https://fns-prod.azureedge.net/sites/default/files/foodsafety_storage.pdf

be changed often. Fresh fish and fresh, shucked shellfish can be kept at about 32°F (0°C) and 65% relative humidity.

f. Sous vide food or vacuum-packed foods must be stored in refrigerators or freezers according to the manufacturer's recommendations.

g. The following are notes for alcoholic beverages.

　i. Beer in kegs must be stored at 38°F (3°C) because it is not pasteurized. Beer in cans and bottles are normally pasteurized so they can be stored in a cool, dark dry goods storeroom or in the refrigerator.

　ii. Wine should not be exposed to direct sunlight and does best without excessive light of any type. Wine bottles with cork stoppers should be stored on their sides so the cork is in contact with the wine, lessening the chance of the cork drying out. If the cork dries out, oxygen will get into the bottle and spoil the wine. Storage temperature should be consistent and between 50 to 60°F (10 - 15°C). Higher humidity is not a problem for wines.

　iii. Liquor can be stored in a dry storage area.

8. *Reserve a storage shelf for any food items that are being returned to a vendor and label the shelf.* Any dented cans, out-of-date products, etc., should be placed here. The health department often requires a separate labeled shelf for this purpose.

8.3 MANAGE INVENTORY INCLUDING CALCULATING FOOD/BEVERAGE COST

To manage inventory, foodservice managers must do the following.

- Decrease inventory losses due to waste, theft, and spoilage, by, for example, keeping storage areas locked and issuing foods to employees as needed.
- Keep inventory as lean as possible, such as by ordering close to when items are used (known as just-in-time ordering).
- Ensure that inventory records are accurate, including how much is in stock and its approximate dollar value.

Accurate inventory records are essential for managers when deciding on how much to order. Inventory records are also used to establish an operation's food costs, so if the records are not accurate, the food costs will not be correct. By having *accurate* food cost information, a manager can take action to control food costs that could be high due to waste, theft, or overportioning.

It is important to have a large enough inventory to avoid running out of items between deliveries (called stockouts—which can lead to unhappy guests), but you also need to avoid having excess items sitting in storage for the following reasons.

1. When the inventory is larger than it needs to be, the foodservice is tying up money in the inventory instead of investing the money somewhere else, such as making improvements or hiring a new employee. For frequently used items, it is okay to have some safety stock—a small amount of inventory to meet higher-than-expected customer demand.
2. The space for the inventory costs money. The less inventory space needed, the less expensive the storage costs.
3. It takes longer to count up the stock when the inventory is larger than necessary.
4. If food is stored too long, there is a greater chance that it will spoil. Every food has a shelf life, in other words, the length of time the food (such as produce) can be stored before its quality or safety lessens.
5. Excess food may encourage theft or waste by employees.

PHYSICAL INVENTORY AND PERPETUAL INVENTORY

Let's look at a small restaurant with a dry goods storage room, walk-in refrigerator, and reach-in freezer. When the cooks or other production employees need ingredients, they simply look for the items they need in the storage areas and take them back to their work stations. These storage areas are referred to as open storerooms because employees can always access them. (Liquor storage areas are locked because they are of high value and a prime target for theft.) When the chef/owner prepares to place purchase orders, first he/she checks the storage areas to see what is on hand.

In this operation, the chef/owner does a physical inventory every month, meaning that every food item in inventory is counted up and entered into inventory management software or a spreadsheet such as Excel. Then the dollar value of the inventory is calculated by multiplying each food item, such as 50 pounds of hamburgers, by the price paid (usually from the most recent order). The chef/owner in this operation knows exactly how much is in stock only once a month after doing the physical inventory.

Meanwhile, in a large foodservice operation with multiple dry goods storage rooms, walk-in refrigerators, and freezers, employees must request the items they need from inventory using a form called a stock requisition, which may be generated by production software. When a foodservice maintains this type of inventory, called a perpetual inventory it keeps a running balance of each inventory item, as displayed in **Table 8-3**.

Product(GTIN)/ Unit	Date	Invoice/ Requisition	Quantity In	Quantity Out	Balance on Hand
Hamburgers, 4 oz., 10 pound box	10/20/2020	INV	80 lbs.		80 lbs.
	10/21/2020	RQ 2259		10 lbs.	70 lbs.
	10/23/2020	RQ 2305		25 lbs.	45 lbs.
	10/24/2020	RQ 2344		15 lbs.	30 lbs.
	10/25/2020	RQ 2401		10 lbs.	20 lbs.
	10/27/2020	INV	80 lbs.		100 lbs.

Table 8-3 Perpetual Inventory Records for 4 oz. Hamburgers

In this manner, the purchasing agent can check on the computer to see how much is on hand in real time for almost every inventory item.

Keeping a perpetual inventory requires a lot of work—namely that *purchases* must be entered into the software (although software that places orders often enters the purchases into the software) along with every item that is *removed* from inventory to make meals and provide beverages. So, in this foodservice, employees can't just walk into a storeroom and take what they need off of the shelf. Instead, they must fill out stock requisitions, which, in some operations, are filled out and handed in the day before the food is needed. Issuing foods not only leads to better inventory control but also requires personnel to oversee the requisition process and to do the issuing. In most operations, issuing foods is only done during certain time periods, not all day, so employees have to plan ahead (although managers are often given the authority to issue supplies, if needed).

Even in an operation with a perpetual inventory, a physical inventory needs to be done periodically (such as monthly) to see if the physical inventory matches what the computer says is on hand. When there is a discrepancy, adjustments to on-hand inventory must be documented.

A physical inventory, including counting and valuing all of the items in storage, may be done weekly, biweekly, twice a month, or monthly. Inventory should be taken on the same day, not date. For example, a manager may choose to do the monthly inventory on the last Wednesday of the month; then, you are assured to have the same number of food delivery days in between inventories. Also, the food purchases will more closely reflect the amount of food sold. In some really large operations, a monthly physical inventory of everything would involve so much time that the inventory is split up into four sections, for example, and one section is inventoried each week during a month. Taking a physical inventory is a time-consuming process but having the inventory dollar value is helpful to see if your inventory costs are high or low and also to calculate food costs.

To take a physical inventory, the inventory should be completely put away in each of the storage areas and each storage area should be tidied up. To begin the process, an employee needs either a printed list of inventory items or a laptop/tablet with the inventory list. The inventory list should show products in the order they are stored in each storage area. Each item is counted and the total entered into the correct column. If the unit for canned peaches, for example, is a case (containing 6 cans), and there are two full cases and three cans, that is counted as 2.5 cases. A case that is not full is referred to as a **broken case**.

Taking a physical inventory goes faster if two people do it. Then one person is in charge of counting and the other in charge of recording the data. Some operations let employees use a handheld barcode scanner to scan the boxes, and this information (both quantity and cost) is transferred to the inventory management system. To control inventory and prevent employee theft, a manager, or someone from another department may help do inventory. For example, the chef may work with the beverage manager to do the inventory of liquor, wine, and beer.

To calculate the food cost for a certain period, managers need to know the dollar value of each inventory item. The dollar value is calculated using this formula.

$$\text{Item amount} \times \text{Item cost} = \text{Item inventory value}$$

Example: 12.5 cases tomato sauce $\times$ \$15.00/case = \$187.50 (Inventory value)

Determining the dollar value for each inventory item can be a little tricky because it is very possible that you paid different prices for an item. For example, five cases of oranges are in stock, of which three cases cost \$18.50 each and the most recent two cases cost \$19.15 each. Ideally, you would want to value each case at the price you actually paid, but that is quite complex and time-consuming to do without a good software program. Therefore, many operations simply use the most recent price paid. Using the most recent price is referred to as the FIFO price method because it assumes the "First in" items (oldest products) are used first.

Once you know the dollar value for all items, they are added up to give the total inventory value. **Table 8-4** shows part of an inventory that has been costed out. A person who helped with counting and totaling the inventory value should not also be in charge of evaluating the inventory levels. That responsibility should be given to someone else.

Some restaurants have state-of-the-art point of sale (POS) computerized systems that deduct items from inventory in response to customer orders entered into the software. For example, every chicken breast and bun ordered at Chick-fil-A is deducted from inventory. The same is true for hamburgers at McDonald's. With this software, a manager can compare sales to inventory on a daily basis. For example, if 40 quarter-pound hamburgers (10 pounds) were pulled from inventory one day, a manager can check how well that matches the number of quarter-pounders that were sold. If the cash register POS says that only 34 quarter-pounders were sold, the manager would need to look into issues such as waste, theft, or mistakes. Although managers still have to enter actual inventory amounts into the software, these systems are very helpful for keeping track of waste and theft, tracking sales trends, suggesting ordering quantities based on par levels and inventory, and giving low inventory alerts so the restaurant does not run out of any menu items.

ABC INVENTORY METHOD

When a monthly physical inventory is costed out, as shown for a few items in Table 8-4, managers can see which items are the most valuable, such as steaks and liquor. By comparison, sugar packets and many seasonings are inexpensive. The **ABC inventory**

Table 8-4 Part of a Physical Inventory Costed Out				
Item Description/ GTIN	Unit	Amount on Hand	Item Cost	Total Item Value
GM Honey Nut Cheerios/ 016000119888	Case (4/case)	2.5 cases	\$51.99	\$129.98
Kellogg's Raisin Bran/038000008917	Case (4/case)	1.25 cases	\$56.99	\$ 71.24
Quaker Granola/025555807010	Case (3/case)	1 case	\$38.99	\$ 38.99
Kellogg's Corn Flakes/001912953107	Case (4/case)	1.75 cases	\$30.08	\$ 52.64
GM Trix Cereal/011963205861	Case (4/case)	2.25 cases	\$51.78	\$116.51

method classifies inventory into one of three categories based on their dollar value and usage so managers can pay more attention to higher value items.

- Category A items are expensive or high in value, such as meat, poultry, seafood, liquor, and wine. In terms of number of items, they make up only about 20% of your inventory but account for closer to 75 to 80% of your inventory in dollars.
- Category B items are of average or moderate value, and include items such as many types of produce. These items comprise about 30% of your inventory in volume and represent 10 to 15% of your total inventory value.
- About half of the items in inventory fit into Category C and are relatively low in value or cost. These items are only worth 5 to 10% of your total inventory value (Dopson & Hayes, 2016).

To figure out which inventory items belong in each category, you have to multiply the purchase price for each item by its monthly usage. Then rank the items from highest dollar usage to lowest. If you had only 100 items, the top 20 items would be in Category A, the next 30 in Category B, and the last 50 items in Category C.

This type of categorization helps to set inventory priorities. Category A items will include most of your entrées or "center of the plate" items. These items drive sales and repeat business. It is smart to give these tight controls such as being protected and inventoried frequently. Category B items are important as they may be used in many dishes, so are important menu staples like potatoes, eggs, and sliced or grated cheese. Category C items can be managed with basic controls such as monthly physical inventories. **Table 8-5** lists more guidelines on managing ABC inventory items.

HOW TO CALCULATE COST OF GOODS SOLD

If a foodservice manager knows how much food costs each month to produce that month's sales, the manager can then calculate important metrics such as cost/meal and **food cost percentage** to help determine if financial/profitability goals are being met. Food cost percentage is the cost of food divided by total sales, and a manager likes to keep that number within a range, such as under 30% for some quick-service restaurants.

To calculate how much it costs to produce sales for a certain period, managers can use the following formula. The **cost of goods sold** is the cost to purchase the foods and

Table 8-5 Guide to Managing ABC Inventory Items	
Category	**Inventory Management Techniques**
A	1. Order only on an as-needed basis. 2. Conduct perpetual inventory on a daily, or at least, weekly basis. 3. Have a clear idea of purchase point and estimated delivery time. 4. Conduct monthly physical inventory.
B	1. Maintain normal control systems; order predetermined inventory (par) levels. 2. Monitor more closely if the sale of this item is tied to the sale of an item in Category A (such as flounder stuffed with spinach—a B item). 3. Review status quarterly for movement to Category A or C. 4. Conduct monthly physical inventory.
C	1. Order in a large quantity to take advantage of discounts if the item is not perishable. 2. Stock constant levels of product. 3. Conduct monthly physical inventory.

Reproduced from *Food & Beverage Cost Control* (6th ed.), p. 118, by Lea Dopson and David Hayes, 2016, Hoboken (NJ): John Wiley & Sons, Inc. Reprinted with permission.

beverages used to generate sales. Cost of goods sold can be calculated for all food and beverages purchased, or separately for any groups of items, such as alcoholic beverages or meat.

$$\begin{aligned}
&\text{Beginning inventory} \\
&\underline{+ \text{ Food Purchases}} \\
&= \text{Cost of food available} \\
&\underline{- \text{ Ending inventory}} \\
&= \text{Cost of goods sold}
\end{aligned}$$

By adding the value of the inventory at the beginning of a period (often a month) to the value of purchases during that period, you have the total value of food available for sale. Then by subtracting the value of the ending inventory for the period, you get the cost of food used during the period.

Example 8.1 shows how the cost of goods sold was calculated for the month of May. First, the inventory on May 1st was added to the purchases made throughout the month of May. The food and beverages available for sale during May was $131,000. When you subtract the value of the May 31st inventory from $131,000, you have the cost of goods sold during May, which is $99,000. If sales during that period were $282,000, the food cost percentage is 35% (divide $99,000 by $282,000).

If a foodservice requires requisitions for all foods and beverages in storage, the manager can actually calculate a daily food cost by adding together the dollar value of the stock requisitions with the dollar value of any direct issues (such as bread or milk). The daily food cost can then be compared with the sales, and a food cost percentage can be calculated.

HOW TO CALCULATE INVENTORY TURNOVER RATE

Inventory turnover measures how often a company uses and replaces its inventory during a given period, such as a month or quarter (three consecutive months). If your turnover rate is much lower than the industry average, you are probably overstocked and have some old inventory. For example, if inventory turnover is 1.5 in a school foodservice, that is low when many schools have an inventory turnover of 3 or higher. A low turnover rate may also occur when sales are slower. It is generally desirable to have a higher turnover rate as long as you are not so understocked that you frequently run out of items.

To calculate inventory turnover for a period of time, use the following formula.

$$\frac{\text{Cost of goods sold}}{\text{Average inventory value}} = \text{Inventory Turnover Rate}$$

EXAMPLE 8.1 HOW TO CALCULATE COST OF GOODS SOLD

Beginning Inventory + Food Purchased − Ending Inventory = Cost of Goods Sold	
Example:	
Beginning Inventory - 5/1/2021	$34,000
Purchases for May	+ $97,000
Food/Bev. Available for Sale During May	$131,000
Ending Inventory - 5/31/2021	− $32,000
Cost of Goods Sold (May)	$99,000

EXAMPLE 8.2 HOW TO CALCULATE INVENTORY TURNOVER

$$\frac{\text{Cost of good sold}}{\text{Average inventory value for the period}} = \text{Inventory Turnover Rate}$$

$$\text{Example: } \frac{\$99,000}{\$33,000} = 3.0 \text{ Inventory Turns}$$

In the prior section, you learned how to calculate the cost of goods sold for a period, the top half of the fraction.

To calculate the average inventory value for a period, you add the beginning inventory and the ending inventory, then divide by 2. Following is an example.

Beginning Inventory + Ending Inventory ÷2 = Average Inventory

Beginning Inventory (May 1st) $34,000

Ending Inventory (May 31st)   + $32,000

$66,000 ÷ 2 = $33,000

Now you are ready to calculate inventory turnover using the cost of goods sold calculated in **Example 8.2** and the average inventory value just computed. Using those numbers, the inventory turnover rate is 3.0 for the month of March.

An **inventory turnover rate** can also be calculated for alcoholic beverages or one inventory category, such as meats. This is done by dividing the cost of goods sold by the average inventory or ending inventory for those items and can be helpful to locate specific inventory items with low turnover rates.

Inventory turnover is best calculated on a regular basis, such as monthly, and compared over time as shown in **Figure 8-9**, which also includes a target turnover rate. It is also a good idea to compare inventory turnover with the industry average and industry standards. For example, an average restaurant inventory turnover rate (across segments) is 4.0 while turnover rates range from 2.5 to 4.0 for foodservices in healthcare or education (Reynolds, 2013, p. 197).

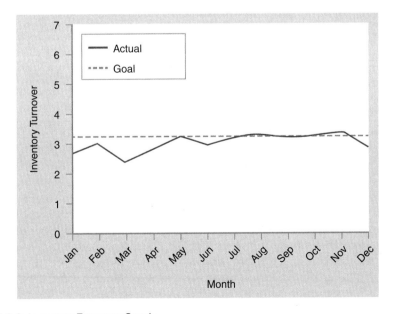

FIGURE 8-9 Inventory Turnover Graph

SPOTLIGHT ON KEEPING INVENTORY SECURE

Theft of items in inventory is quite common. Many employees would never steal money but will steal food. They may not take that much, perhaps just some sliced deli meats to take home, but over time, this will have a financial impact. Here are ways to keep inventory secure.

1. Use suppliers you can trust and develop an approved list of vendors for everyone to use. Ask vendors if they perform criminal background checks on delivery personnel.
2. Lock up storage areas and limit who gets the keys to access these areas. Change locks or codes periodically.
3. Open storage areas at scheduled times for cooks and other production personnel to get what they need, and keep records of all issued items. If locking up all of the storage areas is too difficult, management can lock up only the most valuable foods and beverages and issue them at scheduled times. This way, the operation can maintain a perpetual inventory of the most expensive items.
4. Don't allow only one person in the foodservice for a period of time unless inventory is locked up and the employee doesn't have the key or code.
5. Make sure ordering, receiving, and taking inventory are done during normal business hours whenever possible.
6. Don't let the same person do the purchasing and receiving. This prevents the person who is ordering to work with the supplier to get any type of **kickback**. For example, the purchasing agent may get a kickback (in money or products) by allowing the supplier to bill for more items than were received (incomplete shipments) or bill for lower-quality items at a higher price.
7. Have a manager periodically recheck a recently received order to ensure that the quantities and quality are appropriate.
8. Move products from receiving to storage as quickly as possible.
9. Keep delivery people out of storage areas.
10. Watch out for employees who get very friendly with a supplier or have relatives working for the supplier.
11. Don't let the same person do the purchasing and pay the bills. Have an independent person check and pay the bills.
12. Keep the loading dock, food storeroom, refrigerator and freezers, and exit doors under video surveillance.
13. Keep an eye on what is inside trash pails and consider using clear trash bags.
14. Some operations have a policy that discourages employees from bringing duffel bags, backpacks, etc., to work and warns employees that these items may be inspected when they leave the facility.
15. Compare daily food/beverage cost to sales/orders to monitor possible theft. Check stock requisitions for how many lobster tails, for example, were pulled from storage and compare to the number of lobster tail entrées that were sold. If kitchen staff know they are responsible for foods they get from inventory, they are less likely to steal.

8.4 ISSUE PRODUCTS

As mentioned in the discussion on perpetual inventory, larger foodservices often keep some or all of their inventory locked up. Employees who need supplies must first fill out a Requisition Form (**Table 8-6**) with the items they need and how much is needed. It is helpful for employees to review the menu and recipes a day in advance and identify the items they will need to requisition for the next day. The amount requisitioned should be based on the production schedule, which states how many servings to prepare for each menu item. In most operations, the employee needs a signature from a supervisor or other authorized employee before handing in the requisition. Once the requisition is handed to a storeroom employee, the items are issued. Note in Table 8-6 that a requisition must be signed by someone who reviews and approves the order as well as the person who issues and the person who receives the food.

Foodservices sometimes use a Dutch door to secure the storage areas while issuing foods. A Dutch door is split into two halves, making an upper door and a lower door.

Table 8-6 Stock Requisition Form

Requisition Form	Date: 6/20/2020			Number: 2273	
Item/GTIN	Unit	Number of Issue Units	Cost/Issue Unit	Total Cost
Del Monte Peaches, sliced, light syrup	#10 can	4	$8.50	$34.00
L. Leaf Butterscotch pudding	#10 can	3	$4.99	$14.97
Nabisco Chocolate Chip Cookie	Sleeve (12 sl/case)	3	$1.66	$ 4.98

Approved by: _____ Issued by: _____ Received by:_____

The lower door is kept closed and locked, and the upper door is kept open. A cook who needs supplies for the lunch meal, for example, brings the requisition up to the Dutch door and hands it to a storeroom employee who gets the needed items.

Smaller operations may require a requisition only for food and beverage items that are the most expensive (such as meat and alcoholic beverages). Any unused items should be returned to the storage area and their return recorded in the inventory records.

A major advantage of issuing foods is that it leads to better inventory control and fewer opportunities for theft. A disadvantage of issuing is that it requires personnel to handle the requisitions and issue foods. Since most foodservices are open for long hours, issuing hours are generally set for specific time periods, such as at the start of a shift, so employees can requisition what they need for the day. This can lead to problems when someone needs something in storage but they are closed. In this situation, a manager may have the key or code to open up a storage area and issue the needed foods.

A foodservice can go a step further than issuing foods. In this situation, storeroom personnel continue to issue foods, but they also weigh and measure the ingredients for each recipe. This is referred to as an **ingredient room**. Ingredient rooms work best in large, high-volume operations. By having ingredient room employees who are tasked with gathering and measuring ingredients for each recipe, chefs and cooks can spend more time cooking. Also, employees who regularly weigh and measure ingredients are usually more accurate and measuring equipment can be centralized for their use.

Another advantage of an ingredient room is that there is less waste because cooks get only what they need. Ingredient-room employees print out each recipe, which has already been adjusted for the correct number of servings. Then they assemble and measure those ingredients, and each ingredient is labeled. If only part of a gallon of milk is needed for a recipe, for example, the milk will be returned to the refrigerator in the ingredient room and used again when needed for another recipe. It is more advantageous for ingredient-room personnel to keep a partially used can or carton rather than have several all around the kitchen. It decreases waste and keeps food safe.

Depending on the operation, ingredient-room employees may also do some preparation tasks such as washing fruits, slicing vegetables, or breading fish. If three different recipes for the day call for chopped onions, it is more efficient to have one ingredient-room employee prepare them for all of the recipes than for three different cooks. It is also less wasteful because each cook will likely wind up with extra chopped onions.

SUMMARY

8.1   Receive products.

- A receiving clerk needs a loading dock and space to check in orders, as well as a desk/table, scales, barcode scanners, equipment to move deliveries such as pallet trucks, and tools such as thermometers and date stamp.
- When receiving an order, the receiving clerk usually uses invoice receiving to check the name and quantity of each item delivered. Distributors normally tag each case with a label containing a barcode (which includes the GTIN) so the receiving clerk may use a barcode scanner to keep track of what has been received.
- When checking quantities, the clerk also takes temperatures on potentially hazardous foods and visually inspects for quality issues (such as frozen precut salad) including outdated products.
- If some items are to be returned, the delivery person will submit a request for credit for the returned items often using a handheld device so the foodservice will get a credit memo.
- In some operations, the receiving clerk also checks the foodservice's purchase order against the supplier's invoice to make sure the right items were delivered along with the correct quantity and price.
- The final step is for the receiving clerk to sign the invoice. By signing the invoice, the foodservice is acknowledging receipt of the items. The receiving clerk may be required to maintain a receiving log.
- Indicators of quality for many foods are listed in Table 8-1.
- When putting foods away, the receiving clerk should make sure all incoming food is marked with the date it was received, all foods are rotated using the first-in, first-out method, the box or can label is face out, and raw protein foods are stored separately from ready-to-eat foods.
- Direct issues are foods, such as cakes and pies, which go directly from receiving to production.

8.2   Store products safely.

- All foods need to be labeled with their product name and date. Any food not in its original container, such as flour that has been put in a bin, must be labeled with the name of the food. Any ready-to-eat TCS food that will be held for more than 24 hours must be marked with a use-by date that is no more than seven days beyond when it was received.
- All foods need to be stored at proper temperatures. Dry storage areas should be maintained between 50°F (10°C) and 70°F (21°C). TCS foods must be kept under refrigeration and at an internal temperature below 41°F (5°C). Freezers must be able to keep frozen food solid, meaning a temperature at or below 0°F (−18°C). To keep frozen goods at proper temperatures, it is important to use open shelving, not overload the shelves, and watch for frost buildup.
- Storage areas must have at least one thermometer that measures air temperature and it must be accurate to within ± 3°F (± 1.5°C). Thermometers are placed in the warmest part of refrigerators and freezers (generally by the door). Temperatures should be checked twice daily and recorded.
- Certain fruits and vegetables do *not* need to be refrigerated and should be stored at room temperature, such as potatoes, sweet potatoes, onions, garlic, winter squash, and bananas.
- Keep onions away from other foods that may absorb odors such as butter, cheese, milk, and cake frosting.
- Ethylene-producing fruits should be stored in the refrigerator as far from vegetables and ethylene-sensitive fruits as possible (Figure 8-8). Allow space for air circulation.
- Food storage areas must be kept clean and dry. Food must be stored at least 6 inches above the ground and 6 inches away from the wall. Never store food near dirty linens, cleaning chemicals or pesticides, exposed waste or sewer lines, or under anything that could drip moisture. Also, never store food in a room such as a locker room, restroom, or garbage room.

8.3   Manage inventory including calculating food/beverage cost.

- To manage inventory, managers must take actions to decrease inventory losses due to shrinkage, keep inventory as lean as possible, and ensure that inventory records are accurate because inventory records are used to calculate food cost.

- When the inventory is larger than necessary, the foodservice is tying up money in the inventory instead of investing the money somewhere else. Also, space for inventory costs money, and too much stock increases chances of spoilage and theft.
- Issuing foods not only leads to better inventory control but also requires personnel to oversee the requisition process and do the issuing.
- Even when a foodservice maintains a perpetual inventory (by recording all incoming food purchases and issues/requisitions), it must periodically do a physical inventory.
- Taking a physical inventory goes faster if two people do it. Then one person is in charge of counting and the other is in charge of recording the data. Some operations let employees use a handheld barcode scanner to scan the boxes, and this information (both quantity and cost) is transferred to the inventory management system. To control inventory and prevent employee theft, a manager or someone from another department may help do inventory.
- To determine the dollar value of the inventory, many foodservices use the most recent price paid or FIFO price method.
- The ABC inventory method classifies inventory into one of three categories based on their dollar value and usage so managers pay more attention to higher-value items (Category A especially).
- Table 8-5 lists guidelines on managing ABC inventory items.
- Example 8.1 shows how to calculate Cost of Goods Sold. Example 8.2 shows how to calculate Inventory Turnover Rate.

- An average restaurant inventory turnover rate (across segments) is 4.0 while turnover rates range from 2.5 to 4.0 for foodservices in healthcare or education (Reynolds, 2013, p. 197).
- The Spotlight lists ways to keep inventory secure.

8.4 Issue products.

- Table 8-6 shows an example of a Requisition Form. It is helpful for employees to review the menu and recipes a day in advance and identify the items they will need to requisition for the next day. The amount requisitioned should be based on the production schedule.
- A major advantage of issuing foods is that it leads to better inventory control and fewer opportunities for theft. A disadvantage of issuing is that it requires personnel to handle the requisitions and issue foods. Since most foodservices are open for long hours, issuing hours are generally set for specific time periods.
- In an ingredient room, storeroom personnel continue to issue foods but they also weigh and measure all the ingredients used in the recipes. Ingredient rooms work best in high-volume operations.
- With an ingredient room, chefs and cooks can spend more time cooking. Also, employees who regularly weigh and measure ingredients are usually more accurate and measuring equipment can be centralized for their use. Another advantage of an ingredient room is that there is less waste because cooks get only what they need. Depending on the operation, ingredient-room employees may also do some preparation tasks such as washing fruits or slicing vegetables.

REVIEW AND DISCUSSION QUESTIONS

1. Describe three tools a receiving clerk uses frequently.
2. Outline the basic steps a receiving clerk goes through when a delivery is made.
3. Name three rules for putting received foods into storage areas.
4. What is a direct issue?
5. How does a receiving clerk know if the foods stored at ambient temperature or in the refrigerator or freezer are being stored correctly and safely?
6. Distinguish between physical and perpetual inventory. What are their advantages and disadvantages?
7. As a foodservice manager, how do you decrease inventory waste and theft as well as make sure you have the items when you need them while keeping a lean inventory?

8. Explain the ABC inventory method. What foods would be in the A category?
9. How do you calculate cost of goods sold?
10. How do you calculate average inventory?
11. What are the advantages and disadvantages of issuing foods?
12. What is an ingredient room? In which type of foodservice would it work best and why?
13. What knowledge, skills, and abilities would you want in a receiving clerk?
14. How does a well-planned and well-executed receiving and storage program contribute to a foodservice operation?

SMALL GROUP PROJECT

For the foodservice concept that you created, go through all of your recipes to find the names of 12 fruits and vegetables. If you have fewer than 12 fruits and vegetables, add the names of common fruits and vegetables to get up to 12. Then you can do the following.

1. Develop guidelines for *receiving* each of the 12 fruits and vegetables in which you describe the quality characteristics the receiving clerk should use when checking in produce orders.
2. Develop guidelines for optimal storage for each of the fruits and vegetables. To develop the guidelines, feel free to use the following USDA publication, which is available online: *The Commercial Storage of Fruits, Vegetables, and Florist and Nursery Stocks* (Agriculture Handbook #66, 2016).
3. Given the following inventory figures and food purchases for your operation, calculate the Cost of Goods Sold during February and also the Inventory Turnover Rate.

   Beginning Inventory (2/1): $14,000
   Ending Inventory (2/28): $12,500
   February Food Purchases: $43,000

REFERENCES

Dopson, L.R. & Hayes, D.K. (2016). *Food & beverage cost control* (6th ed.). Hoboken, NJ: John Wiley & Sons, Inc.

Maras, E. (2015) RFID: A tool for tracking products, assets and more. *Food Logistics*. Retrieved from https://www.foodlogistics.com/technology/article/12141721/rfid-a-tool-for-tracking-products-assets-and-more

National Food Service Management Institute, University of Mississippi. (2012). Inventory management and tracking: Reference guide. University, MS: Author.

O'Boyle, T. (2016). RFID: A taste of traceability. *Food Quality and Safety*. Retrieved from https://www.foodqualityandsafety.com/article/rfid-taste-traceability/

Reynolds, D. & McClusky, K.W. (2013). *Foodservice management fundamentals*. Hoboken, NJ: John Wiley & Sons, Inc.

U.S. Public Health Service and U.S. Food and Drug Administration. (2017). *Food Code 2017*. Retrieved from https://www.fda.gov/Food/GuidanceRegulation/RetailFoodProtection/FoodCode/ucm595139.htm

© Denis Val/Shutterstock

Quantity Food Production

LEARNING OUTCOMES

9.1 Choose appropriate cooking methods.

9.2 Forecast production quantities.

9.3 Write a production schedule.

9.4 Use portion control.

9.5 Monitor quality of meals.

9.6 Identify sustainable practices.

INTRODUCTION

Food production includes all of the activities involved in preparing food and beverages to be served to customers. To produce excellent food, you have to start with standardized recipes and continue with quality ingredients (mostly fresh), preparation, and handling. From the moment food arrives in the operation, employees also need to pay attention to storing it properly and quickly at the correct temperatures both before *and* after preparation. The ideal situation is that food is prepared at the peak of freshness and served immediately whenever possible.

We often split up food production into either hot or cold production, as each meal component is either hot or cold when served. Many entrées, such as spaghetti and meatballs, fall into the hot food category, whereas cold foods include some appetizers and many salads, sandwiches, and desserts. In any operation, a hot or cold food may be prepared from scratch, purchased in a ready-to-eat form, or fall somewhere in between scratch cooking and convenience food. For example, an operation may prepare its lasagna from scratch, use precut and bagged romaine lettuce for Caesar salad, and purchase its desserts from an excellent local artisan bakery.

You can also look at hot and cold foods from the perspective of when they are prepared relative to when they are ordered or picked up by the customer. Some foods are:

- Completely made to order (such as over-easy eggs that are cooked only when the order comes in),
- Prepared ahead of time and dished up when the order is placed (such as mashed potatoes staying warm on the steam table or a pudding or cake staying cold in the refrigerator).

- Partially prepared ahead of time, held, and then finished when the order comes in (such as a hamburger or grilled chicken breast that has been partially cooked, then refreshed on the grill for a few minutes before serving),
- Prepared completely ahead of time (especially for cold foods) in single portions (like pudding or Cole slaw) and put in an open refrigerator or vending machine for customers to grab and go (self-service).

Keep in mind that in some operations, food is prepared and then transported to where it will be served.

Whichever way food is prepared, successful cooks need to utilize the concepts of mise en place and batch cooking. **Mise en place** is a classical French cooking term that refers to all of the preparation and organization of ingredients that must be done *before* a recipe is made. A good example of this is when you order an omelet at a display station, and you see all of the vegetables, cheeses, and meats already chopped and ready to add to the sauté pan with the eggs. Or a grill cook gets the grill station all set up with raw meats, chicken, and fish, as well as makes the accompaniments (onions, peppers, etc.) for each dish. This is all done before the orders start coming in.

When hot foods are kept warm for a period of time, such as on a steam table, they lose quality, meaning they lose color, flavor, and texture. To prevent this problem, cooks often use **batch cooking**—cooking small quantities as needed during the meal service. Vegetables are frequently batch cooked as they lose color and texture and develop odors when held hot for too long.

To begin this chapter, we will look at choosing appropriate cooking methods and healthy cooking techniques. We will then discuss scheduling production as well as portion control and how to monitor quality throughout the meal. The chapter ends with an in-depth discussion of how to reduce food waste as well as energy and water use in food production areas.

9.1 CHOOSE APPROPRIATE COOKING METHODS

When cooking, heat is transferred to food in one of three ways: by conduction, convection, or radiation.

- **Conduction** occurs when heat is transferred from something hot to something touching it that is cooler. For example, heat moves directly from the top of the range to a pot of soup on the range. Another example of conduction is when the outer edges of a roast start to cook, the heat is then conducted from the outside to the interior of the roast.
- **Convection** occurs when heat is spread by moving air, steam, liquid, or hot fat. For example, in a convection oven, fans force heated air to flow to and around the foods. Convection also occurs in a pot of soup. When the liquid at the bottom of the pot is heated, it becomes lighter and rises to the top. The cooler, heavier liquid then sinks down and becomes heated. In any pot of liquids or in a deep-fat fryer, a constant circulation spreads heat.
- **Radiation** is the transfer of heat through energy waves from a source to the food. Two kinds of radiation in the kitchen include microwave radiation and infrared radiation. Microwave ovens contain a magnetron that converts electrical power into high-frequency energy waves called microwaves. These waves penetrate the food placed in the oven, causing the water molecules in the food to vibrate, which creates heat. Infrared radiation is given off by the heating element in a broiler, for example, which cooks food.

Probably the most important consideration in applying heat in cooking is whether the heat is moist, dry, or a combination of both. **Dry-heat cooking methods** transfer heat without the use of water or steam. Instead, they rely on hot air (such as in an oven), hot fat (such as in a deep-fat fryer), hot metal (such as cooking on a griddle), or radiation (such as using a microwave or a ceramic infrared burner). Dry heat cooking methods include roast/bake, smoke-roasting, broil, grill, griddle, pan-broil, sauté, stir-fry, pan-fry, and deep-fry. At first glance, you might think that frying is a moist-heat method, but fat does not contain moisture. In addition, it does not interact with the food in the way that liquids do in moist-heating cooking. In deep-fat frying, some fat is absorbed in the food's coating. Dry-heat cooking methods allow for the browning of foods (such as via the Maillard reaction), which add flavor.

Moist-heat cooking methods involve water, a water-based liquid, or steam as the vehicle of heat transfer. Examples include poaching, simmering, boiling, steaming, and braising. Compared with most dry-heat cooking methods, moist-heat cooking does not add the flavor that dry-heat cooked foods get from browning, deglazing, or reduction. For foods that use moist-heat cooking to be successful, you will need seasonings and flavorings as well as good fortified stocks as the cooking liquid.

DRY-HEAT COOKING METHODS

Roasting, cooking with heated dry air, is an excellent method for cooking larger, tender cuts of meat, poultry, and fish that will provide multiple servings. When roasting, always place meats and poultry on a rack so that the drippings fall to the bottom of the pan and the meat, therefore, doesn't cook in its own juices. Also, cooking on a rack allows for air circulation and more even cooking. To develop flavor in meats, poultry, and fish, use rubs and marinades. Also, season and/or sear the food before cooking.

Baking is the same as roasting—cooking foods by surrounding them with heated dry air. The difference is simply that baking applies to breads, cakes, and other baked goods, as well as vegetables and fish.

Smoke-roasting, also called pan-smoking, is done on top of the stove. Smoke-roasting is both a cooking method and a way to flavor foods. Smoke-roasting is popular nowadays as a way to add flavor to meat, poultry, and seafood. Don't confuse smoking with smoke-roasting. Smoking, an ancient method used to preserve foods, often takes place at a temperature in the danger zone, so you can only smoke meats, poultry, and seafood that have been cured first. Curing adds salt and reduces available water needed by bacteria. Smoke-roasting for too long can cause undesirable results. Practice, experience, and training are needed to become proficient and knowledgeable at smoke-roasting.

Broiling, cooking with *radiant heat from above*, is wonderful for single servings of steak, chicken breast, and fish such as salmon, tuna, and swordfish, which are tender and can be served immediately. The more well done you want the product or the thicker it is, the longer the cooking time and the farther from the heat source it should be to ensure that it is properly cooked.

Grilling, cooking *with a heat source under the food*, is an excellent method for cooking vegetables as well as meat, poultry, and seafood that are tender. Like broiling, grilling browns foods, and the resulting caramelization adds flavor. Once considered a tasty way to prepare hamburgers, steaks, and fish, grilling is now used to prepare a wide variety of dishes from around the world. For example, chicken is grilled to make fajitas (Tex-Mex style of cooking) or to make jerk barbecue (Jamaican style of cooking). Grilling is also an excellent method to bring out the flavors of many vegetables. Grill them dry to avoid burning, then marinate with a light dressing consisting of a little oil, vinegar, or lemon juice and selected spices and fresh herbs. A charbroiler is a favorite piece of equipment used to grill foods. Although the name includes "broiler," the charbroiler uses heat from below.

Grilling foods properly requires much cooking experience to get the grilling temperature and timing just right. Here are some general rules to follow:

1. Cook meat and poultry at higher temperatures than seafood and vegetables.
2. If thicker cuts are used, start on the grill and finish in the oven to avoid burning.

3. Don't try to grill thin fish fillets, such as striped bass, tilapia, or flounder, because they tend to fall apart. Firm-fleshed thicker pieces of fish, such as salmon, grouper, or swordfish, do much better on the grill.

4. Don't turn foods too quickly or they will stick and tear. Add char marks to foods by turning the food about 90 degrees before turning over to finish cooking.

To flavor foods that will be broiled or grilled, consider marinades, rubs, herbs, and spices.

When broiling or grilling, turn foods with tongs instead of a fork. When you stab meat with a fork, juices are lost and the meat will be less moist and tender. Also keep the grill clean and properly seasoned to prevent sticking. The broiler must also be kept clean and free of fat buildup to avoid smoke and excess flames and avoid discoloring the food with soot or carbon residue.

Cooking hamburgers or pancakes on a solid, flat griddle (**Figure 9–1**) is referred to as **griddling**. Some fat is usually used to prevent sticking. When you use a griddle, the temperature is adjustable and much lower than on a grill. Other foods can be cooked on a griddle, such as grilled cheese and scrambled eggs. **Pan-broiling** is similar to griddling, except that it is done in a sauté pan or skillet. Any fat that accumulates while pan-broiling must be poured off, otherwise the cooking method would be pan-frying.

Sautéing, cooking food quickly in a small amount of fat over high heat, is used to cook tender foods that are either in single portions or small pieces. Sautéing can also be used as a step in a recipe to add flavor to foods such as vegetables. Sautéing adds flavor in large part from the caramelization (browning) that occurs during cooking at relatively high temperatures.

When sautéing, use a shallow pan to let moisture escape and allow space between the food items in the pan (**Figure 9–2**). Use a well-seasoned or nonstick pan and add a vegetable oil (just enough to cover the bottom of the pan) or two sprays of oil per serving after preheating the pan. Vegetable-oil cooking sprays come in a variety of flavors, such as butter, olive, Asian, Italian, and mesquite. To use these, spray the preheated pan *away* from any open flame (the spray is flammable) and then add the food. Pump spray bottles are also available that you can fill with oils of your choice.

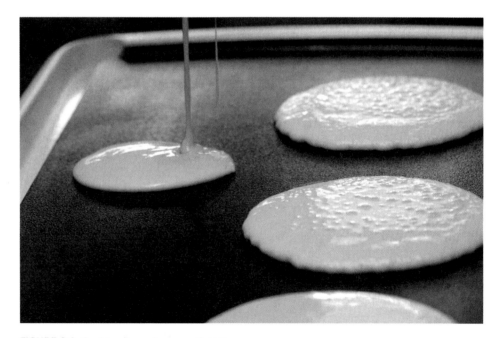

FIGURE 9-1 Cooking Pancakes on a Griddle

© BrandonKleinPhoto/Shutterstock

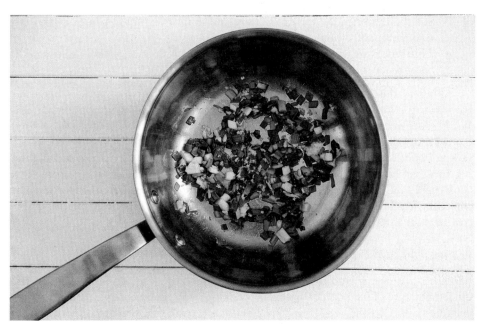

FIGURE 9-2 Sautéing

© Spring song/Shutterstock

To sauté, the food should be consistent in size to ensure even cooking. As food cooks, it releases steam—so some space between the pieces of food help that steam get released. For even cooking, stir frequently (but not constantly) when sautéing. If sautéing one portion of meat or other protein, turn it only once.

Dry sauté is a low-fat method of browning and reheating. To use this technique, heat a nonstick pan, spray with vegetable-oil cooking spray, then wipe out the excess with a paper towel. Heat the pan again, then add the food. If browning is not important, you can simmer the ingredient in a small amount of liquid such as wine, vermouth, flavored vinegar, juices, or defatted stock to bring out the flavor. Vegetables naturally high in water content, such as tomatoes and mushrooms, can be cooked with little or no added fluid at a very high heat, but do not add salt as this draws moisture out of the vegetables, which produces steam.

When you have finished sautéing, add shallots, garlic, or other seasonings, then deglaze the pan with stock, wine, or another liquid and reduce to a sauce consistency or add a previously reduced sauce to accompany your dish. **Deglaze** means to swirl a liquid in the pan to dissolve cooked particles of food remaining on the bottom of the pan.

Stir-fry, cooking bite-size foods over high heat in a small amount of oil preserves the crisp texture and bright color of vegetables and cooks strips of poultry, meat, or fish quickly. Typically, stir-frying is done in a wok, which today comes in nonstick versions. Steam-jacketed kettles and tilt frying pans can also be used to make large-quantity, stir-fry menu items. Cut up the ingredients as appropriate into small pieces, thin strips, or diced portions. Thick vegetables may need to be blanched to ensure even cooking. Proteins are cooked separately, then combined. The following are additional tips.

- Coat the cooking surface with a thin layer of oil. Peanut oil works well because it has a strong flavor and a high smoking point.
- Have all of your ingredients ready (mise en place) so you can execute this process quickly.
- Preheat the equipment to a high temperature.
- Foods that require the longest cooking times—usually meat and poultry—should be the first ingredients you start to cook.

- Stir the food rapidly during cooking and don't overfill the pan or cook items separately and combine at the end of the process.
- Thin sauces are usually thickened with cornstarch slurry, creating a silky smooth consistency.

Whereas sautéing and stir-frying use small amounts of fat and high temperatures, **pan-frying** cooks food in a moderate amount of fat in a pan over a moderate heat. While sautéing and stir-frying are used to cook smaller, evenly sized pieces of food; foods for pan-frying can be larger and thicker, such as a fish fillet, because cooking is slower. Foods to be pan-fried are often breaded, and then flipped once during cooking.

In **deep-fat frying**, food is completely surrounded by hot fat, where it tends to cook evenly and quickly. Foods, such as poultry or fish, are breaded or dipped in batter before frying. The breading or batter, once fried, adds color, crispness, and flavor. The coating does absorb some fat from the fryer.

MOIST HEAT COOKING METHODS

Poaching, simmering, and boiling all take place in a pot of liquid. What is different is the temperature of the liquid. **Poaching**, cooking a food submerged in liquid at a temperature of 160° to 185° F (71° to 85°C), is used to cook fish, tender pieces of poultry, eggs, fresh chicken or fish, sausages, and some fruits and vegetables. Liquids for poaching could include stock, wine, or fruit juices with flavoring such as fresh herbs, spices, ginger, or garlic.

Simmering is cooking a food in a liquid that is bubbling gently at a temperature of about 185° to 200° F (85° to 94°C). There is some action in the liquid, but it is not agitated, as in a boil, and the surface is fairly quiet. **Boiling** is cooking a food in a liquid that is bubbling rapidly. Water and most other cooking liquids, except liquid fats, boil at 212° F (100°C) at sea level.

Steaming has been the traditional method of cooking vegetables in many high-quantity kitchens because it is quick and retains flavor, moisture, and nutrients. It provides a balanced healthy alternative, because it requires no fat. The best candidates for steaming include vegetables and proteins with a delicate texture such as fish or chicken breasts. Steamed foods also continue to cook after they come out of the steamer, so allow for this in your cooking time. It is possible to introduce flavor into steamed foods (as well as poached foods) by adding herbs, spices, citrus juices, and other flavorful ingredients to the water.

Braising is excellent for cooking meats that are not very tender. It involves two steps: searing or browning the food (usually meat) in a small amount of oil or its own fat (to seal the outer layer and maintain moisture inside) and then adding liquid and simmering until done. Foods to be braised are also often marinated before searing to develop flavor and tenderize the meat. When browning meat for braising, sear it in as little fat as possible without scorching and then place it in a covered braising pan to simmer in a small amount of liquid. To add flavor, place roasted vegetables, herbs, spices, and other flavoring ingredients in the bottom of the braising pan before adding the liquid. Stewing is the same as braising, it is just that stewing usually refers to smaller pieces of meat or poultry.

SPOTLIGHT ON HEALTHY COOKING

With so many customers demanding healthy food options, most foodservices are considering nutrition when developing or updating menu items. Chefs are no longer relying on salt, sugar, and butter for flavor. Instead, they are building flavor through the appropriate use of ingredients, preparation techniques, and cooking methods. The following are 10 listed ingredients, preparation techniques, and cooking methods to help produce tasty and healthy menu options (Drummond & Brefere, 2017).

SPOTLIGHT ON HEALTHY COOKING (continued)

1. Ingredients: Fresh, quality ingredients are imperative. In addition, the use of seasonings and flavorings, such as the following, are excellent flavor builders.
   a. Herbs (fresh and dried). Fresh herbs are superior and more versatile for creating recipes and adding a fresh taste. Fresh herbs can only withstand about 30 minutes of cooking, so they work best for finishing dishes.
   b. Spices. Mostly available in dried forms, spices are used in savory and sweet dishes to enhance an existing flavor or add a new flavor. Some spices, such as salt, pepper, and paprika, are available smoked to add more flavor.
   c. Herb and spice blends. Combining herbs and spices creates infinite possibilities. Many international flavor profiles use both herbs and spices. For example, Chinese 5-spice is a base seasoning mix used in Chinese cooking. It usually includes herbs such as peppercorns and spices such as star anise, fennel seeds, cinnamon, and cloves. Lemon pepper, Old Bay seasoning, and Montreal steak seasoning are common spice blends.
   d. Flavorful and infused oils. Extra virgin olive oil is full of flavor and is wonderful in salad dressings or drizzling to finish a dish. Other oils, such as peanut oil, can be used to add flavor to cooked dishes. In addition, oils can be infused with ingredients such as ground and whole spices, fresh herbs, and more.
   e. Vinegars. Vinegars such as wine vinegars or balsamic vinegar can be used to add flavor to a wide variety of dishes. Like oils, vinegar can also be infused with ingredients such as chili peppers and herbs. Vinegar (as well as lemon or lime juice) are acidic and speed the cooking process but discolor vegetables.
   f. Reduced liquids. Ingredients, such as wine and fruit juices, can be reduced to a smaller volume, making a product with an intense flavor and syrupy texture that can be used in sauces, salad dressings, and more.
   g. Aromatic vegetables. Aromatic vegetables are often used as a flavor base and include ingredients such as onions, celery, carrots, and shallots.
   h. Grilled, roasted, smoked, pureed, and dried vegetables. Grilling, smoking, and other techniques are ways to enhance the flavor of vegetables.
   i. Citrus fruits. Citrus juices, reduces juices, and grated citrus rinds can be used in a number of recipes, such as salad dressings, to add flavor.
   j. Condiments. Condiments, such as mustards, sriracha sauce, and hoisin sauces, insert flavors into many of our favorite foods.
2. Preparation techniques: Chefs have a variety of techniques to use both before and during cooking to add flavor.
   a. Rubs. Dry rubs are a mixture of ground spices. Wet rubs, also called pastes, are mixed with liquid ingredients such as vinegar and mustard. Rubs are patted on the surface of meat, poultry, or fish either just before cooking (for delicate items such as a fish fillet) or 24 to 48 hours before cooking (for large cuts of meat). See **Figure 9–3**.
   b. Marinades. Marinating adds flavor and can also tenderize tough proteins.
   c. Reduction. By reducing a soup or sauce to a smaller volume, you can eliminate using thickeners (that may contain butter) and increase flavor.
   d. Searing. Searing meats and other proteins not only gives color but produces a distinctive flavor.
   e. Sweating. Sweating is when a food, usually a vegetable, is cooked over a low heat with a small amount of fat to soften the food and develop flavor. Instead of using fat, stock, juice, or wine can be used.
   f. Puréeing. Puréed vegetables or starchy foods can be used to thicken soups, sauces, and more without using fat.
   g. Caramelizing. Caramelizing can cook and brown the natural sugars in meat, fruits, and vegetables. For example, caramelizing is the essential step for cooking onions in a French onion soup recipe.
   h. Toasting. By toasting nuts, whole spices, and grains, flavors are brought out and developed.
   i. Smoking. Smoking meat, poultry, and fish adds new flavors.
   j. Deglazing. Deglaze means to swirl a liquid in a pan to dissolve cooked particles of food remaining on the bottom of the pan. The browned bits of food are scraped up and add flavor and color to the liquid, which will be used as a sauce.

(continues)

SPOTLIGHT ON HEALTHY COOKING (continued)

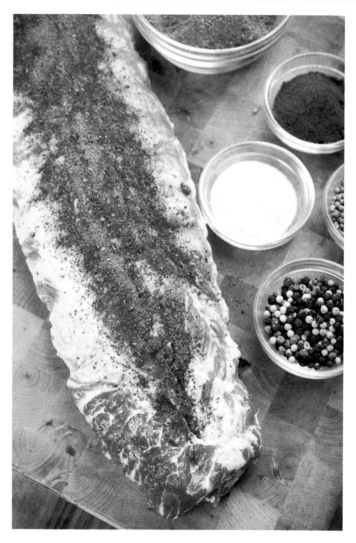

FIGURE 9-3 Baby Back Rib with Spices Used in Rub Seasoning (Spices are ground and sometimes toasted before used in rubs.)

© Msheldrake/Shutterstock

3. <u>Cooking methods</u>: All cooking methods work in healthy cooking except those using large amounts of fat or oil.
   a. <u>Sauté</u>
   b. <u>Dry sauté</u>
   c. <u>Stir-fry</u>
   d. <u>Roast</u>
   e. <u>Smoke-roast</u>
   f. <u>Broil</u>
   g. <u>Grill</u>
   h. <u>Steam</u>
   i. <u>Poach, simmer, boil</u>
   j. <u>Braise</u>

Reproduced from Drummond, K. E., & Brefere, L. M. (2016). Nutrition for foodservice and culinary professionals. John Wiley & Sons.

9.2 FORECAST PRODUCTION QUANTITIES

The production staff is told daily how much to produce of various menu items for different day parts—such as lunch or late-night meals. These estimates are determined by **forecasting**—a process in which a prediction is made of how much of each menu item will be needed for a specific time period or meal. If the forecasted numbers are accurate, there will be very little (or no) food leftover and every customer's order will be filled (instead of being told that "We are out of ...."). So accurate forecasting decreases overproduction (making too much) and underproduction (making too little), and, therefore, helps tremendously in controlling food and labor costs and keeping customers satisfied.

Forecasting is a necessary skill in every foodservice manager's toolbox and is a cooperative process that cannot be done in a vacuum. The managers and chefs who plan and write the menu are thinking about the number of sales each menu item will generate. The purchasing manager forecasts how much of each ingredient to purchase. The manager or chef in charge of food production forecasts how much of each item to prepare. Then the manager in charge of the schedule needs to schedule enough staff to produce and serve the required number of portions. There needs to be a true team effort if you want to get things right.

So, how do you accurately forecast the number of servings of chicken fajitas needed for Friday dinner? Sales forecasting is based on a number of factors but the most important factor is the historical sales numbers for that specific day and meal—including how many total customers were served and how much of each menu item was sold or served. For a foodservice that uses a cycle menu, you need the historical data for the specific day and meal in the cycle, such as Wednesday breakfast in Week 2. **Table 9-1** gives you examples of typical data saved in restaurants, colleges and universities, schools, and hospitals. Keep in mind that historical records are also useful to change or update menu choices.

Forecasting the *total* number of customers to be served can vary depending on the segment.

- Healthcare facilities, colleges, schools, business and industry, and the military have cycle menus and very specific meal times. In a hospital, the patient census

Table 9-1 Examples of Typical Data Saved in Different Foodservice Industry Segments

Restaurants
- Number of customers served during each time period (such as lunch from 11–3 PM)
- Number of each menu item sold during each time period
- Amount and type of beverages sold during each time period

Colleges and Universities
- Number of students who have purchased each meal plan
- Number of students served at each dining location during each time period
- Number of servings of each menu item used at each dining location

Schools
- Number of students in the school
- Number of meals (breakfast or lunch) planned and produced
- Number of meals served (including number of paid meals and the number of meals to be reimbursed partially or fully by the federal school breakfast and lunch programs)

Hospitals
- Daily inpatient census (number of patients in the hospital each day at a specific time such as midnight)
- Number of patients on modified/therapeutic diets
- Number of servings of each menu item used for patient meal service
- Number of servings of each menu item sold for nonpatient meals (cafeteria)

(how many patients are in a hospital at midnight) is used to forecast the number of patient trays to be served. The number of student meal plans sold in a university or the number of students in an elementary school would be used to forecast the total number of meals in universities and schools. In some small hospitals or other healthcare facilities where patients choose meals ahead of time, an employee may simply count up or "tally" the number of patients who want each lunch entrée for tomorrow's service, and then add a little to those numbers (called **padding**) to anticipate changes and avoid running out. (Keep in mind that cooks like to pad the number of portions to make because it creates a lot of work for them if they run out—but too much padding creates over production.)

- Quick-service restaurants serve food throughout the day with specific rush periods. They have excellent historical records for rush periods and nonrush periods.
- Full-service restaurants have specific meal periods and can use reservations and historical data to predict the number of customers.

Once you have a good idea of the total number of customers, it is a matter of estimating how much of each entrée will be needed. To manually forecast the number of servings of chicken fajitas, you may use a simple average, a moving average, or percentage forecasting. To get the average, you would look back at dinner sales for the past 10 Fridays—assuming there were no holidays, poor weather, or special events in the mix. You can add up how many servings of chicken fajitas were sold each week and then divide by 10 to get the average number of servings of chicken you can expect to sell this Friday.

Another forecasting method that is more sophisticated is the **moving average** method. If calculating a five-day moving average, for example, first you calculate the average of five days. This provides the first data point. Then, the oldest day is dropped off and the new day is added, and an average is again calculated. In this manner, the moving average shows a true average over time that smooths out any spikes in demand. The following is an example.

Day	Number of Chicken Fajitas five-Day Moving Average	Sold at Friday Dinner
1	44	
2	63	
3	51	
4	59	
5	49	53
6	66	58
7	55	56
8	59	58
9	51	56
10	60	58

Another forecasting method is known as **percentage forecasting**. One thing to keep in mind is that if the same five entrées are offered each Friday to 100 customers, you will likely notice patterns, such as the steak entrée accounts for about 20% of orders each Saturday. Being familiar with the popularity of each item on your menu is important and can be used to calculate a rough estimate of the number of items needed. For example, if you expect 300 customers and 20% of the orders are usually for steak, there will be about 60 steak orders (0.20×300).

Today, all foodservice segments use some type of computerized tracking of sales and production that is often available from your primary food supplier. For example, Sysco and US Foods have programs that include food production and inventory software. Sysco also offers Point of Sale (POS) or cash register systems that track the individual items sold. POS systems track sales hourly throughout the day to keep management informed of how much food needs to be purchased, thawed, prepped, and available during different phases of the lunch or dinner rush or other dayparts. Ideally, this would interface with labor scheduling software to assure that adequate staff is available at peak production and service times. Using data collected from a POS system, you can review detailed sales reports from your foodservice's history to make forecasting easier.

In fact, some software will do the forecasting for you using mathematical models that are much more sophisticated than you could do yourself. Forecasts are typically generated using historical sales or guest-count data as a starting point; they are then adjusted as necessary for current variables. For example, a system might go through the following process in creating a forecast:

1. Review the actual sales trends for the previous four weeks (or operator set value).
2. Use floating averages (means over time periods) and determine if sales are increasing or decreasing.
3. Adjust to reflect the most recent trends and operator input. Operator input is crucial when recent sales have either been hurt or helped by extraneous events. For example:
   - You are located in a college town and the students are on break.
   - You are near a convention center that was closed for renovations
   - It's a national holiday—depending on the circumstances, this could increase or decrease your sales.
   - Beef and pork sales drop dramatically because of Ash Wednesday or Good Friday.
   - Lunch sales are down due to daytime fasting holidays like Yom Kippur or Ramadan.
4. Adjust if your daily specials adversely affected the sales of regular menu items. For example, last week you offered a sustainable fish special or free-range Amish Chicken, and these pulled sales away from your regular fish and chicken menu items.
5. The system will then come up with the coming week's forecast, and assist you and your managers with your purchasing, production, and staffing decisions.

Keep in mind that your software cannot know everything. Forecasting becomes an "Art" once you get to know your customer base and use your own skills and intuition as a foodservice manager to make adjustments on the fly. Food sales around holidays like Thanksgiving, Christmas, and New Year's will never be normal. If you do not have televisions above your bar (or no liquor license) and a championship game is broadcast, your sales will be reduced. If you work for a child-themed restaurant like Chuck E. Cheese's, and the circus or Disney on Ice comes to town, your sales will be lower. And if you are near a multiplex theater and the new Marvel movie is premiering on three screens and they all let out at 9 PM, you need to be aware and ready with plenty of food and staff. A well-run operation requires planning, and forecasting is one of the "planning" keys to success.

9.3 WRITE A PRODUCTION SCHEDULE

Now that you can forecast how much to make for each menu item, you must communicate this to each station in the kitchen and/or café using a **production schedule** and a **production meeting** with appropriate staff. Also called a food production worksheet or prep sheet, production schedules are documents that communicate to employees which menu items need to be prepared and how many along with pertinent instructions, etc. But production schedules are not just to inform employees. Once the cooking is done, employees also enter information on production schedules—specifically how many portions were prepared and served, and whether too much or too little was prepared—and this information goes back to management to inform future forecasting. Good production planning should reduce problems, such as running out of food and help you serve quality meals.

Production meetings, also called pre-shift meetings, are normally held by production managers or chef managers before the meals are made. This is the time to discuss recipes, how to handle possible missing ingredients, give any special instructions, and get feedback from the cooks and other employees on what is working and what could be improved. Perhaps the cooks are having problems with an oven that is not keeping temperature properly or there is a timing issue that needs to be discussed.

Although production schedules are very individualized, most contain the following information (see **Table 9-2**). Keep in mind that there are often several production sheets

Table 9-2 Production Schedule

Production Sheet - Main Kitchen-Hot Food   Day/Date: Sunday December 1, 2019
Meal: Dinner
Weather: Sunny, cold
Special Events: End of Thanksgiving holiday weekend
No. Customers: 225

| Menu Item | Recipe Number | Portion Size | NUMBER OF PORTIONS | | | | Note time if ran out | Assignments, Instructions, Comments |
			Forecast	Prepared	Served	Leftover		
Prime Rib	59	6 oz.	40					Slice to order.
Chicken Milano	75	6 oz.	47					Do not hold more than 30 minutes on line.
Roast Turkey Breast	101	6 oz.	28					No more than four servings on the line at a time.
Lasagna	164	1 each	25					
Asian Stir-Fry	216	1 cup	27					Use wok range.
Chicken Fajitas	99	6 oz.	35					
Grilled Salmon	123	6 oz.	42					
Macaroni and Cheese	188	1 cup	110					
Broccoli	204	½ cup	175					Batch cook every 20 minutes during service.
Carrots	210	½ cup	175					Batch cook every 20 minutes during service.
Steamed Red Potatoes	232	½ cup	150					
White Rice	250	½ cup	180					Batch cook every 20 minutes during service.

PRE-PREPARATION

Employee	Menu Item	Instructions
Jim K.	Chicken Noodle Soup	Make chicken stock for tomorrow's soup.
Mike H.	Roast Beef	Pull out 80# eye round from freezer and put in refrigerator.
Anthony D.	Hard-Boiled Eggs	Make 40 hard-boiled eggs for breakfast.

for each meal—such as one for hot food production staff, one for cold food production staff, and one for the bakery staff.

1. Date
2. Day of the week
3. Daypart (such as lunch, dinner, or afternoon snacks)
4. Number of customers expected
5. Other events going on
6. Menu items
7. Portion sizes
8. Forecasted number of portions needed
9. Number of portions prepared (for various reasons—such as pan size—cooks may not make the exact number of portions forecasted—they may make a few more or a few less)
10. Number of portions served
11. Number of portions left over or what time ran out of product (and what was substituted once the product ran out)

In addition, some operations will list the recipe number or the product (such as canned peach halves) when a recipe is not needed. The cooks/food preparation staff are responsible for filling in #9 through #11.

Some managers will also use the production schedule to:

- Assign menu items to different employees
- Give special instructions (such as timing of the cooking/preparation)
- List prepreparation tasks (such as pulling meat from the freezer to put into the refrigerator to thaw or putting beans into water to soak overnight).

At the end of each day, the completed production schedules are records of how many portions were produced and served, as well as which items were overproduced or underproduced. As such, these numbers become part of the historical records used for future forecasting. Employee notes/comments on the production schedules can also be useful in communicating issues and improving production.

Figure 9-4 is another example of a production schedule, this one being for a university. It contains important considerations for forecasting. This production sheet includes the following.

Drummond University Dining	Hall	Meal	Prep	Sheet			Date	9/14/2019
Day: M Z W T F S Su	Meal	B L D	Leader: Sara	Weather	Sun Cloud	Warm Cold	Event? Orient 26	
Station and Menu Item	Recipe	H-High	H-Low	Forecast	Prepped	Dumped	Over/Under	POS Check
Salad: Rst. Beets Filberts Gorgonzola	S277	76	51	70				
Soup 1 - Beef Pho Noodle Bowl	B127	152	122	150				
Soup 2 - Italian Wedding	C079	168	111	125				
Grill: Chicken Steak	C112	108	78	90				
Grill: Corned Beef Reuben	B161	89	62	70				
Grill: Pork Banh Mi	P041	77	48	60				
Sauté: Day Boat Scallops Egg Risotto	F163	63	39	50				
Sauté: Oyster Mushrooms & Pak Choi	V038	31	17	25				
Pasta: Almond Agnolotti Black Truffle	V206	43	26	35				
Pasta: Vodka Rigatoni Vegan Sausage	V089	56	42	50				
Veg; Savoy Cabbage w Sunchokes	V091	77	51	60				
Veg; Broccoli Rabe w Garlic Pancetta	P109	46	29	40				
Dessert: Nutella Banana Pizza	D048	195	124	160/20				
Dessert: Meyer Lemon Ricotta Cake	D135	86	66	60/8				
Dessert: Blood Orange Sorbet	D204	89	53	70/25sl				

FIGURE 9-4 University Production Schedule

A.   Date: The date helps you see if it is the beginning or end of the term or if students are on break.

B.   Day of Week: The day of the week is also important, as students may go home a lot on weekends and commuter students are certainly not around on weekends.

C.   Meal Period: The number of students eating at each meal period varies. For example, a number of students don't eat breakfast.

D.   Weather: Indoor dining halls do better in bad weather, and food trucks and take-out service do better when sunny. Some customers will not go out in wind and rain and instead will order food delivery. (Gingerella, 2018)

E.   Events: Orientations and "prospective student days" add volume. BYO Sundaes add volume. Free-food events at other outlets decrease sales. Home football games at noon will reduce lunch traffic.

F.   H-High and H-Low: This column includes information on historical high and historical low sales for each item. This is important for bulk-produced items like soups and stews, which take several hours to prepare. A general rule is that it takes the same amount of time to make 10 gallons of soup (80 portions) as it does to make 20 gallons (160 portions). So if you run out and end up making two batches of 10 gallons each, you have doubled your labor cost for soup on that day.

G.   Forecast: This is the best guess based on history, recipe scaling, and type of day. This usually includes your pad (planned extra to prevent running out). Where you see the forecast for Nutella Pizza, it calls for 160 servings or 20 pies at eight slices each.

H.   Prepped: This is what the cook actually made with the ingredients provided to them.

I.   Quality Dumping: This is not overproduction but a quality monitor. When food is displayed on a hot line, it overcooks, dries, degrades, and changes color. Dumped means that you took the food out of service while there was still demand for more of this same item. When you see timers on coffee pots, the old coffee is dumped after it loses flavor and becomes more acidic, and new coffee is brewed. When display pizza dries and curls on the edges, you remove it before replacing it with a fresh pie. Tracking this will help you adjust your serving pan sizes and how much product you put out at one time.

J.   Over/Under: Over is what you have left at the end of the meal service and is considered your waste. For Under, you list the time you run out of a product or if you have an exact tally of the demand, the number you were short.

K.   POS Check: If your cash register system tracks the sales of each individual item, it is good to compare actual sales with your prepared portions. If you prepare 120 portions and only sell 85 portions at the register yet the production schedule shows there was none leftover, this is an indicator of several possibilities that are costing the business money such as the following.

   1.   Staff is overportioning the product on the serving line.
   2.   The product does not hold up well during service and is being dumped frequently.
   3.   Many customers are sampling the product, but not purchasing it.
   4.   Your cooks are not following the recipes or your recipe is not giving the proper yield.
   5.   You have a theft problem.

Another variation of a production schedule may be used for a station that makes items to order, such as a deli station in a café, or a grab-and-go refrigerator. These production sheets may simply list levels of ingredients (such as five lbs. of sliced cheddar cheese) that need to be stocked at the station before service. This type of production sheet may be called a prep sheet and the par levels are usually different depending on the meal or whether it is for a weekday or weekend (such as in a hospital café that is not as busy on weekends due to lower staffing). **Table 9–3** gives an example of a prep sheet for

Table 9-3 Prep Sheet for University Dining Hall

Prep Sheet: <u>Grill Station—Dinner</u>

Item	On Hand	Par Level Sunday–Thursday	Par Level Friday and Saturday	Comments
4 oz. hamburger patties		80	40	
4 oz. rib eye sandwich steaks		40	20	
2 oz. hotdogs		20	10	
4 oz. chicken breast		35	20	
4 oz. beer battered fish		15	8	
4 oz. Garden Burger		10	5	
BLT setups		20	10	
Cheddar cheese—1 oz.		100	50	
White American—1 oz.		100	50	
Swiss cheese—1 oz.		50	25	
Provolone cheese—1 oz.		50	25	
Sautéed onions		Half pan	Quarter pan	
Sautéed mushrooms		Half pan	Quarter pan	
Bacon strips		Half pan	Quarter pan	
French fries		8 bags (5#)	4 bags (5#)	
Onion rings		4 bags (2#)	2 bags (2#)	

a university dining hall. The person in charge of the grill station first checks what is on hand and fills that amount on the sheet. Then the employee gets enough of each item to come up to the par level. The par level is lower on Friday and Saturday because students return home or eat off campus more on those days.

THE BIG PICTURE

As you have seen, production schedules can look quite different from one another depending on the type of foodservice operation and how foods are prepared and served (such as self-service or table service). Any production schedule should be designed to clearly *communicate* what an employee, or a group of employees, need to get ready or prepare for a given meal or time period. When production schedules and production meetings allow ample communication among production managers, chefs, cooks, and food preparation workers, the foodservice is much more likely to control food costs and keep customers happy by not running out of foods.

9.4 USE PORTION CONTROL

Just as a child is unhappy when a sibling gets a bigger piece of cake, a customer will be unhappy when getting a smaller portion and paying the same price as someone enjoying a larger portion. Serving standard portion sizes is very important for overall customer satisfaction. Whether a customer is a repeat customer or visiting a chain restaurant in a different city, it is important to manage customer expectations by providing a consistent product. **Portion control** refers to serving standard portion sizes that have previously been decided on by managers and chefs. Without portion control, it is really impossible to control food costs. For instance, when cafeteria employees serve larger portions that costs the foodservice money. Lastly, portion control is necessary to ensure adequate calories and nutrition, particularly in hospitals, long-term care facilities, schools (K–12), and other programs where menus must meet specific calorie and nutrient guidelines. For example, serving appropriately sized portions to elementary students ensures that nutritional values per serving are accurate and students receive adequate nutrients.

For effective portion control, managers take the following steps.

1. A list of portion sizes is developed for all items that are served. Recipes include a portion size but you also need portion sizes for an item such as a fresh 9-inch pie (will it be cut into six or eight slices?) or canned fruit (will a serving of peach halves include one or two halves?). When determining the size of a portion, it is important to consider how it will look on the plate, the calories and nutrients it provides, and where it is listed on the menu. There are no absolute rules for portion sizes but dinner menu items tend to be larger than lunch items, and main courses are larger than appetizers.
2. Portion sizes are communicated to employees via posted sheets, recipes, production sheets, and so on.
3. Appropriate tools, such as scales and scoops, are available for employees to accurately measure and serve appropriate portions.
4. Portion control is monitored by supervisors and managers in the kitchen and serving areas.

If any of these steps are not implemented, the operation is likely having portion control problems.

Portions are measured in one of three ways.

1. <u>Count</u>: Examples of portion sizes using count include one banana or two eggs. Tongs or spoons may be used to serve foods portioned by count.
2. <u>Weight</u>: Weight is frequently used for solids and is measured in pounds and ounces (kilograms and grams in metric) such as 4 ounces of meat and 1 oz. of cheese in a sandwich. Weight is more *precise* than volume for solid ingredients. Portion control scales are either mechanical or digital (**Figures 9–5** and **9–6**).
3. <u>Volume</u>: Volume, such as 1 quart of soup, measures the amount of space occupied by the soup. Units of volume measurement are teaspoons, tablespoons, fluid oz. (often just called oz.), cups, pints, quarts, and gallons. Common metric

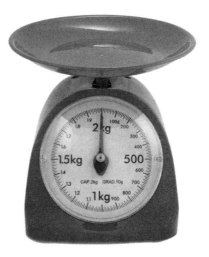

FIGURE 9-5 Mechanical Scale

© Ratthaphong Ekariyasap/Shutterstock

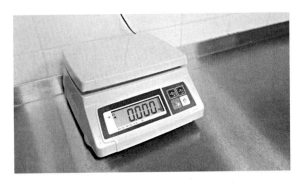

FIGURE 9-6 Digital Scale

© FabrikaSimf/Shutterstock

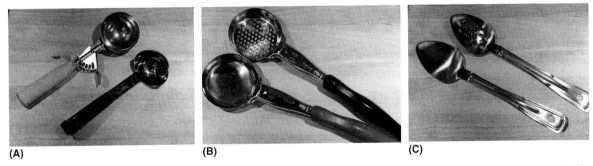

(A)   **(B)**   **(C)**

FIGURE 9-7 (A) Scoop and Ladle, **(B)** Perforated Spoodle (top) and Solid Spoodle (bottom), **(C)** Perforated Spoon (top) and Solid Spoon (bottom)

measures of volume are milliliters and liters. Volume is measured using utensils such as portion scoops.

Of course, many foods in a foodservice are purchased already preportioned—such as an 8-oz. steak or a 3-oz. potato.

The following tools may be used when measuring by volume (See **Figure 9–7**).

1. <u>Scoops</u> (also called dippers or dishers): Every scoop size has a specific number, such as a #8 scoop. The size or number is based on the number of level scoops it takes to fill a 32–fluid ounce container (a quart). So if a #8 scoop has to be filled eight times to fill a quart container, divide 32 by 8 and you will see that each full scoop contains 4 fluid oz. **Table 9-4** shows the volume for different sized

Table 9-4 Scoop Sizes and Capacity

Scoop Size #	Volume (fl. oz.)	Volume (cups)	Handle Color
#40	¾ fl. oz.	3/32 cups	Purple
#30	1	⅛	Black
#24	1⅓	1/6	Red
#20	1⅝	7/32	Yellow
#16	2	¼	Blue
#12	2⅔	⅓	Green
#10	3¼	⅜	Ivory
#8	4	½	Gray
#6	5⅓	⅔	White

For 25 servings, cut 5 x 5

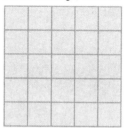

FIGURE 9-8 Cutting Diagram for Portioning

scoops. To push the food out of many scoops, just squeeze the handle with your hand. For scoops with a thumb press, you dispense the product by simply pushing down on the thumb press with your thumb. Scoops can be used to measure mashed potatoes, cooked rice, cookie dough, and many other foods.

2. Spoodles: Spoodles are part spoon and part ladle. Each one holds a certain amount of food, such as 4 fluid oz. or 6 fluid oz., and may be solid or perforated (to let liquid drain out before serving). The bowl may be round or oval. They measure portions much better than serving spoons and are excellent for serving vegetables.

3. Ladles: Ladles are used to measure fluids such as salad dressings, sauces, gravies, or soups. Like spoodles, they are labeled according to the number of fluid ounces they hold.

4. Serving spoons: Serving spoons do not measure capacity so they are more useful for self-service. They may be solid, slotted, or perforated.

When using scoops, spoodles, or ladles, employees must not overfill them. To get an accurate portion size, each should be leveled off.

Keep in mind, for example, that an 8-oz. spoodle or ladle holds 8 *fluid ounces* (volume), not 8 ounces (weight). *The only time that 8 fluid oz. (or 1 cup) equals 8 ounces is when you are measuring water.* For comparison, 1 cup of all-purpose flour weighs 4.25 ounces and 1 cup of honey weighs about 12 ounces. The weight of one cup varies depending on the density of the food/liquid you are measuring.

In addition to being able to measure portions by weight or volume, employees also have to be trained on how many portions are in a menu item such as lasagna or cornbread so they can cut up the item into the right portion. For example, a lasagna may be cut 5 by 5 (**Figure 9-8**). For cakes, employees can use a round cake marker that scores the top of a cake so that it can then be evenly sliced. A portion-control tool used for pies is a pie cutter. The pie cutter should be the same diameter as the pie and when you push it down, it slices the pie into even slices (such as six slices from a 9" pie). Tongs can also be useful for serving menu items measured by the count.

9.5 MONITOR QUALITY OF MEALS

Every foodservice needs to establish quality standards for its menu items. Quality standards look at several attributes.

- Flavor (includes taste and smell)
- Appearance (outside and inside)
- Texture
- Temperature

Figure 9-9 looks at how you can use these attributes to evaluate an egg dish.

Managers, supervisors, and employees can use a number of methods to ensure that meals are high quality.

Quality Score Card for Eggs

Date: _____   Name of Menu Item: _____

Proudly Prepared by _____

Quality Scored by _____

Directions: When the food is ready to serve, use this Quality Score Card to evaluate the quality. Mark YES when the food meets the standard and NO when it does not. Mark NA (Not Applicable) when a specific quality standard does not apply to the food being evaluated. Use the COMMENTS section to explain why a food does not meet a standard.

Remember, if a food does not meet the quality standards, it should not be placed on the serving line.

Quality Standard	Yes	No	NA	Comments
Appearance				
Product appears moist, but not watery.	○	○	○	
No oil or fat is visible.	○	○	○	
Egg yolk is bright yellow and white is opaque, with no evidence of greening.	○	○	○	
Texture or Consistency				
Product is fork tender.	○	○	○	
Product is moist, not dry.	○	○	○	
Food items within the product have a defined texture.	○	○	○	
Egg mixture is soft, without accumulated water (weeping).	○	○	○	
Flavor and Seasoning				
Ingredients have a balanced taste.	○	○	○	
Product is free from a burned taste or off-flavor.	○	○	○	
Seasonings are well blended.	○	○	○	
Service Temperature				
135 °F or higher.	○	○	○	

FIGURE 9-9 Quality Score Card for Eggs

Reproduced from National Food Service Management Institute. (2009). *Culinary techniques for healthy school meals: Preparing cakes, cookies, and pastry* (2nd ed.). University of Mississippi: Author.

- Use photos of plated items to guide production and serving personnel to produce an attractive, consistent product.
- Chefs, cooks, and other personnel should taste products before service. By using disposable forks or spoons that are thrown out immediately after one use, they can taste test without contaminating any food. Another way to taste test food is to use the two-spoon method. In this method, one spoon is designated as the

sampling spoon, and this spoon is used to dip into the pot to get a sample of food. The contents of the sampling spoon are then transferred to the tasting spoon and then usually to a small plate or bowl for tasting. The two spoons should not touch one another as the tasting spoon is contaminated.

- Food temperatures should also be tested before service. *When foods are not served immediately, you must hold hot foods at an internal temperature of 135°F (57°C) or higher and cold foods at an internal temperature of 41°F (5°C) or lower.* Temperatures must be checked (and documented) at the start of service and at least every four hours (preferably every two hours). If you check temperatures every four hours and a hot food is now below 135°F (57°C), you have to throw out the food. However, if you check the temperature every two hours and find that a hot food is below 135°F (57°C), you can reheat it up to 135°F (57°C) and put it back into the hot-holding unit.

- For certain menu items that are prepared and held (such as coffee), there need to be standards about the amount of time each item is held before being discarded. For example, at a quick service restaurant, French fries may be cooked and held for seven minutes. If not served in that time, they are discarded.

Appendix C gives examples of Quality Score Cards for many categories of menu items such as sandwiches, cooked vegetables, and cakes and cookies.

9.6 IDENTIFY SUSTAINABLE PRACTICES

This section will look specifically at how to reduce wasted food from being thrown out and also how to reduce energy and water use in foodservices. While much of the discussion involves food production, other operational areas (such as serving) are included.

WASTE REDUCTION

Food waste is defined as food that is produced for us to eat but is never consumed. Food waste is a big problem in the United States, and the Natural Resources Defense Council (2017) reports that up to 40% of food in the United States is wasted. If you look at how much food is wasted by each consumer in the United States, it amounts to almost a pound of food per person daily (Conrad et al., 2018). Food waste starts on farms where some crops are left in the fields, to the supply chain where food is processed and distributed, to retail stores and foodservices, and finally in homes where food is thrown into the trash. Another research study found that food that was not eaten contributes to about 28% of the overall carbon footprint of the average American diet (Heller & Keoleian, 2015). Nearly 80% of wasted foods are perishable foods, such as fruits, vegetables, dairy, bread, and meat (ReFED, 2016). There are many reasons and places where food is wasted, from the overplanting of crops to overproduction in a foodservice.

According to ReFED, a nonprofit using economic and other data to rethink food waste, restaurants and other foodservices could save $1.6 billion in food purchasing by reducing food waste (ReFED, 2016). Reducing wasted food also helps the environment because it means less food is rotting in landfills (and producing methane, a greenhouse gas) and it also saves water, gas, and other natural resources that go into growing and delivering foods. There are still more reasons to reduce wasted food (EPA, 2015).

1. Reduces labor costs by preparing only the food you need.
2. Reduces disposal costs.
3. When excess food is given to food banks or soup kitchens, it reduces hunger.

Thanks to the work of the Environmental Protection Agency (EPA), the Food Waste Reduction Alliance, the Food Recovery Network, the Natural Resources Defense Council (NRDC), and documentaries like: *Wasted! The Story of Food Waste* (2017) hosted by a bevy of high-profile celebrity chefs, awareness and action toward reducing food waste is increasing. In addition, in 2015, the U.S. Department of Agriculture and the EPA set the first-ever national food loss and waste goal to reduce food waste by 50% by 2030.

The first step to reduce waste is to measure and track the amount and type of food being discarded and why it is being thrown out. For example, the Waste Not program, developed by Compass for its accounts, asks employees to measure and track production waste (such as vegetable trimmings), over production (when too much food has been made), and out-of-date foods. To create targeted and successful interventions that reduce wasted food, it is important to understand more than just the quantity of waste produced. Information on the waste type (such as bell peppers or chicken breast) and reasons for loss (such as overproduction or improper cooking) is important to make meaningful changes. Additionally, tracking *when* the excess is generated can also provide useful information to target specific causes for wasted food.

Most waste reduction programs use a combination of daily paper tracking (see **Table 9-5**) and spreadsheets that automatically generate graphs and data summaries. On a daily basis, data are collected and then entered into spreadsheets. The resulting graphs and data summaries are then analyzed to identify patterns and track where the biggest issues are. Software is available to track waste, such as the Conserve program (National Restaurant Association), LeanPath 360 (LeanPath), or the Food and Packaging Waste Prevention Tool (Environmental Protection Agency).

The Food Recovery Hierarchy (**Figure 9-10**) shows what foodservices can do to prevent and divert wasted food so that it doesn't end up in a landfill. At the top of the food recovery hierarchy is the most preferred way to deal with food waste: source reduction. **Source reduction** means to eliminate waste before it is created so that less is thrown out. Source reduction may be as simple as using up leftovers at another meal or using carrot trimmings in a vegetable puree. The top levels of the hierarchy are the best ways to prevent food from being wasted, such as source reduction and feeding hungry people. At the bottom of the hierarchy is the least

Table 9-5 Food Waste Tracking Sheet

Date: _____   Weather: _____   Notes: _____

| | | | | | Due to: | | |
Time	Recorded By:	Food Type	How Much? (pounds, quarts, or # portions)	Stored Food Expired	Prep. Waste	Cooking Error	Plate Waste
	TOTAL:						

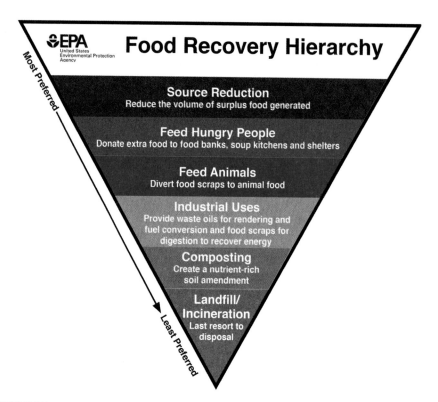

FIGURE 9-10 Food Recovery Hierarchy (EPA)

Reducing Wasted Food & Packaging: A Guide for Food Services and Restaurants, p. 3, by the Environmental Protection Agency, 2015. https://www.epa.gov/sites/production/files/2015-08/documents/reducing_wasted_food_pkg_tool.pdf

preferred way to deal with food waste: throwing it out. **Table 9–6** shows many different ways a foodservice can implement the concept of source reduction, from menu planning to serving.

The next step to take after source reduction is to use excess food to feed hungry people. Many foodservices distribute unspoiled, perishable and prepared foods to hungry people in their communities. Some local food banks will pick up food donations free of charge. Check with your local food bank or food rescue operation (soup kitchens, pantries, and shelters) to find out what items they will accept. To find your local food bank, check out Feeding America online. To find your local pantry, go to the website of Finding Pantries, and to find local homeless shelters, go to the website of Homeless Shelter Directory. Also check with your state or local health department for more information on how to safely donate food.

Feeding animals is the third level of the Food Recovery Hierarchy. With proper and safe handling, food scraps for animals can save farmers money. Regulations vary by state and some states ban food donations for animal feed. Other states regulate what can be donated (often no meat or dairy). For information, contact your local solid waste office, county agricultural extension office, or public health agency for information. Also, become familiar with the federal Swine Health Protection Act, which protects human and animal health by ensuring that food scraps fed to swine are free of active disease organisms. This law requires that meat-containing food scraps are heat-treated to kill disease-causing bacteria. An excellent resource for using leftovers for animals is *Leftovers for Livestock: A Legal Guide for Using Food Scraps as Animal Feed* (2016).

The fourth level of the Food Recovery Hierarchy is industrial uses. Fats, oil, and grease can be used to make biodiesel and other products. Liquid fats and solid meat products are materials that should not be sent to landfills or disposed of in the sanitary sewer system. Fats, oils, and grease can clog pipes and pumps both in the public sewer lines as well as in wastewater treatment facilities. Fats, oils, and grease should be sent to

Table 9-6 Source Reduction Strategies

Menu Planning
- Revise menus on a regular basis to keep up-to-date with what customers want to eat and how big portion sizes should be to satisfy customers and reduce waste.
- Offer different meal sizes/portions.
- Leave a space for a "Daily Special" on a menu that can be used for leftovers that will be made into a new recipe, such as making beef stew with leftover roast beef.
- Check plate waste in the dish room to see which menu items are not being fully consumed.

Purchasing and Storage
- Implement a "just-in-time" purchasing system to only order what is needed when it is needed.
- Buying imperfect produce, also known as "ugly" produce, can save a foodservice money and prevent it from being wasted. Some imperfect produce doesn't have a great shape or color, while other imperfect produce may need to be used quickly because it's ripe.
- Monitor inventory levels to identify overpurchased food items.
- Ensure that foods are stored under the proper conditions (temperature, humidity, air flow), freezer and coolers are well-maintained, and older products are used first. Some fruits and vegetables last longer at room temperature and with good ventilation.
- Use see-through storage containers so employees can see what is available and keep an eye on freshness. Do not cover containers if good circulation is needed.
- Date products and rotate so that the oldest product is used first (FIFO).
- Create menu specials to prioritize the use of older products.

Production
- Keep records of how much was forecast, then prepared, and left over. Use these records to forecast more accurately.
- Use as much of each food as possible. For example, don't peel potatoes. Train staff on knife skills to make more efficient knife cuts to use more of the food (especially fruits and vegetables) being prepared.
- Train staff on root-to-stalk cooking in vegetables.
- Creatively repurpose leftovers and trimmings to efficiently use excess food as long as proper food safety practices are followed. For example, leftover fruit can be used to make smoothies or a topping for desserts, or stale bread can be used to make croutons or breadcrumbs. Vegetable trimmings can be used to make stock or pureed to use in soups, sauces, or smoothies.
- Batch cook and practice "just in time" cooking to keep food fresh and prevent overproduction.

Serving
- Offer tastings to customers of different menu items. This prevents someone getting a serving of something they don't like and won't eat.
- Don't automatically put bread or water on the table when customers sit down. Have servers ask customers if they would like bread or water. Also ask if a customer wants a side item instead of automatically providing sides.
- In all-you-can-eat facilities, such as many university dining halls, using smaller plates and no trays reduces the amount of food students take, which reduces food waste and can reduce the amount of purchased food. Trayless dining also eliminates the cost of washing the trays (saving water, cleaning chemicals, and energy) as well as the cost of the trays themselves.
- On hot or cold food bars, identify which items are regularly wasted and reduce the quantity of those items prepared and reduce the size of the container in which they are served.
- Offer to-go containers and encourage customers to take their leftover food with them.

the rendering industry to be made into another product, converted to biofuels, or sent to an anaerobic digester.

- *Rendering:* Liquid fats and solid meat products can be used as raw materials in the rendering industry, which converts them into animal food, cosmetics, soap, and other products. Many companies will provide storage barrels and free pick-up service.
- *Biodiesel:* Fats, oils, and grease are collected and converted by local manufacturers into environmentally friendly biodiesel fuel. Biodiesel is an alternative fuel produced from renewable resources such as virgin oils (soybean, canola, palm), waste cooking oil, or other biowaste feedstock. Biodiesel significantly reduces

greenhouse gases and sulfur dioxide in air emissions. Along with creating less pollution, biodiesel is simple to use, biodegradable, and nontoxic.

- *Anaerobic Digestion:* Fats, oils, and grease can be added to anaerobic digesters at wastewater treatment plants to generate renewable energy in the form of biogas.

The fifth level of the Food Recovery Hierarchy is composting. **Compost** is organic material that can be added to soil to help plants grow. All composting requires three basic ingredients.

- Browns: This includes materials such as dead leaves, branches, and twigs.
- Greens: This includes materials such as vegetable waste, fruit scraps, coffee grounds, eggshells, tea bags, and grass clippings.
- Water: Having the right amount of water, greens, and browns is important for compost development.

A compost pile should have an equal amount of browns to greens, and you should also alternate layers of organic materials of different-sized particles. The brown materials provide carbon for your compost, the green materials provide nitrogen, and the water provides moisture to help break down the organic matter. Food scraps need to be handled properly so they don't cause odors or attract unwanted insects or animals.

Composting can be small scale or large scale, on-site or off-site. Foodservices can have their own composting pile or simply contribute food scraps to community composters. Findacomposter.com is a website for locating a composting facility near your business.

The foodservice industry is full of examples of operations that have reduced waste. For instance, two business and dining facilities in Oregon, serving about 12,000 meals per week, tracked how much food was thrown out in the kitchen and why for 1 year. With the data, the chef and cooks looked at how to reuse some of the wasted food and came up with ideas such as turning leftover fruit into chutney and pureeing certain starches to use as thickeners. The changes resulted in a reduction of food waste by 47% and a reduction in food costs per meal by 13% (Environmental Protection Agency, 2015b).

ENERGY CONSERVATION

Compared with other businesses, foodservices use a lot of energy—about 5 to 7 times more energy per square foot than other commercial buildings (Environmental Protection Agency, 2016). How many businesses have refrigerators the size of a bedroom or ovens that can cook 12 trays of food at the same time? While food preparation accounts for about 35% of energy used in a restaurant, about 28% is used for heat, ventilation, and air conditioning, 18% for sanitation, 13% for lighting, and 6% for refrigeration (Environmental Protection Agency, 2015a).

When foodservices replace old appliances, or buy new ones, managers should seriously consider buying equipment that have earned the ENERGY STAR certification. ENERGY STAR certified equipment is energy-efficient and offers energy savings of 10 to 70% over standard models (depending on the product category) without sacrificing features, quality, or style (Environmental Protection Agency, 2016). While high-efficiency appliances could cost more up front, significantly lower utility bills (sometimes more than 50% lower) can quickly make up for the price difference. Keep in mind that the purchase price is often a small portion of the total cost when you take into account the amount of energy (and possibly water) a piece of equipment uses.

The following are ways to conserve energy.

Refrigeration and Other Equipment

- Regular maintenance and servicing of all equipment optimizes performance and saves energy. Personnel should be trained to report issues such as worn gaskets on convection oven doors or a broiler that is missing knobs.
- Select ENERGY STAR certified appliances whenever buying new equipment. You can compare specific appliances, such as ENERGY STAR dishwashers, on the EPA website.

- Choose the appropriate size for refrigeration and other equipment. Larger units often require more energy.
- Recalibrate to stay efficient. For example, thermostats and control systems can fail, fall out of calibration, or need to be readjusted. Take the time to do a regular thermostat check on your appliances such as ovens and fryers, refrigeration, dish machines, and hot water heaters and reset them to the correct operating temperature. Most of this will be done for you if you have a good preventative maintenance contract with a reputable equipment repair service such as one with CFESA certification and CFESA-certified technicians. CFESA stands for the Commercial Food Equipment Service Association, a trade association of professional service and parts distributors, which offers certification of companies and technicians after meeting strict requirements.
- Cut idle time. If you leave your equipment "on" when it is not being used, it wastes energy and costs money. Implement a startup/shutdown plan to make sure you are using only the equipment you need.
- Refrigerators use a lot of energy, so keep doors closed as much as possible, use air curtains or strip curtains, replace worn gaskets, and keep condensers and evaporators clean. Also make sure that there is adequate airflow in and around the unit.
- Use LED lighting for refrigerated food and beverage case displays. They give off less heat and use less electricity.

Heating, Ventilation, and Air Conditioning (HVAC)

- A yearly tune-up of heating, ventilation, and cooling systems can improve efficiency and comfort.
- Properly sized HVAC equipment dramatically cuts energy costs, increases the life of the equipment, and reduces greenhouse gas emissions.
- Install a programmable thermostat so that you are not heating/cooling spaces (such as the dining room) when not in use.
- Switch off kitchen extraction hoods when not needed or consider a demand-based exhaust control system for hoods that uses sensors to monitor cooking and then varies the exhaust fan to match the ventilation needs.
- Ventilation units and extractor hood grease filters should be cleaned regularly and part of the master cleaning schedule.
- Heat water with an ENERGY STAR-certified commercial water heater and set appropriate hot water temperatures.

Lighting

- Turn off lights in unoccupied areas.
- Install occupancy sensors in closets, storage rooms, break rooms, and restrooms. Occupancy sensors are indoor motion-detecting devices that detect the presence of a person to automatically turn on lights.
- In some areas, bi-level switching will help reduce energy. Bi-level switching allows you to turn off some of the lights in a room when full illumination is not needed.
- Replace traditional light bulbs with ENERGY STAR-certified LED bulbs or compact fluorescent lamp bulbs when possible. An ENERGY STAR-certified light bulb uses 70–90% less energy than traditional bulbs, lasts 10–25 times longer, and produces 70% less extra energy as heat (2015a).
- Use ENERGY STAR-certified light fixtures in the production and dining areas.
- Dim the lights. Dimmers are available for both LEDs and CFLs (make sure you have *dimmable* CFLs). Daylight dimmers are special sensors that automatically dim room lights based on the amount of natural daylight coming in.
- ENERGY STAR-certified commercial signage displays can be used for digital menu boards, and are, on average, 15% more energy efficient than conventional models.
- Swap your old "Open/Closed" and "Exit" signs with LED technology for additional energy savings.

WATER CONSERVATION

Using water more efficiently preserves water supplies, saves money, and protects the environment. By conserving hot water, for example, you not only trim one but two costs: one for the water and sewer and another for the electricity or natural gas required to heat the water used in bathroom faucets, kitchen sinks, prerinse spray valves, and dishwashers.

But before you even goes into the kitchen to prepare a meal, many gallons of water have been used to produce each of the ingredients used to produce your menu. For example, beef and pork require many more gallons of water to produce than chicken, eggs, cheese, peanuts, or dry beans (Culinary Institute of America & Harvard T.H. Chan School of Public Health, 2017, p. 42).

When choosing equipment, three categories of ENERGY STAR-certified equipment save water as well as energy: dishwashers, ice machines, and steam cookers. ENERGY STAR-certified steam cookers actually use 90% less water than standard steam cookers (Environmental Protection Agency, 2012).

Similar to the ENERGY STAR label, WaterSense is a partnership program sponsored by the Environmental Protection Agency that identifies water-efficient products. WaterSense-labeled products are mainly residential but do include a growing number of commercial products such as prerinse spray valves (the handheld sprayers that are used to rinse dishes, pots, etc.).

Foodservices can save water in a number of ways, as described next. In addition, one of the most effective ways to conserve water is to train and motivate your employees to help reduce water use.

<u>Sinks and Dishwashers</u>

- Check regularly for leaks and fix leaks as quickly as possible.
- Reduce sink and tap usage.
- Often, sinks use up to eight gallons per minute (gpm) while sinks with high-flow aerators use around 2.2 gpm. Aerators make faucets use less water. Sinks with WaterSense-labeled aerators have a maximum flow rate of 1.5 gpm, which can save significant amounts of water.
- Use automatic sensors on bathroom sinks and toilets to avoid unnecessary water use. Also install WaterSense-labeled toilets.
- A WaterSense-labeled commercial prerinse spray valves (at the dishwasher or potwashing stations—see **Figure 9-11**) is one of the most energy- and water-saving devices available to the foodservice operator. The water flow is slower but these spray valves are just as effective at cleaning food from dishes.
- Upgrade dishwashers to ENERGY STAR-certified models to save water and energy.
- Do regular cleaning and maintenance of dishwashers including, for example, doing frequent temperature checks and cleaning rinse-arm nozzles as well as replacing them when worn. Also check the pressure gauge—if it is above 25 psi, you may be using more water than needed.
- Operate the dishwasher close to or at the minimum flow rate recommended by the manufacturer. Set the rinse cycle time to the manufacturer's minimum recommended setting and periodically verify that the machine continues to operate with that rinse cycle time.
- Run fully loaded dish racks through the dishwasher. Educate employees on how to load dish racks properly and scrape dishes prior to loading racks.

<u>Equipment</u>

- Any kitchen equipment that uses water needs to be periodically maintained.
- When using steam kettles, steamers, or combination steamer-convection ovens, keep the door/lid closed, make sure the gaskets are in good condition, use the timer, and turn the equipment off or down between uses.

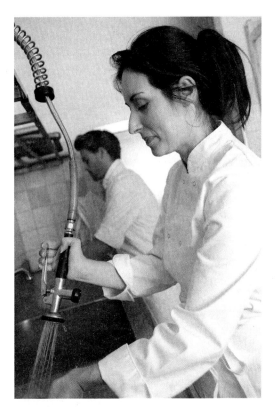

FIGURE 9-11 Using a Pre-Rinse Spray Valve

© ALPA PROD/Shutterstock

- Boiler-based steam cookers and combination steamer-convection ovens use a lot more water than a closed system steamer. A closed-system steamer recycles its own water supply by reusing condensation that would otherwise be lost.
- ENERGY STAR–certified ice machines reduce water and energy usage. Bigger ice machines are usually more efficient than smaller ones, yet the price difference is not that big. Avoid water-cooled ice machines because of their high water cost.
- For optimal ice-machine efficiency, keep the lid closed, keep the coils clean, and periodically clean the entire machine.
- Food disposal systems use a lot of water (2 to 15 gallons per minute when in use) so new equipment may be needed to maximize efficiency. As an alternative to a traditional garbage disposal, some facilities use **food pulpers** to collect and dispose of food scraps. Food pulpers are located where the grinder would otherwise be located. Unlike a traditional garbage disposal with a grinder, food pulpers crush food waste into a pulp (i.e., slurry), extract excess water from the pulp, and send the pulp waste to a bin for later disposal or composting. In many food pulper systems, the extracted water can be recycled.
- Dipper wells (used in ice cream stores) discharge water continually. Replace older equipment for more efficient models and turn off when not in use.

Serving

- Have servers ask customers if they would like water.

Managers should track their energy and water usage. The Environmental Protection Agency created ENERGY STAR Portfolio Manager®, an online tool managers can use to measure and track energy and water consumption, as well as greenhouse gas emissions.

The Grey Plume, a restaurant in Omaha, Nebraska, is known for its efforts in saving energy and water. In the kitchen, water-efficient aerators are installed on all handwashing and preparation sinks and a high–efficiency, prerinse spray valve is also used. Both the ice machine and dishwasher are ENERGY STAR qualified. Instead of using a garbage disposal, food waste is composted. Kitchen grease is converted to biodiesel through the Omaha Biofuels Coop. Almost all lights are LEDs and programmable thermostats are used in all areas of the restaurant.

SUMMARY

9.1   Choose Appropriate Cooking Methods

- Successful cooks utilize the concepts of mise en place and batch cooking.
- Heat is transferred to food by conduction (heat moves from something hot to something touching it that is cooler), convection (moving air, steam, liquid, or hot fat), or by radiation (such as microwave or infrared).
- Dry-heat cooking methods transfer heat without the use of water or steam. Instead, they rely on hot air (oven), hot fat (deep-fat fryer), hot metal (griddle), or radiation (microwave). Dry heat cooking methods include roast/bake, broil, grill, griddle, pan-broil, sauté, stir-fry, pan-fry, and deep-fry.
- Moist-heat cooking methods involve water, a water-based liquid, or steam as the vehicle of heat transfer. Examples include poaching, simmering, boiling, steaming, and braising (includes browning and simmering in a small amount of liquid). Compared with most dry-heat cooking methods, moist-heat cooking does not add the flavor that dry-heat cooked foods get from browning, deglazing, or reduction.
- Chefs are no longer relying on salt, sugar, and butter for flavor. Instead, they are building flavor through the appropriate use of ingredients, preparation techniques, and cooking methods. The following are ingredients that are excellent flavor builders: herbs, spices, herb and spice blends, flavorful and infused oils, vinegars, reduced liquids, aromatic vegetables, grilled and roasted vegetables, citrus fruits, and condiments such as sriracha sauce. Preparation techniques can also add flavor, such as rubs, marinades, reduction, searing, caramelizing, toasting, and deglazing. All cooking methods work in healthy cooking except those using large amounts of fat or oil.

9.2   Forecast Production Quantities

- When forecasted numbers are accurate, there will be very little (or no) food leftover and every customer's order will be filled. In addition, accurate forecasting helps tremendously in controlling food and labor costs.
- Sales forecasting is based on a number of factors but the most important are the historical sales numbers for that specific day and meal—including how many total customers were served and how much of each menu item was sold or served. You also have to take into account extraneous factors such as holiday weekends (which may increase or lower your business) or that it is orientation week for college freshmen. You can do forecasting manually by calculating averages, moving averages, or using percentage forecasting.
- In some small hospitals or other healthcare facilities where patients choose meals ahead of time, an employee may simply count up or "tally" the number of patients who want each lunch entrée for tomorrow's service, and then pad those numbers to anticipate changes and avoid running out.
- Today, all foodservice segments use some type of computerized tracking of sales and production that is often available from your primary food supplier. Using data collected from a POS system, you can review detailed sales reports from your foodservice's history to make forecasting easier.
- Some software will do the forecasting for you using mathematical models that are much more sophisticated than you could do yourself.

9.3   Write a Production Schedule

- Also called a food production worksheet or prep sheet, production schedules are documents that communicate to employees which menu items need to be prepared and how many, along with pertinent instructions, etc. But production schedules are not just to inform employees. Once the cooking is done, employees also enter information on production schedules—specifically how many portions were prepared and served, and whether too much or too little was prepared—and this information goes back to management to inform future forecasting.

- Table 9-2 shows a typical production schedule.
- Good production planning should reduce problems, such as running out of food, and help you serve quality meals.
- Another variation of a production schedule may be used for a station that makes items to order, such as a deli station in a café or a grab-and-go refrigerator. These production sheets (sometimes called a prep sheets) simply list par levels of ingredients (such as 5 lbs. of sliced cheddar cheese) that need to be stocked at the station before service.

9.4   Use Portion Control

- Serving standard portion sizes is very important for customer satisfaction, to control food costs, and to ensure adequate nutrition.
- For effective portion control, managers must have a list of standard portion sizes for all menu items served, communicate with employees, have portion control tools such as scales available, and monitor serving.
- Portions are measured by count, weight, or volume. When measuring by weight, mechanical or digital scales are used. When measuring by volume, employees use scoops, spoodles (part spoon and part ladle), or ladles and level them off. Serving spoons do not measure capacity so they are more useful for self-service.
- Every scoop size has a specific number, such as a #8 scoop. The size or number is based on the number of level scoops it takes to fill a quart container (see Table 9-4).
- An 8-oz. spoodle or ladle holds 8 *fluid ounces* (volume), not 8 ounces (weight). *The only time that 8 fluid ounces (or 1 cup) equals 8 ounces is when you are measuring water.* For comparison, 1 cup of all-purpose flour weighs 4.25 ounces and 1 cup of honey weighs about 12 ounces.
- Employees also need to know how to cut up a pan of lasagna or a pie in order to get the correct number of portions.

9.5   Monitor Quality of Meals

- Quality standards for menu items look at flavor, appearance, texture, and temperature.

Figure 9-9 illustrates quality standards for an egg dish.

- To assure quality meals, managers can use photos of plated items to guide employees, taste products before service (using a disposable utensil or the two-spoon method), test temperatures, and have rules about how long to hold an item before being discarded.

9.6   Identify Sustainable Practices

- Food waste refers to food that winds up not being eaten. Reducing wasted food saves money, helps the environment because it means less food is rotting in landfills (and producing methane, a greenhouse gas), and saves water, gas, and other natural resources that go into growing and delivering foods.
- The first step to reduce waste is to measure and track the amount and type of food being discarded and why it is being thrown out. Most waste reduction programs use a combination of daily paper tracking (see Table 9-5) and spreadsheets that automatically generate graphs and data summaries. The resulting graphs and data summaries are then analyzed to identify patterns and track where the biggest issues are.
- The Food Recovery Hierarchy (Figure 9-10) shows what foodservices can do to prevent and divert wasted food so that it doesn't end up in a landfill: source reduction, feed hungry people, feed animals, industrial uses (such as using fats and oils to make biodiesel), and compost. Source reduction means to eliminate waste before it is created so that less is thrown out. Table 9-6 lists source reduction strategies.
- Foodservices use a lot more energy and water than other businesses. Ways to save energy and water are discussed. For example, when foodservices replace old appliances, or buy new ones, managers should seriously consider buying equipment that have earned the ENERGY STAR certification. ENERGY STAR-certified equipment is energy-efficient and ENERGY STAR dishwashers, ice machines, and steam cookers also save water.
- Managers can track their energy and water usage by employing programs such as ENERGY STAR Portfolio Manager®, an online tool that measures and tracks energy and water consumption.

REVIEW AND DISCUSSION QUESTIONS

1. How would a chef describe mise en place and batch cooking, and why would they use these techniques?
2. Give an example of a cooking method that uses conduction, convection, or radiation.
3. List dry-heat and moist-heat cooking methods. Give an example of a food cooked using each method.
4. What is the difference between baking and roasting, broiling and grilling, sautéing and pan-frying, poaching and simmering, and browning and braising?
5. Describe three preparation techniques used to develop flavor.
6. For forecasting, what is the difference between using a simple average, moving average, or percentage method?
7. What does a production schedule communicate and why is it important?
8. Name one food that is best served with a scoop, a spoodle, a ladle, or a serving spoon.
9. What is portion control and why is it important?
10. Quality standards for served food include what aspects of menu items? How does a manager ensure that the food being served meets those standards?
11. To reduce wasted food, briefly describe how a foodservice manager can use each level of the food recovery hierarchy.
12. What does it mean when a piece of equipment is ENERGY STAR-certified?
13. Describe four ways that a manager can be a good role model in terms of saving energy and water.

SMALL GROUP PROJECT

For the foodservice concept that you created in Chapter 1, develop the following.

1. Write production schedules (like Table 9-2) for your foodservice for one lunch OR dinner meal. Develop one production schedule for hot food and one production schedule for cold food. First determine how many total people you will be serving. Next, determine the percentage of customers who will pick each item. Then use percentage forecasting to forecast the number of portions for every item and pad each item. Also list special instructions for any menu item, such as to batch cook broccoli.
2. Recommend portion control tools for each menu item noted on your production schedules.
3. Develop a quality score card for two of the menu items being served.

REFERENCES

Conrad, Z., Niles, M. T., Neher, D. A., Roy, E. D., Tichenor, N. E., & Jahns, L. (2018). Relationship between food waste, diet quality, and environmental sustainability. *Plos ONE, 13*(4). Retrieved from https://doi.org/10.1371/journal.pone.0195405

Culinary Institute of America & Harvard T.H. Chan School of Public Health. (2017). *Menus of Change: The business of healthy, sustainable, delicious food choices.* Retrieved from http://www.menusofchange.org/images/uploads/pdf/2017_Menus_of_Change_Annual_Report_FINAL.pdf

Drummond, K., & Brefere, L. (2017). *Nutrition for foodservice and culinary professionals.* Hoboken, NJ: John Wiley & Sons, Inc.

Environmental Protection Agency. (2012). WaterSense at work: Best management practices for commercial and institutional facilities. Retrieved from https://www.epa.gov/sites/production/files/2017-02/documents/watersense-at-work_final_508c3.pdf

Environmental Protection Agency. (2015a). ENERGY STAR Guide for Cafés, Restaurants, and Institutional Kitchens. Retrieved from https://www.energystar.gov/sites/default/files/asset/document/CR%20ES%20Restaurant%20Guide%202015%20v8_0.pdf

Environmental Protection Agency. (2015b). *Reducing wasted food & packaging: A guide for food services and restaurants.* Retrieved from https://www.epa.gov/sites/production

/files/2015-08/documents/reducing_wasted_food_pkg_tool.pdf

Environmental Protection Agency. (2016). *Energy saving tips for small businesses: Restaurants*. Retrieved from https://www.energystar.gov/buildings/tools-and-resources/energy_star_small_business_restaurants

Gingerella, B. (2018). How restaurants are forecasting customer traffic. *Restaurant Business Magazine*. Retrieved from http://www.restaurantbusinessonline.com/operations/how-restaurants-are-forecasting-customer-traffic

Heller, M. C., & Keoleian, G. A. (2015). Greenhouse gas emission estimates of U.S. dietary choices and food loss. *Journal of Industrial Ecology, 19*(3), 391–401. doi: 10.1111/jiec.12174

Natural Resources Defense Council. (2017). Wasted: How America is losing up to 40 percent of its food from farm to fork to landfill (2nd ed.). Retrieved from https://www.nrdc.org/resources/wasted-how-america-losing-40-percent-its-food-farm-fork-landfill

ReFED. (2016). *A roadmap to reduce U.S. food waste by 20 percent*. Retrieved from https://www.refed.com/downloads/ReFED_Report_2016.pdf

© Denis Val/Shutterstock

Distribution and Service

LEARNING OUTCOMES

10.1 Compare and contrast different service styles.

10.2 Manage meal assembly, distribution, and service in healthcare.

INTRODUCTION

In most restaurants, once a meal is ordered, it is prepared (or finished) and then plated and served to the customer. Some foods (such as hamburgers and sandwiches) can be likewise prepared, plated, and served in onsite foodservices such as a business and industry café. However, many onsite foodservices cook menu items in bulk before a meal and then serve multiple meals. For example, the food for an elementary school may be prepared in a kitchen ten miles away and then transported to each school in the district. At each school, employees get the cafeteria ready for meal service with all appropriate hot and cold foods. Once students start coming in for lunch, the food must be kept hot or cold during service, which can last for over two hours.

Distribution is the name for the process of getting food from where it was produced to where the customer will be served (also known as the **point of service**). **Assembly** is putting components of a meal together on plate(s) to be served. When a restaurant prepares meals for customers in the same building, distribution and assembly are not an issue. Assembling and distributing meals to patients in 200 rooms in a large urban hospital will be a lot more challenging. All foodservices must use one or more styles of service. A **style of service** is how the food is presented to the guest. For example, using table service, a server places meals on the guest's table. This chapter will discuss service styles and assembly, distribution, and service in healthcare facilities.

10.1 COMPARE AND CONTRAST DIFFERENT SERVICE STYLES

This section discusses service styles including table service, counter service, drive-through service, take-out and delivery service, cafeteria service, self-service, and tray service. Regardless of which service style is used, certain elements must be present to ensure customer satisfaction. For example, in the SERVQUAL model developed by Parasuraman, Berry, and Zeithami (1991) the following dimensions of service quality are key components of service delivery that result in customer satisfaction.

1. Reliability (consistency of service; doing it right the first time)
2. Responsiveness (prompt service and quick response to customer questions/complaints)
3. Assurance (competent and courteous service while keeping customers informed)
4. Empathy (connecting with customers and getting to know their needs/wants)
5. Tangibles (appearance of foodservice and its employees)

In this model, the gap between what a customer expected and perceived is a measure of the quality of the service. This model has been criticized mostly due to difficulties scoring this gap (Pizam & Ellis, 1999), however, the components of service delivery are very relevant. More on customer satisfaction is discussed later in this chapter.

TABLE SERVICE

Table service is most common in commercial foodservices such as restaurants. Table service involves a server or waitperson who places food and beverages on the guest's table or counter, as seen in **Figure 10-1**. In most restaurants, guests are first seated by a host or hostess and given menus. Next, servers take orders (in some restaurants, orders are entered on a touchscreen) and deliver items to the table. A dining room often has additional employees, known as bussers or buspersons, who fill water glasses, remove used dinnerware and flatware, and clear and reset tables. In some foodservices, guests eat at a counter rather than a table, and they are served in the same manner as guests at tables (Figure 10-1). In onsite foodservice, table service is used, for example, in dining rooms

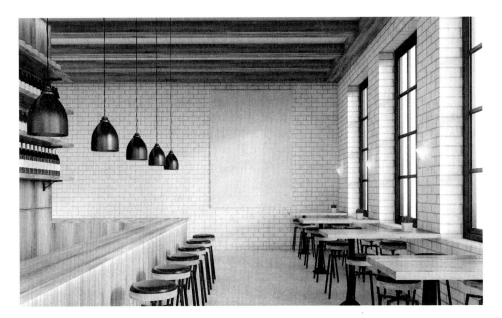

FIGURE 10-1 Restaurant with Tables and Counter Seats

© ImageFlow/Shutterstock

for independently living seniors in retirement communities as well as executive dining rooms in business and industry foodservices.

There are different styles of table service. Most restaurants use **American-style service** in which food is arranged on plates in the kitchen and then placed in front of each guest. Another style of table service is called **family-style service** in which large serving platters and bowls of food are placed on the guests' table, and they are passed around the table for diners to serve themselves. The platters and bowls may also be placed on a Lazy Susan, which is turned so each guest can serve themselves. In some foodservices, appetizers, entrées, and side dishes are served family style, while other foodservices plate the entrée individually and serve the appetizers, salads, and/or side dishes family style.

Using **English service**, the server holds a large dish of food and serves each guest individually, starting with the host. It is like a formal version of family-style dining. **French service** is yet another style of table service distinguished by some food being prepared (sometimes just partially prepared) and served table-side such as carved prime rib, Caesar salad, or a flambé dish such as crêpes Suzette or steak Diane.

Banquet service is another style of table service. With **banquet service**, guests are all seated at tables (as for a wedding) and served a preset menu at the same time. Using banquet service, servers often put the first course on the tables before the guests come in, then clear that course and serve the main entrée next. Often, there are two or more choices for the entrée. Sometimes, banquets include a self-service buffet or food stations (such as a cake station or a cookie station for dessert) for one or more of the courses.

Whenever table service is used, each guest requires a place setting, with plates, glasses, napkin, and flatware put into the proper places, as seen in **Figure 10-2** for a formal multicourse meal with wine. The dinner plate is always placed directly in front of

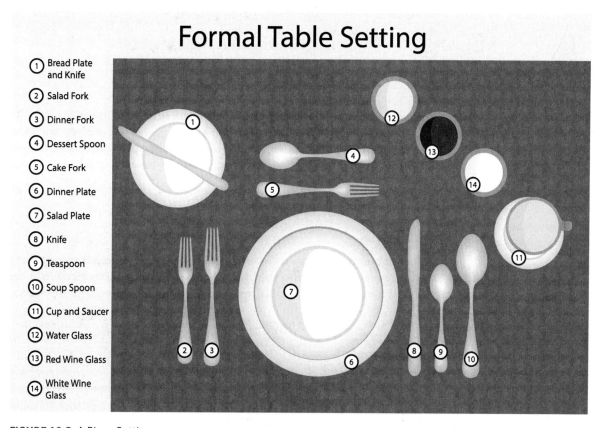

Formal Table Setting

1. Bread Plate and Knife
2. Salad Fork
3. Dinner Fork
4. Dessert Spoon
5. Cake Fork
6. Dinner Plate
7. Salad Plate
8. Knife
9. Teaspoon
10. Soup Spoon
11. Cup and Saucer
12. Water Glass
13. Red Wine Glass
14. White Wine Glass

FIGURE 10-2 A Place Setting

© Sakurra/Shutterstock

the guest, and the place setting should be one inch up from the edge of the table. Food is always served from the guest's left side and dishes removed from the right.

COUNTER SERVICE

Counter service has two meanings. Restaurants, like those shown in Figure 10-1, serve customers at tables and also at a counter. Counter service also has another meaning. It occurs any time a guest walks up to a counter and orders food from a person or from a touchscreen. Payment is made and the food is assembled and given to the guest. In most cases, the guest can choose whether to eat in the foodservice (when seating is available), in which case the food is usually put on a tray, or eat elsewhere (in which case the food is placed in a bag). Counter service is most common in quick-service and fast casual restaurants, such as Wendy's, Panera Bread, or Chipotle. Counter service is also used in some cafeterias as, for example, when a guest asks a grill worker for a cheeseburger. In a cafeteria, payment is not normally made at the counter but at a central cashier's station.

DRIVE-THROUGH SERVICE

Many quick-service restaurants, and some fast casual restaurants, offer the convenience of drive-through service. The COVID-19 pandemic pushed many consumers to favor drive-through service as a safer option. The customer generally drives up to a menu board and orders into a microphone. The customer then pulls up to a window(s) to pay and receive the food. Not having to get out of the car is a real plus for customers who want to avoid getting children in and out of the car, escape any bad weather, and save time. Drive-throughs do require a lot of space and service must be monitored to make sure it is speedy.

TAKE-OUT SERVICE AND DELIVERY SERVICE

Take-out service and delivery service are growing in popularity. Take-out food is any purchased food that is not eaten on premises. We have already discussed two instances when food is not eaten on premises (drive-through and some counter service). In both of these examples, the guest *orders at the foodservice* and goes elsewhere to eat the food.

Take-out service also occurs when the guest *orders take-out food at home, at work, or almost anywhere* by using a foodservice's app on a mobile phone, ordering on the foodservice's website, or making a phone call directly to the foodservice. When ordering, the guest finds out when the order will be ready for pick up. Some restaurants, such as Panera Bread and Zoe's Kitchen, have a pick-up location (actually a shelving unit) in the store where guests can check for their name on the appropriate bag and leave with their meal. In other foodservices, you have to go to a counter to pick up or you may be able to do curbside pickup.

Many consumers like to order take-out service but don't want the bother of picking up the food. To order food and have it delivered (for a delivery fee), you can either order directly from a foodservice that offers delivery or order from a delivery company such as Grubhub, Uber Eats, or DoorDash. Each of these companies has a website that shows you which local foodservices and menu items are available for delivery. Consumers then use the delivery company's website or a phone app for easy ordering and payment. Some of the restaurants that the delivery company represents are actually **ghost kitchens** or **virtual kitchens**. Ghost kitchens don't have a storefront or dining room but only have a kitchen space (possibly shared) to produce meals for delivery (Marston, 2019).

Ordering and delivery services such as Grubhub are still quite young but growing rapidly. In the past, it was mostly pizza chains that made deliveries because a driver could go out and deliver multiple orders on one run (which helped reduce delivery costs). When a delivery company delivers an order from a restaurant, the

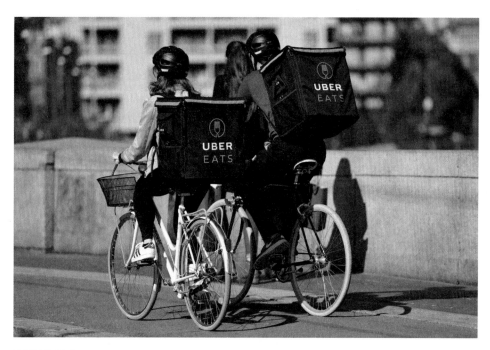

FIGURE 10-3 Thermal Insulated Bags Being Used to Deliver Meals

© DELBO ANDREA/Shutterstock

restaurant must pay them a commission of 15% to as high as 30% on each order (Isaac & Yaffe-Bellany, 2019), so profitability must be seriously considered. For some foodservices, the commission is simply too high and they will lose money.

Some foodservices provide their own delivery service, such as sweetgreen, and others use one or more delivery services, such as Uber Eats, to deliver their orders. Within each market, there are often several delivery services, with one being dominant, although this could change as this business matures. One thing that probably will not change is the fact that most consumers only want to put one or two delivery apps on their phones because apps take up space.

Consumers also want their food delivered at the right temperature, and that is more of a challenge for hot foods than for cold foods (although cold foods must be kept cold!). To deliver hot foods, many companies use thermal insulated bags (**Figure 10-3**) and keep hot foods separate from cold. It is important to pick the right size and shape bag for the job it has to do. Too much extra room in the bag can cause problems. Quality closures are also important. A good insulated bag will maintain food temperature as well as control moisture. Steam from hot foods, such as pizza, can cause condensation and will make a pizza crust soggy if the steam can't escape. Nylon-lined delivery bags are more expensive than vinyl-lined bags but nylon allows steam to escape better. Delivery bags with polyurethane or polyester foam insulation are lightweight, breathable, and won't trap odors. Food is often delivered by car or van, but bicycles are popular in urban areas.

CAFETERIA SERVICE

In many on-site foodservice operations, from the Army dining hall to a workplace café, cafeterias are used to feed a lot of customers with a minimal number of employees. If you need to feed lunch to 250 middle school students, you would certainly not offer table service with servers. Instead, the students go through a cafeteria line and, for example, pick up a carton of milk and salad (self-service) and ask a server to give them a slice of pizza and green beans (counter service). So, in most cafeterias, service is a mix of self-service (such as for beverages) and counter service (getting a sandwich made to order).

Because cafeterias serve meals for longer periods of time, special equipment will be needed to keep foods hot or cold, and some items (such as hamburgers) may be cooked to order during service to keep food fresh. Keeping food hot for too long can cause changes in appearance, color, consistency, and flavor.

Many cafeterias in business and industry, colleges and universities, and healthcare use a **scramble (scatter) system**, also called a **hollow square** or food court cafeteria. In a scramble system, customers pick up a tray and then walk around and look at the foods offered at each station before deciding on what to eat. Some stations, such as a salad bar, may be self-service, while other stations have an employee who will make a sandwich to order, grill a hamburger, or stir fry a custom order. While scramble systems require more space, service is generally faster, the variety of food is better, each station can be as big or small as needed, and there may be room for exhibition cooking. The scramble concept also allows the manager to see the popularity of each station and change the menu to maximize or balance traffic flow.

SELF-SERVICE

Self-service includes any situation in which guests pick up what they want to eat, by for example, making a salad at a salad bar or filling a soft drink cup with iced tea. *Self-service is found in settings such as cafeterias (just discussed), buffets, convenience stores, vending machines, and micromarkets.* It is also used in quick-service restaurants where customers are given a beverage cup to fill up themselves.

Catering sometimes involves the use of self-service buffets. In a **buffet**, equipment such as chafing dishes (**Figure 10-4**), refrigerated food wells, and platters are placed on one or more tables. Guests pick up plates and walk along the table(s) and help themselves to what they want to eat. In some buffet lines, staff may be present to portion and serve certain items such as freshly sliced prime rib, or prepare and serve items such as omelets made to order. Buffet style service is used, for example, on cruise ships and at hotel breakfasts. A hot food bar or salad bar are buffets for certain menu items. Buffet service is typically faster than table service and allows the guests more choices. For management, buffet service does not require as many employees as table service does.

Convenience stores, such as 7-Eleven, Speedway, or Casey's General Store, are retail outlets that sell made-to-order and grab-and-go foods, snacks, and beverages, along with tobacco products, newspapers, a limited selection of household staples, and often gas for the car. In the eastern United States, Wawa is a leader in food and beverage, offering a wide variety of fresh sandwiches, bowls, salads, soups, and beverages. In addition to offering a wide selection of self-service grab-and-go foods, customers can use touch screens to order food and beverages such as custom paninis and coffee beverages.

Vending machines have been used for over 100 years to sell beverages, foods, and other items. They are the ultimate self-service device as the user puts coins or bills into the vending machine and then hits a button to dispense the item. Nowadays, many vending machines also accept cashless payments such as credit cards, debit cards, or mobile wallet payments using a smartphone. Students often use their identification card as a debit card at vending machines as long as they have money set up in an appropriate account. Likewise, employees at work may be able to use their identification cards. With some vending machines, users can scan their fingerprints on biometric readers.

Vending machines are commonly used and very useful for onsite foodservices because they offer the opportunity for customers, such as hospital employees who work around the clock or college students who are up late at night, to purchase items 24/7. Vending machines are also great for foodservices located in a business that is spread out in a number of different buildings so employees don't have to walk too far to get something to eat.

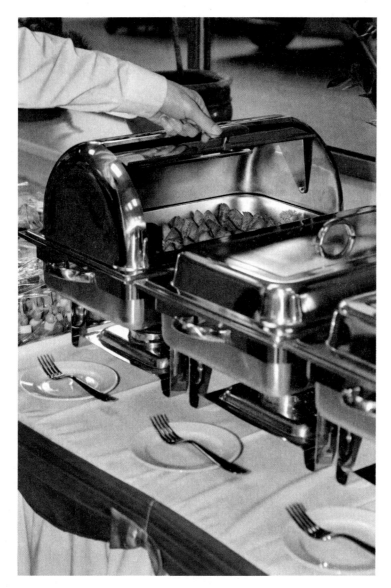

FIGURE 10-4 Chafing Dishes

© Serghei Starus/Shutterstock

There are a number of types of vending machines: those serving sodas and beverages, snacks, cold foods such as sandwiches and salads, coffee and other hot beverages, frozen foods such as ice cream, or even some hot foods. Instead of offering hot foods in a vending machine, with its potential food safety issues, many foodservices prefer to offer the same foods in a refrigerated vending machine and have a microwave available for the customer to heat up the food.

Many foodservices with vending machines contract with a vending company, such as Canteen, to properly stock and maintain the machines. Foodservice contract companies, such as Aramark, often have a vending division so they can run the vending program in their own accounts. If a vending contractor is used, the foodservice must negotiate a favorable contract including commission rates and how the commission is tracked, amount of liability insurance required, cleaning and stocking schedule, compliance with regulations, and how quickly common issues such as the machine didn't dispense a soda, will be resolved.

Running a vending program is not as simple as just stocking machines with soda and chips. You have to figure out where the machines should be located and then what your customers want to buy. Temperatures in machines holding perishable foods must be carefully monitored and recorded. Stock must be replenished in a timely manner and rotation procedures followed. Outdated products must be promptly removed. Customer service is also very important and needs to be dealt with on a timely basis.

Vending companies sometimes replace a bank of vending machines with **micromarkets**, a fairly recent innovation found at colleges and universities, healthcare facilities, workplaces, and other locations (**Figure 10-5**). Micromarkets are small self-service retail stores in a secure area where customers can choose grab-and-go foods, meals that can be heated up, snacks, and beverages. They pay at self-checkout kiosks that accept cash and cashless payments. Most micromarkets do not have a foodservice employee present so they are truly self-service.

Micromarkets have a number of advantages compared with vending machines. Customers like the retail environment of the micromarket more and see it as more personal. Also, micromarkets offer a wider variety of food and beverage choices (including sandwiches, salads, and foods that need to be heated) that are customized to the location. The menu for entrée items often changes daily or weekly. Customers are happier when they can pick up items and look at them before purchase. Because customers perceive food from a micromarket as being higher in quality than vending machine food, they are willing to pay more and sales in micromarkets are indeed higher than the vending machines they replace (Parlevel, 2017). Since there are no coin jams or food that gets stuck in the machine, costs are lower. Also, micromarket open shelves can be refilled quicker than products in vending machines so that also saves money.

Because most micromarkets are unmanned, there is a concern about theft. The entrance to the micro-market is often restricted (customers often need a card or badge

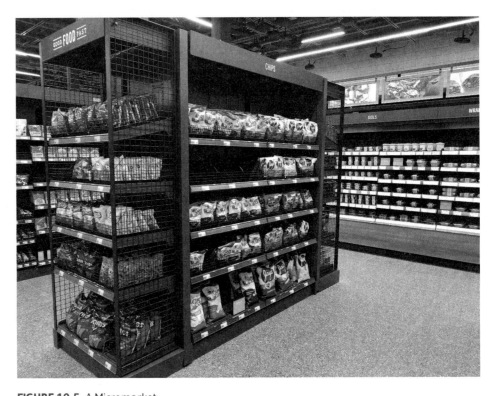

FIGURE 10-5 A Micromarket

© ChicagoPhotographer/Shutterstock

to gain access) and some micromarkets have an employee present at certain times for stocking and monitoring. Other deterrents include the following.

- Webcams and closed-circuit television
- Frequent inventorying to monitor product sales
- Signage

Another way to decrease theft is to offer beverages such as soda in a can or bottle rather than a soda fountain. If foods need to be heated up, it is helpful to put the microwave in a separate area so a customer doesn't heat and eat the meal before leaving.

TRAY SERVICE

Tray service is seen in several settings: healthcare, hotels, and airlines. Tray service is useful when the guest can't come to the foodservice, so the foodservice has to bring the meal to them. In hospital settings, a meal is assembled on a tray in a kitchen and then delivered by foodservice employees to the patient's room (**Figure 10-6**). In hotels, the guest orders room service delivery by phone or electronic device. The tray is delivered, usually within a certain timeframe, by hotel employees. Airline meals are usually made at a commissary kitchen near the airport, then blast-chilled. The meals are transported to the airplane, placed on board under refrigeration, and reheated at the appropriate time. Meal trays are then passed out to passengers during the flight.

Each of these types of tray service presents distribution concerns because the meals are prepared and assembled at a distance from where they are served. Similar to the problems delivering food to someone's home or office, maintaining food temperature and food quality is crucial to successful tray service. Hotels, for example, use plate covers (also called domes) on plates with hot food to trap the heat. Lids help keep heat in and also protect the food from contamination during transport. Popular lids used in hotels are made of stainless steel or polycarbonate. Polycarbonate lids are clear and lighter in weight compared with stainless steel. Lids may be vented, meaning that they have a

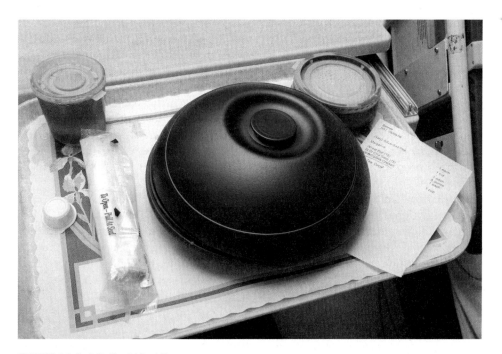

FIGURE 10-6 A Patient Meal Tray

© Rob Byron/Shutterstock

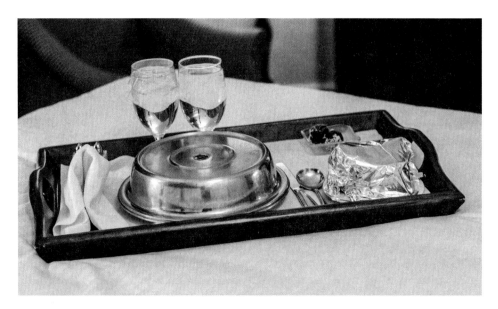

FIGURE 10-7 Hotel Room Service Tray

© Cabeca de Marmore/Shutterstock

small round hole in the middle, so that moisture can escape (**Figure 10-7**). Too much moisture ruins crispy foods such as French fries or toast. Hotels often use insulated carts that are pushed up to the guest's room.

10.2 MANAGE MEAL ASSEMBLY, DISTRIBUTION, AND SERVICE IN HEALTHCARE

In this section, we will look at foodservice in hospitals, assisted-living facilities, and long-term skilled nursing facilities (also called nursing homes). One unique feature of preparing meals for patients/residents in most of these settings is that some meals are modified to meet dietary requirements, such as a low-sodium diet for someone with high blood pressure or a carbohydrate-controlled diet for someone with diabetes. In most of these facilities, each patient/resident has a **diet order** based on their medical needs that details any restrictions on what someone can eat. For many patients/residents, the diet order will be for a "regular" diet, meaning that there are no restrictions on what they can eat. For other patients/residents, they may be placed on a modified diet such as a low-sodium or soft diet (soft in texture). A **modified diet** is a diet that has been adjusted with regard to its nutrient content or its texture.

Whether someone is in a hospital, assisted-living facility, or nursing home, tasty and healthy foods are very important for overall well-being and good health. When patients/residents are not feeling well, their appetite is reduced, resulting in poor nutrient intake and weight loss. Increased pressure to provide high-quality meals, increase patient satisfaction with meals, and also contain and reduce food and labor costs have long been challenges faced by healthcare foodservice managers.

HOSPITALS

There are many types of hospitals that provide medical and surgical treatment for ill patients. Most hospitals are acute-care hospitals, meaning that treatment is short-term. The average number of days that a patient spends in a hospital is 4.6 (Freeman, Weiss, & Heslin, 2018). Because the length of a patient's stay is relatively short, many hospital foodservices use a restaurant-style menu or one-week cycle menu.

When looking at patient meals, how the food orders are taken and how the food is prepared, assembled onto a tray, and distributed to the patients will vary. Some of the considerations that any hospital foodservice director considers when designing a tray service system include the following.

- The number of beds in the hospital, the percentage of beds that are normally occupied, and the average length of stay
- How spread out the hospital buildings are (how vertical and how horizontal) and the distance that must be traveled to get to patient rooms
- Availability of elevators for meal transport
- The type of foodservice operation (conventional, ready-prepared, assembly/serve, and commissary)
- The physical design of the kitchen
- The foodservice budget
- Staffing

The further the distance from where meals are assembled to where they will be served, the bigger the challenge to deliver a fresh, hot meal. It can also be a challenge to deliver hot meals when elevators have to be relied upon to get meals up to patients. In some facilities, at meal delivery hours, one elevator may be designated *only* for foodservice employees to deliver meals.

Three systems for tray service in hospitals will be discussed: traditional trayline system, room service program, and spoken menu system. Many hospitals use one of these systems but not always exactly as described here.

Traditional Trayline System

The **traditional trayline system**, which is still used in some hospitals and nursing homes, starts with handing a paper menu (**Figure 10-8**) to patients to circle their choices for the next day's meals (sometimes just lunch and dinner). The patients circle their choices, and someone from the foodservice department picks up the menus (and also helps a patient make choices as needed) later in the day. With the traditional trayline

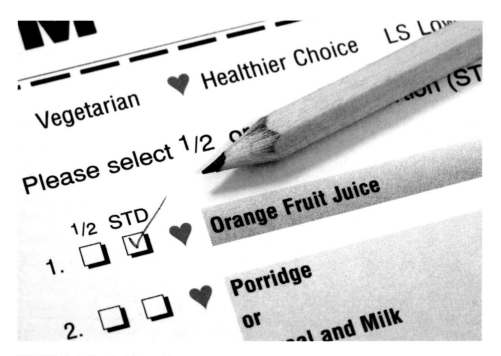

FIGURE 10-8 Hospital Paper Menu

© Empato/iStock/Getty Images Plus/Getty Images

system, the menu is usually a one- or two-week selective menu, but a nonselective menu could certainly be used. If the dinner meal on a nonselective menu is fish, for example, the patients who don't eat fish will be given a substitute item. Records must be kept of each patient's likes and dislikes when there is a nonselective menu (which may be used in some long-term care facilities).

When all of the menus for the next day are collected, foodservice employees line up the menus by floor and room, then check to see if any new patients were admitted, current patients were discharged, or if a patient was transferred to a different room or their diet order was changed. The menus of patients on modified diets, such as a diabetic diet, are reviewed to make sure the choices are appropriate. If not, changes are made. In some hospitals, an employee(s) uses the menus to come up with a count of how many of each menu item was ordered to use for the Production Sheet for the cooks for the next day. Before each meal, foodservice employees again check for new admissions and discharges to be sure that a meal gets delivered to each patient who is allowed to eat.

When it is time to assemble meals, the patient menus are given to the trayline personnel. A trayline, shown in **Figure 10-9**, is like an assembly lines that builds cars. Each patient tray starts down a belt or roller conveyor (which may be straight or oval, powered or manual) with the menu visible at what is called the "starter" station. The starter is an employee who places the placemat, menu, utensils, and appropriate condiment pack (some patients cannot have salt or sugar packets) on the trays. As the tray moves down the line, each employee places certain items on the tray, such as entrées and hot side dishes, hot beverages, or cold salads and desserts. The employee in charge of entrées and

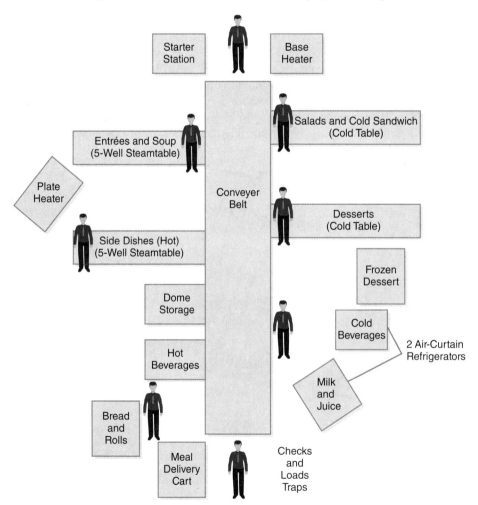

FIGURE 10-9 Trayline

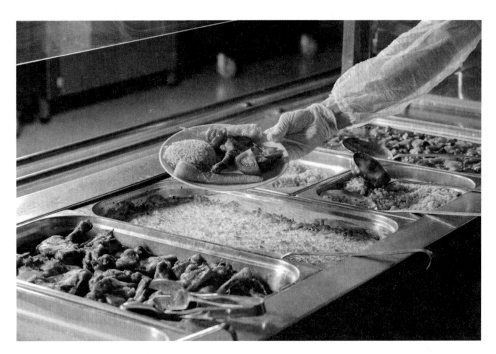

FIGURE 10-10 Steam Table

© Ercan senkaya/Shutterstock

hot side dishes, for example, stands behind a steam table (**Figure 10-10**), looks to see which menu items were chosen, places them on a heated plate, puts a lid on the plate, and places it on the tray. Once all of the items are on a tray, the employee at the last station (often called the checker) checks the tray to make sure the items are correct and places the tray in a meal delivery cart.

Before the trayline can assemble trays, each station has to have all of its items ready to serve. For example, the cooks fill the steam table with the appropriate menu items and the starter station will have its supply of placemats, utensils, condiment packs, etc., refilled from the last meal. Cold items, such as milk cartons or puddings, are commonly placed in air-curtain refrigerators that use a curtain of air to keep food cold while allowing employees to easily grab items with the refrigerator door open (**Figure 10-11**). Much of the trayline equipment, such as steam tables and air-curtain refrigerators, is mobile (on rollers or casters) and can be moved around for cleaning. During meal service, hot food is replenished with fresh items. Some made-to-order items may also be prepared, such as grilled cheese.

Let's take a look at some of the foodservice equipment used on a trayline.

1. *Fiberglass tray and tray dispenser.* Fiberglass trays are strong and come in a number of colors. Often a paper tray cover (disposable) is put on top of the tray to help keep items from sliding and improve the appearance. Nonskid trays are now available with a print design if the foodservice does not want to use tray covers. Trays are stacked on a tray dispenser that is self-leveling.
2. *Steam table.* The space where a hotel pan fits into the steam table is called a well, which is either sealed or open. You can add water into a sealed well to get moist heat that is good for items like soups, vegetables, pasta, and rice. Sealed wells (also called dry wells) are time consuming to clean and get lime scale buildup. You can create moist heat in a open well by using a spillage pan or chafing dish with water and place that under the food. Open wells are easier to clean and good for maintaining temperatures below that of boiling water. Some high-efficiency sealed wells use convected air to maintain even food temperatures (Sherer, 2019).

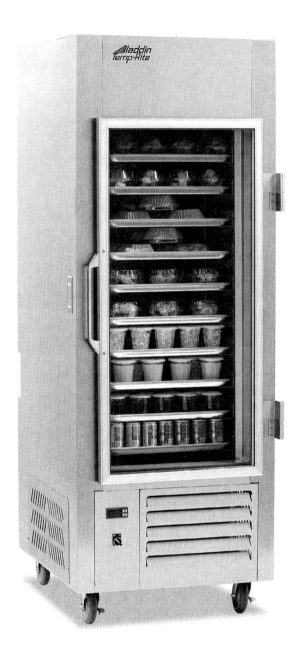

FIGURE 10-11 Air-Curtain Refrigerator

Courtesy of Aladdin.

3. *Convection plate heater.* To keep food hot during delivery, you will need hot plates and a base (next item). A convection plate heater heats the plates to a temperature of about 170° F (77°C) in approximately two hours.

4. *Bases and domes.* To keep the plate and the food nice and hot, the plate is placed on top of a hot **base** (**Figure 10–12**). Most bases can keep food warm for 45 to 60 minutes as long as a dome (shown in Figure 10-6) is placed over the food. Some bases can keep food warm for a little longer. The best and quickest way to heat up a base is by using an induction charger (Figure 10–12). The base heats up very fast and stays cool to the touch. Cool bases are also available and can freeze in just two hours. A small number of institutions use an insulated tray with individual molded compartments that hold hot and cold items. Each time the insulated tray is used, an employee puts either a reusable or disposable dish into each compartment. Then an insulated lid is put on top to maintain temperatures.

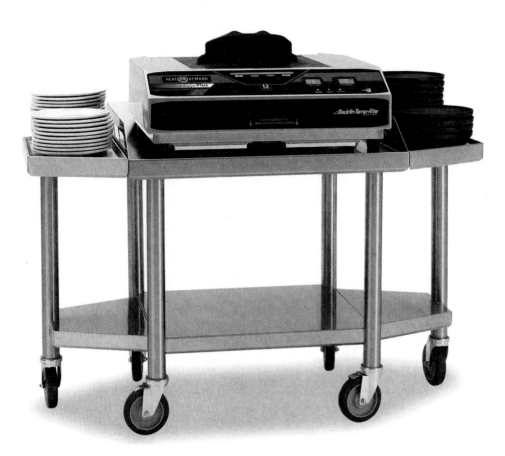

FIGURE 10-12 Induction Base and Charger

Courtesy of Aladdin.

5. *Insulated mugs and bowls.* Mugs and bowls used for both hot and cold foods such as soups, oatmeal, or salad, are insulated to maintain appropriate temperatures. They are shown in Figure 10-6.
6. *Air-curtain refrigerator.* During trayline service, the door on these refrigerators can be kept open. A horizontal air screen keeps the contents of the refrigerator cold and allows easy access for the trayline employee to grab beverages, salads, desserts, and other cold items.
7. *Delivery cart.* Delivery carts come in a variety of sizes and some are insulated to help maintain food temperatures. Better delivery carts are quiet, lightweight, easy to maneuver, easy to clean, and have wraparound bumpers. Some carts have a railing on the top to secure accessories such as a coffee pot or condiment carrier (**Figure 10-13**). Conventional traylines usually use larger carts while smaller carts work best in room service and host/hostess programs. Some carts are motorized so they just have to be guided. Some hospitals use **automated guided vehicles (AGV)**, or robotic vehicles, for meal delivery and tray pickup. To successfully use AGV in hospitals, there are many considerations such as corridor space and elevators. Although it is easiest for the AGV to have their own dedicated space to roam, it is not always needed with large enough corridors. AGVs also need a space where they can sit on the patient floor, often called a send-and-receive station. For example, when Reading Hospital (Pennsylvania) opened a new building, the distance from the kitchen to the patients was quite a distance so they purchased some AGVs, which actually control specific elevators and send a text message to the host/hostess when it is close to its destination (Buzalka, 2017).

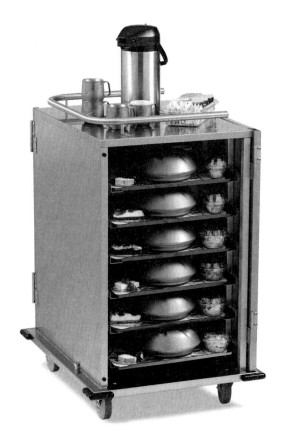

FIGURE 10-13 Delivery Cart

Courtesy of Aladdin.

In a small hospital located in one building, you will typically find a trayline located close to the production area. This is known as **centralized meal assembly** because assembly takes place in one central location (this is also the case for many restaurants) before meals are distributed for service. However, as a hospital gets bigger and expands from one building, it becomes harder to get fresh, hot meals to all patients. In this situation, the foodservice may use a **decentralized meal assembly** system in which food is transported in bulk from the production area to a location(s) closer to the point of service where the meal trays will be assembled.

Some hospitals actually use both centralized and decentralized meal assembly. For example, patient trays for the main building on a hospital campus are assembled next to the production area (centralized assembly) and transported to patient rooms. Meanwhile, a cardiac unit is located a distance from the main building with a long corridor connecting it with the main building. So as mealtime approaches, a steamtable loaded with the hot foods (in bulk) for the cardiac unit, along with cold items such as salads and desserts, are transported from the main kitchen down the corridor to a **satellite kitchen** (sometimes called a **galley kitchen**). When the food is transported, it must be covered. Once in the galley kitchen, the meals are assembled (decentralized assembly) and then delivered to the cardiac patients. Some items, such as condiments and beverages, are stocked in the satellite kitchen. Satellite kitchens typically have refrigerators, warming equipment, coffee equipment, toasters, a trayline (or shortened trayline), and sometimes cooking equipment such as a griddle to make fresh, popular items like grilled cheese.

Having a centralized meal assembly area allows for better supervision, consistent portions and presentation, and less labor and space than when meal assembly is decentralized. However, decentralized meal assembly is better for serving meals at appropriate temperatures (because the meals don't have to travel as far) and may allow for more attention to each meal. Also, several decentralized galley kitchens can feed patients in a shorter period of time than a centralized trayline.

While a majority of hospital kitchens produce fresh food each day, some do use cook-chill systems. Cook chill is a production system in which food is prepared in advance, blast chilled, and held for service at a later time. Using cook-chill menu items, meals are plated *cold* on a trayline and then reheated in special equipment just prior to service. The foods are rethermalized (heated) either in the foodservice kitchen or transported by carts to the patient floors and rethermalized there.

Figure 10-14 shows a cart full of trays that has been pushed into a **docking station**, a specialized piece of equipment that can rethermalize cook-chill foods and, at the same time, keep cold foods cold. Because trays for this system are divided into a hot section and a cold section, they are put into a cart with a center divider to separate hot from cold. The docking station provides the controls for refrigeration and heat as required, and can rethermalize trays/meals automatically or manually at the touch of a button. While the plates are heated in the hot section, the refrigeration continues in the cold section of the tray. After rethermalization, the cart is pulled away from the docking station and serves as the meal delivery cart. To use this type of system, you must use the manufacturer's carts, docking station, trays, and dishes.

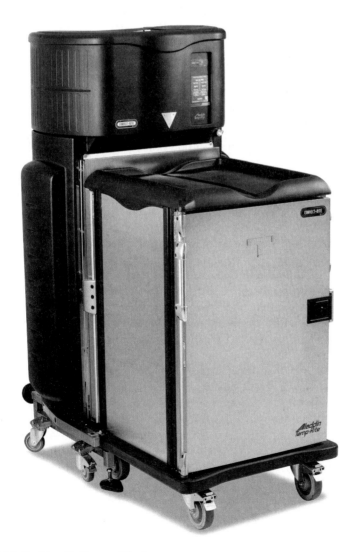

FIGURE 10-14 Docking Station and Cart

Courtesy of Aladdin.

Table 10-1 Steps in Traditional Trayline System
1. Patients receive a menu for upcoming meals and are asked to circle their choices.
2. Later in the day, a foodservice employee (or sometimes nursing) picks up the menus (making sure the patient's name and room number are correct), and assists patients who may require assistance. If a patient is not available to complete the menu, the employee will choose menu items based on the patient's record of likes and dislikes.
3. In the foodservice department, the menus are lined up by floor and room number with attention given to new admissions and discharges. Staff review each menu to make sure the menu choices are appropriate given the patient's diet. Then staff can tear or separate the menu for Breakfast, Lunch, and Dinner.
4. Between meals, changes are made to menus to accommodate new admissions, discharges, transfers, and diet orders.
5. Before each meal, the menus, separated by patient unit or floor, are sent out by patient floor to the trayline to assemble.
6. The trayline swings into operation at set times and an employee at each station puts the appropriate items onto each tray.
7. The trays are put on a cart for delivery to patients.
8. Foodservice employees (sometimes it is a nursing employee) deliver the trays to the patients. The delivery sequence (the order in which trays are assembled and delivered) is often the same for each meal. Some hospitals may change the delivery sequence a little so that certain floors don't always get meals so early or late. However, most patient units want to feed their patients at the same times daily to accommodate the administration of medications such as insulin, and the normal schedule of therapy sessions and procedures.
9. Often within 60 minutes of delivery, employees pick up trays from the patients' rooms starting with the patients served the earliest. Trays are returned to the dish room to be washed, sanitized, and used at the next meal time. Meal carts are also cleaned and stored.

Table 10-1 summarizes the steps in traditional trayline systems. There are certain advantages and disadvantages to this system. The system is precise and, when implemented correctly, ensures that every patient who can eat will get a tray. However, the trayline is labor-intensive and not very efficient. The trayline can only move as fast as the slowest employee. Most traylines produce from two to three trays/minute so, depending on the number of trays, it may require over two hours. No doubt that some patients are eating much earlier than they normally would, and others are eating much later. But if the trayline is having problems at one meal, everyone is eating late. A smaller and more efficient type of trayline, referred to as a **pod**, has since been developed and has replaced a number of traditional traylines.

Another problem with the traditional trayline system is that patients generally order food one day ahead, which can be a concern because some patients don't remember what they ordered and then complain that they want something else when their tray arrives. This could be due to the stress of being in the hospital, medications, or other factors. In addition, newly admitted patients or patients who didn't fill out a menu won't have any choices and will receive a preselected meal.

Another problem revolves around the menu. If the menu offers two entrées, a number of patients will request something outside of those entrées, so the foodservice usually establishes what is called write-ins or approved substitutions. **Write-ins** are menu items that can be written on the menu when a patient needs to eat something not on the menu. Common write-ins are items like chicken tenders, hamburger on a bun, or macaroni and cheese. While it is nice to offer patients additional items, they do require additional time and labor and they tend to slow down the trayline.

Room Service Programs

As computers were being integrated into hospitals in the 1990s, software was developed to support **room service programs** for hospital patients to order meals using a menu in their room. Then the meal would be delivered, often within 30 to 45 minutes. The room service programs were seen as a way to improve patient meal satisfaction by allowing patients to order what they want (within diet restrictions) and when they want. The following are the steps in a typical room service program.

1. Patients view a menu in their room. The menu is restaurant-style and may also include some rotating menu items for lunch/dinner. The menu may offer the same items for lunch and dinner, but, for example, one of the eight hot entrées changes each day of the week (like a Chef's Special at a restaurant).

2. The patient can use the room phone, or an in-room television in some hospitals, to order a meal. Many room service programs offer meals throughout the day, such as from 7:00 AM to 7:00 PM and promise delivery within 30 to 45 minutes of the order. Even though meals are offered throughout the day, there is a cut-off time for each meal, such as breakfast is no longer served at 11:00 AM. Some foodservices offer a limited menu all the way up to midnight or later, but they are in the minority.

3. The patient's phone call is answered in the "call center" by an employee who takes menu orders and keeps in mind any diet restrictions. The call center also helps guide patients as to how room service works. If a patient has not put in a meal order by a certain time, foodservice must call the patient's room, or other mechanism, to offer a meal. The foodservice department must be able to verify that all patients are offered meals three times a day (due in part to regulations). The call center usually has one employee for every 50 to 60 meal orders.

4. Once the call center has the order, an order ticket is printed so the cookline, cold food area, and assembler can get the order ready. Instead of using a trayline with at least five to six employees, trays are usually assembled in a pod. A pod is a mini-trayline with about two or three employees who have everything within reach, or a couple of steps, to assemble trays (**Figure 10-15**). Hot items are prepared to order, such as a flatbread sandwich or omelet, or simply finish cooked. Rapid-cook ovens are useful as they can heat up items, such as pizza, quickly.

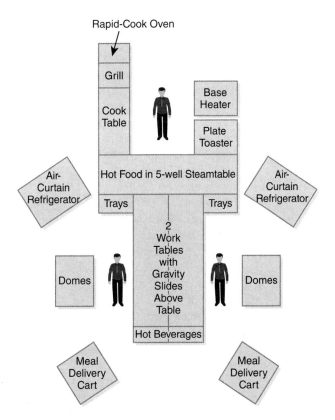

FIGURE 10-15 Sample Layout of a Pod Containing Two Mini-Traylines

Cold food, such as salads and sandwiches, may be prepared fresh and some cold items, such as desserts, fruits, and beverages, are already portioned and ready to put on the tray. One position, the **assembler**, collects the hot and cold food items for each tray and checks the food for quality and accuracy of the diet order. Whereas a hospital using a traditional trayline usually has just one trayline operating at each meal, a hospital using pods has more than one mini-trayline operating at the same time.

5.   Next, the assembler puts the tray into a cart. Many foodservices set a timer for eight to 10 minutes once the first tray is put into a cart. When the timer goes off, an employee, often called a **runner**, leaves with the cart (generally with five to 10 trays) and delivers the trays. At peak service times, each cart is for an assigned nursing unit. At nonpeak times, trays for several floors that are close to each other can be put on one cart.

6.   The host/hostess on the receiving floor is notified that a cart is coming. Some carts have insulated coffee/decaffeinated coffee/water dispensers on top, so the host/hostess pours any hot beverages before delivering the tray, and checks in with patients shortly after tray delivery to see if everything is okay and offers additional hot beverages or condiments.

7.   Trays are picked up from patients' rooms by the host/hostess. Because mealtimes in room service are quite long (compared with the traditional trayline) and there is no sequence in which trays are delivered, the foodservice must have a system to track meal tray pickup.

The use of pods to assemble trays has been evolving for over 15 years. As mentioned, conventional traylines are not very efficient. With the emphasis in business and healthcare to continuously improve work processes and increase productivity, the development of an alternative to the trayline was inevitable. With pods, workflow is reorganized, employee duties are changed, and principles such as motion economy are used to increase efficiency. Equipment such as gravity-fed condiment bins and beverage slides that tilt down are also critical to pods being successful.

Most pods actually contain two mini-traylines as seen in the pod in Figure 10-15. Figure 10-15 shows a T-shaped pod (they can come in a number of different shapes) with a steamtable at the top and a cook's table alongside it with a counter griddle and rapid-cook oven. This will be the station for the production employee to get the hot food orders ready. In addition to the production employee, the assembler starts by grabbing a tray and tray cover and then adding flatware, napkins, condiments, and the cold/ambient temperature items. Each assembler has a worktable with gravity-feed shelves full of condiments and some menu items. An air-curtain refrigerator keeps salads, desserts, and beverages cold. The cook will give the hot food items to the assembler and a base and dome are used to maintain heat. Hot beverages are usually put on last, if not served on the floor, and the tray is checked for accuracy and placed in a cart.

Most pods have two or three employees. To keep the pod moving at a good speed, it is important to design each job so that each job has an equal amount of work. Much of the equipment used in pods is mobile, meaning that it has caster wheels and employees can easily move them for cleaning or to reconfigure a station. The equipment should be able to be restocked while the system is being used, so restocking is done from the back.

Pods have a number of advantages. First, pods save time so trays get to patients in a timelier manner. If a conventional trayline slows down, all the trays yet to be made will be late. Some hospitals have three or even four pods working at a time (which means from six to eight mini-traylines humming) so even if one pod slows down, it isn't going to delay the majority of trays going out. With only two or three people assembling trays, accuracy tends to improve as fewer employees are involved and there is increased employee accountability. Another advantage is that a hospital serves a variable number of patient meals each day. When the number of patients is particularly high or low, the foodservice director can choose to utilize more or fewer pods at mealtime (you can't do that with a conventional trayline), which is more labor-efficient. Overall, many food-services find pods to be more efficient, resulting in faster tray delivery, and some report labor savings (Rezendes, 2015; Sherer, 2011).

Potential advantages of room service include the following (Norton, 2006).

1. Increased patient satisfaction with meals (Doorduijn et al., 2016; Klein & Webb, 2012; McCray et al., 2018)
2. Decreased food costs because the kitchen is sending only what patients want (Klein & Webb, 2012; McCray et al., 2018)
3. More made-to-order foods and improved freshness
4. Improved nutritional intake by patients (Doorduijn et al., 2016; McCray et al., 2018)

In addition, because most programs send meals up all day, there are no *late trays*. In the traditional trayline system, each meal is sent up to the floors during a certain time span, such as from 11:15 AM to 1:15 PM for lunch trays. For various reasons, a patient may not have received lunch and can't wait until dinner so they request a meal at 2:30 PM. In that case, a *late tray* is sent up to the patient's room. Late trays are time-consuming plus there is usually not much variety in what can be sent to the patient between meals.

Some of the disadvantages of room service are that the menu can get boring for patients who are in the hospital for longer periods of time. Also, moving to a room service program involves a *lot of work*: changing menus, changing employee schedules, and finding money for new equipment and renovations are only some of things that have to be done. Moving to room service requires many months for planning and also for implementation.

Tips for successful room service programs include the following.

- Call center employees need to be friendly and very customer-service oriented.
- Training is very important for all employees involved in room service.
- Employees who deliver meals and interact with patients should have an upscale uniform for an enhanced image and so everyone recognizes the employee as part of the room service program.
- Instant communication is essential for everyone.

Spoken Menu System (Host/Hostess)

As room service programs became more popular, another program developed that is really a variation on room service. In the **spoken menu system**, instead of the patient contacting the call center with meal selections, a foodservice employee (called a host or hostess or sometimes a nutrition ambassador) goes to the patient's bedside. The host/hostess reviews the food choices with each patient (before lunch and before dinner) and takes the meal order on a tablet or smart device. The menu for this system could be a restaurant-style menu, a cycle menu, or a combination of restaurant-style and cycle menu. Some hospitals also like to offer a Chef's Special for lunch and dinner, which changes from day to day. Patients will often pick the Chef's Special, but if they want to pick something else, additional items are always available such as baked chicken, grilled chicken sandwich, grilled cheese, or Chef's salad (Schilling, 2009).

A patient's tray ticket is then sent electronically from bedside to the kitchen pod where it prints out. In many hospitals, the host/hostess helps assemble the trays after taking orders. The following is an example of what a host/hostess will do during the day.

1. The host/hostess will start work in the morning and first help assemble and then deliver breakfast trays (the breakfast order was taken the day before).
2. Then the hosts/hostesses make rounds to retrieve finished meal trays and place them in carts to be returned to the main kitchen for cleaning and sanitation.
3. After getting lunch orders from patients, they help assemble and deliver the lunch trays.

THE BIG PICTURE

We have discussed different ways that a hospital distributes, assembles, and delivers trays to patient's rooms. If you were to walk into a hospital foodservice today, you could use the following questions to find out exactly how patient meals are handled, from cooking to serving.

1. What type of menu is used? (such as restaurant-style or cycle or a combination, selective or nonselective)
2. How is food prepared? (conventional scratch cooking, cook-chill, commissary, or a combination)
3. How and when are meal orders taken? (a patient contacting the call center or a host/hostess getting a meal order before meals)
4. Where are the trays assembled? (centralized or decentralized)
5. How are the trays assembled? (traditional trayline or pod)
6. Who delivers the trays? (the host/hostess who took the meal order, an employee who just delivers trays, or nursing)
7. Who picks up the trays? (the host/hostess who delivered the tray or nursing)

4. Next, they retrieve finished lunch trays to be returned to the kitchen.
5. In the afternoon, they will get the dinner and breakfast orders from each patient.
6. Then they will help assemble and deliver the dinner trays.
7. Last, they retrieve finished dinner trays and return them to the kitchen.

In many hospitals, the host/hostess is scheduled for a longer shift than the traditional eight hours. For example, at one Pennsylvania hospital, hosts/hostesses work a 10.5-hour day and serve all three meals for the same patients (Boss, 2016).

The spoken menu is very helpful to the patient as they communicate with the same employee all day and get to order meals within a few hours of service. With this system, the host/hostess is more accountable for excellent patient service. In addition, nursing likes having a host/hostess take the orders and see the same patients all day as the improved communication helps relieve nursing of resolving food issues. A critical piece of this program is the ratio of hosts/hostesses to patients. If the host/hostess takes meal orders, helps assemble the trays, and then delivers the trays, each host/hostess can only handle about 30 to 40 patients (Rezendes, 2015; Sherer, 2011).

ASSISTED LIVING FACILITIES

Assisted living facilities provide residents with housing, food, housekeeping, and daily assistance with tasks such as dressing and bathing. Many facilities also offer laundry services, recreational and religious activities, and part-time nursing help. Assisted living is useful for individuals who need help with what are called the "activities of daily living" such as eating, bathing, dressing, or getting out of a bed or chair. Some, but not all, assisted living facilities offer services specifically designed for people with dementia (memory issues).

Assisted living bridges the gap between living independently and living in a nursing home. If a resident develops serious medical problems that require daily nursing care by a Registered Nurse, the resident will likely be transferred to a skilled nursing facility where round-the-clock nursing care is available.

Assisted living is *not* regulated by the federal government unless the facility accepts Medicaid payments. In that case, it is regulated like a skilled nursing facility (to be discussed in a moment). Each state has licensing and certification requirements for assisted-living facilities. For example, assisted-living facilities and personal-care facilities in Pennsylvania are actually licensed separately. They both offer the same basic services but the assisted-living facilities must allow residents to have a private apartment, age in place, and receive more skilled nursing services than are found in personal-care facilities.

In most assisted-living facilities, the foodservice uses a cycle menu that offers two or more entrée choices for each meal. The kitchen is often adjacent to the dining room where most residents come for meals. If desired, a resident may eat in his/her room. Depending on the size of the facility, there may be more than one dining room or more than one seating for each meal. A printed menu is available for the residents to review. Using table service, servers take the resident's food choices and bring meals and beverages to the table. Sometimes buffet service may be used, such as for a breakfast meal. Some assisted living facilities also have a small café or bistro that is used for between-meal snacks or small meals. Grab-and-go foods may also be available.

LONG-TERM SKILLED NURSING FACILITIES

Long-term skilled nursing facilities, also known as nursing homes, provide health-related care and services needed on a daily basis due to a physical or mental condition such as dementia. Because most skilled nursing facilities accept Medicare and Medicaid payments, they are subject to federal requirements for acceptable quality. The Centers for Medicare and Medicaid Services (CMS) have many requirements that affect the foodservice department. The following are some examples.

- Established national nutrition guidelines must be used to confirm that the menus meet the residents' nutritional needs.
- Menus must also meet residents' religious, cultural, and ethnic needs.
- Residents have the right to make personal food and beverage choices. Options for those who ask for a different meal or beverage choice must be appealing to the resident and be of similar nutritive value.
- Alternative meals and snacks must be provided to residents who want to eat outside of scheduled times.
- Meals must be provided in a safe and sanitary manner and in a timely fashion.
- Staff must be available during meals to assist residents as needed.
- Residents can eat foods from outside of the facility.

Nursing facilities are moving from a traditional culture in which residents had to comply with the staff about when to go to bed, eat meals, etc., to a more *person-directed culture* in which residents are making their own decisions as much as possible about their individual routines.

Residents value control and making choices improves their well-being. Residents who feel they can make their own food choices, such as being able to grab a snack between meals, can improve their quality of life (Carrier, West, & Ouellet, 2009). As stated by the Academy of Nutrition and Dietetics, "Involving individuals in choices about food and dining, such as diet and supplement orders, texture and consistency modifications, food selections, dining locations, and meal times, can help them maintain a sense of dignity, control, and autonomy in every post-acute care setting." (Dorner & Friedrich, 2018, p. 727). Modified diets are often liberalized as much as possible to offer meals that taste better and are more likely to be eaten. This is especially helpful to prevent unintended weight loss, malnutrition, and dehydration.

Long-term skilled nursing facilities are increasingly focused on upgrading dining and offering more choices of what to eat, when to eat, and where to eat. Many residents eat in a dining room environment that resembles a home dining room (not a restaurant). Each resident is served the foods and beverages that they desire from the choices available, and modified diets are often liberalized. If a resident prefers to eat elsewhere, such as in his/her room, a meal tray will be delivered.

Meals are served in a variety of ways depending on the specific nursing home.

- Table service where staff take resident orders. Often, this takes place in what looks like a home kitchen that is outfitted with equipment to hold foods (hot and cold) and make some items to order (such as a sandwich or eggs). Plating and delivery of the meal is completed in front of the residents. Some facilities have established the "neighborhood" concept in which a small number of residents come together and share meals in this homelike environment.

- Buffet style where residents serve themselves, or if that is not possible, staff will get the food items the resident wants.
- Family style where residents serve themselves and staff assist.
- Tray service may be used in smaller facilities.

Group meals in a home-like dining room supports engagement between individuals and reduces isolation. Group meals are also helpful for residents who need assistance eating, as a Certified Nursing Assistant can sit at a table and help two or three residents at a time.

In addition to looking at service style, another facet of foodservice is when residents can dine. There may be set times to come to the dining room to eat, or open dining in which meals are available during a certain time frame, such as lunch from 11:30 AM to 1:30 PM, and residents can come when they choose. Some foodservices offer 24-hour dining where residents can order food at any time.

SUMMARY

10.1 Compare and Contrast Different Service Styles

- Distribution is the process of getting food from where it was produced to where the customer will be served (also known as the point of service). Assembly is putting components of a meal together on plate(s) to be served.
- Service styles include table service, counter service, drive-through service, take-out and delivery service, cafeteria service, self-service, and tray service. Regardless of which service style is used, certain elements must be present to ensure customer satisfaction, such as reliability/consistency, responsiveness, assurance, and empathy.
- Table service is most common in commercial foodservices. There are different styles of table service including American-style service, family-style service, English service, French service, and banquet service.
- To deliver hot foods, many companies use thermal insulated bags (Figure 10-3) and keep hot foods separate from cold. It's important to pick the right size and shape bag for the job it has to do.
- Many cafeterias in business and industry, colleges and universities, and healthcare use a scramble (scatter) system or hollow square cafeteria. Most cafeterias use a combination of self-service and counter service.
- Self-service is also found in settings such as buffets, convenience stores, vending machines, and micromarkets.
- Tray service is used in healthcare, hotels, and airlines.

10.2 Manage Meal Assembly, Distribution, and Service in Healthcare

- Most hospitals are acute-care hospitals. Because the length of a patient's stay is relatively short (4 to 5 days), many hospital foodservices use a restaurant-style menu or one-week cycle menu.
- Factors that influence the tray service delivery system include the size of the hospital, how vertical and horizontal the buildings are, the distance to get to patients' rooms, availability of elevators for meal transport, budget, etc.
- Most hospitals use one of these three tray service systems: traditional trayline, room service, or spoken menu (a variation of room service).
- Figure 10-9 shows a traditional trayline that can produce approximately two to three trays/minute.
- Table 10-1 summarizes the steps in traditional trayline systems.
- Traylines and pods use equipment such as steam tables, convection plate heaters, bases and domes, insulated mugs and bowls, air-curtain refrigerators, and delivery carts.
- Centralized meal assembly takes place in one central location. Decentralized meal assembly is when food is transported (usually in bulk) from a central production kitchen to a location (called a satellite kitchen) closer to the point of service and trays are assembled there so food is served hot and fresh.
- In the case of a cook-chill system, meals are plated *cold* on a trayline and then reheated in a docking station just prior to service.

The foods are either rethermalized in the foodservice kitchen or transported by carts to the patient floors and rethermalized there.

- Steps for a room service program are given. Room service programs were developed in large part to increase patient meal satisfaction. The menu is usually restaurant-style.
- Potential advantages of room service include increased patient satisfaction with meals, decreased food costs, fresher meals, and improved nutrient intake by patients.
- In the spoken menu system (a variation of room service), instead of the patient contacting the call center with meal selections, a foodservice employee (called a host or hostess or sometimes a nutrition ambassador) goes to the patient's bedside. The host/hostess reviews the food choices with each patient (before lunch and before dinner) and takes the meal order on an electronic device such as a tablet. The host/hostess then helps assemble these trays and performs their delivery and pick-up.
- Both room service programs and spoken menu programs often use pods (mini-traylines) instead of a traditional trayline. Figure 10-15 shows a sample layout of a pod containing two mini-traylines. Many foodservices find pods to be more efficient, resulting in faster tray delivery, and some

of the foodservices also find they save some labor costs.
- Assisted living bridges the gap between living independently and living in a nursing home. It is not regulated by the federal government unless the facility accepts Medicaid payments. In most facilities, the foodservice uses a cycle menu that offers two or more entrée choices for each meal. The kitchen is often adjacent to the dining room where most residents come for meals. Other eating options, such as a bistro, may be available.
- Long-term skilled nursing facilities (nursing homes) provide health-related care and services needed on a daily basis due to a physical or mental condition such as dementia. Because most skilled nursing facilities accept Medicare and Medicaid payments, they are subject to federal requirements (as listed) for acceptable quality.
- Long-term skilled nursing facilities are increasingly focused on upgrading dining and offering more choices of what to eat, when to eat, and where to eat. Many residents eat in a dining room environment that resembles a home dining room (not a restaurant). Each resident is served the foods and beverages he/she desires from the choices available, and modified diets are often liberalized.

REVIEW AND DISCUSSION QUESTIONS

1. How is table service different from counter or cafeteria service? Think in terms of how the order is given and how the food is served.
2. What is a ghost kitchen and why would a foodservice owner want to start one?
3. What are the pros and cons of a restaurant chain having its own delivery service or using a company such as Door Dash? As a consumer, which do you prefer and why?
4. Give three examples of settings where self-service is used and why self-service is appropriate.
5. What are the advantages and disadvantages of having a micromarket in a building that has business space for several large businesses?
6. Discuss considerations for serving quality meals to patients on five different floors in a hospital.
7. How is food kept hot once it leaves a hospital kitchen?
8. What are the advantages and disadvantages of a centralized and decentralized meal assembly? Can a healthcare facility use both?
9. How does a room service program work in a healthcare facility? What are its advantages and disadvantages compared with a traditional trayline with a cycle menu?
10. What is a pod and why would a foodservice manager choose to use pods instead of a trayline?
11. Why is the spoken menu system popular? How does it affect staffing?
12. Describe the variety of ways in which meals are served in skilled nursing facilities.
13. What does it mean to have a more person-directed culture in healthcare facilities and why is it important?

SMALL GROUP PROJECT

For the foodservice concept that you created, complete the following.

1. Pick and justify an appropriate distribution/service system for your foodservice concept.

Describe how the system will operate including any equipment that will be needed.

REFERENCES

Boss. D. (2016). Game changers in healthcare foodservice. *Foodservice Equipment & Supplies.* Retrieved from https://fesmag.com/features/foodservice-issues/13525-game-changers-in-healthcare-foodservice

Buzalka, M. (2017). Robots ease tray delivery to far-flung hospital wings. *Food Management.* Retrieved from https://www.food-management.com/healthcare/robots-ease-tray-delivery-far-flung-hospital-wings

Dorner, B. & Friedrich. E. K. (2018). Position of the Academy of Nutrition and Dietetics: Individualized nutrition approaches for older adults: Long-term care, post-acute care, and other settings. *Journal of the Academy of Nutrition and Dietetics, 118*(4): 724–735. doi: 10.1016/j.jand.2018.01.022

Doorduijn, A. S., van Gameren, Y., Vasse, E., & de Roos, N. M. (2016). At Your Request® room service dining improves patient satisfaction, maintains nutritional status, and offers opportunities to improve intake. *Clinical Nutrition, 35*(5), 1174–1180. doi: 10.1016.j.clnu.2015.10.00-

Fourth. (2019). Fourth unveils first annual "Truth About Dining Out" survey results, revealing Americans' eating-out habits, the rise of third-party delivery apps and favorite celebrity chef. Retrieved from https://www.fourth.com/press-room/fourth-unveils-first-annual-truth-about-dining-out-survey-results/

Freeman, W. J., Weiss, A. J., & Heslin, K. C. (2018). Overview of U.S. hospital stays in 2016: Variation by geographic region (Statistical Brief #246). *Healthcare Cost and Utilization Project, Agency for Healthcare Research and Quality.* Retrieved from https://www.hcup-us.ahrq.gov/reports/statbriefs/sb246-Geographic-Variation-Hospital-Stays.pdf

Isaac, M. & Yaffe-Bellany, D. (2019). The rise of the virtual restaurant. *The New York Times,* p. B1.

Klein, B. & Webb, J. (2012). Room service continues to deliver for hospitals. *Foodservice Equipment & Supplies.* Retrieved from https://fesmag.com/features/foodservice-perspectives/6074-room-service-continues-to-deliver-for-hospitals

Marston, J. (2019). A rough guide to ghost kitchens according to Chowly CEO Sterling Douglass. *The Spoon.* Retrieved from https://thespoon.tech/a-rough-guide-to-ghost-kitchens-according-to-chowly-ceo-sterling-douglass/

Maze, J. (2019). As delivery evolves, so do restaurant chains' approaches to the service. *Restaurant Business.* Retrieved from https://www.restaurantbusinessonline.com/financing/delivery-evolves-so-do-restaurant-chains-approaches-service

McCray, S., Maunder, K., Krikowa, R., & MacKenzie-Shalders, K. (2018). Room service improves nutritional intake and increases patient satisfaction while decreasing food waste and cost. *Journal of the Academy of Nutrition and Dietetics, 118*(2), 284–293. doi: 10.1016/j.jand.2017.05.014

Negrete-Rousseau, R. (2018). Trays in transition. *Foodservice Equipment Reports.* Retrieved from https://www.fermag.com/articles/8511-trays-in-transition

Norton, C. (2006). Room service: The nuts and bolts (Part I). *Healthcare Foodservice TRENDS Magazine, 8*(2), 6–19.

Parlevel. (2017). Infographic: The impact of micro markets. Retrieved from https://www.parlevelsystems.com/2017/03/08/infographic-impact-micro-markets/

Pioneer Network Food and Dining Clinical Standards Task Force. (2011). New dining practice standards. Retrieved from https://www.pioneernetwork.net/wp-content/uploads/2016/10/The-New-Dining-Practice-Standards.pdf

Rezendes, A. (2015). Equipping pods. *Foodservice Equipment Reports.* Retrieved from https://www.fermag.com/articles/7751-equipping-podspo

Rollins, C., Dobak, S. (2018). Creating a great patient experience: Improving care with food and nutrition services. *Journal of the Academy of Nutrition and Dietetics, 118*(5), 805–808.

Ryu, K, & Jang, S. C. (2008). DINESCAPE: A scale for customers' perception of dining environments. *Journal of Foodservice Business Research, 11*(2), 2–22.

Schilling, B. (2009). Pod-tastic. *FoodService Director Magazine.* Retrieved from https://www.foodservicedirector.com/operations/pod-tastic

Sherer, M. (2019) Advantages of dry hot wells. *Foodservice Equipment Reports.* Retrieved from https://www.fermag.com/articles/9375-equipment-comparison-dry-hot-wells/

Sherer, M. (2011). Anatomy of a pod. *Foodservice Equipment Reports.* Retrieved from https://www.fermag.com/articles/966

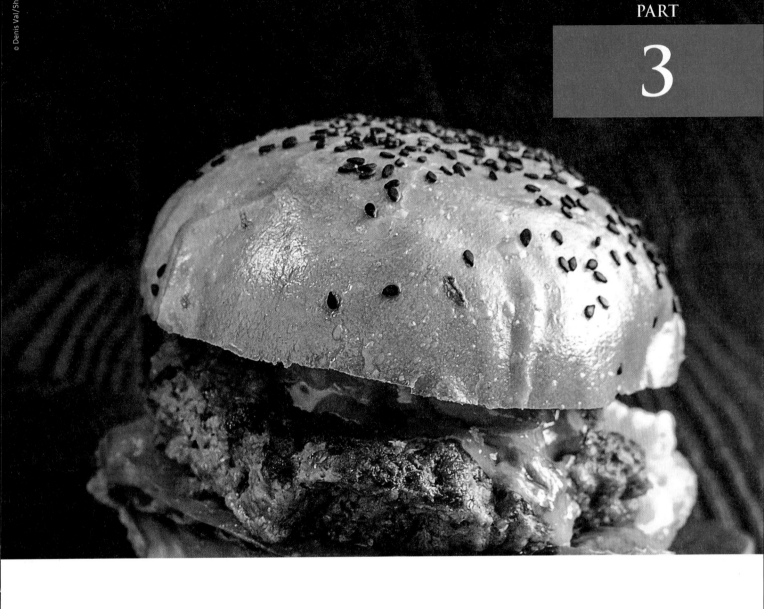

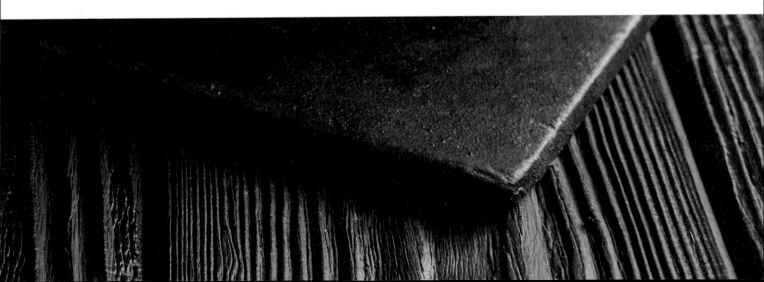

© Denis Val/Sh

Management and Leadership

© Denis Val/Shutterstock

Introduction to Management

LEARNING OUTCOMES

11.1 Describe management skills, functions, and roles.

11.2 Compare and contrast major approaches to management theory.

11.3 Communicate effectively.

11.4 Discuss how to motivate employees.

11.5 Identify effective decision-making techniques.

INTRODUCTION

Hourly employees in a foodservice, such as servers or cooks, come to work each day to complete specific tasks. They often make routine decisions during the work day, but will likely ask a manager if they have any serious questions or encounter unforeseen situations. What makes a management position different from an hourly position is that the **manager** oversees and coordinates the work activities of others to ensure that organizational goals and objectives are being achieved efficiently and effectively.

Efficient managers get the maximum output of goods or services from the smallest amount of inputs. In the foodservice systems model, inputs include people, food and supplies, facilities, money, information, and technology. In management, we like to call inputs **resources** and often split them up into similar groups as follows.

- Human resources: People, meaning their knowledge, skills, and experience, are an organization's most valuable asset.
- Financial resources: Every organization needs money to operate. The size of a manager's budget is very important. In a foodservice, money pays for the human resources as well as food, supplies, equipment, etc.
- Physical resources: For a foodservice, physical resources include the facilities, equipment, food, and supplies.
- Intangible resources: This category includes resources such as information and technology.

When managers do things right, they are being efficient and not wasting resources. For instance, a production manager keeps an eye on menu items that are overproduced and takes steps to reduce overproduction and waste and to recycle overproduced items.

Whereas an efficient manager does things right, an **effective manager** does the right things—meaning that the manager chooses appropriate goals and activities to make a business successful. Effectiveness looks at a business' goals and objectives, including how appropriate they are and the degree to which the business achieves them. For instance, McDonald's decided in 2015 to serve breakfast all day to increase sales, which turned out to be very successful. Unfortunately, during the COVID-19 pandemic in 2020, McDonald's pulled this program back in order to simplify restaurant operations and speed up the drive-through.

You can't discuss management in organizations without mentioning organizational culture. **Organizational culture** encompasses the values, practices, and expectations that guide the actions of managers and employees in an organization or business. Culture is created through behaviors such as how a manager handles an employee who is underperforming. Successful organizational cultures encourage listening to others, learning and growing, living by company values such as service, recognizing team members for achievements such as excellent performance, encouraging strong connections among team members, and personalizing the employee experience.

This chapter will discuss many aspects of being a manager, from skills and functions to roles. In addition, some especially important management skills are discussed including how to communicate and motivate others, and make decisions.

11.1 DESCRIBE MANAGEMENT SKILLS, FUNCTIONS, AND ROLES

This section will describe the skills managers need as well as the traditional functions they perform, including planning, organizing, controlling, and leading. Because managerial work is very dynamic, different roles played by managers will also be described. Lastly, levels of management are explained.

SKILLS

Management skills can be separated into three categories: technical, human or interpersonal, and conceptual.

- **Technical skills** are the job-specific knowledge, methods, and techniques needed to perform tasks. For instance, a foodservice manager overseeing a dining room needs to know the menu as well as understand the tasks performed by the servers, host/hostess, and bussers. Because this manager supervises the work of hourly employees who serve customers, they are known as a **first-line managers** or **supervisors**. First-line managers need to have knowledge of the technical skills of the employees who report to them. These types of technical skills are more important for first-line managers than managers with higher level positions. Managers also need general technical skills such as how to use technology, complete written reports (such as production sheets or financial statements), and determine if food is safe to serve.
- To be effective, **human or interpersonal skills** are vital at all management levels. Human or interpersonal skills look at how well someone relates to and understands other people, both one-on-one and in groups. Communication and motivational skills are examples. Buckingham (2005, p. 72) describes here why interpersonal skills are so important.

  "There is one quality that sets truly great managers apart from the rest: they discover what is unique about each person and then capitalize on it....Great managers know and value the unique abilities and even the eccentricities of their employees, and they learn how best to integrate them into a coordinated plan of attack."

Key to human skills is **emotional intelligence**—meaning being aware of how your emotions drive your behavior and impact other people, as well as managing those emotions. Emotional intelligence not only includes self-awareness and self-management but it also includes your ability to sense how others are feeling and to handle the emotions of others.

- **Conceptual skills** help managers better understand complex and abstract situations to analyze a problem and develop a creative solution. Managers with good conceptual skills think about the "big picture" and understand how different parts of an organization work together so they can analyze situations, draw connections, anticipate problems, and think creatively. Examples of conceptual skills include long-range planning, problem-solving, and decision making.

Whereas lower-level managers use more technical skills, and upper-level managers use more conceptual skills, all levels need good interpersonal skills.

FUNCTIONS

So, what does a manager do? Managers share certain functions or processes in which they are involved: planning, organizing, controlling, and leading (**Figure 11-1**).

- **Planning** involves identifying and selecting appropriate **goals** (a desired outcome such as increased sales) and choosing **strategies** (a course of action) to achieve them. An example of a goal would be to increase sales, and two strategies to achieve this goal could be to utilize social media and offer online ordering. By having goals and strategies, managers and employees have a sense of direction and can pull in the same direction. Other benefits of planning are that good plans can build commitment for the goals and make managers more invested in, and accountable for reaching those goals.
- **Organizing** refers to structuring and coordinating the work of a business into tasks, jobs, and departments to accomplish the business' goals and objectives.

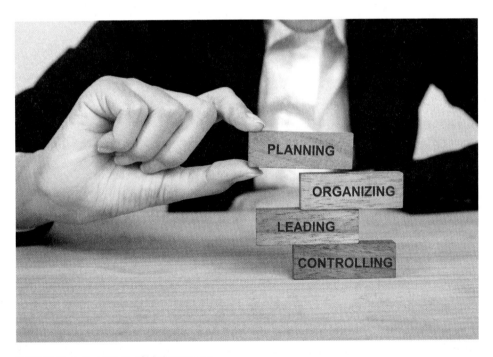

FIGURE 11-1 Functions of Management

© Penguiin/Shutterstock

Organizing also involves allocating and coordinating resources such as salaries, space, and equipment. Organization is seen in the formal lines of authority and relationships among individuals, groups, and departments, in an organizational chart.

- **Controlling** is a process that involves monitoring employees and the department, products being made, and services being delivered, as well as keeping an eye on food costs, sales, and other important indicators. Monitoring is important as it enables you to measure performance and progress against standards (such as servers greeting customers within three minutes of being seated) and organization goals (such as decreasing food cost by 5%). When needed, corrective actions are taken. Organizational goals and standards are also reviewed regularly.
- **Leading** is a process by which managers use motivation and other skills to guide and influence the actions of others to accomplish the business' goals and objectives. When managers motivate subordinates, influence how teams are working, or actively listen to concerns from a group of employees, they are leading. In theory, as a manager, you have **formal authority** over your subordinates—meaning the right to give directions. However, **real authority** is conferred or granted by the subordinates, and you have to earn the right to lead them, in large part by developing trust and positive relationships.

ROLES

Up to this point, you probably think that everything a manager does is related to planning, organizing, controlling, or leading. After observing how managers spent their time, Mintzberg (1973) took a different look at management and described 10 roles that managers perform. The 10 roles fall under three overarching categories.

1. Interpersonal: Many management functions involve using interpersonal skills.
2. Informational: The manager not only processes incoming information but also communicates key information to others.
3. Decisional: Formal authority gives the manager a major role in using conceptual skills to make plans and decisions.

You can think of the 10 roles (**Table 11-1**) as different hats that a manager wears.

LEVELS OF MANAGEMENT

The foodservice industry includes single-unit independent restaurants, chain restaurants, noncommercial foodservices in settings such as universities, and foodservice contract companies. Large businesses, such as multiunit foodservices, often have three levels of management from the top down: the corporate level, the division or business level, and the operational level (**Figure 11-2**). The *corporate level* includes top (upper) management personnel who work in areas such as finance, supply chain, sales and marketing, technology, operations, menu development, human resource management, and corporate communications. Below the corporate level, a large foodservice company is often broken down into *divisions or business units*. For example, Dunkin', which owns the Dunkin' and Baskin Robbins brands, includes divisions such as Dunkin' (U.S. and Canada), Baskin Robbins (U.S. and Canada), and an International Division. Other chain restaurants with both company-owned stores and franchised stores have divisions for each store type. A foodservice contract company has divisions such as Healthcare, Education, and Business and Industry to reflect their different clients. Each division has its own management team. The lowest level of management is the *operational (or functional) level*, which is where you find the actual foodservice(s) and the functional departments such as purchasing, production, and customer service.

Table 11-1 Managerial Roles Identified by Mintzberg		
Type of Role	**Specific Role**	**Description**
Interpersonal	Figurehead	Represents the department/unit/organization in key events/situations.
	Leader	Motivates and encourages employees to reach goals. Exercises formal authority.
	Liaison	Makes contacts and interacts outside of the chain of command or outside of the organization to gain information, etc.
Informational	Monitor	Scans the environment and talks to others to get information.
	Disseminator	Gives information to employees and others, such as about changes or the business' vision/goals.
	Spokesperson	Gives information to people outside of the business, such as launching a new marketing program.
Decisional	Entrepreneur	Develops innovative ideas such as new goods/services.
	Disturbance handler	Takes action during disputes or unexpected problems.
	Resource allocator	Allocates resources such as money and work space.
	Negotiator	Works within and outside of the business to gain agreements/commitments.

Data from Mintzberg, H. (1973). *The Nature of Managerial Work.* New York: Harper & Row.

Within a single-unit foodservice, there are not as many levels of management. The General Manager oversees and is responsible for the foodservice, so they represent upper management. In small to medium foodservices, there is often a manager in charge of the dining areas and also a manager in charge of the back-of-the-house, and they each report to the General Manager. The hourly employees generally report directly to the manager in charge of the dining room or the kitchen. Therefore, there are just two levels of managers.

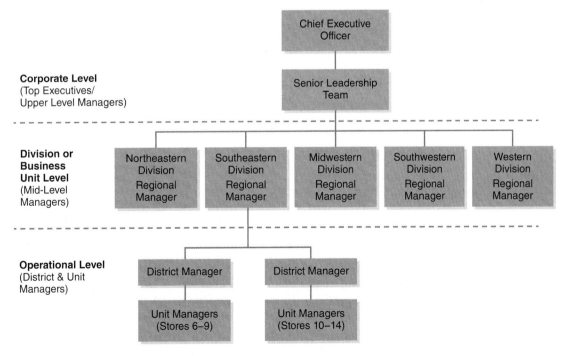

FIGURE 11-2 Levels of Management in a Multiunit Foodservice

In larger foodservices, there may be three levels of managers with the General Manager again at the top. Therefore, the managers reporting to the General Manager would be considered middle management and the managers who report to them would be first-line managers who supervise the hourly employees.

11.2 COMPARE AND CONTRAST MAJOR APPROACHES TO MANAGEMENT THEORY

Management has been practiced for many centuries. Since the early 1900s, there have been different approaches to management theory, each influenced by key researchers and what was happening in history at that time. **A management theory** is a collection of ideas explaining how a manager should act, such as how to motivate employees or implement plans that help accomplish the organization's objectives. We will look at some major approaches to management theory that start in the early 1900s and progress up to present times.

CLASSICAL APPROACHES

The first studies of management, often called the classical approach, focused on jobs and how workers could do their jobs efficiently. The classical approach also looked at the functions that all managers should be doing. In the early twentieth century, when writings on management began to take shape, the work of Frederick Taylor and Frank and Lillian Gilbreth focused on getting tasks done as efficiently as possible. Their work was done at a time when labor was in short supply. They founded the **scientific management school**, which used such procedures as time-and-motion studies to determine the most efficient way to perform a task. They also redesigned jobs, created performance standards, and selected and trained workers to perform the tasks. Taylor and the Gilbreths realized good results: higher productivity and earnings and less worker exhaustion.

While scientific management looked at how to increase worker efficiency, **administrative management theory** focused more on what managers do. Henri Fayol, a French management theorist known as the "father of modern management theory," was another key figure in the classical school of management. Fayol (1841–1925) distinguished between activities related to operations and activities related to management. He had first-hand knowledge of operations and management because he managed a mining company in France. Fayol identified five functions of management that are still used today: planning, organizing, coordinating, controlling, and commanding (to be known later as leading). He also developed 14 principles of management shown in **Table 11–2**.

Another contributor to administrative management theory was Max Weber (1864–1920), a German sociologist. At a time when the number of large businesses was growing, Weber developed an ideal type of organization called a **bureaucracy** with the following characteristics (some were also discussed by Fayol).

- A hierarchy of positions with a clear chain of command.
- A clear division of labor with jobs broken down into well-defined tasks.
- Formal rules that everyone in the organization follows, along with standard operating procedures and norms.
- A clear set of goals that everyone works toward.
- Hiring the best-qualified candidates and promoting based on qualifications.
- Job performance judged by productivity.

The aim of bureaucracy was for employees to be treated fairly in a transparent environment. Although many businesses today incorporate some aspects of a bureaucracy,

Table 11-2 Fayol's 14 Principles of Management
1. <u>Division of work</u>. Divide work up so each employee has a relatively specialized job, so they become more skilled and efficient, as well as less bored.
2. <u>Authority</u>. Managers have the authority to give orders to their subordinates and make sure the orders are completed.
3. <u>Discipline</u>. Managers must maintain discipline among employees while acting fairly.
4. <u>Unity of command</u>. One employee should receive orders from only one superior.
5. <u>Unity of direction</u>. The organization should have a single plan of action that directs and guides everyone, such as with respect to using organizational resources.
6. <u>Subordination of individual interests to the common interest</u>. The best interests of the organization take precedence over individual interests.
7. <u>Remuneration</u>. Employees should receive fair pay for their services.
8. <u>Centralization</u>. Authority should not be completely centralized at the top of the chain of command. Employees can be involved in making decisions.
9. <u>Scalar chain</u>. Each employee should know their place in the organization and address questions or concern with their immediate supervisor.
10. <u>Order</u>. Positions should be arranged within the organization to provide the greatest benefit to the organization and also give employees possible career opportunities.
11. <u>Equity</u>. Employees should be treated fairly and with respect by their superior.
12. <u>Stability of tenure of personnel</u>. Employees who stay for many years in important and positions must be filled quickly once they are vacant.
13. <u>Initiative</u>. Supervisors should encourage employees to take initiative and act on their own without supervisory direction.
14. <u>Esprit de corp</u>. Managers should promote a sense of unity or team spirit.

Data from Fayol. H. (1984). *General and Industrial Management*. New York: IEEE Press.

the environment in which businesses work is constantly changing and fast-moving, so greater flexibility is needed. Opportunities for employees to take on more responsibility, work in teams, and be more creative is also more important nowadays.

BEHAVIORAL APPROACH

Instead of looking at the workers' efficiency and how managers should manage, the behavioral approach puts the focus squarely on people, specifically how managers can work with people to get things done. The behavioral approach was the early beginning of the field of **organizational behavior (OB)**: the study of how people act and behave in the organizational setting. The goals of organizational behavior are to understand, explain, and influence behavior. When managers can influence others, they have the potential to improve job performance, job satisfaction, customer service, and more.

Contributors to the behavioral approach included Mary Parker Follett, Elton Mayo, and Douglas McGregor. Mary Parker Follett (1868–1933) would have preferred that Frederick Taylor focused more on people and groups than doing time-and-motion studies. She felt employees were capable of determining the best, most efficient way to accomplish tasks and that supervisors should act more like coaches. Follett also thought that managers with more knowledge and expertise should do more leading regardless of other managers' formal authority. She also believed in resolving conflicts so the resolution was a win–win for each party, rather than win–lose. At that time, her approach was considered to be quite radical; however, she clearly influenced modern management theory.

Probably the most well-known behavioral study was the Hawthorne study, which took place at Western Electric Company in Illinois from 1924 to 1932. Engineers did a research study on the level of lighting under which employees performed their tasks. The engineers wanted to measure productivity at different levels of lighting, hypothesizing that more light would mean more productivity. The results were very intriguing—productivity increased whether the lighting increased or decreased (except when it became too dark to see).

To help determine what was going on, Elton Mayo, a Harvard psychologist, worked with the researchers to do another set of experiments that also looked at how aspects of the work environment, such as the length of breaks, affected job performance and fatigue. Again, they saw productivity increase even under circumstances when that would not be likely. The researchers concluded that because workers were given a lot of attention during these studies and the workers interacted a lot with the researchers (who acted more like managers), it improved productivity and morale. What is now called the **Hawthorne effect** is the experience in which performance of employees is influenced by the people they are working with—including fellow employees, groups, and managers. Employees performed better when they felt managers cared about their workplace and gave them a chance to be heard. Mayo's research helped put emphasis on how groups of employees affect both individual behavior and output. For example, many employees resisted incentive pay if they felt that producing more would negatively affect their relationships with fellow employees when those relationships were important and satisfying.

Douglas McGregor elaborated on the contrasting beliefs of the scientific management and the behavioral approach in his own work, published in 1960, which he called Theory X and Theory Y. Each theory explains basic assumptions of human nature that managers hold about the way employees view work and also about how they can be motivated. **Theory X managers** hold that the average employee is lazy and will work as little as possible. Therefore, employees need to be closely supervised and controlled through work rules (including rewards and punishments). In contrast, **Theory Y managers** hold that employees are motivated (not inherently lazy) and will contribute to the organization when trusted and empowered, such as having appropriate resources and opportunities to exercise self-direction. Theory Y managers offer support and advice to employees, while Theory X managers offer rules, standard operating procedures, rewards, and punishments. McGregor felt Theory Y was not the answer to a manager's problems but can be the basis for improved management and organizational performance.

Today, the behavioral approach is used in organizations and more research is being done, although we now prefer to call it the behavioral science approach. The behavioral science approach involves a number of disciplines, including psychology, sociology, economics, and organizational behavior. According to Robbins and Coulter (2018, p. 37), "The behavioral approach has largely shaped how today's organizations are managed. Much of what the early organizational behavior (OB) advocates proposed and the conclusions from the Hawthorne Studies have provided the foundation for our current theories of motivation, leadership, group behavior and development."

The behavioral science approach is useful to help engage employees. Engaged employees look forward to going to work every day and are committed to their job and workplace. Gallup has regularly tracked the number of "engaged" employees in the United States since 2000. The percentage of engaged employees was at its highest in March of 2020—at 38%. Unfortunately, once the COVID-19 epidemic hit, the number fell to 31% in June of 2020 (Harter, 2020). In any case, even at 38%, the number of engaged employees in the United States is not stellar, especially when you consider that employee engagement is directly related to an organization's performance.

QUANTITATIVE APPROACH

The quantitative approach to management uses quantitative techniques (such as statistics, computer modeling, or queuing theory) to help managers solve problems, make decisions, and use resources wisely. Also called the management science approach, the quantitative approach emerged from statistical and mathematical techniques used during

World War II to solve military problems. After the war (late 1940s to 1950s), businesses started to use quantitative techniques in several areas.

- Operations management works to convert inputs into goods and services as efficiently as possible, as well as improve goods and services.
- Operations research uses analytical methods to transform data into insights to make better decisions. It emphasizes mathematical model building, employed nowadays to develop algorithms used by businesses to promote products and understand consumers.
- Management information systems (MIS) provide internal and external data for businesses. Whereas **data** are unorganized facts and numbers, **information** are data that have been organized and can be used to do a job or make decisions. MIS transforms data into information that is usable and timely.
- Total quality management (TQM) is a management philosophy that focuses on responding to customer needs and expectations while continuously examining and improving organizational processes and empowering employees. TQM examines work processes to make improvements and uses accurate measurements and statistical techniques to measure process performance.

CONTEMPORARY APPROACHES

Two contemporary approaches to management theory will be discussed here, including the open-systems approach and the contingency approach. Up to this point, most approaches looked inside an organization. In the 1960s, management researchers expanded their view to look outside of the organization and investigate the environment in which the organization functioned.

Systems theory is one of the contemporary approaches to management. Systems theory was originally developed in the sciences, and then researchers started to apply it to organizations in the 1960s. An organization is an example of an **open system**, meaning that it interacts with the environment outside of the organization. An open system receives various inputs and transforms them in different ways to generate outputs. Inputs, transformation, and outputs are the major parts of the system. In the foodservice industry, inputs include, for example, people, materials (such as food), and facilities. The work of an organization is transformation—meaning using the inputs to create the outputs. In foodservice, the operations and management subsystems are used to transform inputs to outputs, such as quality meals (tangible) and customer satisfaction (intangible).

In an open system, the boundary between the organization and its environment is considered permeable, meaning that information, raw materials, products, services, and more can flow freely to and from the environment. Organizations certainly can't respond to everything going on in the environment, but a foodservice company would certainly want to pay attention to regulatory agencies, competitors, suppliers, customers, and labor availability, as examples.

Researchers are interested in how the inputs are converted to outputs and how the various parts of the system work together. Are they efficient? Are they effective? Is there synergy? When an open system is steadily transforming inputs into outputs and responding to feedback from internal and external environments, it is said to be in a state of dynamic equilibrium. Management is in charge of maintaining balance while reacting to changes and forces in the internal and external environments. Over time, organizations do change and evolve.

Contingency theory was developed in the 1960s. According to contingency theory, each organization needs to manage and organize itself differently and this depends on the external environment and technology. A number of researchers have discussed key characteristics of two organizational forms: **mechanistic (bureaucratic)** or **organic** (Burns & Stalker, 1994; Lawrence & Lorsch, 1967b; Morand, 1995). Most organizations are somewhere on the continuum between mechanistic and organic and lean more toward one or the other (**Table 11-3**).

Table 11-3 Continuum from Mechanistic to Organic Organizations	
Mechanistic ◄————————————————► Organic	
Rigid departmentalization	Loose organizational structure
More specialized jobs	More broadly defined jobs
Tall, strict chain of command	Short chain of command
Narrow span of management	Wide span of management
Centralized authority	Decentralized authority
Many management levels (tall organization)	Fewer management levels (flat)

The characteristics of mechanistic organizations are best for companies operating in a fairly stable environment in which each day has a steady routine and well-defined tasks, such as foodservice operations. The flexibility of **organic organizations** works best in uncertain environments so that they can stay open and respond to environmental changes. When trying to innovate, the looser structure and free-flowing information of a more organic organization works well. For an example of an organic company, consider the technology companies like Apple or Google. These companies tend to have fewer levels of management and employees often work in teams that have quite a bit of authority. Many of the jobs are more professional (and creative) than those found in bureaucratic companies and the employees are expected to act professionally and handle diverse types of problems. The employees don't need a lot of rules or supervision, so a manager can have quite a large number of subordinates (wide span of management).

11.3 COMMUNICATE EFFECTIVELY

Within a foodservice organization, **communication** is the act of transmitting information, ideas, and meaning through various channels and is the cornerstone of any organization's success. Communication takes places between individuals, within groups, and within the entire organization, as well as up, down, and across the organizational chart. Communication is vital to planning, organizing, controlling, and (especially) leading, and benefits both employees and customers.

THE COMMUNICATION PROCESS AND CHANNELS

Even in its simplest form, communication is a two-way process in which several things typically happen.

1. The person who initiates the communication (the sender) must decide on the contents of the message and the communication channel. The **communication channel** is the means by which a message is transmitted. The sender has a choice of oral, written, electronic, and/or nonverbal channels.
2. The sender transmits the message via the chosen communication channel(s).
3. The receiver listens or reads, interprets, and personalizes the message. In the case of oral communication, the receiver also attends to the nonverbal cues. The receiver decides whether to give **feedback** (information to clarify or verify a message) or transmit a new message.
4. When the receiver responds, they now become the sender.

During the communication process, the sender and receiver repeatedly change roles as the conversation goes on. At any point, there may be some **noise**, referring to anything that hinders the process such as a sender who speaks too fast or a receiver who isn't listening.

Verbal communication refers to messages composed of words that are either spoken (oral communication) or written. **Oral communication** includes face-to-face conversations, phone conversations, meetings, and presentations. Face-to-face conversations are thought to be the richest form of communication because both parties can take advantage of verbal and nonverbal communication. Along with phone conversations, face-to-face conversations are faster and more effective than email or texting. Examples of **written communication** include letters, memos, reports, newsletters, and posters. **Electronic communication** uses electronic media to transmit messages, such as texts; email; Skype, Zoom, or other videoconferencing software; or social networking sites such as Facebook, Twitter, LinkedIn, or YouTube. Some electronic communication is written and some is oral.

Nonverbal communication is the transfer of information using mostly body language and no words. Body language can be expressed through facial expressions (such as piercing eye contact or a frown), gestures (such as nodding the head or pointing at something), posture (such as leaning forward or crossing arms), and the way that words are said (such as urgently or loudly). Clothing and accessories also have significance and convey nonverbal clues about a person's age, background, and financial status. Nonverbal communication is only possible when the sender and receiver can see each other, so you don't have this advantage when talking on the telephone or using email. Examples of nonverbal cues are given in **Table 11-4**. Advantages of oral, written, electronic, and nonverbal channels are shown in **Table 11-5**.

Table 11-4 Nonverbal Cues

Indicators of . . .

Boredom	• Slouching in one's seat • Yawning • Staring out the window • Lack of eye contact • Neutral expression • Fidgeting • Closed posture • Drifting attention • Slowness to respond • Neutral or "flat" speech
Frustration	• Rubbing forehead with hand • Tense, worried expression • Throwing hands up in the air
Agreement, Enthusiasm	• Leaning toward the speaker • Making eye contact • Nodding head • Relaxed, open posture • Smiling or laughing • Faster speech • Higher pitch
Disagreement, Confusion	• Frowning • Shaking head • Leaning back or away • Pursing lips • Tightened jaw and closed posture • Staring elsewhere • Shallow, rapid breathing • Limited facial expression and hand gestures • Slower speech • Lower pitch

U.S. Department of Homeland Security (FEMA). 2014. *Effective Communication: Instructor Guide.* https://training.fema.gov/emiweb/is/is242b/instructor%20guide/ig_complete.pdf

Table 11-5 Advantages and Disadvantages of Different Communication Channels

Communication Channel	Advantages	Disadvantages
Oral	• Builds relationships • Immediate feedback • Includes nonverbal messages (except on telephone) • For meetings—gets message out to many and saves time	• Not always possible or practical • Can be time-consuming due to small talk
Written	• Can be well thought out and organized • Provides hard documentation	• Can be impersonal • No feedback—often, it's a one-way communication • More chance for misunderstanding
Electronic	• Fast • Efficient • Can reach a large or small audience	• Impersonal and does not provide a way to express emotion • Waiting for feedback/reply and delayed decisions • Does not include nonverbal component • Security/privacy issues • Because it is fast, sometimes a message is sent that needs to be recalled but usually cannot be taken back.
Nonverbal	• Can reinforce verbal message • Fast	• May contradict verbal message • Easily misinterpreted because nonverbals are vague, imprecise, and vary between cultures • Distortion of information

FUNCTIONS AND TYPES OF COMMUNICATION

Communication is a necessity. We communicate to accomplish many things, such as the following.

- Ask questions
- Express ideas, feelings, etc.
- Give information
- Give directions
- Persuade/influence
- Motivate
- Control
- Socialize

In an organization, **formal communication** among people occurs based on lines of authority set up in an organizational chart, such as a manager speaks to a subordinate. **Informal communication** occurs among people independent of their organizational relationship, level of authority, or job functions. One of the main forms of informal communication in an organization is more commonly known as the **grapevine**. Since the grapevine comes out of social interactions, it is as fickle and varied as the people involved. Features of the grapevine include its fast pace and unusual ability to get information from the most secret of places. Some managers would prefer to ignore or cut out the grapevine, neither of which is a wise idea. Managers can learn much from the grapevine, such as what employees are excited about, what they are griping about, and what the current rumors are (some may need to be addressed).

Formal communication can be either vertical or horizontal. **Vertical communication** goes either up or down the organization's chain of command. Upward vertical communication occurs when a subordinate speaks about something with his/her supervisor. An employee may, for example, discuss concerns or make suggestions. Effective upward communication moves up through levels of management to possibly solve a problem or address a concern. Many organizations have an **open-door policy**, which encourages employees to discuss matters of concern with their supervisor. An open-door policy is a good way to encourage upward communication, and it helps employees feel that management is listening.

Downward vertical communication such as when managers create policies and procedures and communicate them to lower-level employees, is often of an informative or directive nature. Downward communication helps to link the different levels of the organization together. Employee meetings and emails are frequently used to communicate decisions, changes, and other news. Feedback is another downward communication, such as when managers discuss performance.

Horizontal (or lateral) communication is when information flows among people at approximately the same level in an organization. As organizations become flatter (with fewer management levels), horizontal communication is more common. An example of horizontal communication is when a manager needs to consult with a human resources manager or when a management team includes managers from different departments. Organizations with a collaborative environment encourage lateral communication.

OBSTACLES TO GOOD COMMUNICATION

There are many reasons why managers fail to send messages effectively or receive messages correctly.

1. Poor communication channel chosen. An example of this problem can be seen when a manager uses email instead of face-to-face communication. Because of instant feedback and the ability to see nonverbal language, face-to-face communication helps reduce misunderstandings and is quite efficient. A sender should carefully consider which channel is best for their message.

2. Noise in the environment. Noise is anything in the environment that interferes with communication. Managers should plan oral communications in environments that are free from distractions. One of the biggest distractions in organizations are personal cell phones and the computer. Companies often have policies about using electronic devices while working.

3. Poor listening. Hearing what someone says is a sensory experience. We can hear something without choosing to listen. Listening is a voluntary activity that involves interpreting or processing. **Active listening** is being engaged and attentive to what the speaker is saying, including nonverbal messages. It is discussed in more depth in the next section.

4. Emotions and biases. Emotions and biases make it hard for you to be objective. For example, if you are unhappy or stressed, you are more likely to overreact to a situation or get defensive if someone offers you advice. If you have a bias against younger workers, such as their not wanting to work hard, that will definitely create problems when communicating with younger employees. By being aware of our own emotions and biases, we are more likely to stay objective.

5. Information overload. Information overload, especially via email, adds stress and interruptions, so it becomes harder to really focus on what is important (Hemp, 2009).

6. Mixed messages. Mixed messages occur when spoken words don't match the nonverbal cues. Mixed messages can occur when the speaker is not being sincere or is not committed to the message.

The next section will discuss skills to overcome these concerns.

ACTIVE LISTENING AND OTHER COMMUNICATION SKILLS

Good communication is many things: honest, accurate, timely, responsive, and empathetic. Listening is a very important communication skill. There are many roadblocks that keep us from really listening well. Sometimes, we hear only what we want to hear. At other times, we are tuning out because our biases, such as stereotyping, come into play or we are simply resistant to ideas and change.

Managers need to practice the skill of active listening by doing the following (**Figure 11-3**).

1. Look at the speaker and concentrate on the main ideas or points that they are talking about. Give your undivided attention (put down your phone).
2. Listen for feelings and look for nonverbal communication clues for additional clues about how they are feeling.
3. Don't make any judgments about the speaker or what they are saying. Be empathetic and understand how things look from the speaker's point of view.
4. Give the speaker some cues that you are really trying to listen, such as making eye contact and nodding your head.
5. Ask probing or open-ended questions at the appropriate time to clarify information. Focus each question on a single issue. Don't turn off to information that is new, difficult to understand, or complex.
6. Confirm if you are understanding the speaker with mirroring statements such as "Am I hearing that you feel it was unfair that Jamal got next week off as vacation and you didn't." You may also paraphrase or restate what the speaker has said.

Also react to the ideas, not the speaker.

The following are communication tips for _when managers **send** messages_.

1. <u>Think before you speak and send clear and complete messages</u>. In other words, plan your message. Consider factors such as who is going to receive the message, what the goal of the message is, and when the message should be sent. Then select the appropriate words. To send clear messages, avoid the use of **jargon** (special words or expressions used in a profession or group) if you are not sure that the audience will understand it.
2. <u>Choose an appropriate communication channel for the message</u>. Written communication is best for routine matters and impersonal messages. Messages that

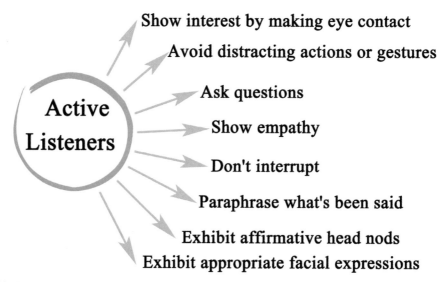

FIGURE 11-3 Active Listening Skills

© Arka38/Shutterstock

are more likely to be misunderstood or that will elicit questions should be delivered face-to-face. Exceptional news, such as meeting sales targets, or bad news, such as layoffs, should also be done face-to-face. If a matter needs an immediate response, don't use email. Instead, pick up the phone.

3. <u>When sharing information, make sure the information is accurate and hasn't been filtered</u>. **Filtering** is the withholding of information because the sender thinks the information is either not needed or the receiver doesn't want to receive it. Sometimes, managers filter the information they give because they don't have a lot of trust in someone or they are afraid of losing some of their own power. People also tend to filter bad news, especially when it is moving upward in an organization.

4. <u>Incorporate ways to get feedback in every message and check for understanding</u>. Don't assume that everyone understands what you have communicated. Encourage questions and answer any questions in a thoughtful and patient manner. You can also ask questions to see if the message got through accurately. For example, you can ask someone to paraphrase what you have said—meaning they will restate the message in their own words. In written communications, you can request comments and ideas, perhaps in a future meeting or in a follow-up using the phone.

5. <u>Avoid sending messages if you or the receiver are emotionally upset</u>. For a communication to be effective, both the sender and the receiver must be open to speaking and listening to each other. When upset, we are less likely to send a clear, effective message and will be more likely to ignore or distort information.

The following are communication tips for *when managers **receive** messages*.

1. <u>Be a good listener (as just discussed) and be empathetic</u>.
2. <u>Don't let someone's different linguistic style affect how you interpret messages</u>. **Linguistic style** refers to a person's characteristic speaking pattern. For example, a person's accent is part of their linguistic style. Your linguistic style can vary by gender, geographic region, country, or culture.
3. <u>Don't jump to any conclusions</u> until you have heard the entire message, discussed it, and evaluated it.
4. <u>As the receiver, pick an appropriate response style</u> (Lussier, 2019).
   a. Advise: Advising responses are often given to subordinates who need direction or evaluation of a situation. Often, the employee can be asked to give input on the situation.
   b. Probe: Probing responses, often questions, ask for more information or clarification.
   c. Reassure: Sometimes you need to reassure someone and give them the confidence to do something.
   d. Reflect: Reflective statements assure the speaker that you are understanding them.
   e. Divert: Sometimes you need to switch to a new message and change the subject.

Table 11-6 gives basic communication tips.

CROSS-CULTURAL COMMUNICATION

Culture is a shared system of meanings that drives how we act and what we value. Culture influences how you view and relate to others, including how you communicate and even something as simple as how close you stand to others when talking. Some cultures rely mostly on words for communication; whereas other cultures convey messages mostly through nonverbal cues such as body language. Just think about how the following cultural factors can complicate communication: the use of slang,

Table 11-6 Basic Communication Tips

Speaking	• Think before you speak. • Make your messages clear, accurate, and complete. • Speak loud enough to be heard. • Speak clearly. • Don't speak too fast and slow down for important points. • Vary the pace of your speech. • Pause from time to time to encourage others to speak up.
Listening	• Show interest. Pay attention. • Give a nonverbal cue that you are listening such as nod your head. • Listen for the central themes. • Be empathetic. • Consider the speaker's nonverbal behaviors. • Don't start formulating a rebuttal. Hear the person out before making a decision or judgment. • Be aware of your own emotions and biases. • When appropriate, use probing questions for more specific information, open-ended questions for general feedback, and mirroring statements or paraphrasing to increase understanding and connect with the speaker. • Acknowledge responses in a positive manner.
Nonverbal Communication	• Maintain eye contact. If there is a group, continually scan the group with your eyes. • Position your body so you face the person(s) you are talking to and you are not too far away. • Stand or sit with good posture. • Smile and relax. • Use natural gestures that are not seen as judgmental or negative.
Writing Emails	• Do not use emails for matters that will need clarification or personal matters. • Use a professional greeting and a clear subject line. • Don't overuse emojis or exclamation points. • Only use abbreviations or jargon that is commonly understood. • Be careful with humor, which often goes over better when spoken. • Don't rush to press the send button. You may have incorrect or incomplete information or you may be sending an angry email that you will regret later. • Always proofread your emails before sending. • Include a signature block with your full name, title, company name, and contact information. • Sign off on your emails. • Think twice before hitting "Reply All."

euphemisms (such as "let you go" meaning to fire someone), humor, and choice of topics for small talk. American businesspeople tend to discuss neutral topics such as sports or weather while other cultures talk about religion or politics.

To communicate effectively with people from other cultures, you can do the following.

- Learn the customs of different cultures. For example, learn the cultural rules about touching and how far away to stand when you are talking.
- Respect personal space.
- Pay attention to body movements and body language.
- Be an active listener.
- Avoid slang, jargon, and euphemisms.
- Summarize points to check on agreement and understanding.
- Note that a "yes" response does not necessarily indicate that someone has understood.
- Deliver feedback in an appropriate manner.
- Be supportive and encouraging toward anyone who speaks English as a second language.

11.4 DISCUSS HOW TO MOTIVATE EMPLOYEES

Motivation is a force inside us, such as needs, that energizes us to engage in persistent goal-directed behavior. Motivation is not a trait, and what motivates one person may not motivate another person. Even your own motivation level changes from situation to situation. In the workplace, motivating high levels of employee performance is important.

At work, we may be motivated by a reward of getting a pay raise, bonus, or simply being recognized. These are examples of **extrinsic motivation**. It is called extrinsic because the reward is external to the work itself. On the other hand, **intrinsic motivation** is when you do something because it is internally satisfying and you enjoy it. Intrinsic rewards at work could be feeling competent, using your own judgment to accomplish your work, progressing in the right direction, or having an overall sense that your work is meaningful. When employees are able to make decisions about their work, many are intrinsically motivated to perform well.

When speaking about motivation, it is important to also explain the concept of attitudes and job satisfaction. **Attitudes** are a learned tendency to evaluate people, situations, etc., in a positive or negative manner. Attitudes are important because they affect behavior, such as when a server with a negative attitude is hasty and inattentive with customers. Attitudes are not permanent—they can change. Perhaps your attitude toward a new employee at work became more positive as you got to know each other. Attitude is important because it can affect how well you perform at work and influence the performance of the people you work with. When a group of employees has mostly positive attitudes, it is easier to work together and get work done. Likewise, a manager with a positive attitude who encourages open communication and makes employees feel appreciated helps employees to be productive.

Job satisfaction is your attitude toward your job, meaning the degree to which you feel positive or negative about work. The following are examples of factors that may affect your job satisfaction.

1. Safety, health, and physical conditions of workplace
2. Relations with co-workers
3. Reasonable/unreasonable workload
4. On-the-job stress
5. Utilization of your skills and talents
6. Frequency and quality of feedback from the supervisor
7. Level of support from the supervisor
8. Recognition given
9. Fairness of performance evaluation and pay raises
10. Flexibility of hours
11. Training available
12. Communication and collaboration within the organization
13. Feeling valued
14. Chances for a promotion
15. Respect for senior leaders
16. Salary
17. Benefits (including paid time off)
18. Job security

Keep in mind that no one is 100% satisfied with their job—there are always going to be some aspects that are seen as undesirable yet job satisfaction can still be high.

Employees with positive attitudes and higher job satisfaction are more likely to perform well, be engaged in their work, and exhibit organizational citizenship behaviors. **Organizational citizenship behaviors** are seen when someone takes an action that goes beyond the call of duty. For example, a foodservice manager is starting to close up the kitchen at the end of the night when a regular customer comes in and needs to pick up several meals. Instead of saying the kitchen is closed, the manager prepares the food for the customer and winds up staying an hour late, for which he will not get any compensation. On the other hand, employees with low job satisfaction are more likely to disrupt the workplace with behaviors such as calling in sick frequently, taking shortcuts, sabotaging efforts, instigating conflict and confusion among employees, or stealing.

EARLY THEORIES OF MOTIVATION

The foundation for today's theories of motivation came from early theories such as Maslow's Hierarchy of Needs theory. These early theories are referred to as needs theories because early researchers focused on understanding what people need. Early theories had simple approaches to the relatively uncomplicated work environment of the time, but contemporary theories are more complex due to today's more complicated workplace.

In the 1940s, Abraham Maslow developed what he called a **Hierarchy of Needs Theory** (**Figure 11-4**), in which people are motivated by five types of needs: physiological, safety, social or belonging, esteem needs, and self-actualization. Maslow felt the lower needs, such as physiological and safety, must be satisfied before the higher needs become active sources of motivation. Examples of these needs are as follows.

1. Physiological: food, water, and shelter.
2. Safety: physical safety, security from harm, psychological/emotional safety.
3. Social or belonging: social acceptance, friendship, belongingness, affection.
4. Esteem: status, recognition, self-respect, achievement.
5. Self-actualization: growth, self-fulfillment, self-realization, achievement.

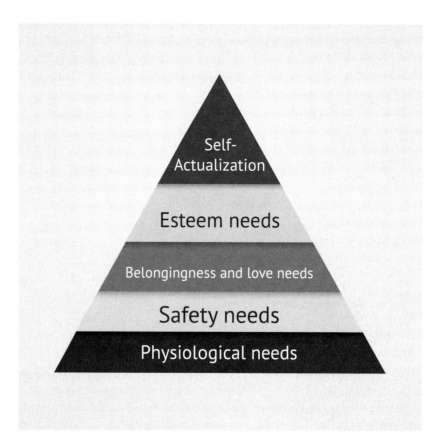

FIGURE 11-4 Maslow's Hierarchy of Needs

© Voin_Sveta/Shutterstock

Self-actualization can be described as a need to realize one's own potential. The need for self-actualization can never be fully satisfied, as there are always new challenges and opportunities for growth.

To use this theory, you need to understand which level an employee is at so you can focus on satisfying needs at or above that level. For example, for an employee who has their physiological and safety needs met, you can focus on meeting some social needs by having them participate on a work team or being involved in company-sponsored after-hours events. Despite little research supporting Maslow's theory, it was popular during the 1960s and 1970s, in part because it was easy to understand and makes some sense. Another short-coming of the theory is that it is only applicable to the American culture.

In the 1950s and 1960s, Frederick Herzberg developed what he called a **two-factor theory**, also called the motivation-hygiene theory. His theory separated factors that increase motivation, referred to as satisfiers or motivators, from those whose absence leads to job dissatisfaction, referred to as hygiene factors (**Figure 11-5**). Hygiene factors, such as salary and working conditions, do not themselves motivate employees but without them, employees are likely to be dissatisfied. Motivators include, for instance, achievement, growth, and work itself, and managers can use these to engage employees and increase job satisfaction. When comparing the hygiene factors to the motivators, it is clear that hygiene factors are extrinsic motivators and deal with job context, while motivators are intrinsic motivators and deal more with job content.

In his 1961 book, "The Achieving Society," David McClelland built on the work of Maslow and developed a motivational theory known as the **three-needs theory**. The theory identifies three needs that are learned—they are not innate.

1. Need for achievement: the drive to set and meet challenging goals, to excel.
2. Need for affiliation: the need to belong to a group and have friendly, interpersonal relationships and camaraderie.
3. Need for power: the need to influence others.

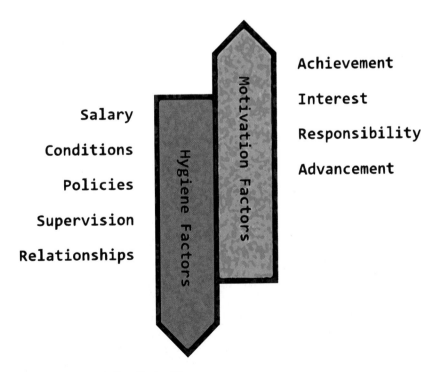

Salary
Conditions
Policies
Supervision
Relationships

Hygiene Factors

Motivation Factors

Achievement
Interest
Responsibility
Advancement

FIGURE 11-5 Herzberg's Two Factor Theory

© Badproject/Shutterstock

The need for power can either be a need for personal power, in which an individual wants to influence others for personal gain, or a need for institutional power, in which an individual wants to influence others for the good of an organization.

McClelland investigated and wrote in depth about the need for achievement. From his research came a profile of the characteristics of the high achiever.

- Wants to do something better or more efficiently.
- Wants to be personally responsible for a task/job.
- Takes on moderate challenges and risks.
- Wants to receive immediate feedback to be able to improve.
- Feels satisfied with accomplishment itself—no need for external rewards.

Indeed, McClelland's research showed that employees can learn to achieve if they are put in a situation in which they are asked to take a moderate risk, be personally responsible, and are able to receive regular feedback (Miron & McClelland, 1979).

Contemporary Theories of Motivation

This section will discuss more contemporary theories. In contrast to the earlier theories, these are all supported by research. In this section, we will look at goal setting theory, expectancy theory, equity theory, and reinforcement theory.

In the 1960s, research that became known as **goal setting theory** by Edwin Locke updated our knowledge of how goal setting can positively affect performance at work. Along with Gary Latham, Locke showed that working toward a clear goal (along with getting appropriate feedback) is a major source of motivation and motivated employees perform better. The following is their guidance on setting and meeting goals to increase motivation and commitment (Locke & Latham, 2002).

1. Set clear and specific goals that are well-defined.
2. Set challenging goals that are difficult to achieve but not too difficult or too easy. Make sure the work isn't too complex or overwhelming.
3. Give employees frequent feedback on how they are doing so they can make corrections when needed.

As a manager, it is important to either set goals for employees or involve them in setting their own goals. For many employees, being involved in setting goals gets them to buy into and achieve the goal.

Locke and Latham's research confirms the usefulness of SMART goal setting in improving performance. SMART objectives are specific, measurable, achievable, realistic, and time-bound (**Figure 11-6**). By making each objective specific rather than vague, everyone will be clear about what needs to be accomplished. Next, each objective must be able to be measured and have a deadline so that the people involved in achieving it are accountable and more likely to work hard. Lastly, each objective should be attainable and realistic. As already mentioned, employees perform better when the objective has some difficulty but is attainable than when the objective is too difficult or too easy.

According to Victor Vroom's **expectancy theory** (1964), motivation to behave or perform in a certain way is a function of three factors: expectancy, instrumentality, and valence (**Figure 11-7**). Vroom said that in order for a reward (or other desired outcome) to work, employees first have to believe that an increase in effort will result in a high level of performance (expectancy). Second, employees have to believe that a higher level of performance will be noted and rewarded (instrumentality). Lastly, employees have to actually want the reward that is being promised (valence). Whether a certain reward or outcome is desirable enough to motivate someone will vary from individual to individual. If expectancy, instrumentality, or valence is low, motivation is also likely to be low.

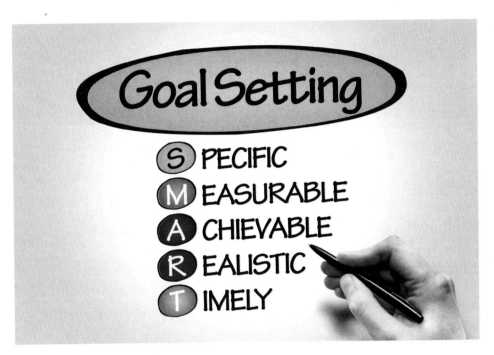

FIGURE 11-6 SMART Goal Setting

© Dizain/Shutterstock

Another contemporary motivational theory is known as **equity theory**. In the early 1960s, behavioral psychologist J. Stacey Adams suggested that employees compare what they give to an organization (inputs such as time, effort, experience, etc.) against what they receive (outputs such as pay, status, recognition, etc.), and then compare their outputs/inputs with others in the organization (**Figure 11–8**).

If an employee feels that their output-to-input ratio is similar to employees in comparable positions, there is no problem and no effect on motivation. However, if an employee finds that a coworker with similar experience and effort earns a higher salary or gets more recognition, that employee will feel that something is not fair, in other words—an inequity. Equity theory is obviously based on the concept of fairness and how the employee perceives their outputs/inputs (which may or may not be viewed accurately). We are all sensitive to being treated fairly, and not being treated fairly at work is a common experience for many, such as minorities and women. When inequities occur, employees may take actions such as to call in sick, perform at

Expectancy Theory

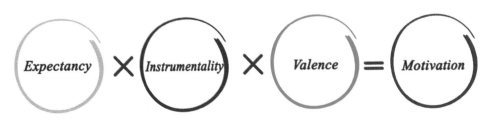

FIGURE 11-7 Expectancy Theory

© Arka38/Shutterstock

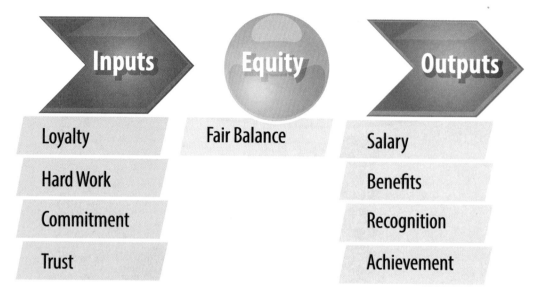

FIGURE 11-8 Equity Theory

© Kheng Guan Toh/Shutterstock

less-productive levels, or find another job. Equity theory shows managers the importance of being fair (no playing favorites), equitable (especially with outputs such as pay, rewards, and recognition), and transparent.

The final theory, called **reinforcement theory**, says that how people behave depends on the consequences—whether they are rewarded, ignored, or punished. Reinforcement theory is quite different because it does not consider a person's needs, intentions, or goals. It was developed by the behaviorist B.F. Skinner as a way to explain what motivates behavior.

Behavior may result in **positive reinforcement**, in which there are pleasant consequences or it could be followed by punishment—unpleasant consequences. The purpose of positive reinforcement is to increase a behavior, so a manager may give praise or a small bonus to employees after they complete a certain action or set of actions. The purpose of punishment is to decrease the behavior. Another type of reinforcement is **negative reinforcement**, in which someone is rewarded for desired behavior by having something unpleasant removed. For example, if an employee comes to work on time, they are not subject to the boss's ridicule for being late, or if the staff finishes all their work on time, they will not have to stay late to finish.

Managers can use positive reinforcement in the workplace to influence employees' behaviors to complete tasks and reach organizational goals. **Table 11-7** gives examples

Table 11-7 Examples of Positive Reinforcers in the Workplace
1. Bonus or raise
2. Recognition awards such as gift cards
3. Positive verbal feedback that is frequent and timely
4. Opportunities for advancement
5. Flexible work hours
6. Free meals, beverages, and/or snacks
7. Flexible dress code
8. Better office space
9. Onsite gym or paid club memberships
10. Learning opportunities including college tuition reimbursement

of positive reinforcers. Using punishment only has a short-term impact and can result in negative side effects such as absenteeism, so it is rarely used.

USING MOTIVATIONAL THEORIES

When considering the topic of keeping employees engaged and motivated, two important considerations are the uniqueness of each employee and flexibility. Each employee has different needs, wants, and drives when they go to work, so it is important to *not* try a "one size fits all" approach. This is where flexibility comes in. A manager has to be flexible in what to offer different employees to increase engagement. Also, motivating professionals is going to be different from motivating minimum-wage frontline workers. Professionals are more likely to be motivated by challenging work, while frontline workers, who rank lower in motivation (McGregor & Doshi, 2018), are more likely to be motivated by on-the-job training and rewards. There are also cultural differences, such as individual accomplishment is valued in the United States, but other cultures (such as China and Japan) value group accomplishments more.

Almost all employees are looking for some basics when they come to work, such as respect, fairness, and interesting work. **Table 11-8** gives examples of actions managers can take to increase employee motivation and engagement.

Table 11-8 Types of Actions to Increase Employee Motivation	
Category	**Examples of Actions**
1. Rewards and Recognition (financial and nonfinancial)	• Offer good/fair compensation. • Pay-for-performance (links rewards to performance)—including merit pay increases, bonuses, profit sharing, stock options. • Give appreciation for a job well done. • Have an employee recognition program with awards such as "Employee of the Month." • Give frequent small rewards such as gift cards. • Base rewards on what the employee wants. (wide variety of rewards such as flexible work schedule, educational opportunities, or bonuses) • Make rewards continuous or intermittent.
2. Feedback and Praise	• Make feedback as positive as possible. Don't focus on shortcomings or scare people into action. • Give specific praise for a behavior. Explain why it is important and encourage more of the same.
3. Job Design and Performance Management	• Make work challenging. • Make work interesting. • Make work meaningful. • Provide a reasonable work schedule. • Invest in employee training and development. • Engage employees in goal setting. • Increase employee autonomy. • Be fair in annual performance appraisals. • Help employees see the end result of their work.
4. Organizational Culture	• Listen. • Foster interpersonal relationships and camaraderie among employees. • Promote collaboration and teamwork. • Build trust by being just and transparent in assigning work, giving rewards and recognition. • Treat employees fairly and consistently. • Provide a safe and clean work environment.

11.5 IDENTIFY EFFECTIVE DECISION-MAKING TECHNIQUES

Foodservice managers make many decisions in an average day at work. Many of those decisions have obvious solutions, such as getting someone to mop up a spill in the kitchen. Other decisions are more serious and will require a lot more thought. We often talk about problem-solving and decision making together. **Problem-solving** is the process of identifying a problem and considering and taking corrective action. The **decision-making process** involves selecting a course of action to: solve a problem (such as decrease labor costs), take advantage of an opportunity (such as expand a business), or simply make a management decision (such as set long-term goals). The decision-making model depicted in **Figure 11-9** shows the six steps in the process.

In the first step of the decision-making process, it is important to classify the type of decision and consider the conditions under which a decision will be made.

1. Decisions can be classified as programmed or nonprogrammed. **Programmed decisions** are concerned with relatively routine problems (often repetitive) such as an employee with a lateness issue, that can be dealt with by using policies and procedures. Since these decisions are relatively simple and affect only small segments of the organization, there is no need to follow all of the decision-making steps and lower-level managers often make these decisions. On the other hand, **nonprogrammed decisions** are concerned with unique or unusual situations that need to be addressed because they could have major consequences. The situations are usually nonrepetitive and more complex, and

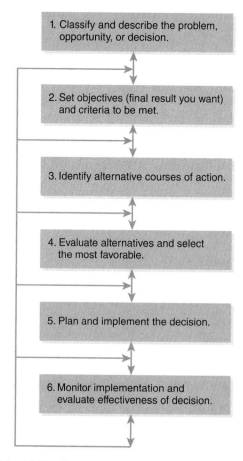

FIGURE 11-9 The Decision-Making Process

information is more likely to be ambiguous or incomplete. Higher-level managers usually make these decisions, such as deciding whether to adopt a new technology, purchase costly new equipment, or how to expand a business.

2. When preparing to make a decision, it is a good idea to consider the degree of risk. **Risk** is the probability that the predicted outcomes of a course of action will occur, and it varies on a continuum from certainty to uncertainty. Under conditions of *certainty*, enough information is available so you can assign a probability for each course of action, and you are more likely to make a good decision. Under conditions of *uncertainty*, a lack of necessary information or the impossibility of getting comprehensive and reliable data make the outcome of each alternative unpredictable. This can happen, for example, when the environment changes constantly and is unpredictable. Under conditions of uncertainty, since the probability for each course of action can't be determined, it is more likely that a poor decision is made. Lower-level managers are more likely to make decisions under conditions of certainty, and higher-level managers are more likely to make risky decisions.

3. Most people use one of two approaches (or sometimes a mix of both approaches) when making decisions (March & Simon, 1993). Managers who use **maximizing** want to make the optimal decisions, so they don't think twice about spending a lot of time evaluating a wide range of alternatives or options, especially if the decision outcome is very important. Maximizing is more useful for nonprogrammed decisions when risks are hard to calculate. Another decision-making style is known as **satisficing** (combining satisfy and suffice). When managers satisfice, they are usually working fast and want to find an acceptable decision rather than the optimum decision (Simon, 1957). They may be under time pressure or just don't want to be bothered with thoroughly checking out each option. Satisficing works best for more programmed decisions when the decision outcome is not as important.

When starting the decision-making process, managers must also think about who should participate and who should make the final decision. Group decision making is employed quite often, and groups often yield more innovative solutions, better decisions, and greater commitment to the decision. Although trends are moving toward more group decision making, there are certainly situations where a manager, often with input from others, will be responsible for the process.

The *first step* in the decision-making process involves consideration of the four points just discussed. Then, the problem, opportunity, or decision needs to be described. In the case of a problem, it is important to identify the real cause of the problem and distinguish it from the symptoms. If a foodservice is having difficulty being profitable, that is a symptom, not a cause. The foodservice may not be as profitable as it once was because of new nearby competitors siphoning business away.

The *second step* is to set an objective or purpose. The objective should state what you want to accomplish or the final result that you want. For example, if the problem is that a pandemic has closed down your dining room to only 50% of capacity, a restaurant may have an objective to increase revenue. Once you set an objective, it is useful to create criteria to judge the quality of the alternative solutions. You could set criteria such as the desired level of sales dollars you want to bring in as well as how much money can be used to make this happen.

The *third step* is to identify alternative courses of action to solve this problem or take advantage of the opportunity. Because many managers find it hard to see many problems from a fresh perspective, using groups of employees to help foster creativity is helpful. The following are some techniques that can be used to help identify creative and innovative solutions.

1. **Brainstorming:** When a group brainstorms ideas, individuals are encouraged to call out any ideas they have. Each idea is recorded and there is no criticism or

discussion of ideas during the session, so as to encourage free expression of ideas. Combining, modifying, or expanding ideas is encouraged.

2. **Synectics:** Synectics is a form of brainstorming that uses analogies, imagery, and role playing to generate creative ideas.

3. **Nominal grouping:** Nominal grouping is a more structured type of brainstorming that still encourages everyone to contribute ideas. Each person writes down their ideas and then presents their best idea to the group and it is recorded. Each idea can be discussed and each person then ranks their top three choices. Discussion continues and a secret vote(s) is taken to decide on the top ideas. During this process, the purpose of discussion is to explain and clarify ideas—not to influence others.

A **decision tree** is a diagram of the possible outcomes for each alternative. It is an excellent management tool to depict the possible directions that actions might take. Possible outcomes are included, with a notation about the probabilities associated with each outcome. **Figure 11-10** is a decision tree for a restaurant in Pennsylvania that was forced to close half of its dining room during a pandemic. In order to get the restaurant closer to its monthly sales level of $160,000, they first plan to streamline the menu and then they want to expand service options that don't involve the dining room. The decision tree lists alternatives to expand service options and gives information about the costs and outcomes for each alternative. The outcomes are given in sales dollars along with the probability of each happening. Although computers are commonly used to calculate the probability of events when such detailed information is available, it is also possible to use intuition. A decision tree is helpful in the next step when you need to evaluate alternatives.

After alternatives have been proposed, the *fourth step* is to evaluate the alternatives and select the most favorable. It is important to keep the process of generating alternatives separate from the process of evaluating and picking one. Doing both steps 3 and 4 at the same time typically leads to satisficing (Lussier, 2019). The most favorable alternative should be the one that has at least acceptable outcomes, but just as important, it must be doable. If one of the alternatives has excellent outcomes but is going to be really hard to pull off, pick another alternative that is more feasible. When analyzing alternatives, also compare each one to the objective(s) and criteria set in step two, and compare alternatives to each other.

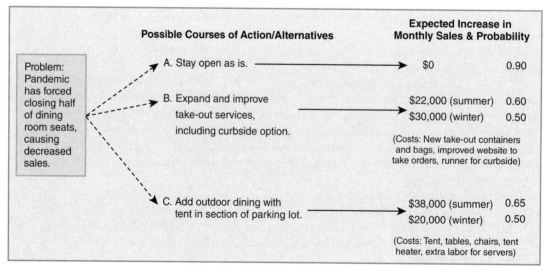

FIGURE 11-10 Example of Decision Tree

SPOTLIGHT ON METHODS TO EVALUATE ALTERNATIVES

A popular way to evaluate alternatives is to rate how well each alternative meets the criteria you set in the second step. You have probably used this process when making a big purchase, such as buying a laptop. You likely set criteria such as cost, memory, and battery life, and then rated each laptop on those criteria. Whichever laptop overall rated the highest was the one you purchased.

The following are additional methods to evaluate alternatives. Some are more qualitative in nature, such as using intuition, while others are more quantitative and use math. Many of the quantitative methods work best in certain situations.

- Pros and cons: For each alternative you have, list the advantages and disadvantages.
- Intuition: Intuitive decision making means making decisions based on past experiences, judgment, and feelings. Using intuition along with more quantitative methods can be quite useful and is referred to as informed intuition.
- Cost-benefit analysis: **Cost-benefit analysis** is a way to compare the costs and benefits of an alternative, where both are expressed in dollars. For example, the decision tree in Figure 11–10 shows the benefits of each alternative in terms of revenue. The extra costs for each alternative are also listed. By attaching a dollar value to the costs, you can calculate net benefits as follows.

Alternative B. Benefits ($22,000 in sales) – Costs ($8,000) = Net Benefits ($14,000)

- Break-even analysis and cost/volume/profit analysis: **Break-even analysis** is a useful tool to determine at what point your business, or a new product or service, will be profitable. It can tell you how much you need to sell to at least cover your costs. To determine how much revenue you need in order to make a certain profit, you can use the **Cost-Volume-Profit formula**. Chapter 15 explains how to use formulas to calculate the break-even point or the revenue required for a certain profit level.
- Capital budgeting techniques: A capital budget allocates money for major investments such as equipment. Capital budgeting techniques help in decisions such as fix-or-replace or buy-or-lease. Two methods used to evaluate capital investments include **payback period** (length of time required to earn back the value of an investment from profits or net annual savings) and **net present value**. The payback period is calculated by dividing the cost of the investment by the net annual savings or profits. The net present value (NPV) of a capital investment is the value of the total revenues (over the life of the equipment) discounted to today's dollars, minus the cost of the capital investment. When the net present value is above zero, the capital investment is desirable. Chapter 15 explains how to use these techniques.
- Use of big data: According to Oracle (2020), **big data** is "larger, more complex data sets, especially from new data sources......these massive volumes of data can be used to address business problems you wouldn't have been able to tackle before." Analyzing big data is useful when managers ask the right questions and recognize patterns and opportunities in the data. For example, multi-unit foodservices use big data to select new store locations.
- Probability theory: **Probability** is the likelihood that a particular event will occur. The probability of an event can only be between 0 - 1. If the probability is 0.45, that can also be stated at 45%. Probability theory lets us analyze chance events in a logically sound way, such as to help evaluate the possible outcomes of decisions. You can weigh the possible outcomes by assigning a probability to each outcome and finding expected values. Expected value is the return, such as profit, you can expect for some kind of action.

The *fifth step* is to plan and implement the decision. Once an alternative has been chosen, it is important to first make a detailed plan/schedule that shows how the alternative will be put into action along with a schedule for implementation. Employees should be involved and good communication will ensure that everything is implemented according to plan. Managers should keep an eye on any changes in the environment that might change an aspect of implementation.

Managers often use a **Gantt chart** developed by Henry Gantt, a pioneer in scientific management. A Gantt chart has the format of a bar chart and depicts the tasks that must be completed for a project to be finished, along with when they must occur and how long each task or activity lasts. It also shows who is responsible for completing each task. As the work progresses, shading is used to show which activities have been completed. The calendar legend is placed at the top or the bottom of the chart. Checkpoints should be put into the Gantt chart so you can evaluate how things are going at several points in the process.

Checkpoints will help with the *final and sixth step:* Monitor implementation and evaluate the outcome and effectiveness of the decision. To evaluate how well things went, the manager can refer back to the original objective and criteria.

SUMMARY

11.1 Describe Management Skills, Functions, and Roles

- Efficient managers get the most output of goods or services from the smallest amount of inputs.
- Inputs include human resources, financial resources, physical resources, and intangible resources (such as information and technology).
- Whereas an efficient manager does things right, an effective manager does the right things—meaning the manager chooses appropriate goals and activities to make a business successful.
- Organizational culture encompasses the values, practices, and expectations that guide the actions of managers and employees in an organization or business.
- Management skills are technical, human or interpersonal, or conceptual.
- Managers share certain functions or processes in which they are involved: planning, organizing, controlling, and leading.
- Managers have roles, including interpersonal, informational, and decisional roles.
- Levels of management include upper management, middle management, and first-line managers (supervisors).

11.2 Compare and Contrast Major Approaches to Management Theory

- The first studies of management, often called the classical approach, focused on jobs and how workers could do their jobs efficiently. Frederick Taylor and Lillian Gilbreth helped found the scientific management school that focused on designing jobs and training workers to function as efficiently and productively as possible.
- Administrative management theory (still part of the classical approach) looked at the functions that all managers should be doing. Henri Fayol distinguished between operation and management activities and was the first to identify the management functions of planning, organizing, coordinating, controlling, and commanding (leading). Table 11-2 shows Fayol's 14 principles of management.
- Max Weber also contributed to administrative management theory with his ideas about bureaucracies with a clear chain of command and set of goals and rules.
- The next approach, the behavioral approach, moved away from a focus on productivity to a focus on the people themselves. Mary Parker Follett felt employees were capable of determining the best way to accomplish tasks and that supervisors should act more like coaches.
- The Hawthorne study, the most well-known behavioral study in which Elton Mayo was involved, showed that the performance of employees is influenced by the people with whom they are working—including fellow employees, groups, and managers. Employees performed better when they felt managers cared about their workplace and gave them a chance to be heard.
- Douglas McGregor held that managers either think the average employee is lazy and will work as little as possible (Theory X) or that employees are not inherently lazy and will contribute to the organization when trusted and empowered (Theory Y).
- Today, the behavioral approach is used in organizations to engage employees and more research is being done, although we now prefer to call it the behavioral science approach. The behavioral science approach involves a number of disciplines including psychology, sociology, economics, and organizational behavior.

- The <u>quantitative approach</u> to management uses quantitative techniques (such as statistics, computer modeling, or queuing theory), to help managers solve problems, make decisions, and use resources wisely.
- <u>Contemporary approaches</u> include the open-systems approach and the contingency approach.
- An open system receives various inputs and transforms them in different ways to generate outputs. Inputs, transformation, and outputs are the major parts of the system. In the foodservice industry, inputs include, for example, people, materials (such as food), and facilities. The work of an organization is transformation—meaning using the inputs to create the outputs. In foodservice, the operations, and management subsystems are used to transform inputs to outputs such as quality meals (tangible) and customer satisfaction (intangible). In an open system, the boundary between the organization and its environment is considered permeable.
- According to contingency theory, each organization needs to manage and organize itself differently and this depends on the external environment and technology. A number of researchers have discussed key characteristics of two organizational forms: mechanistic (bureaucratic) and organic.
- The characteristics of mechanistic organizations are best for companies operating in a fairly stable environment in which each day has a steady routine and well-defined tasks, such as foodservice operations. The flexibility of organic organizations works best in uncertain environments so that they can stay open and respond to environmental changes.

11.3 Communicate Effectively

- Communication is vital to planning, organizing, controlling, and (especially) leading, and benefits both employees and customers.
- Components of communication include the sender, communication channel, receiver, feedback, and noise.
- Table 11-5 lists advantages and disadvantages of communication channels: oral, written, electronic, and nonverbal. Table 11-4 gives examples of nonverbal cues.
- Within an organization, communication can be formal or informal (grapevine).

- Formal communication can be either vertical (upward or downward) or horizontal.
- Obstacles to good communication include poor choice of communication channel, noise in the environment, poor listening, emotions and biases, information overload, and mixed messages.
- Figure 11-3 shows skills needed to actively listen.
- When managers send messages, they need to think before they speak, send clear and complete messages, choose an appropriate communication channel for the message, make sure the information is accurate and has not been filtered, ask for feedback, check for understanding, and avoid sending messages when emotions are high for either party.
- Table 11-6 lists communication tips. Tips are also given for communicating effectively with people from other cultures.

11.4 Discuss How to Motivate Employees

- Extrinsic motivation is when the reward is external to the work itself. Intrinsic motivation is when you do something because it is internally satisfying and you enjoy it.
- Early theories of motivation are referred to as needs theories because early researchers focused on understanding what people need. For example, Abraham Maslow's Hierarchy of Needs Theory (Figure 11-4) felt the lower needs in his hierarchy (physiological and safety) must be satisfied before the higher needs (such as belonging or esteem) become active sources of motivation.
- Herzberg's two-factor theory separated factors that increase motivation, referred to as satisfiers or motivators, from those whose absence leads to job dissatisfaction, referred to as hygiene factors (Figure 11-5). Hygiene factors, such as salary and working conditions, do not themselves motivate employees but without them, employees are likely to be dissatisfied. Motivators include, for instance, achievement, growth, and work itself.
- McClelland's three-needs theory identified three needs that are learned—need for achievement, need for affiliation (belonging to a group), and need for power (personal power or institutional power). McClelland's research showed that employees can learn to achieve if they are put in a situation in which they are asked to take a moderate risk, be

personally responsible, and are able to get regular feedback.

- Contemporary theories, supported by research, include goal setting theory, expectancy theory, equity theory, and reinforcement theory.
- In goal setting theory, Locke and Latham showed that working toward a clear goal is a major source of motivation. They recommended setting clear and specific goals that are not too difficult or too easy, as well as giving employees frequent feedback on how they are meeting their goals. Locke and Latham's research confirms the usefulness of SMART goal setting (Figure 11-6).
- Vroom's expectancy theory states that in order for a reward (or other desired outcome) to work, employees first have to believe that an increase in effort will result in a high level of performance (expectancy). Second, employees have to believe that a higher level of performance will be noted and rewarded (instrumentality). Lastly, employees have to actually want the reward that is being promised (valence).
- Adams' equity theory suggests that employees compare what they give to an organization (inputs such as time, effort, experience, etc.) against what they receive (outputs such as pay, status, recognition, etc.,), and then compare their outputs/inputs with others in the organization. When inequities occur (such as someone with a comparable background gets paid more), employees may take actions such as to call in sick, perform at less-productive levels, or find another job. Equity theory shows managers the importance of being fair (no playing favorites), equitable (especially with outputs such as pay, rewards, and recognition), and transparent.
- Reinforcement theory says that how people behave depends on the consequences. The purpose of positive reinforcement is to increase a behavior, so a manager may give praise or a small bonus to employees after they complete a certain action or set of actions.
- When considering how to keep employees engaged and motivated, two important considerations are the uniqueness of each employee and flexibility. Each employee has different needs, wants, and drives when they go to work, so it is important to *not* try

a "one size fits all" approach. Table 11-8 gives examples of different ways to engage and motivate employees.

11.5   Identify Effective Decision-Making Techniques

- Figure 11-9 gives the steps in the decision-making process.
- Programmed decisions are concerned with relatively routine problems (often repetitive), such as an employee with a lateness issue, that can be dealt with by using policies and procedures. Nonprogrammed decisions are concerned with unique or unusual situations that need to be addressed because they could have major consequences. The situations are usually nonrepetitive and more complex, and information is more likely to be ambiguous or incomplete.
- When preparing to make a decision, it's a good idea to consider the degree of risk. Under conditions of *certainty*, enough information is available so you can assign a probability for each course of action, and you are more likely to make a good decision. Under conditions of *uncertainty*, a lack of necessary information or the impossibility of getting comprehensive and reliable data make the outcome of each alternative unpredictable.
- Most people use one of these approaches to decision making: maximizing or satisficing. Managers who maximize want to make optimal decisions and spend a lot of time evaluating a wide range of alternatives. Maximizing is more useful for nonprogrammed decisions when risks are hard to calculate. When managers satisfice, they are usually working fast and want to find an acceptable decision rather than the optimum decision. This works best for more programmed decisions.
- A decision tree is an excellent management tool to depict the possible directions that actions might take (Figure 11-10). Possible outcomes are included, with a notation about the probabilities associated with each outcome.
- When analyzing alternatives, compare each one to the objective(s) and criteria set in step two, and compare alternatives to each other. Additional methods for evaluating alternatives include pros and cons, informed intuition, probability theory, break-even analysis, capital budgeting techniques, and analysis of big data.

- When planning implementation, a Gantt chart may be useful. Using a bar chart, it depicts the tasks that must be completed for a project to be finished, along with when they must occur and how long each task or activity lasts. A calendar legend is at the top or bottom.

REVIEW AND DISCUSSION QUESTIONS

1. How are managers different from hourly employees? Why are they important to hire?
2. Compare an effective manager with an efficient manager. What are a manager's resources?
3. Describe the three categories of management skills and give an example from each category.
4. Give an example of how a manager plans, organizes, controls, and leads.
5. What are the three levels of management? How many levels of management would you find in a typical one-unit, small to medium restaurant? What would be the titles of managers at each level?
6. Why is it important to study management history?
7. What is a bureaucracy? Do they exist today?
8. How does the behavioral approach differ from the scientific management approach?
9. What has the quantitative approach contributed to management practices?
10. Have the two contemporary approaches, systems theory and the contingency approach, made managers better at what they do? Explain your answer.
11. List the four channels of communication and give an example of when each channel is used most effectively.
12. Contrast formal and informal communication.
13. What is the grapevine and how should managers deal with it?
14. What are some steps you can take to become a better listener and overall better communicator?
15. What is motivation? How is it different from job satisfaction?
16. How do you motivate an employee using goal-setting, expectancy, equity, and reinforcement theory?
17. Which types of decisions can be made using maximizing? Using satisficing?
18. Describe the steps in decision making.
19. When is a decision tree useful and how is it helpful?
20. Why do good managers sometimes make poor decisions? How can a manager improve their decision-making skills?

SMALL GROUP PROJECT

For the foodservice concept that you created in Chapter 1, develop the following.

1. A policy and procedure on communication within the foodservice.

2. Identify a problem within the foodservice that you want to solve. Describe how you went through the decision-making process to solve this problem. Include a decision tree.

REFERENCES

Adkins, A. (2015) Report: What separates great managers from the rest? Gallup. https://www.gallup.com/work place/236594/report-separates-great-managers-rest .aspx

Beck, R., & Harter, J. (2015). Managers account for 70% of variance in employee engagement. Gallup. https://news.gallup.com/businessjournal/182792 /managers-account-variance-employee-engagement .aspx

Buckingham, M. (2005). What great managers do. *Harvard Business Review, 83*(3), 70–79.

Burns, T. and Stalker, G. (1994.) *The management of innovation* (3rd ed.). Oxford (U.K.): Oxford University Press.

Fayol. H. (1984). *General and Industrial Management*. New York: IEEE Press.

Gino, F. (2017). To motivate employees, show them how they're helping customers. *Harvard Business Review,* https://hbr.org/2017/03/to-motivate-employees-show-them-how-theyre-helping-customers

Harter, J. (2020). Historic drop in employee engagement follows record rise. Gallup. https://www.gallup.com/workplace/313313/historic-drop-employee-engagement-follows-record-rise.aspx

Hemp, P. (2009). Death by information overload. *Harvard Business Review, 87*(9), 82–89.

Lawrence, P. R. and Lorsch, J. W. (1967). *Organization and environment*. Boston: Harvard Business School, Division of Research.

Locke, E. A., & Latham, G. P. (2002). Building a practically useful theory of goal setting and task motivation: A 35-year odyssey. *American Psychologist, 57*(9):705–717.

Lussier, R.N. (2019). *Management fundamentals: Concepts, applications, and skill development*. Thousand Oaks (CA): Sage Publications, Inc.

Magee, J. F. (1964). Decision trees for decision making. *Harvard Business Review, 42*(4):126–138.

March, J. G., & Simon, H. A. (1993). *Organizations* (2nd ed.). New York: John Wiley & Sons, Inc.

McGregor, L, & Doshi, N. (2018, Aug 30). How to motivate frontline employees. *Harvard Business Review,* https://hbr.org/2018/08/how-to-motivate-frontline-employees. Review.

Mintzberg H. (1989). Mintzberg on Management: Inside our Strange World of Organizations. New York: Free Press.

Mintzberg, H. (1973). *The Nature of Managerial Work*. New York: Harper & Row.

Miron, D., & McClelland, D. C. (1979). The impact of achievement motivation training on small businesses. *California Management Review, 21*(4), 13–28. doi: 10.2307/41164830

Morand, D. A. (1995). The role of behavioral formality and informality in the enactment of bureaucratic versus organic organizations. *Academy of Management Review, 20*(4), 831–872. doi:10.5465/amr.1995.9512280023

Nohria, N., Groysberg, B., & Lee, L-E. (2008). Employee motivation: A powerful new model. *Harvard Business Review, 86*(7-8), 78–84.

Oracle. (2020). Big data defined. https://www.oracle.com/big-data/what-is-big-data.html

Robbins, S.P., and Coulter, M. (2018). *Management* (14th ed.). New York: Pearson Education Inc.

Sharot, T. (2017). What motivates employees more: Rewards or punishments? *Harvard Business Review,* https://hbr.org/2017/09/what-motivates-employees-more-rewards-or-punishments

Simon, H. (1957). *Models of man*. New York: John Wiley & Sons, Inc.

U.S. Department of Homeland Security (FEMA). (2014). *Effective communication: Instructor guide.* https://training.fema.gov/emiweb/is/is242b/instructor%20guide/ig_complete.pdf

Planning and Organizing

LEARNING OUTCOMES

12.1 Use the strategic planning process.

12.2 Plan for risk and emergencies/disasters.

12.3 Plan your own time.

12.4 Interpret organizational structure.

12.5 Analyze and design jobs.

12.6 Create and manage groups and teams.

INTRODUCTION

Planning and organizing are important management functions that are also important for college success. As a college student, you have to carefully plan which courses to register for each semester in order to complete your degree on time. Then you have to plan and organize your time each week to be prepared for classes plus take care of commitments such as jobs and families.

Planning involves identifying and selecting appropriate **goals** (a desired outcome such as increased sales) and choosing **strategies** (a course of action) to achieve them. An example of a goal would be to increase sales, and two strategies to achieve this goal could be to utilize social media and offer online ordering. By having goals and strategies, managers and employees have a sense of direction and can pull in the same direction. Other benefits of planning are that good plans can build commitment for the goals and make managers more accountable for reaching goals. Indeed, businesses are more likely to perform better when they perform strategic planning (Miller and Cardinal, 2017).

Organizing refers to structuring and coordinating the work of a business into tasks, jobs, and departments to accomplish the business' goals and objectives. Organizing also involves allocating and coordinating resources such as salaries, space, and equipment. Organizing is essential to establish formal lines of authority and relationships among individuals, groups, and departments, as seen in an organizational chart. This chapter will start with a discussion on planning and then move on to organizing.

© Denis Val/Shutterstock

12.1 USE THE STRATEGIC PLANNING PROCESS

Before discussing the strategic planning process, let's look at what strategic planning is as well as other types of plans.

DIFFERENT TYPES OF PLANS

In a foodservice, you hear about plans such as a single-use plan or a long-term plan. Plans vary depending on these factors.

1. Length of time the plan is in effect. A **short-term plan** usually covers one year or less, such as a one-year budget. A **long-term plan** may cover five years, but could be as short as three years or as long as 10 years. An **intermediate-term plan** (or medium-term plan) fits in between a short-term and a long-term plan. Depending on the organization, an intermediate-term plan could be nine months, a year, or 18 months (Houlder & Nandkishore, 2016).

2. How often the plan will be used. Sometimes an organization will develop a **single-use plan**. A single-use plan, such as a budget or development of a new advertising campaign, is used just once to address a unique situation and achieve a particular goal. Once that goal is met, it is unlikely that the exact situation will reoccur. In contrast, a **standing plan** is used frequently and is designed to provide a blueprint or set of procedures to be used in a recurring or repetitive situation. A menu is a standing plan for the food to be prepared. A policy and procedures manual for the dining room is a standing plan for how to greet guests, take orders, and other dining room protocol. A **policy** is a guideline for decision making that is expressed in fairly broad terms, such as "employees will receive written performance evaluations once a year and verbal evaluations as needed." Policies help ensure that decisions are consistent with the business' objectives. **Procedures** are step-by-step descriptions of actions required to carry out the policy. For example, the procedures for employee evaluations would explain when written evaluations take place and what form is to be used. Procedures often include **rules** such as employees must wash their hands after using the rest rooms.

3. The degree of flexibility in the plan. **Specific plans** clearly define objectives and don't allow any flexibility or room for interpretation. For example, an objective in a specific plan would be to increase patient meal satisfaction (in a hospital) by 25% within 12 months. In contrast, a **directional or options-based plan** is a flexible plan that defines general guidelines. These plans give direction but not a precise goal or exactly how to accomplish it. For example, an objective in a directional plan would be to decrease food waste in the kitchen. It does not state how to do so or how much, that will be left up to the production employees, but they have a clear direction in which to go.

4. Which level of the business develops the plan. Multiunit restaurant chains and foodservice contract companies often have three levels of management from the top down: the corporate level, the division or business level, and the operational level (**Figure 12-1**). The corporate level includes upper-level managers in areas such as finance and supply chain management (purchasing and distribution). Below the corporate level are divisions or business units, such as healthcare or schools for a foodservice contractor, or franchise stores and company stores for a restaurant chain with both types of stores. The lowest level of management is the operational (functional) level where you find the individual foodservice(s) with their functional departments such as production and customer service. With three levels of management, upper and middle managers (at the corporate and division levels) are more involved in **strategic planning** while lower level managers are more involved in **operational planning**. Within a single-unit

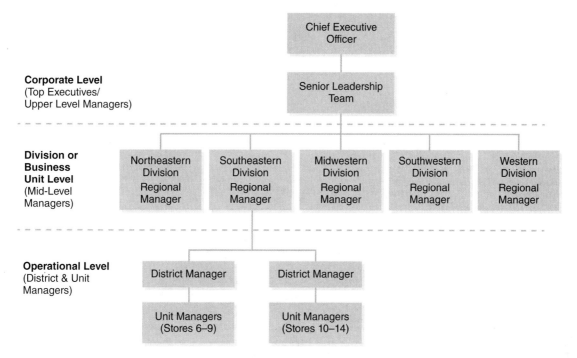

FIGURE 12.1 Levels of Management in a Multiunit Foodservice

foodservice, upper-level managers (such as the owner, general manager, or unit manager) generally perform the strategic planning, while department heads (such as the chef/production manager) do more operational planning.

So, what are strategic and operational planning? **Strategic planning** refers to establishing the overall mission, goals, and long-range objectives and strategies for the entire business. **Operational planning** involves setting short-range objectives and strategies to improve the ability of each subsystem (such as production or service) to perform its activities while supporting the overall strategic plan. When comparing these types of planning, strategic plans are often broader, longer in duration, and more directional.

STRATEGIC PLANNING PROCESS

Strategic planning is a step-wise process that starts when top management develops the mission statement for the foodservice or reviews an existing mission statement. **Figure 12-2** shows the steps in the strategic planning process. In a large foodservice company with three management levels (corporate, divisions, operations), each *division* needs to develop its own mission (building on the corporate mission), do its own SWOT analysis (assessing its Strengths, Weaknesses, Opportunities, and Threats), and set objectives and strategies, *just as the corporate level does*. In a single foodservice or a restaurant with several locations—*the corporate and division levels are the same*.

A **mission** is a broad statement describing what the business does, why the business exists, and what purpose it serves for its customers. For example, a restaurant's mission may be "to provide a relaxing and enjoyable dining experience with distinctive food, drinks, and service for our guests, as well as offer a cooperative, rewarding environment for our employees." Although mission statements are sometimes only one sentence, they can be longer (such as a few sentences).

To expand on their mission statements, many companies nowadays are also listing their **core values**. For example, the Sweetgreen restaurant chain has six core values,

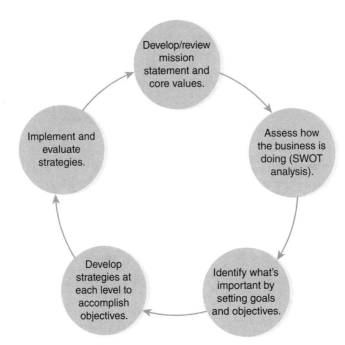

FIGURE 12-2 The Strategic Planning Process

which emphasize the importance of helping customers, helping the community, and acting sustainably. Other values may be listed such as having a team spirit or being accountable. A mission statement and core values are excellent ways to communicate and guide managers and employees as to what is most important.

Some organizations also have a **vision statement**, which describes their future expectations, including how the organization wants to impact the communities or areas it serves. For example, the vision for the Alzheimer's Association is a "world without Alzheimer's."®

The next step in the strategic planning process is to look at how the business is doing and where it is at the present moment. To be successful, any business needs to have a competitive advantage over its competitors. A **competitive advantage** is something unique that is different from and better than what your competitors offer, such as outstanding value, food, or service. An excellent tool for analyzing your business is to do a **SWOT analysis** in which you identify the strengths and weaknesses inside your business and also the opportunities and threats in the external environment. Another tool for analyzing a business as part of strategic planning is the balanced scorecard developed by Kaplan and Norton.

In a SWOT analysis, *strengths* look at what your foodservice does well, such as having excellent service, or other qualities that separate you from your competitors. *Weaknesses* force you to look at what your foodservice lacks or could be doing better such as lowering food costs or getting help with marketing. When looking at the external environment, *opportunities* are possible areas for you to do more business, such as underserved markets or an increased need for some of your products. Opportunities include any external factors, such as consumers supporting sustainable foods, that could positively impact your foodservice. External *threats*, such as increasing competition, a downturn in the economy, increasing food prices, or new/revised regulations, can disrupt your foodservice. **Table 12–1** gives an example of a SWOT analysis for a university foodservice.

Using the SWOT analysis, the next step is to develop goals and objectives showing what is important and needs to be achieved. If the organization had developed goals and objectives previously, they should be reviewed and updated and new ones may be

Table 12-1 SWOT Analysis for University Foodservice		
Internal Factors	**Strengths** • High satisfaction ratings from students, faculty, and administration in self-operated foodservice. • Cutting-edge menu. • Newly renovated production facilities. • Qualified employees. • Supportive administration.	**Weaknesses** • Retention of quality cooking personnel can be challenging. • Food costs a little higher than desired. • Outdated POS (point of sale) system.
External Factors	**Opportunities** • More local farms offering organic products. • Availability of employees due to high unemployment in your area. • Expansion of commissary to serve local clientele.	**Threats** • College-age population/enrollment in decline. • Area colleges being approached by foodservice contract companies. • Increasing threat in food supply of foodborne illness.

added. Managers should consider goals/objectives that flow from the mission statement and build on strengths, correct weaknesses, exploit external opportunities, and counter threats identified in the SWOT analysis.

Whereas a **goal** is a desired result or broad outcome to be achieved, **objectives** also describe what must be accomplished but are more specific. Objectives are more measurable than goals because they identify how and when the goal is to be accomplished. Goals usually have multiple objectives. Some typical foodservice goals might be to increase net profit, develop new menu items, be more environmentally responsible, improve service, or increase customer retention.

If a foodservice sets a goal to become more environmentally responsible, here are some possible objectives they may choose.

Objective 1. Reduce food waste by 20% within one year.
Objective 2. Decrease water consumption by 10% by the end of 2022.
Objective 3. Double local and organic food purchases by January of 2022.

These objectives are written using a format known as a SMART objective. SMART objectives are specific, measurable, achievable, realistic, and time-bound. By making each objective specific rather than vague, everyone will be clear about what needs to be accomplished. Next, each objective should be able to be measured and have a deadline so that the people involved in achieving it are accountable and more inclined to work hard. Lastly, each objective should be attainable and realistic. Employees perform better when the objective has some difficulty but is attainable than when the objective is too difficult or too easy.

The next step in the strategic planning process is to develop strategies or action plans. **Strategies** are the steps needed to accomplish each objective and help get a business to where it wants to be. For a large restaurant company, such as Darden Restaurants, with a corporate level and many business units (such as Olive Garden and Red Lobster restaurants), the corporate office develops corporate-level strategies. Corporate-level strategies often revolve around growth, stability, or renewal. **Growth strategies** could involve increasing sales within restaurants, opening new restaurants, or entering new lines of business, which could be related or not related to existing ones. Growth could also involve a **merger** (when two companies form one company) or an **acquisition** (when one company buys all or part of another). A **stability strategy** involves either slow growth or staying the same. A **renewal strategy** is called for when a company has declining performance. When this happens, a company will normally need to cut costs and restructure operations such as the menu and service model.

Each division or business must develop its own business-level strategies, which often focus on adapting to the external environment (adaptive strategies) and using tactics to beat the competition (competitive strategies). **Adaptive strategies** look at how a business reacts to changes in the business environment. If a business sees opportunities in the environment, it may decide to expand or enter new markets with existing or new products and services. Other businesses may react to the environment by sticking to what they do best, while others cautiously try out new menu items and consider new markets. These strategies correspond to the corporate strategies of growth and stability.

Porter (1980) identified the following three business-level **competitive strategies**, which can be used to beat the competition and make higher profits.

1. **Differentiation strategy**: A differentiation strategy requires a business to create products or services that are unique and valued by customers. In other words, the business has to develop a competitive advantage. For example, when Buffalo Wild Wings® started its business as a sports bar and casual restaurant, it considered other sports bars and how to offer a better experience. They decided to focus attention on the variety and quality of its menu and beer selection along with making the restaurant a fun place for fans to watch sports on any of its numerous TVs. With an emphasis on the guest experience, the chain continues to grow. Other differentiation strategies could focus on, for example, authentic foods/ingredients or allowing the customer to customize their order. Customization is the hallmark of chains such as QDOBA Mexican Eats or Chipotle where meals can be made that fit into a variety of diets such as paleo or gluten-free. Some businesses with a competitive advantage due to their premium products, such as Starbucks, have higher costs and will, therefore, charge higher prices.

2. **Low-cost strategy**: When using a low-cost strategy, a business focuses on driving costs lower than rivals so that products can be sold at lower prices, a useful way to attract more customers. Of course, huge foodservice companies, such as McDonald's, can buy food at better prices because of the volume they purchase. Combined with paying minimum wage to many of their employees, McDonald's can really keep costs down. Retail stores such as Walmart have also been successful with a low-cost strategy.

3. **Focused differentiation or focused low-cost strategies**: In a focused strategy, the business develops low-cost or unique products for a specific regional or niche market. For example, Whole Foods opened 12 smaller stores mostly on the west coast, called Whole Foods 365, that had lower prices and more of a local flavor.

Finally, at the operational level, each functional department (such as Production, Customer Service/Dining Room, Purchasing, or Marketing) develops strategies to achieve the mission and objectives. For example, each department needs its own standing plans, such as policies and procedures, to handle everyday situations, as well as single-use plans, such as budgets and programs, to address situations that don't repeat in exactly the same way. A policy is a guideline for making decisions, such as a policy on safe food handling. Policies are derived from the organization's mission, goals, and objectives. Procedures describe how each policy will be put in action and give acceptable ways of accomplishing a specific task.

Programs are a set of activities to fulfill an objective during a specific period of time. The program could be to develop a new menu item, engage in a sustainability initiative, develop a new marketing campaign, or open a new location. Departments must also plan for emergencies and disasters. This topic is discussed next.

So, the business has gone through some important steps in the strategic planning process from developing the mission to selecting strategies. Now it is time to implement the strategies and let some time pass before evaluating how well they are working. There is never an "end" to strategic planning. Managers have to continually review how well objectives are being met as well as refine and update any steps in the process as needed.

SPOTLIGHT ON POLICY AND PROCEDURE MANUALS

Policies and procedures function like a road map for managers and supervisors because they describe how work is done as well as how employees and customers are to be treated. Within a foodservice, each department often has its own policy and procedure manual, or at least its own section in a master manual. For example, a *human resources policy and procedures manual* will include policies and procedures on topics such as employee pay, discipline, and cell phone use. An *operations policy and procedures manual* will include policies and procedures on topics such as how foods are purchased and received, as well as how employees are to interact with customers.

A good policy and procedures manual is:

- Simple and easy to read and understand.
- Developed through a collaborative effort.
- Thorough and includes all critical topics.
- Contains procedures that are clear and specific.
- References other pertinent materials such as an Employee Handbook or Production Training Manual.
- Is not put on a shelf to collect dust (it should be reviewed yearly and revised as needed).

A policy and procedures manual should also include forms, such as a Production Schedule or Request for Vacation Time Off.

12.2 PLAN FOR RISK AND EMERGENCIES/DISASTERS

On a daily basis, you run the risk of having your identity stolen, your credit card number stolen, or being involved in a vehicular accident. Most people take actions to reduce these risks by, for example, storing personal information securely or driving in a safe vehicle. Foodservices also run risks, such as serving food that makes customers sick or having to provide meals to hospital patients when a hurricane has hit and there is no electricity. **Risk** is the possibility of injury, damage, or loss. To decrease risks, foodservices and other businesses utilize risk management techniques.

Risk management is a process in which potential risk events are managed proactively to minimize outcomes such as injuries, damages, or loss. For example, hospitals in hurricane-prone regions use emergency plans (set up in advance) including when to make emergency food purchases before a hurricane hits and how to prepare cold meals when hot meals can't be made. Restaurants don't have to stay open during weather emergencies (although some community-minded ones do), but many onsite foodservices (such as healthcare, universities, and military bases) have customers who cannot evacuate and must be served meals. An excellent resource for any foodservice manager is the Foodservice Industry Risk Management Association, a professional group of risk professionals in the hospitality and foodservices industries.

MANAGING RISKS

Foodservice managers concern themselves with risks such as the following.

1. <u>Food safety risks</u>: Foodborne illness in customers/employees, foreign materials in food, pests in foodservice, poor ratings on health department inspections.
2. <u>Employee/customer risks</u>: Injuries of customers/employees due to accidents or fire, an employee harassing other employees or customers, an infectious disease that affects both employees and customers.
3. <u>Weather risks</u>: Tornadoes, hurricanes, earthquakes, floods, excessive snow, drought.

4. Environmental risks: Poor water quality, poor air quality.
5. Financial risks: Decreased sales and revenue loss, poor purchasing practices, employee theft, changes in inflation or stock prices, access to capital, loss of lease, foreclosure, cash flow problems, increasing insurance costs.
6. Legal risks: Lawsuits due to accidents, food poisoning, fraud, theft, or employment law violations (as examples).
7. Technological risks: Not investing in new software or innovative cooking equipment, social media slamming, failure to protect confidential customer information such as financial transaction data from cyberattack.

There are also positive risks. A **positive risk** is when you invest time or money into new programs, equipment, personnel, or systems that could result in the long-term saving of money (decreased costs), or gaining a competitive edge over your competition (increased revenue).

According to Kaplan & Mikes (2012), you can classify potential risks into these risk categories (Kaplan & Mikes, 2012).

1. Preventable Risks: These are risks from within the business that can be eliminated or prevented. Many of these risks are prevented every day simply because employees follow policies and procedures and comply with food safety regulations. A strong company culture also helps make clear that employees need to comply with standards and controls.
2. Strategy (Calculated) Risks: A foodservice may take a calculated risk to expand its dining room or parking lot in order to generate more sales. This is an example of a positive risk.
3. External Risks: These are risks due to events outside of the foodservice (such as natural disasters or an economic recession) and the foodservice can only control how it reacts. Monitoring these risks relies on the knowledge, experience, and intuition of managers.

Businesses that frequently take risks are said to be "risk tolerant." Nonprofits, healthcare, and on-site operations tend to be "risk averse," or reluctant to take risks.

When developing your risk management plan, it is good to start a dialogue with all of the people involved. Your goal is to prevent harmful events that will negatively affect your customers, employees, facilities or reputation. Work together to identify all of the potential risks to which your business may be vulnerable.

Most risk-management processes follow the same basic four to six steps, which is very similar to the continuous quality improvement cycle. If you run each of your identified risks through this cycle, you will have helped your organization reduce its vulnerability.

1. Assess: Identify and describe each risk that might affect your organization or its ability to function and to achieve its goals and objectives. Determine the probability of each risk (a fall or burn, a food poisoning, a robbery, liability, or lawsuit), and the potential consequences (financial, reputation, quality).
2. Evaluate: Rank each risk by considering how likely it could happen along with the seriousness of its potential consequences. Use this to decide which risks are serious enough to require a plan of action.
3. Manage: Manage each risk. During this step, you must develop a plan to reduce the possibility of the negative event. In the case of bad weather or utility problems, which you obviously cannot control, you can develop emergency plans. Plans to reduce the possibility of preventable risks may include strategies such as staff education, manual and wireless monitoring of temperatures, frequent cash removal from registers, improved lighting or ventilation, or a new preventive maintenance program for equipment.
4. Monitor and review. For this step, you monitor negative risk events (incidents) that do occur and evaluate your risk management failures and successes.

Understanding risk helps a business to thrive. When you are proactive with your risk management plan, you keep the business safe by reducing potential threats to your customers, patients/residents, employees, stakeholders and the reputation of your brand.

EMERGENCY/DISASTER PLANNING

According to the World Health Organization (2019), a **disaster** is "a serious disruption of the functioning of a community or a society causing widespread human, material, economic or environmental losses, which exceed the ability of the affected community or society to cope using its own resources." Disasters can be due to natural hazards, such as flooding, or manmade hazards, such as terrorism. **Emergencies** are similar to disasters but generally occur on a much smaller scale and the affected community/business can often handle the problem without asking for outside help. Examples of emergencies include local power outages, gas leaks, water main break, fire, flood, loss of Internet service, security breach of computers/software, active shooter incidents, robbery, or the fire suppression system in the kitchen going off accidentally and covering everything with foam. Disasters are of a greater magnitude and are more likely to result in widespread destruction of property and infrastructure and have the potential to cause loss of life, evacuations, and *extended* power and water shortages.

Foodservices need to develop plans to deal with disasters and emergencies. For foodservices located in a state such as Florida, plans should be developed to deal with hurricanes. Even if a foodservice does not need to remain open during a hurricane, there should be a plan for shutting down, informing the employees, and protecting the building and food supplies. The Food and Drug Administration's *2017 Food Code* and the Small Business Administration (2019) recommend that your emergency/disaster plans address the following situations.

1. Loss of power. This includes electric and gas, which affect cooking, lighting, and your ability to keep foods cold and out of the temperature danger zone. You may not be permitted to operate without electric power if your ventilation and fire suppression systems rely on electric. Some foodservices do maintain backup generators to remain open or to at least maintain refrigerator and freezer temperatures (preventing food loss).
2. Lack of clean water. If you lose your water supply, you lose your restrooms, handwash sinks, and beverage dispensing systems including coffee makers and soda fountains. You will also lose your dishwashing and sanitizing capabilities. You may not operate under these conditions. If you experience contaminated water, you will have to disinfect all of your water-fed equipment before reopening.
3. Fire. Employees should all be trained on procedures for when there is a fire, including how to call the fire department. Training on how to use alarm stations, fire extinguishers, the fire suppression systems and blankets should be done at least once a year.
4. Medical emergencies. Employees need to know how to react to falls, cuts, choking, burns, heart attacks, workplace violence, allergic reactions, and other medical emergencies. Some should be familiar with first aid, choking prevention, cardiopulmonary resuscitation, and the use of defibrillators (if available).
5. Infectious disease/pandemic. Infectious diseases, such as colds or measles, are caused by organisms such as viruses, bacteria, fungi, or parasites. Whereas an epidemic is when a disease affects a large number of people within a community or region, a **pandemic** is when a new disease spreads around the world. COVID-19, the coronavirus disease discovered in 2019, started a pandemic. Symptoms of the disease typically include fever, cough, and shortness of breath and the illness can vary from mild to severe. Because of infectious diseases such as COVID-19, foodservices may not be able to remain open, and when open, they must employ a variety of techniques to limit its spread.

For example, since COVID-19 spreads mainly from person-to-person when within about 6 feet of each other, employees need to wear masks and stay at least 6 feet apart to avoid infection from respiratory droplets when an infected person coughs or sneezes.

6. <u>Sewage back-up or inadequate trash removal</u>. The presence of sewage or infectious waste is considered an immediate health hazard and will force you to cease operations. Excessive trash will draw vermin (flies and rodents), which are an immediate health hazard.

7. <u>Outbreak of foodborne illness or act of food terrorism/sabotage</u>. Any apparent outbreak of foodborne illness, or the suspected presence of toxic, infectious, or poisonous substances in foods will constitute an imminent health hazard and you will be forced to close. You may not reopen until you get permission from the public health authority. According to the Johns Hopkins Center for Public Health Preparedness, **food terrorism** is "an act or threat of deliberate contamination of food for human consumption with chemical, biological, or radionuclear agents for the purpose of causing injury or death to civilian populations and/or disrupting social, economic, or political stability" (Johns Hopkins Center for Public Health Preparedness, 2019). Protecting the food supply is of utmost importance. Appendix F contains a checklist for foodservices to see how vulnerable they may be to a possible food terrorism threat.

8. <u>Severe weather/earthquake</u>. Severe weather or earthquakes can cause problems already discussed, such as loss of power or clean water. If your foodservice will not operate under these conditions, the person in charge must be responsible for making the decision on when to close and then when to reopen.

9. <u>Interruption in communication (phones) or Internet/online access</u>. This will affect ordering, deliveries, wireless monitoring, and credit card sales. Job one is to put an alternate communication system in place with a means to communicate with staff.

10. <u>Active shooter situations</u>. Plan how to react to someone presenting with a gun or other weapon. The Federal Emergency Management Agency has excellent resources on this topic.

11. <u>Evacuation or shelter-in-place plan</u>. Ensure staff safety by having guidelines for when to stay and when to leave the building(s) that house your business. Plan for where to meet outside the building, choose the most secure rooms to shelter in place, and set up a building lockdown procedure. Recorded instructions can be sent over public address systems as well.

Appendix F includes a form that can help guide you through the process of developing an emergency response plan.

Your emergency/disaster plan should be thorough and available on paper and posted online so employees can access it from home. Once you activate all or a portion of your emergency plan, you need to determine if it is legal for you to continue operation. The *2017 Food Code* states that you may not operate if you have an imminent health hazard, such as sewage backup, fire, or extended loss of water or electrical service.

Emergency/disaster planning for healthcare facilities is even more detailed. The primary objective of the plan is to continue to provide nutritionally adequate meals and water for patients/residents, employees, and anyone else who may enter the facility. Both the Centers for Medicare and Medicaid Services and The Joint Commission, who perform inspections of many healthcare facilities, require an "all hazards" approach to assess risk for patients, staff, and visitors during a disaster or emergency (CMS.gov, 2016). The CMS guidelines require that each facility do the following (CMS.gov, 2019).

- Perform a risk assessment and develop an emergency plan for possible emergencies and geographic disasters (such as hurricanes, earthquakes, etc.).

- Develop policies and procedures for these emergencies/disasters, including emergency meal plans that meet the needs of all diets as well as potable water (generally 1 gallon/person/day), arrangements with vendors to receive food and other supplies *before* the emergency, and the ability to provide three to 10 days of meals and beverages (depending on the severity of the emergency/disaster). Policies and procedures must be reviewed annually.
- Include a communication plan that complies with federal, state, and local health departments.
- Have alternate sources of energy (such as backup generators) to keep food at safe temperatures, provide lighting, and detect and extinguish fires.
- Post emergency procedures.
- Provide annual training including practice drills.
- Evaluate and improve your emergency/disaster plan yearly.

In many situations, the foodservice will change over to an emergency menu that is easier to prepare than the regular menu and has fewer choices, although it must still meet nutritional requirements. For example, instead of offering eggs, pancakes, fruit juice, toast, cold cereal, and milk at breakfast, the menu may just offer fruit juice, cold cereals, milk, and muffins or bagels—all cold foods. Lunch menus often offer cold sandwiches and dinner menus may offer easy-to-heat up entrées, such as lasagna. The menu is determined in part by how many employees will be available, which equipment is on emergency power, and the number of modified diets that must continue to be served. A disaster plan often includes standing orders with vendors to deliver predetermined amounts of supplies to your facility with a phone call. Many facilities will also have some emergency meal supplies on hand at all times.

SPOTLIGHT FOODSERVICE OPERATIONS DURING THE COVID-19 PANDEMIC

When the coronavirus crisis hit in March 2020, some restaurants closed completely while others remained open for takeout, curbside service, or delivery. Depending on the local or state government, some restaurants were able to reopen with some table service if they made some changes to it. Meanwhile on-site foodservices in hospitals, retirement facilities, assisted-living facilities, nursing homes, and other healthcare facilities continued to serve meals but with many changes to menus, styles of service, and more. Even though K–12 schools were mostly closed, many school foodservices made to-go breakfasts, lunches, and snacks for families to pick up.

Some changes that foodservices had to make during this time are described here.

1. Employee health had to be managed differently. Employees were informed not to come to work if they were sick or had any symptoms associated with COVID-19. If an employee was sick at work, they were sent home right away. Many foodservices also prescreened employees as they came to work by taking temperatures and asking about symptoms. Employees were also encouraged to self-monitor for signs and symptoms. If an employee came down with COVID-19, others who may have been in contact with this infected employee were informed as well as authorities responsible for contact tracing if required.

2. **Social distancing** (keeping six feet away from other people) had to be implemented and **Personal Protective Equipment (PPE)** used. Foodservices had to make it possible for employees to be six feet apart from each other while working or taking a break and at least six feet from customers. Customers in a line or waiting area had to be kept from getting too close and tables had to keep groups of customers six feet apart. To help customers maintain social distancing, self-serve food bars, buffets, and beverage stations were also discontinued. Self-service was especially a problem if customers used common utensils or dispensers. Technology, such as tablets for ordering or contactless payment options, as well as physical barriers such as Plexiglass at a bar or cash register, also helped maintain social distancing. In addition, signs were posted to remind everyone to social distance. Many employees were also required to use PPE such as masks (or face coverings) and sometimes

(continues)

SPOTLIGHT FOODSERVICE OPERATIONS DURING THE COVID-19 PANDEMIC (continued)

gloves to prevent disease spread. If not required by law, the Centers for Disease Control and Prevention (CDC) recommended the use of face coverings (which should be cleaned daily if not disposable). Healthcare foodservice employees had to wear gloves and masks when handling trays, dishes, and utensils of patients with COVID-19.

3. <u>Handwashing and sanitizing surfaces became more important than ever</u>. Handwashing is always important for foodservice employees, but even more important during a pandemic. Handwashing or using a 60% alcohol-based hand rub (when handwashing is not available) is a simple yet effective way to remove or inactivate the virus and prevent its spread. Employees were also reminded to avoid touching their faces, cover coughs or sneezes with a tissue, and use gloves to touch ready-to-eat foods. Cleaning and disinfecting became all important as employees needed to spend more time disinfecting surfaces touched by employees or customers such as door knobs, digital ordering devices, check-out counters, and even menus (some foodservices switched to electronic menus or paper menus to be used once). Equipment used for deliveries, such as coolers and insulated bags, were routinely cleaned and sanitized. Hand sanitizer was made available to customers.

4. <u>Menus were often revised</u>. To streamline operations, some menu items were taken off the menu. Because of food supply shortages and increased prices for some ingredients, additional menu items were either removed or modified. Especially during periods when Americans were told to stay home, many foodservices focused their menus on what worked well for pickup and delivery, and also offered new items such as family meals or cocktails to go. Hospital foodservices benefited by switching to a simplified menu because many hospitals had to prepare more meals with less staff.

5. <u>Service included more remote ordering, pickup, and delivery</u>. The safest way to get food to restaurant customers was by having customers order and pay online or through a phone app, and then use either curbside delivery (place the bag in the car away from the driver) or "contactless" delivery (no face-to-face between the customer and delivery driver). Often, a text, phone call, or doorbell was used to alert a customer that the food was on their doorstep. To make customer pickup safer, outside (or inside) areas were designated for pick-up and often used floor markings to keep customers apart. In many healthcare environments, taking menu selections by phone was safer than face-to-face.

As with any disaster, each foodservice handles its challenges in a way that works best for their operation. When you consider the wide variety of foodservices, each has its own unique challenges. For example, many college and university foodservices closed up or fed smaller numbers of students due to COVID-19, so they had to make a lot of decisions on what to do with all of the food in their storerooms, refrigerators, and freezers. Meanwhile, many K–12 foodservices had to scramble to get food supplies to make two brownbag meals plus snacks for each student and then figure out how to distribute the meals to the students. Providing meals to hospital patients in their rooms did not change much, but long-term care foodservice, which had always focused on dining room service, suddenly had to make meal trays to be delivered to residents' rooms. This required employees to transition to trayline assembly and deliver trays. In addition, new equipment had to be purchased, such as domes for plates so the food was covered during transport.

12.3 PLAN YOUR OWN TIME

Time is a valuable resource that many managers and employees waste without even realizing it. **Time management** refers to techniques that help you accomplish more and get better results, which can be very helpful when building a career.

Before you can manage your time better, the first thing you need to do is learn how you are really spending your time. This can be done by filling out a daily time log (**Table 12–2**) for one to two weeks, noting all activities honestly in the 30-minute slots. At the end of each day, calculate the length of time you spent in each activity noted, such as 20 minutes to coach an employee or two hours in meetings. You can also learn how much time you spend on tasks by using an app, such as Toggl, on your mobile device. This step, whether using paper or your smartphone, helps make

Table 12-2 Daily Time Log

Daily Time Log

Day and Date: _____

Starting Time	Description of Activities	Length of Time	Evaluation of How Time Was Used
8:00 AM			
8:30 AM			
9:00 AM			
9:30 AM			
10:00 AM			
10:30 AM			
11:00 AM			
11:30 AM			
12:00 PM			

you aware of the activities you are doing that waste time so you can better control or eliminate those activities. Major wastes of time for managers and employees include the following.

- Checking/using personal phone frequently.
- Checking corporate email/chat service constantly.
- Surfing on the Internet (YouTube, social media, fantasy football, etc.).
- Excessive socializing with coworkers.
- Time spent trying to find written or electronic files due to poor/no filing system.
- Time spent on tasks that you should have said "no" to or should have delegated.
- Time spent handling interruptions (when many could have been prevented).

Once you have maintained a time log for a week or two, you can analyze the data. Here are some questions to consider.

1. How much time do you spend each day on important or high-priority tasks?
2. How much time do you spend on low-priority tasks?
3. Can you identify any tasks where you spend too much time?
4. Can you identify any tasks where you spend too little time?
5. Are you frequently interrupted during the day? Are those interruptions necessary? Is there some action(s) you could take to decrease interruptions?
6. Are there any distractions or activities that you could decrease or eliminate to enable you to be more productive? If you look at emails too much, perhaps you could check your email only at *two or three designated times each day*.

Many years ago, the Italian economist and sociologist Vilfredo Pareto conjectured that 80% of wealth belonged to 20% of the population and later found that his 80-20 split also worked in other situations. From his work came what is now known as the **80-20 principle**, which states that 80% of results come from just 20% of the actions taken. Applied to time management, the 80-20 principle says that you spend 20% of your time getting 80% of your results, and 80% of your time getting 20% of your results.

To increase the amount of time you spend getting results, you need to set your own time management plan. The first step is to identify your overall objectives and the tasks to accomplish each objective. Divide large tasks into smaller parts in order to get started and keep moving. For example, if an objective is to write next year's budget, break it down into small chunks you can fit it into your schedule.

The second step is to set priorities, a key element to making your time management plan work. A common method for prioritizing tasks is the ABC method, which ranks each task with the letter A, B, or C. The most important and time-urgent tasks on your time management plan are given the letter A, less important tasks the letter B, and the least important tasks the letter C. If you do not need to be personally involved in a certain task and can delegate it to someone else, do so.

So now, you know what you need to do and what tasks are most important. The next step is to plan what to accomplish each day for the week using a daily planner (**Table 12-3**) using either paper or an electronic device (**Figure 12-3**). First, schedule in meetings and appointments that are already set, as well as any blocks of time when you know you will be helping with meal service or other normal responsibilities. Then write in tasks you want to accomplish for each day. Do not fill up all the time slots. Leave some free time to deal with unexpected issues and so on. At the end of the week, when you prepare your time management plan for the next week, look at any outstanding tasks from the current week and add them to next week's plan. As time goes on, you also need to update your objectives/tasks list as some items get accomplished and new ones appear.

The following are additional tips to help use your time more efficiently.

1. Do the most important tasks first. It may also be helpful for you to do the tasks you don't want to do first, because they are the ones most likely to be put off indefinitely.
2. Do the hard tasks when you are fresh. Some people work best in the morning, so that's the time for them to work on harder jobs. Others may work best later in the day.
3. If you need a large block of uninterrupted time, such as two or three hours, try to schedule it at a quiet time of day. If necessary, hide away somewhere.
4. Schedule an hour or so each day when you don't want to be interrupted—unless of course there is a real emergency—and tell your coworkers in advance.
5. Organize your work area and handle paperwork and email efficiently. Use equipment such as letter trays and file sorters to keep track of papers. Under the desk is the most important file: the wastebasket. Don't hesitate to trash or

Table 12-3 Day Planner

Day Planner

Day/Date _____

Time	Task	Priority	Delegated To:
8:00 AM			
9:00 AM			
10:00 AM			
11:00 AM			
12:00 PM			
1:00 PM			
2:00 PM			
3:00 PM			
4:00 PM			
5:00 PM			
6:00 PM			

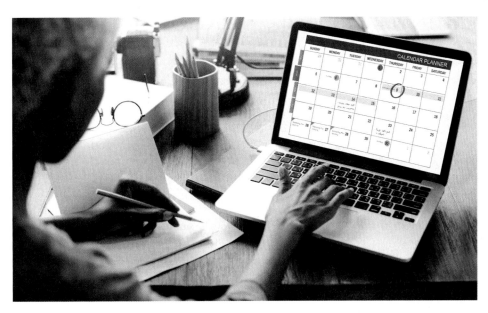

FIGURE 12-3 Keeping an Electronic Calendar

© Rawpixel.com/Shutterstock

file emails. All papers and emails should be handled once and then put where they belong. Keep the desk clear of everything except the current task.

6. During the day, ask yourself frequently "What would be the best use of my time right now?"

7. To cut down on the number of coworkers and employees who drop into your office, close the door when necessary. When someone does come in, stand up and remain standing until the conversation is over. Some people set up certain times when others can come in to discuss something.

8. Have someone screen your telephone calls.

9. When you have a meeting, plan an agenda to pass out to everyone. Also start and end the meeting on time.

10. Avoid digital distraction. Some people schedule two or three times each day to check and reply to email so they can focus on other tasks.

11. Strive to remove distractions from your work day, such as stopping for snacks, making personal phone calls, surfing the Internet, sending personal emails, or playing computer games. Instead, consider completing lower priority tasks on your time management plan if you need a change of pace.

12. Keep socializing to a minimum. Ask friends and family to contact you at work only if there is an emergency.

13. Learn to say no to requests for time when they are unreasonable or unjustified.

14. Train your subordinates well and do not do their work for them.

15. Take regular breaks and take time to eat lunch each day. Having a break from work makes you more productive.

16. If you are a perfectionist and take a lot of time to finish a project, let colleagues evaluate parts of your work so you can get some constructive feedback before the final submission. If you are a procrastinator, focus on *doing (not avoiding)* and keep in mind that your managers are there to help you (Berglas, 2004).

To be efficient at work, you also need to take care of yourself outside of work. Make sure you recharge by getting enough sleep, exercising regularly, spending time outdoors, engaging with others, doing hobbies, and taking a real vacation.

12.4 INTERPRET ORGANIZATIONAL STRUCTURE

Organizational structure refers to the formal arrangement of jobs and positions within an organization, including reporting relationships that will help the people in the organization achieve its mission and goals. A **job**, such as cook, is a group of tasks and responsibilities that an employee is required to perform. A foodservice may have four cooking positions, and each position is either filled or empty. A position is not the same as a job, as each **position** is held by one person and the positions are specific to a given department.

Organizational design is the process of creating the formal arrangement of jobs and positions within the organization so it runs efficiently and effectively. According to **contingency theory**, there is no one best way to design an organization (Burns & Stalker, 1973; Lawrence & Lorsch, 1967a). Duncan (1979) identified factors that can seriously influence organizational design such as the stability of the external environment, size of the organization, and how closely parts of an organization must coordinate with each other. *Managers must consider a number of questions to develop a formal arrangement of jobs/positions.*

1. How do we organize into units and departments so that we can implement our mission and objectives? Related activities, such as food production, need to be grouped together, which is referred to as **departmentalization**. The operations subsystems in the foodservice systems model—procurement, production, distribution and service, and safety/sanitation—provide guidance on how to set up units and departments for a foodservice. Many restaurants split up their activities into two basic departments: front-of-the-house (service) and back-of-the-house. The back-of-the-house department includes several related units: purchasing, receiving, and storage; production; distribution; and sanitation. Organizations often create departments based on functions performed (such as production), which is called a **functional structure**. Organizations may also create departments based on their product (service) lines, geographic regions, or type of customer.

2. How should we divide up the work? Once departments are set up, work activities (such as preparing meals) need to be divided into separate job tasks, which is referred to as **work specialization** or **division of labor**. Employees have specialized jobs in their functional area. For example, the production staff in an upscale restaurant includes an executive chef, sous chef, pastry chef, and several line cooks and assistant cooks. Each of these jobs includes different tasks, such as the pastry chef makes desserts and line cooks prepare hot foods. There are times when work specialization is good for productivity, but there are also times when work specialization leads to boredom for employees. When that happens, foodservices may choose to cross-train employees, meaning they train employees to perform several jobs. For example, hosts can be trained to be servers and servers to be hosts; a drive-through employee can be trained to do other positions in a fast-food restaurant; or a grill cook can be trained to also work as a prep cook.

3. To whom does each position report? In other words, "Who's my boss?" The **chain of command** is the line of authority from the top of an organization down to the lowest position, which can be seen in the organizational chart portrayed in **Figure 12-4**. An **organizational chart** is a "graphic illustration of the organization's management hierarchy and departments and their working relationships" (Lussier, 2019, p. 212-213). Solid lines connecting the boxes show the chain of command. As you can see from this organizational chart, each position reports to just one person, a concept known as **unity of command**. There are additional concepts to understand about organizational charts.

   a. The organizational chart shows the departments and levels found in an organization. The top level encompasses top managers, such as the owner

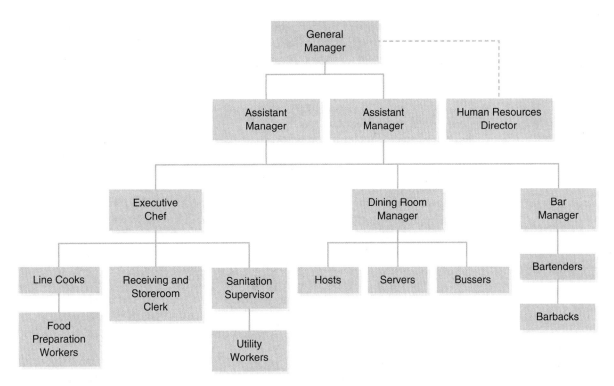

FIGURE 12-4 Example of an Organizational Chart

or general manager in Figure 12-4. Mid-levels managers include the assistant manager, executive chef, bar manager, and dining room manager. At the lowest level of management is where you find **first-line managers** (also called **supervisors**), such as the sanitation supervisor, who supervises the hourly employees. Servers are **hourly employees**, meaning they are paid by the hour and are entitled to overtime pay if working over 40 hours in a week. **Salaried employees**, such as the bar manager, are not paid by the hour and instead earn a yearly salary. In most cases, salaried employees are not eligible to collect overtime pay.

b. On the organizational chart, authority and responsibility are handed down the chart from the top, while accountability travels up the chart. **Authority** is the right of a manager to direct others at work (generally people who are lower on the organizational chart), to make decisions, and to use resources. Authority is not the same as power. **Power** is the ability to influence others' behavior. **Responsibility** refers to the obligation that each employee, at any level, has to carry out certain activities or tasks or see that someone else has done so. When responsibility to complete a task is delegated (assigned) to someone, so is accountability. For example, if the executive chef delegates preparing a catered luncheon to a line cook, the line cook is accountable to get the job done (but the executive chef is ultimately accountable as well).

c. Most of the authority seen on an organizational chart is considered **line authority**, meaning that a manager's position is in the direct chain of command and they direct the work of subordinates. A line authority relationship is shown with a solid line on the organizational chart, whereas a staff authority relationship is shown with a dashed line. In a **staff authority** relationship, the person(s) has responsibility to advise, assist, or support other people instead of having formal authority over people. For example, in Figure 12-4, you see that the Human Resources director has a staff authority relationship. Staff people, such as those who work in human resources, public relations, research and development, or information technology, are not directly responsible for the daily operations. Instead, their job is to help line personnel do their jobs, such as by helping them hire new employees or fully utilize new computer software.

    d. Organizational charts also portray **lateral relationships** in an organization. Each position that appears on the same horizontal line is often on a similar level in the hierarchy.

4.   <u>How many people should report to a manager?</u> Of course, there are many factors that affect this decision. An upper-level manager with well-trained, responsible subordinates can obviously accommodate more employees than a first-line manager with inexperienced subordinates who need close supervision. The **span of control** (also called **span of management**) is the number of subordinates a manager has. The span of control should not be so wide that the manager can't effectively get the job done or so narrow that it is inefficient. The span of control depends on considerations such as the nature of the work, employees' abilities, and organizational policies. Organizations have been trending toward a wider span of management (more subordinates under a manager), which has been found in some organizations to lead to empowered employees, faster decision making, and lower costs. A wider span of management decreases the number of levels needed in the organization, which can indeed speed up the decision-making process.

5.   *At what level should decisions be made?* When top management makes more of the key decisions with little or no input from lower levels, authority is said to be more centralized. On the other hand, when lower-level managers and employees are more involved in making key decisions, authority is said to be more decentralized or distributed across all levels. On a continuum from centralized to decentralized authority, most organizations try to find a balance somewhere in between the two extremes. There are certainly situations when centralized authority is more appropriate, such as when an organization is facing a crisis or lower-level managers lack the experience or desire to be involved in decision making. Decentralized authority works better when lower-level managers are skilled and want to be empowered and/or the organization needs to respond quickly to changes in the environment, such as competitors offering lower prices. Since first-line foodservice managers and their employees are closer to the customer, they are often in the best position to understand and remedy service issues.

6.   <u>How do we get all levels and all employees to work together?</u> Lawrence and Lorsch (1967a) found that organizations must balance differentiation (organizing into departments) with integration to be successful. **Integration** is the need to coordinate efforts throughout the organization to create a smooth workflow and meet goals. Cross-functional teams and liaison roles are two examples of integration. A **cross-functional team** includes employees from different functional areas (departments) of the company who work on a common project/ goal. For example, Shake Shack has used teams with members from operations, culinary, supply chain, marketing, design, and real estate to develop new business opportunities ("Shake Shack Shuffles," 2019). A manager may also be given a task to act as a **liaison** between their department and other managers in other departments. Through meetings, these managers help coordinate activities and keep communications open. Coordination and collaboration between individuals, groups, and departments are necessary so everyone is working together toward common goals.

A number of researchers have discussed key characteristics of two organizational forms: **mechanistic (bureaucratic)** or **organic** (Burns & Stalker, 1994; Lawrence & Lorsch, 1967b; Morand, 1995). Most organizations are somewhere on

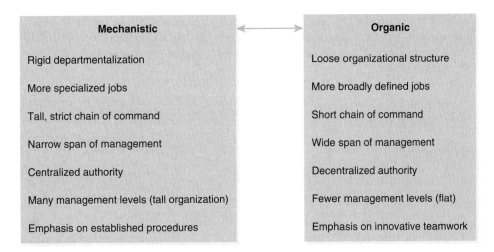

Mechanistic	Organic
Rigid departmentalization	Loose organizational structure
More specialized jobs	More broadly defined jobs
Tall, strict chain of command	Short chain of command
Narrow span of management	Wide span of management
Centralized authority	Decentralized authority
Many management levels (tall organization)	Fewer management levels (flat)
Emphasis on established procedures	Emphasis on innovative teamwork

FIGURE 12-5 Continuum from Mechanistic to Organic Organizations

the continuum between mechanistic and organic and lean more toward one or the other (**Figure 12–5**).

For an example of a mechanistic (bureaucratic) organization, consider when you have visited your local motor vehicle office to get a driver's license or register a car. From the moment you get there, you can see that many of the employees are specialized and only handle certain types of transactions, such as taking the photo for your driver's license. The employees follow strict procedures to handle your request and do not hesitate to call their supervisor if they are not sure about how to handle something.

For an example of an organic company, consider the technology companies like Apple or Google. These companies tend to have fewer levels of management and are quite flexible compared with the rigid mechanistic organization. Jobs are more broadly defined and employees often work in teams that have quite a bit of authority. Many of the jobs are more professional (and creative) than those found in bureaucratic companies and the employees are expected to act professionally and handle diverse types of problems. The employees don't need a lot of rules or supervision, so a manager can have quite a large number of subordinates (wide span of management).

The characteristics of mechanistic organizations are best for companies operating in a fairly stable environment in which each day has a steady routine and well-defined tasks, such as foodservice operations. The flexibility of organic organizations works best in uncertain environments so that they can stay open and respond to environmental changes. When trying to innovate, the looser structure and free-flowing information of a more organic organization works well. A highly organic organization would not be able to put out 500 meals a day. Although a multiunit restaurant chain could be more organic in its upper- and mid-level management levels, it needs to lean toward being more bureaucratic at the unit level due to the steady routine and well-defined tasks.

12.5 ANALYZE AND DESIGN JOBS

Job analysis involves examining an existing job to get a picture of exactly what is involved, including tasks or work activities, responsibilities, work conditions, interactions with others, equipment used, supervision needed, and qualifications. There are a number of job analysis methods, such as a work diary or log, questionnaire, interview, or observation to learn about which tasks are performed, how often they are done, their relative importance, and skills needed for the job. The use of several methods increases the reliability of the data. Job analysis should always focus on the job itself, not the actual person doing the job. The primary purpose of job analysis is to write or revise **job descriptions** (responsibilities and tasks of a job) and **job specifications** (minimum qualifications for a job); important documents used to guide hiring, training, and evaluation of employees.

A job description (**Table 12–4**) lists the responsibilities and tasks that a job entails and describes the job setting. The job description is very helpful when recruiting applicants and gives them a clear understanding of what is required and what a day on the job may look like. It also shows where the employee fits into the organization, sets clear expectations, and helps to set an appropriate rate of pay. You should not base the job description on the capabilities and skills of the person in the job but should base it on the department's needs. Every position in a foodservice needs a job description and they should be reviewed periodically to make necessary changes.

A job description generally includes the following information.

1. Job identification. Some basic information is normally given at the beginning of the job description, such as the job title, the department the job is in, the position that supervises this job, exempt or nonexempt status, and salary information. An exempt job is exempt from federal minimum wage and overtime pay requirements. A nonexempt job is paid hourly and receives overtime pay when more than 40 hours are worked in one week.
2. Job summary. A job summary should be one paragraph long, but may need to include two paragraphs for some jobs. It need not go into specific tasks but should include a summary of key responsibilities and tasks and any other pertinent

---

Table 12-4 Job Description with Job Specification

Job Description

1. Job Identification

Job Title: Host

Department: Dining Room

Reports to: Dining Room Manager

Exempt or Nonexempt: Nonexempt

Grade: 5

2. Job Summary

Communicates effectively and courteously with guests and coordinates efficient guest seating. Works evenings and weekends.

3. Responsibilities and Tasks

Responsibility: Communicates effectively and courteously with all guests to make them feel welcome.	
Tasks:	1. Answers the phones and takes reservations and answers questions. 2. Greets guests in a friendly and upbeat manner and bids goodbye as they leave. 3. Replies to guest questions quickly, accurately, and politely. 4. Resolves guest concerns and provides service recovery as needed.

Responsibility: Coordinates seating of guests to provide service as quickly as possible.	
Tasks:	1. Keeps accurate reservation records. 2. Maintains an accurate wait list when needed. 3. Promotes efficient seating of guests and minimizes wait times. 4. Directs staff to seat guests and bus tables when needed to expedite service. 5. Provides direction for guests attending private parties.

Responsibility: Provide feedback to management.	
Tasks:	1. Listens and observes the surroundings to pick up on any guest complaints or service issues. 2. Communicates problems to management immediately.

Performs other appropriate tasks as needed and directed by the dining room manager.

4. Job Setting

Works in air-conditioned building, which becomes congested at meal times. Stands and walks throughout most of the shift. Some lifting required. Almost constant interaction with other employees, guests, and management.

5. Level of Supervision

Immediate supervision is received from the dining room manager. This position has no reports (subordinates).

6. Job Specification

Education/Knowledge:

- Must speak fluent English; additional languages are desirable.
- Excellent reading and writing abilities to record reservations.
- Basic math skills.

Work Experience:

- At least one year of customer service experience in a retail or restaurant setting.

Skills and Abilities:

- Demonstrated ability to interact effectively and courteously with guests, employees and third parties.
- Must be able to read, review, and understand seating charts.
- Works quickly and accurately with an attention to detail.
- Set priorities. Use discretion and exercise good judgment.
- Works with frequent interruptions.
- Maintains a positive, professional attitude.
- Carries or lifts items weighing up to 40 pounds.
- Requires standing for long periods, walking, kneeling, bending, pushing/pulling, holding/lifting, twisting, and reaching.
- Must be able to stay in one location, such as at the entrance, for long periods of time.
- Must be able to work evenings and weekends.

information such as working weekends. The job summary is often used in job postings.

3. <u>Responsibilities</u>. Responsibilities are listed next, as seen in Table 12-4. Most jobs have anywhere from two to six areas of responsibility, such as receiving incoming food and supplies, preparing soups and sauces for lunch and dinner, or serving guests. It is important to separate out the job's responsibilities and then list them in order from most important to least important.

4. <u>Tasks</u>. Under each responsibility, there is a list of tasks that must be performed. Each task should begin with an action verb such as "monitor" or "prepare." Tasks includes details on the "what" and "how" of the job. The "what" refers to the nature of the specific tasks that make up the overall responsibilities. "How" refers to the techniques and methods, resources, guidelines, and controls involved in a job. Employees use various resources in performing job duties, such as tools, equipment, and other work aids. Guidelines are the policies and procedures and standard practices followed in a foodservice. Controls refer to the amount of supervision from above that the job requires. When the job tasks are well written, they communicate the scope, complexity, and impact of a job.

5. <u>Job setting</u>. The working conditions should be described along with any physical or lifting requirements. For example, the job description may mention that most work is completed in an air-conditioned kitchen that is busy and noisy during peak meal times. This section also details the level of communication this position has with others in the organization. For example, it may state that the position has frequent contact with delivery drivers, the chef, and kitchen staff.

6. <u>Level of supervision</u>. It should be noted how much supervision this position receives as well as if the position has subordinates (and if so, how many).

Many organizations also like to put a statement at the bottom of the job description that states that an employee must complete "other duties as assigned" to cover other possible situations.

Some job descriptions also include **performance standards**—in other words, how well parts of a job must be completed. Performance standards provide a basis for measuring performance. For example, if a server is responsible for stocking the service station in the dining room before meals, the performance standard may be to "stock the station according to standard procedures completely and correctly in 10 minutes or less at least 30 minutes prior to the start of service." In a healthcare foodservice, the ability of a foodservice director to contain food costs could be measured by the food cost percentage each month. Performance standards must be specific and clear as well as measurable.

Job specifications list the minimum qualifications for a specific job and are often stated at the end of the job description (as seen in Table 12-4) or in a separate document. When developing a job specification, you have to consider what knowledge, skills, and abilities (referred to as KSA) are needed to do the job. Knowledge consists of a body of information an employee must have to successfully perform the job and its components. A skill is an individual's proficiency at performing a task, such as forecasting production needs or preparing a budget. Whereas skills are learned, abilities are more innate—such as the ability to prioritize, work well with others, or communicate well verbally. Job specifications often include sections such as the following.

- Minimum education (such as high school or college degree)
- Additional knowledge requirements (such as legal interviewing practices)
- Minimum relevant work experience (such as two years as restaurant server)
- Skills and abilities (such as lift 50 pounds, analyze financial reports, utilize Microsoft Office programs, work independently, or have excellent interpersonal skills)
- Other requirements (such as must have valid Driver's License, pass criminal background checks or child abuse clearance)

When *new jobs* are created, **job design**—the process of identifying tasks and responsibilities to form a complete job—is used. How jobs are designed is so important because it affects both employee productivity and satisfaction. While improving efficiency is one goal of job design, another is to consider the employee's well-being. A manager can also use job design methods to redesign *existing jobs*. Job design methods include job expansion and job simplification. **Job expansion** is when jobs are made less specialized, and this is accomplished through job enlargement, job enrichment, or job rotation.

- **Job enlargement**, also called horizontal loading, widens the scope of a job by asking an employee to perform a greater number of tasks. The tasks are similar to the current ones but offer more variety. The hope is that adding tasks will decrease boredom or downtime. An example of job enlargement is evident in a Subway store where each employee can bake the bread, take orders, make sandwiches, and handle the payment. Keep in mind that you want to add more variety to a job—not simply more work to be done in the same period of time.
- In **job enrichment**, also called vertical loading, the employee is given more freedom, control, and/or responsibility over their work to make the job more challenging, rewarding, or interesting. Vertical loading refers to adding to a job such elements as allowing the employee to become more responsible for a total job cycle, from planning and organizing to evaluating results. For example, an assistant cafeteria manager may be asked to plan and implement special theme days. Some organizations use flexible work arrangements, such as flextime or telecommuting, to enrich jobs. Flextime allows employees to determine when they start and finish each workday as long as they meet their required hours and work within certain hours.

- **Job rotation** refers to employees who do different jobs on a rotating schedule. For example, crew members in quick service restaurants are often trained to handle several different positions. This helps decrease employee boredom and also increases scheduling flexibility for the manager.

Job design can also involve **job simplification**. Job simplification, reducing the number of tasks that each employee performs, is evident in an assembly line where each employee performs a key task. This improves efficiency. In healthcare kitchens that use traylines to assemble patient meal trays, each employee on the trayline has one task, such as put the entrée on a plate, which then goes on the tray, or pour hot beverages and place on the tray. Job simplification also refers to when a task, such as making hoagies, is broken down into separate steps with the intention of eliminating steps, combining steps, or changing the sequence of steps to work smarter, not harder.

12.6 CREATE AND MANAGE GROUPS AND TEAMS

As a college student, you have no doubt been asked to join other students in a group to answer questions or complete a project. Companies are adopting more organizational designs such as groups and teams at work (**Figure 12-6**). For example, in a healthcare foodservice, a Meal Satisfaction Committee (including the executive chef, several dietitians, tray passers, and dishroom employees who see what foods are returned uneaten) meets monthly to review survey results on how well patients enjoyed their meals. In addition to evaluating results, the committee may develop and implement plans to increase meal satisfaction as needed. In a restaurant, an assistant manager is in charge of assembling the Food Safety Group each month to perform a sanitation inspection of the facility and take appropriate corrective actions.

WORK GROUPS AND WORK TEAMS

Work groups usually include three or more people (often more) who come together to achieve a specific goal(s), and the group includes a clear leader/manager who usually has decision-making authority. Members of a work group share information,

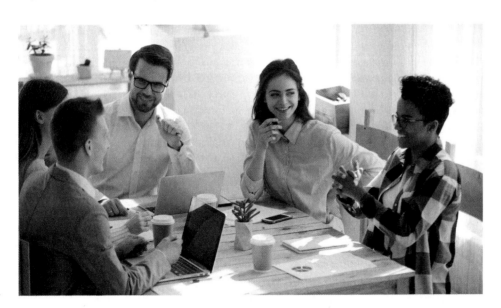

FIGURE 12-6 A Work Group

© Fizkes/Shutterstock

help each other do their jobs more efficiently or effectively, and troubleshoot problems to find solutions or another task. If a work group is in charge, for example, of preparing meals for an elementary school cafeteria, each member performs their part of the process independently until the cafeteria line is ready to open and serve students. Members may help each other out during this process but each job is independent of the other. At the end of the day, the cafeteria manager evaluates how well *each individual* performs.

Work teams are a *very specialized type of group* that are now commonplace in organizations, in part because teams can be more productive than groups (Lorinkova et al., 2013) and can help an organization react quickly to changes in the environment and customer needs, and also stay ahead of the competition. The following is what makes a team different from a work group.

- Work groups can get large in size, but *teams often include just five to nine (sometimes more) members*. If the team is too large, it is difficult to get work done effectively.
- Whereas a group member performs a job mostly independently of other group members, team members *work intensely with each other to complete an entire process*, such as open a new restaurant unit or develop and test new menu items.
- Because team members share tasks and responsibilities, they are evaluated and rewarded for *both how well each person performs and how well the team performs*.
- *Leadership of the team is often shared* among the members. Shared leadership is positively related to team effectiveness (Wang et al., 2014) in part because these teams are more cohesive and encounter less conflict than teams without shared leadership (Northouse, 2016).
- *Leaders of a team empower team members* to work on the task at hand and help the members work together well, whereas group leaders tend to be more directive.

In some cases, there is no clear line between a group and a team. There is certainly a continuum with groups at one end and teams at the other end. However, *the characteristics of shared leadership and working intensely together to complete a process is certainly a team*. In many foodservices, the word "teams" and "teamwork" are frequently used to remind employees to help each other and work together. For example, hourly employees in quick-service restaurants are often referred to as team members (or crew members). Because each employee has an independent job, this is clearly a group, not a team. There is nothing wrong with asking this group to function as a team—but they are not acting as a genuine team. The manager is simply asking the employees to talk to each other and coordinate what they are doing as well as help each other out when possible.

Having groups and teams in the workplace is generally good for performance. According to Jones and George (2018), groups and teams help organizations be more competitive by increasing employee satisfaction and helping companies innovate and respond quickly to its customers. When people work together, often a synergy develops, meaning that the group or team produces something bigger and better than if they had worked individually. The idea of synergy is evident in the saying that "The whole is greater than the sum of its parts." Members of groups and teams bring a wide variety of expertise, experiences, and perspectives to the table so they often come up with more diverse ideas (although they usually take more time to make decisions) than a single individual.

Let's look briefly at some types of groups and teams found in foodservice organizations.

1. **Formal groups** are established by managers for a certain purpose. Every employee belongs to a department so each department is an example of a formal group. A crew of six cooks and cook's assistants who work together are another example of a formal group. Organizations also have **informal groups** that form for social reasons or because members have common interests. For example, several friends who eat lunch together most days are an informal group.

2. A **command group** is made of a manager and the employees they supervise. For example, a bar manager supervises the bartenders and bartender assistants (also called barbacks). This is also known as a functional command group because everyone is from the same department. Most command groups are functional. However, the president of a large organization oversees people in charge of different departments. This command group is, therefore, cross-functional because it includes employees from different functional areas (departments) of the company.

3. **Task groups** (sometimes called task forces) usually include members from different departments (so they are cross-functional) to work on a specific objective. For example, a restaurant may set up a hunger task force with members from front- and back-of-the-house to investigate how to repurpose safe leftovers to needy individuals in the local community. The task force is given the objective and a period of time in which to report back ways to repurpose leftovers. Although task groups often focus on issues that are pretty short-term, sometimes a task group will work on a long-term issue facing the foodservice. When task forces are more permanent, they are often referred to as **standing committees**. Members on this type of group may rotate, so each member is on the committee for a period of time such as one or two years.

4. **Self-managed work teams** are given the responsibility and authority to do what is needed to produce an output with little or no supervision. The team decides how to do the job, who will do the different tasks, and what to do when problems pop up. For example, a product development team for a regional convenience store chain works on developing new products for its customers, such as beverages that reflect current food trends. The team may share leadership, choose a leader, or a leader may emerge over time. Some teams prefer to rotate the leader position.

5. A **problem-solving team** may function as a team, but more often functions as a group, to discuss and come up with solutions for a problem. Quite often, the solutions are presented to a manager for consideration.

6. A **top management team** includes the president and other top executives who develop the mission, goals, and strategy for the organization. This team is definitely cross-functional as it includes people from departments such as finance and operations. It is important for this team to include diverse people with different backgrounds, skills, expertise, and experience. Diversity (including cognitive diversity) helps protect against groupthink. In **groupthink**, group members agree on a course of action that they know is not optimal instead of expressing doubts or disagreeing with the consensus. This can happen when some group members feel a need to conform.

GROUP DEVELOPMENT, STRUCTURE, AND DYNAMICS

So why do some groups and teams perform so well while others are just mediocre at best? There are several sets of factors that influence how well a group or team performs. First, the organization in which a group or team exists can affect it for better or worse. Other important factors include how the group develops over time, how the group is structured, and how the members interact.

First, let's look at how groups develop. Tuckman & Jensen (1977) identified stages that most new groups (and teams) go through over time.

1. Forming stage: As members are together for the first time, they start to get acquainted and are often wary and unsure. Members are trying to figure out what they should be doing (roles), if they will fit in (status), how they will get along (conflict/cohesiveness), and how decisions will be made (decision making). In the case of a work group, a manager will guide members as to what the group

will be working on and what is expected of group members. In the case of a work team, a leader or facilitator may be used to create a welcoming environment and provide guidance.

2. Storming stage: Before a group can work well together, they will go through a stage in which members may question and confront each other's ideas and perspectives on individual roles, acceptable behaviors, leadership, and group direction. Dissatisfaction is common as members are figuring out everyone's relationship to each other as they work on a task. The manager's or leader's ability to listen and deal with conflict or competition is essential in helping the group move forward from this stage. In the case of a self-managed work team with shared leadership, there will likely be conflict about who is functioning as a leader and the hierarchy developing within the team.

3. Norming stage: In this phase, members get to know each other better and relationships develop. Members better understand each other's differences and expectations for each member's role are clearer. Members feel psychologically safe so they are comfortable asking for help and providing ideas and feedback. Although members are enjoying better relationships and uniting around common objectives, disagreements may still re-emerge and the group can definitely slide back to stage two.

4. Performing stage: The group is comfortable working together as cooperation, trust, and a stable structure are well-established. Conflicts still emerge but the group is much better able to deal with them. The group is focused on its goals and working together to achieve them.

5. Adjourning stage: Some groups that are short-term in nature, such as task groups, do end after the task is completed.

Of course, not every group or team will go through these stages exactly as described. Every group or team is different.

Group structure also affects how well a group or team performs. Group structure looks at factors such as the size and composition of the group and the group's formal (appointed) or informal leader. When a group or team is too small, you won't have enough diversity to get lots of ideas and creativity may be more limited too. On the other hand, when a group or team gets too big, it's harder for each member to communicate and maintain a relationship with all of the other members as well as coordinate activities. Members also find it harder to speak up and contribute, which adversely affects motivation and commitment. In response, subgroups or cliques may develop. In a large group or team, it's easier for a member to keep a low profile and put less effort into the group than when working alone (known as **freeriding** or **social loafing**). Creating metrics and tracking data in individual team member performance is a key to controlling this behavior. Making decisions also often takes longer in larger groups.

The size of a group depends largely on what the group needs to accomplish and the variety of expertise and skills needed to do so. Managers need to consider how many group members are needed to complete the group's objectives. The more diverse members are in terms of the capabilities, experiences, and perspectives they bring to a specific project, the better the group or team will perform. More is not always better, as it is definitely easier to share information and coordinate with nine members rather than 19.

The group leader seriously influences the group's structure and whether the group will succeed (Alexander & Van Knippenberg, 2014). To work effectively with group members, a leader needs a number of skills. For example, the leader needs to encourage an open expression of views by asking for and drawing out opinions from all members, not just the ones who speak up frequently. Also, the leader must genuinely want to listen to the members and be an active listener.

Leaders need to develop commitment and enthusiasm among group members for working with each other toward a common objective. Within a group, the abilities of different team members will always vary. When a leader encourages each member to do his or her best, some members will wind up doing more work than others. If the team members are more concerned about the success of the group than keeping tabs on each member, this will not be a problem. To increase commitment, a leader should reward and praise member contributions, show trust and respect to all group members, communicate openly, and be a good role model.

Group dynamics, also called **group process**, is the study of how group/team members interact with each other. Some elements of group dynamics to consider include the following.

1. **Group roles**: A group role is how a group member is expected to perform because of their position in the group. Group roles usually involve how a member works with others to get work done or to maintain good relationships between group members (task and maintenance roles as described next). Sometimes, a group member assumes a disruptive role, which neither helps get work done nor reduces conflict within the group.
   a. **Task roles** are behaviors that help accomplish the group's objectives.
   b. **Maintenance roles** are behaviors that strengthen and maintain the group or team such as giving members support when introducing new ideas.
   c. **Self-oriented roles** are selfish behaviors that disrupt the group such as frequent interrupting.

2. **Norms**: Every group has norms, meaning guidelines or ground rules of how group members will behave. A common group of norms revolve around performance and provide members with cues on how hard to work, how to make decisions, and how to hold members accountable. Other norms address dress, appearance, and social interaction. Examples of norms include "keep an open mind," "treat each other with respect," or "it's okay to not know the answer." A group's norms can strongly influence a member's performance. Members want to conform to norms because they want to be seen as part of the group and not as someone who is "different." Norms are sometimes questioned by members and may need to change over time. Too much conformity is not good and leaders should encourage a balance of conformity and nonconformity to the norms.

3. **Group cohesiveness**: The ultimate purpose of a group is to perform with professionalism and purpose. Groups that are smaller, diverse, and committed to the group's objectives tend to have higher cohesiveness, meaning the team members are connected with each other. Having success as a group also increases its cohesiveness. Because members of a cohesive group actively participate, work together, and recognize member contributions, they can easily outperform an unmotivated group or a group mired in interpersonal conflicts.

4. **Status**: Each person in a group has a status, or perceived ranking, relative to the other group members. That status is based on many different factors, such as how high they are on the organizational chart, seniority, performance, salary, expertise, ability to relate and get along with others, and other factors. Because high-status members tend to have more influence in a group, it's important for a leader to also listen to and include lower-status members in the discussion to keep up group cohesiveness.

5. **Decision making:** Although groups take longer than individuals to make decisions, groups can generate more diverse alternatives than one person alone. A group that makes a decision is also more likely to commit and support it than if they were asked to do so by a superior. Shared decision making, in which all group members have a say and no single person (even the highest ranking) can make the final decision, is becoming more common in organizations. A danger of shared decision making is that some members may go along with a decision even though they do not support it because they feel pressured and/or feel they had to agree with the majority (groupthink).

Understanding group dynamics is important whether you are working in a group or team.

PRODUCTIVE MEETINGS FOR GROUPS AND TEAMS

Planning and having productive meetings is important for both groups and teams. Many people dread going to meetings because they are time-consuming and not always worthwhile. A meeting leader may think the weekly meetings are going well when in fact the attendees think the meetings are too long and are frustrated that a few people constantly take over the discussion. Time wasted on nonproductive meetings costs money as employees could be working on more important tasks. The following are ways to ensure that meetings are an opportunity for employees to share ideas and opinions as well as coordinate and cooperate with one another.

Before the Meeting

- Before calling for a meeting, be sure the meeting is necessary by being able to state a clear meeting purpose and objectives. Don't hold a meeting because "it has always been done that way."
- Get feedback from attendees on when is the best time for the meeting and reserve a room that is conducive to the size of the group. Only ask people who absolutely must be there to attend. If you need someone to attend just one part of a meeting, have them come at a certain time to participate in the relevant segment.
- A few days before the meeting, send out an agenda and let attendees know if they need to read or review anything *before the meeting*. Doing so helps members prepare and know what to expect. The agenda (**Table 12-5**) should list the time and place of the meeting, objectives of the meeting, and the topics in the order that they will be discussed. Some leaders like to list agenda topics as questions the group or team needs to answer (Schwarz, 2015). You may also want to note for each topic whether the purpose is to gather/share

Table 12-5 Meeting Agenda Form			
Meeting Agenda			
Meeting Title / Purpose			
Logistics			
Date:		**Time:**	
Location:		**Conference Details:**	
Meeting Materials Required			
• • •			
Participants			
Facilitator:		**Note taker:**	
Moderator:		**Other:**	
Invitees:			
Objectives:	• • •		

Agenda Topics	Time	Lead

"Facilitation Tip Sheet" by Centers for Disease Control and Prevention. Retrieved from: https://www.cdc.gov/phcommunities/docs/plan_facilitation_tip_sheet.doc

information, gather input for a decision, or make a decision. Sometimes, the facilitator will want to ask a member to take over facilitating a specific topic to which they are closer.

- It is a good idea to put an estimate of how much time will be allotted for each agenda topic as it helps to keep the group on task and lets you know how much total time you need for the meeting. The most important topics should be done earlier in the meeting. This way, if you run out of time, the least important topics are at the bottom of the schedule.

The Meeting Begins

- As attendees file into the meeting room, greet each person and show appreciation for their attendance.
- Start the meeting *on time* by explaining the purpose of the meeting.
- Then you may want to remind attendees of certain meeting rules, such as asking everyone to put aside (or turn off) their phones and laptops. You may also ask for approval of the prior meeting's minutes, appoint someone to take today's meeting minutes, and ask if any agenda topics should be changed or added.
- The leader is supposed to **facilitate** or guide (not direct) the meeting. As a facilitator, you help guide a group through verbal and nonverbal communication, toward the objectives and ensure that all relevant viewpoints are discussed and considered. For example, a facilitator may use a "round robin" technique to get all members (including quiet ones) to take turns giving input on a topic or use body language to signal that a member has spoken enough and others should be given a turn to speak.
- As a facilitator, you must be able to communicate well, listen actively, build rapport with the group, resolve conflicts, build shared commitment to the objectives, develop synergy in the group, and use verbal communication skills such as those listed in **Table 12-6**. The facilitator needs to create an environment in which team members show mutual respect and accept responsibility for their actions.
- When the group needs to make a decision, the facilitator can give their opinion; but the facilitator's main job is usually to have the group reach a **consensus**, meaning that all members can support the decision or at least live with it.

The Meeting Ends

- End the meeting on time and quickly summarize what was accomplished and remind members to complete any assignments for future meetings. Also ask for input on future agenda topics.
- At the end of the meeting, some facilitators like to ask for quick feedback on what the group did well and what could be done differently for the next meeting (known as **plus delta evaluation**).

Table 12-6 Verbal Communication Skills for Facilitators Working with Groups and Teams

Skill Name	Skill Description	Examples
Supporting	Backing a member's right to speak and give opinions.	"Thank you for your comments." "Let's look at and discuss that last comment."
Blending	Finding areas of agreement between two or more members' difference of opinion.	"Let's start from where both of you agree. You do agree that ….."
Accessing	Making sure all members are able to take part in the discussion.	"Bob looks as though he has been trying to get a word in here. Let's hear from him." "Sally, you've discussed several interesting ideas. Could we get some opinions from others now?"
Confronting	Getting the group to discuss a topic it seems to be avoiding. Opposing others' offensive behavior such as putting someone down, dominating a discussion, interrupting, or being negative about an idea before it is fully discussed.	"Nick brought up a topic 10 minutes ago that has so far been ignored." "It appears to me that no one has been able to state more than a few sentences without being interrupted by someone else."
Clarifying	Stepping in to clear up the positions of two or more members disputing a topic.	"I am not sure I understand what Rich and Yuri are saying. I seem to be hearing from Rich that ….."
Processing	Making a statement to get a discussion back on track by calling attention to what is going on.	"Keep in mind that as a team we have decided not to have private conversations during meetings."
Summarizing	Summing up main points, particularly when many ideas are brought up at once.	"Let's state the major discussion points up to now."
Consensus testing	Checking with members for support on an issue.	"Who can support or at least live with this decision?"
Rewarding	Reinforcing contributions and celebrating successes.	"It is time to commend and reward the team for successful project implementation."

Reproduced from Drummond, K. E. (1990). *Human resource management for the hospitality industry.* John Wiley & Sons.

After each meeting, reflect on who participated and how much, how well the group stayed on topic, how attendees behaved or misbehaved, and the level of engagement and energy. Make some notes about what you would might want to work on for the next meeting. Also, consider rotating the leader of each meeting using different group members.

HOW TO DEVELOP EFFECTIVE TEAMS

Much research has been done on team effectiveness. One of the most well-known researchers in this area, J. Richard Hackman, has been studying teams since the 1970s. Many people may think that great teamwork is mostly a result of good leadership at team meetings or members getting along really well. Hackman (2012) suggested that work done by the leader *before the team launches accounts for 60% of team performance*, and the work the leader does after the team launches only accounts for 10% of team performance. Important factors that should be looked at before the first meeting include the following (Hackman, 2012; Wageman et al., 2005).

1.   The mission/purpose of the team needs to clearly laid out and must be able to motivate and challenge members.
2.   The mission or work to be accomplished must make sense for a team to do.

Table 12-7 Questions to Consider to Develop Effective Teamwork

1. Does the team have the resources (such as funding and training) it needs?
2. Does the team have enough authority and responsibility to be truly self-managing?
3. Do the team members agree on the goals and what success will look like?
4. Are the members energized to work toward the goals?
5. Does the team have an appropriate number of members (smaller is usually better) and are members treating others fairly and investing in relationships with one another?
6. Do team members bring a balance of knowledge, skills, and perspectives?
7. Has the team established clear norms on what to do (i.e., get to meetings on time) and what not to do (i.e., withhold important information)?
8. Do the members have a strong cohesiveness?
9. Does the team work together to resolve difficult and controversial issues?
10. Does the team receive coaching and support (not supervision) from a leader/manager?
11. Does the team track its progress and receive honest feedback?
12. Will team members be rewarded for good performance as individuals and as a team?

Data from "The Secrets of Great Teamwork," by M. Haas and M. Mortensen, 2016, *Harvard Business Review 94*, 70–76; "From Causes to Conditions in Group Research," by J.R. Hackman, 2012, *Journal of Organizational Behavior, 33*, 428–444; "Organizations That Get Teamwork Right," 2018, *People & Strategy, 41*(2), 42–45.

3. The size of the team and the mix of their skills, expertise, and personalities should be carefully considered. Bigger is not better. A study by a global management consulting firm, Bain & Company, showed that teams larger than seven people decreased decision-making effectiveness (Larson, 2017).
4. Members should have received teamwork skills training ahead of time. Team members need to be active listeners, effective communicators, committed, flexible, respectful, and problem solvers.
5. Team members should be able to work interdependently to accomplish the mission.
6. The team needs ground rules (norms) that help members work together without friction and support one another.
7. The team approach should be supported within the organization by receiving needed resources (such as information, computers, meeting space, training).
8. Members need to have a similar idea of what success will look like. Then, they are more likely to pull in the same direction.
9. The organization should recognize and reward excellent team members individually and as a group for excellent performance.
10. A team member or external person should be available to keep an eye on the team process (such as task management, communication, decision making, and conflict resolution) and intervene when fine tuning is needed.

Once the team starts meeting, it is also important to build a sense of psychological safety (trust in the team) so members are confident enough to take risks. **Table 12-7** lists questions to consider to develop effective teamwork.

SUMMARY

12.1 Use the Strategic Planning Process

- There are different types of plans depending on the length of time the plan is in effect (short-term, intermediate-term, or long-term plan), how often the plan will be used (single-use or standing plan such as policies and procedures), the degree of flexibility in the plan (specific or directional plans), which level of the business develops the plan (strategic or operational plan).

- Strategic plans are often broader, longer term, and more directional than operational plans.
- Multi-unit restaurant chains and foodservice contract companies often have three levels of management from the top down: the corporate level, the division or business level, and the operational level.
- Strategic planning (Figure 12-2) starts when top management develops the mission statement for the foodservice or reviews an existing mission statement. The mission describes what the business does, why it exists, and the purpose it serves for its customers. Some organizations also have a list of core values and/or a vision statement that describes future expectations. The next step is to do a SWOT analysis to better understand how a business is doing at the present time.
- The next step is to develop goals (broad outcomes) and objectives (more specific and SMART) that flow from the mission statement and build on strengths, correct weaknesses, exploit external opportunities, and counter threats identified in the SWOT analysis.
- The next step is to develop strategies to accomplish each objective. Corporate-level strategies revolve around growth, stability, or renewal. Division-level strategies are adaptive or competitive. Competitive strategies used to beat the competition and make higher profits include the differentiation strategy, low-cost strategy, or a mix of both.
- At the operational level, each department develops strategies to achieve the mission and objectives such as policies and procedures or programs.
- In a large foodservice company with three management levels (corporate, divisions, operations), each division needs to develop its own mission, do its own SWOT analysis, and set goals, objectives, and strategies, just as the corporate level does. In a single foodservice or a restaurant with several locations—the corporate and division levels are the same.

12.2   Plan for Risk and Emergencies/Disasters

- Foodservice managers concern themselves with risks such as foodborne illness, employee accidents, and legal risks. Risks can be categorized as preventable risks, calculated risks, or external risks.
- Managers need to assess, evaluate, manage, and monitor/review risks.
- Emergencies are similar to disasters but generally occur on a much smaller scale and the affected community/business can generally handle the problem without asking for outside help.
- Emergency/disaster planning should address loss of power, lack of clean water, fire, medical emergencies, sewage backup or inadequate trash removal, outbreak of foodborne illness or act of food terrorism, severe weather and earthquakes (as appropriate), interruption in communication, and active shooter situations.
- Emergency/disaster planning for most healthcare facilities requires a risk assessment, emergency plans for each risk, communication plans, alternate sources of energy, the ability to provide three to 10 days of meals, annual training with practice drills, and annual evaluations.
- In many situations, the foodservice will change over to an emergency menu that is easier to prepare than the regular menu and has fewer choices, although it must still meet nutritional requirements. A disaster plan often includes standing orders with vendors to deliver predetermined amounts of supplies to your facility with a phone call. Many facilities will also have some emergency meal supplies on hand at all times.

12.3   Plan Your Own Time

- To manage your time better, you need to keep a daily time log for one to two weeks to gain insight into how much time you spend on important tasks and unimportant tasks such as checking for friends' text messages.
- The 80-20 principle says that you spend 20% of your time getting 80% of your results, and 80% of your time getting 20% of your results.
- To increase the amount of time you spend getting results, you need to set your own time management plan. The first step is to identify your overall objectives and the tasks to accomplish each objective. Divide large tasks into smaller parts in order to get started and keep moving. The second step is to set priorities by, for example, using the ABC method. Finally, use a daily planner to schedule meetings and appointments

and tasks you want to accomplish each day. At the end of the week, when you prepare your time management plan for the next week, look at any outstanding tasks from the current week and add them to next week's plan.

* Additional time management tips are given.

12.4 Interpret Organizational Structure

* Organizational structure refers to the formal arrangement of jobs and positions within an organization, including reporting relationships that will help the people in the organization to achieve its mission and goals. A job, such as cook, is a group of tasks and responsibilities that an employee is required to perform. A position is not the same as a job, as each position is held by one person.
* According to contingency theory, there is no best way to design an organization.
* Managers must consider the following to develop a formal arrangement of jobs/positions.
  * Related activities should be grouped together, which is referred to as departmentalization. Organizations often create departments based on functions performed (such as food production), which is called a functional structure.
  * Once departments are set up, work activities (such as preparing meals) need to be divided into separate job tasks, which is referred to as work specialization or division of labor. Employees have specialized jobs in their functional area, such as line cook or pastry chef.
  * The chain of command needs to be set up so every employee knows to whom they report. In most cases, a position reports to just one person (unity of command). The chain of command is presented in the organizational chart (Figure 12-4), which includes top managers, mid-level managers, and first-line managers (or supervisors) lower down on the chart. On the organizational chart, authority and responsibility are handed down the chart from the top, while accountability travels up the chart. Most of the authority is considered line authority, but some jobs (such as human resources, public relations, or information technology) are considered staff authority because they advise, assist, or support other people instead of having formal authority.

* The span of control (also called span of management) is the number of subordinates a manager has. The span of control should not be so wide that the manager can't effectively get the job done or so narrow that it is inefficient.
* Another aspect to consider is at what level should decisions be made. When top management makes more of the key decisions with little or no input from lower levels, authority is said to be more centralized. On the other hand, when lower-level managers and employees are more involved in making key decisions, authority is said to be more decentralized or distributed across all levels.
* Integration is the need to coordinate efforts throughout the organization to create a smooth workflow and meet goals. Cross-functional teams and liaison roles are two examples of integration.
* Most organizations are somewhere on the continuum between mechanistic (bureaucratic) and organic and lean more toward one or the other. Figure 12-5 demonstrates how these two organizational forms are different.
* The characteristics of mechanistic organizations are best for companies operating in a fairly stable environment in which each day has a steady routine and well-defined tasks, such as foodservice operations. The flexibility of organic organizations works best in uncertain environments so that they can stay open and respond to environmental changes.

12.5 Analyze and Design Jobs

* The primary purpose of job analysis is to write or revise job descriptions (responsibilities and tasks of a job) and job specifications (minimum qualifications for a job), important documents used to guide hiring, training, and evaluation of employees.
* A job description includes a job identification, job summary, responsibilities and tasks, job setting, and level of supervision.
* Job specifications list the minimum qualifications for a specific job and are often stated at the end of the job description (Table 12-4) or in a separate document. They include minimum education, additional knowledge requirements, minimum relevant work experience, skills and abilities, and other requirements.

- When new jobs are created or current jobs are changed, job design—the process of identifying tasks and responsibilities to form a complete job—is used. How jobs are designed is important because it affects both employee productivity and satisfaction.
- Job design methods include job expansion and job simplification. Job expansion is when jobs are made less specialized, and this is accomplished through job enlargement (horizontal loading), job enrichment (vertical loading), or job rotation. In job simplification, the number of tasks an employee performs is decreased, as in an assembly line.

12.6 Create and Manage Groups and Teams

- Work groups usually include three or more people (often more) who come together to achieve a specific goal(s), and the group includes a clear leader/manager who usually has decision-making authority.
- Work teams are a very specialized type of group that are now commonplace in organizations, in part because teams can be more productive than groups and can help an organization react quickly to changes in the environment. The characteristics of shared leadership and working intensely together to complete a process are what distinguishes teams from groups. In addition, teams are evaluated and rewarded for both how well each person performs and how well the team performs.
- Examples of groups and teams in the workplace include formal groups, informal groups, command groups, task groups or task forces, self-managed work teams, problem-solving teams, and top management teams.
- There are several sets of factors that influence how well a group or team performs. First, the organization in which a group or team exists can affect it for better or worse. Other important factors include how the group develops over time, how the group is structured and how the members interact.
- Tuckman & Jensen (1977) identified stages that most new groups go through: forming, storming, norming, performing, and adjourning.
- Group structure looks at factors such as the size and composition of the group and the group's formal (appointed) or informal leader. When a group or team is too small,

you won't have enough diversity to get lots of ideas and creativity may be more limited too. On the other hand, when a group or team gets too big, it is harder for each member to communicate and maintain a relationship with all of the other members as well as to coordinate activities. Members also find it harder to speak up and contribute, which adversely affects motivation and commitment. In response, subgroups or cliques may develop and some members may put little effort into the group (social loafing).

- The more diverse members are in terms of the capabilities, experiences, and perspectives they bring to a specific project, the better the group or team will perform.
- Group dynamics studies how group/team members interact with each other. Some elements to consider include group roles (task and maintenance roles), group norms (ground rules), group cohesiveness (connections between members), status, and decision making.
- Although groups take longer than individuals to make decisions, groups can generate more diverse alternatives than one person alone and are more likely to commit and support it than if they were asked to do so by a superior. Shared decision making, in which all group members have a say and no single person (even the highest ranking) can make the final decision, is becoming more common in organizations. A danger of shared decision making is that some members may go along with a decision even though they do not support it because they feel pressured and/or feel they had to agree with the majority (groupthink).
- Guidelines are given for having productive meetings and important verbal communication skills for facilitators are listed in Table 12-6.
- Many people think that great teamwork is mostly a result of good leadership at team meetings or members getting along really well. Hackman (2012) suggested that work done by the leader *before the team launches accounts for 60% of team performance*, and the work the leader does after the team launches only accounts for 10% of team performance. Important factors that should be looked at before the first meeting are listed.

REVIEW AND DISCUSSION QUESTIONS

1. A plan may vary depending on how long it is in effect. Describe three other ways that plans vary.
2. What is a policy and procedure?
3. Contrast strategic planning with operational planning.
4. Describe the steps in the strategic planning process. What are strategies?
5. What is a mission statement and how is it different from a business' core values?
6. If planning is so important, why do some managers spend little or no time on it?
7. What is a SWOT analysis and what is its purpose?
8. Describe three competitive strategies that can be used to beat the competition and make higher profits.
9. Name four risks that foodservice managers face. Which of these risks are preventable and which are external? Describe the steps in managing risks.
10. Describe the steps you can take to improve your time management skills.
11. Describe four considerations in how to formally arrange jobs/positions in a business.
12. What is a job analysis, job description, and job specification?
13. What are the components of a job description?
14. Give two examples of job design methods.
15. Compare groups and teams. Give an example of two types of groups and two types of teams.
16. Describe the stages that new groups and teams go through.
17. What is group dynamics? Give an example of how it can affect group performance and satisfaction.
18. Give three tips for conducting successful meetings.
19. Give five tips for developing effective teams.

SMALL GROUP PROJECT

For the foodservice concept that you created, complete the following.

1. In Chapter 1, you wrote a mission statement for your foodservice. Now, develop two to three core values for your foodservice.
2. Considering the mission statement and core values, develop one goal for the foodservice along with objectives and strategies to achieve it.
3. Develop two job descriptions (including specifications) for any jobs within the foodservice.
4. Develop an organizational chart for the foodservice.

REFERENCES

Alexander, L., & Van Knippenberg, D. (2014). Teams in pursuit of radical innovation: A goal orientation perspective. *Academy of Management Review, 39*(4), 423–438. doi: 10.5465/amr.2012.0044

Andersson, D., Rankin, A., & Diptee, D. (2017). Approaches to team performance assessment: A comparison of self-assessment reports and behavioral observer scales. *Cognition, Technology & Work, 19*, 517–528. doi: 10.1007/s101111-017-0428-0

Berglas, S. (2004). Chronic time abuse. *Harvard Business Review, 82*(6), 90–97.

Burns, T., & Stalker, G. (1994.) *The management of innovation* (3rd ed.). Oxford (U.K.): Oxford University Press.

CMS.gov (2016). CMS finalizes rule to bolster emergency preparedness of certain facilities participating in Medicare and Medicaid. Retrieved from https://www.cms.gov/newsroom/press-releases/cms-finalizes-rule-bolster-emergency-preparedness-certain-facilities-participating-medicare-and

CMS.gov (2019). Emergency preparedness- updates to Appendix Z of the State Operations Manual (SOM). Retrieved from https://www.cms.gov/Medicare/Provider-Enrollment-and-Certification/Survey CertificationGenInfo/Downloads/QSO19-06-ALL.pdf

Duncan, R. (1979). What is the right organization structure? Decision tree analysis provides the answer. *Organizational Dynamics, 7*(3), 59–80. doi:10.1016/0090-2616(79)90027-5

FIRMA. (2019). Mission statement. Retrieved from https://myfirma.org/history-mission-vision-statement/

Grote, D. (2017). 3 popular goal-setting techniques managers should avoid. *Harvard Business Review Digital Article.*

Haas, M., & Mortensen, M. (2016). The secrets of great teamwork. *Harvard Business Review, 94*(6), 70–76.

Hackman, J. R. (2012). From causes to conditions in group research. *Journal of Organizational Behavior, 33*(3), 428–444. doi: 10.1002/job.1774

Houlder, D., & Nandkishore, N. (2016). All hail medium-term planning. *Harvard Business Review Digital Article.* Retrieved at https://hbr.org/2016/06/all-hail-medium-term-planning

Johns Hopkins Center for Public Health Preparedness. (2019). *Bioterrorism and food safety.* https://www.jhsph.edu/research/centers-and-institutes/johns-hopkins-center-for-public-health-preparedness/tips/topics/food_security.html

Jones, G. R., & George, J. M. (2018). *Contemporary management.* New York: McGraw-Hill Education.

Kaplan, R. S., & Mikes, A. (2012). Managing risks: A new framework. *Harvard Business Review, 90*(6), 48–60.

Larson, E. (2017). 3 best practices for high performance decision-making teams. *Forbes.* Retrieved from https://www.forbes.com/sites/eriklarson/2017/03/23/3-best-practices-for-high-performance-decision-making-teams/#36826fd6f971

Lawrence, P. R., & Lorsch, J. W. (1967a). Differentiation and integration in complex organizations. *Administrative Science Quarterly, 12*(1), 1–47.

Lawrence, P. R., & Lorsch, J. W. (1967b). *Organization and environment.* Boston: Harvard Business School, Division of Research.

Lorinkova, N. M., Pearsall, M. J., & Sims, H. P. (2013). Examining the differential longitudinal performance of directive versus empowering leadership in teams. *Academy of Management Journal, 56*(2), 573–596. doi: 10.5465/amj.2011.0132

Lussier, R.N. (2019). *Management fundamentals: Concepts, applications, and skill development.* Thousand Oaks (CA): Sage Publications, Inc.

Miller, C. C., & Cardinal, L. B. (2017). Strategic planning and firm performance: A synthesis of more than two decades of research. *Academy of Management Journal, 37*(6), 1649–1665. doi: 10.2307/256804

Morand, D. A. (1995). The role of behavioral formality and informality in the enactment of bureaucratic versus organic organizations. *Academy of Management Review, 20*(4), 831–872. doi:10.5465/amr.1995.9512280023

National Restaurant Association. (2017). Be the calm in the storm: Prepare your restaurant for natural disasters. Retrieved from https://www.restaurant.org/Articles/Operations/Prepare-your-restaurant-for-disaster

Nilsen, D., & Curphy, G. J. (2018). Organizations that get teamwork right. *People & Strategy, 41*(2), 42–45.

Northouse, P. G. (2016). *Leadership theory and practice.* Thousand Oaks: Sage Publications.

Pearce, J. A., & Ravlin, E. C. (1987). The design and activation of self-regulating work groups. *Human Relations, 40*(11), 751–782. doi: 10.1177/001872678704001104

Porter, M. E. (1980). *Competitive strategy: Techniques for analyzing industries and competitors.* New York: Free Press.

Reproduced from Alzheimer's Association. Vision statement. Retrieved from https://www.alz.org/about/strategic-plan

Rogelbery, S. G. (2019). Why your meetings stink - and what to do about it. *Harvard Business Review, 97*(1), 140–143.

Schwarz, R. (2015). Design an agenda for an effective meeting. *Harvard Business Review Digital Article.*

Shake Shack shuffles executive team. (2019) *QSR.* Retrieved from: https://www.qsrmagazine.com/news/shake-shack-shuffles-executive-team

Small Business Administration. (2019). Prepare for emergencies. Retrieved from https://www.sba.gov/business-guide/manage-your-business/prepare-emergencies

Tuckman, B. W., & Jensen, M. C. (1977). Stages of small-group development revisited. *Group & Organizational Management, 2*(4), 419–427. doi: 10.1177%2F105960117700200404

U.S. Public Health Service and U.S. Food and Drug Administration. (2017). *Food Code 2017.* Retrieved from https://www.fda.gov/Food/GuidanceRegulation/RetailFoodProtection/FoodCode/ucm595139.htm

Wageman, R., Hackman, J. R., & Lehman, E. (2005). Team diagnostic survey: Development of an instrument. *Journal of Applied Behavioral Science, 41*(4), 373–398. doi: 10.1177/0021886305281984

Wang, D., Waldman, D. A., & Zhang, Z. (2014). A meta-analysis of shared leadership and team effectiveness. *Journal of Applied Psychology, 99*(2), 181–198. doi:10.1037/a0034531

World Health Organization. (2019). Humanitarian health action: Definitions. Retrieved from https://www.who.int/hac/about/definitions/en/

© Denis Val/Shutterstock

Managing Human Resources

LEARNING OUTCOMES

13.1 Apply federal laws affecting human resources management.

13.2 Recruit and select employees.

13.3 Train employees.

13.4 Manage employees' performance.

13.5 Schedule employees.

13.6 Work with unions.

INTRODUCTION

You probably know that a human resources department is involved in attracting and hiring employees. In addition to ensuring that the foodservice has the talented and skilled employees it needs, human resources works to create a positive employment relationship between managers and employees, which is crucial to retain employees and support exceptional work performance. **Human resource management** is an umbrella term that includes how an organization recruits and hires employees, and then manages and develops those employees such that they (hopefully) help the organization meet strategic goals and prosper.

Depending on the size of the foodservice, there may be anywhere from just one person to an entire department responsible for human resource management. However, every foodservice manager gets involves in managing human resources - from interviewing applicants to training new employees and doing annual performance appraisals. Traditional human resource functions include the following.

- <u>Analysis and design of jobs</u>. Human resources can help analyze work and design jobs, including creating job descriptions and determining how the job will fit into the organizational chart and how much it should pay. Every employee who is hired should have a job description.
- <u>Recruiting and selection</u>. This is the overall process of acquiring employees including advertising and otherwise soliciting applicants, screening their qualifications and interpersonal skills, checking references, extending employment offers, and, in some cases, providing orientation to the new job and employer.

- **Compensation**. This is the process of creating and maintaining an internal wage and salary structure and ensuring that this structure is administered fairly and consistently. Specialists in this area also stay current about compensation in other similar businesses in the region and elsewhere.
- Benefits administration. Benefits administration consists of creating benefits packages for employees and assisting employees in understanding and accessing their benefits, such as healthcare, reimbursement for college courses, or a 401K program (company-sponsored retirement account).
- Training and development. This involves teaching employees how to perform their jobs and preparing them for possible promotions. **Employee development** refers to initiatives of both the employer and an employee in which the employee gains more education, skills and abilities, job experiences, and relationships (such as a mentor) to move up the career ladder. Employee development is an ongoing, dynamic process that also involves self-assessment of goals, abilities, and personality.
- Performance management. In most foodservices, supervisors evaluate employee performance at periodic intervals, usually once a year. Performance management includes this annual performance appraisal as well as giving employees feedback and coaching and reviewing performance throughout the year. Performance management may, from time to time, require disciplinary action against an employee when performance consistently falls below standards.
- Employee relations. **Employee relations** is generally described as creating a positive work environment. Employee relations activities range from handling employee complaints and concerns to arranging employee recognition and recreation activities.
- Labor relations. If any employees are represented by a labor union, human resources works on maintaining communication and a healthy working relationship with the union.

As a foodservice manager, you will consult people with human resource responsibilities on any of the above topics. **Figure 13-1** shows the human resource management process from deciding who to hire through to employees being developed to take higher level positions. Human resource personnel are involved in a process called

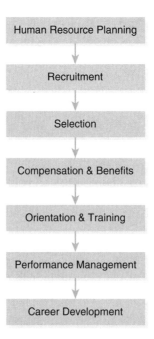

FIGURE 13-1 Human Resource Management Process

human resource planning in which they analyze the present labor supply, forecast how many employees with specific knowledge and skills will be needed in the future, and consistently maintain a skilled workforce that avoids employee shortages or surpluses.

When you consider all of the areas in which human resource managers work, it is easy to understand that they have an important role in building and maintaining an organizational culture. **Organizational culture** encompasses the beliefs, values, practices, and expectations that guide the actions of managers and employees in an organization or business. Organizational culture is created through behaviors such as how a manager handles an employee who is underperforming. The quality of the workplace culture can seriously affect whether an organization succeeds or fails. In successful organizations, the workplace culture encourages listening to others, learning and growing, living by company values such as service, recognizing team members for achievements such as excellent performance, encouraging strong connections among team members, and personalizing the employee experience.

13.1 APPLY FEDERAL LAWS AFFECTING HUMAN RESOURCES MANAGEMENT

From minimum wage laws to age discrimination, there are many federal, state, and even local laws that affect employers. Foodservice managers and supervisors need to be aware of major legislation, as discussed next, and consult with human resources personnel when there are questions. Human resources personnel must ensure compliance with various labor laws.

FAIR LABOR STANDARDS ACT AND THE EQUAL PAY ACT OF 1963

The **Fair Labor Standards Act (FLSA)** establishes minimum wage, overtime pay, and youth employment standards. The federal minimum wage is $7.25 per hour, which was set in 2009. Many states have set higher minimum wage rates that take precedence over the federal rate. The FLSA allows employers to pay less than minimum wage to employees who receive tips, such as servers and bartenders. Businesses are allowed to pay tipped workers as low as $2.13 an hour if those workers earn at least the standard minimum wage of $7.25 an hour once tips are added into their earnings. Be aware that some states set higher minimum wages for tipped workers or ban subminimum wages altogether.

The wage and hour laws specify which employees are considered exempt from the overtime provisions of the law. **Exempt employees** include many executive, administrative, and professional employees who meet special legal requirements, such as being compensated on a salary basis at a rate not less than $684 per week (as of 2020). Employers do not generally require salaried employees to clock in and out each day they work, nor pay them for extra hours worked. On the other hand, **nonexempt employees** are often referred to as hourly employees because they are only paid by the hour for the hours they work. Nonexempt employees must receive overtime pay for hours worked over 40 per workweek at a rate not less than one and one-half times the regular rate of pay. The FLSA does not require overtime pay for work on weekends, holidays, or regular days of rest, unless overtime (over 40 hours in a workweek) is worked on such days.

Child Labor Laws are specific to each state but there are minimum Federal Guidelines. Minors in the age range from 14 to 15 years may work (nonhazardous jobs) no more than three hours on a school day, 18 hours in a school week, and not after 7 PM on a school night. Forty hours is permitted during summer vacation and the day is extended to 9 PM in the summer. There is no limit on the number of hours that 16- and 17-year old employees may work in nonhazardous jobs. The term nonhazardous means that employees under 18 years of age are not permitted to operate or clean any power-driven meat processing machines such as slicers, meat grinders, meat choppers, or patty-forming machines. Employees under 18 years of age are also prohibited from making time-sensitive deliveries, such as pizza deliveries. Fourteen- and 15- year-olds may be employed in restaurants and quick-service establishments outside of school hours in a variety of jobs for limited periods of time and under specified conditions. For example, they are not allowed to perform a number of cooking and food preparation duties, such as they can't cook over an open flame, bake, or operate food slicers, processors, or mixers.

A specific section of the FLSA, as augmented by the **Equal Pay Act of 1963**, requires covered employers to provide equal pay for men and women who are performing the same (equal) work. Work is equal when the skill, effort, responsibility, and working conditions are substantially equal. A higher rate of pay would be allowable under circumstances such as one employee has seniority, works the night shift, or produces more goods. In 1972, coverage of this act was extended beyond employees covered by FLSA to an estimated 15 million additional executive, administrative, and professional employees, including teachers in elementary and secondary schools and outside salespeople.

SOCIAL SECURITY AND BENEFITS LEGISLATION

The **Social Security Act of 1935** established the old-age insurance program, commonly called Social Security, which provides retirement benefits to qualified workers and their family members. The act also established unemployment insurance to help workers who lost their jobs due to no fault of their own and are seeking a new job.

About 90% of American workers are covered by Social Security. Exceptions include railroad employees and employees of federal, state, and local governments who generally have their own retirement plans. Social Security's monthly payments were never supposed to be a person's only income during retirement. They were meant to replace about 40% of someone's preretirement income on average.

To fund this program, employers and employees each pay 6.2% of wages up to the taxable maximum of $137,700 (in 2020) while the self-employed pay 12.4%. The more an employee earns over the years, the more money is paid into Social Security and the Social Security benefit increases.

To be eligible for Social Security benefits, you must generally work at least 10 years. Americans can receive full benefits between the age of 65½, 66, or 67, depending on birth date. They can collect a reduced benefit at age 62 or an increased benefit if they delay taking the benefit up to age 70. If someone collecting Social Security also brings in a substantial income, they will have to pay income tax on from 50 to 85% of the amount from Social Security.

Unemployment insurance is required by the federal government. Each state sets its own eligibility guidelines and administers its own unemployment program using federal guidelines. In order to qualify for unemployment checks, applicants must generally meet the following requirements.

- Work and wage requirements. Most states look at an applicant's time worked and earnings during the "base period"—which is usually the first four out of the last five completed calendar quarters before the claim was filed. Most states also require applicants to have earned at least a minimum amount during the base period.
- Available for work and actively seeking a new job.
- Are unemployed through no fault of their own. An applicant is not eligible for benefits if they quit voluntarily, is out on strike, or was discharged for cause (such as theft or willful misconduct).
- Any additional state requirements.

To fund unemployment insurance, employers pay a small payroll tax to the federal government and also a state unemployment tax. No state imposes the same tax rate on all employers in the state. The size of the unemployment insurance tax is based on the number of laid-off employees a company has had and the cost of providing them with unemployment benefits.

The Social Security Act created the Social Security Administration, which also administers other programs.

- Survivor's Insurance: Established in 1939, Social Security survivor's benefits are paid to widows, widowers, and dependents of eligible workers who have died. The deceased person must have worked long enough to qualify for benefits.
- Disability Insurance: Established in 1956, the Disability Insurance (DI) program provides benefits for workers who become disabled and their families.
- Supplemental Security Income: Established in 1972, the Supplemental Security Income (SSI) program provides financial support to aged, blind, and disabled adults and children who have limited income and resources.

In addition, the Social Security Administration supports national programs administered by other federal and state agencies such as Medicare and Medicaid.

Workers' compensation programs in the United States are state regulated, with laws determined by each state legislature and carried out by a state agency. The programs provide the payment of lost wages, medical treatment, and rehabilitation services to workers suffering from a work-related injury or illness. Employees are not eligible for workers' compensation if the injury resulted from drugs or alcohol or willful disregard for safety rules. Benefits provided are the only benefits available to employees, and employees are not allowed to sue employers for more benefits. Most employers can purchase coverage for workers' compensation through private insurance companies or they can self-fund—meaning they will pay out of pocket when there is a work-related injury or illness. In any case, employees do *not* pay any payroll taxes for workers' compensation. It is considered a cost of doing business.

There are several federal acts that affect health insurance offered by employers for their employees. First, employers who offer medical insurance must meet the requirements of the **Consolidated Omnibus Budget Reconciliation Act (COBRA)** of 1985. Prior to COBRA, employer-provided group health insurance was at risk if an employee changed jobs, was given reduced work hours (and then lost insurance), or got divorced. Under COBRA, employees who lose their health benefits because of these events are able to continue their coverage under the employer's group health plan, usually at their own expense and at the full price (although it is still group rates), for a limited period of time (18 to 36 months). Other possible qualifying events include reduction in the number of hours of employment or termination of an employee's employment for any reason other than "gross misconduct." In addition, if a married employee divorces or separates, the spouse can use COBRA.

The Health Insurance Portability and Accountability Act (HIPPA) of 1996 protects employees' health information while at the same time allowing the flow of health information needed to provide high-quality healthcare and well-being. HIPPA also allows employees who are changing jobs to obtain new group health insurance with preexisting medical conditions (such as cancer) if they had continuous health insurance coverage in the last year (meaning coverage that had breaks of no longer than 63 days).

The Patient Protection and Affordable Care Act of 2010 provides numerous rights and protections that make health coverage fairer and easier to understand, along with subsidies to make it more affordable. State-level insurance exchanges provide a healthcare option for small businesses and consumers. In addition, organizations with 50 full-time employees (or full- and part-time employees equivalent to 50 full timers) must provide essential health coverage that is affordable to at least 95% of their full-time employees or pay a penalty. In addition, organizations with fewer than 25 employees may qualify for tax credits if they buy insurance through the state-level exchanges.

FAMILY AND MEDICAL LEAVE ACT

The **Family and Medical Leave Act (FMLA)** of 1993 makes it possible for an eligible employee (one who has been employed at least 1 year and has worked at least 1,250 hours) to take up to 12 weeks of *unpaid* leave in a 12-month period for certain specified reasons without loss of employment. Qualifying reasons are as follows: the birth of the employee's child or the care of that child up to 12 months of age; placement of a child with the employee for adoption or foster care; care of an employee's spouse, child, or parent with a serious health condition; and the employee's own serious health condition involving the inability to perform the essential functions of the job. Some states provide greater flexibility in defining the caregiver-child relationship. An employee returning to work within the 12-week limit must be returned to his or her original position or to a fully equivalent position in terms of pay, benefits, and overall working conditions.

EQUAL EMPLOYMENT OPPORTUNITY LAWS AND REGULATIONS

Equal employment opportunity (EEO) is a concept that people should be treated equally in employment matters. These laws make it illegal to discriminate against a job applicant or an employee because of the person's race, color, religion, sex (including pregnancy, gender identity, and sexual orientation), national origin, age (40 or older), disability, or genetic information. The laws apply to all types of work situations, including hiring, disciplining, promoting, training, wages, benefits, and harassment. Most employers with at least 15 employees are covered by EEO laws (20 employees in age discrimination cases). It is also illegal to discriminate against a person because the person complained about discrimination, filed a charge of discrimination, or participated in an employment discrimination investigation or lawsuit.

Title VII of the Civil Rights Act of 1964 is a federal law that was a foundation of EEO legislation. As amended by the Equal Employment Opportunity Act of 1972, Title VII prohibits discrimination because of race, color, religion, sex, or national origin in employment decisions. Title VII helps ensure that decisions, such as hiring, firing, promotion, and compensation, are made on job-related criteria.

In another amendment to Title VII, the **Pregnancy Discrimination Act of 1978** forbids discrimination on the basis of pregnancy, childbirth, or a medical condition related to pregnancy or childbirth. Women affected by pregnancy or related conditions must be treated in the same manner as other applicants or employees who are similar in their ability or inability to work.

The **Age Discrimination in Employment Act** (1967) prohibits discrimination in employment decisions against employees who are 40 years of age and older. Complaints about age discrimination is one of the more frequent complaints filed with the Equal Employment Opportunity Commission.

The **Equal Employment Opportunity Commission (EEOC)**, an agency of the Department of Justice, enforces most of the EEO laws, including Title VII, the Pregnancy Discrimination Act, the Age Discrimination in Employment Act, and the Equal Pay Act. The EEOC has the authority to investigate charges of discrimination against employers after an employee files a complaint. The employee is given 180 days from the date of the incident to file charges, and the EEOC has 60 days to investigate the complaint. Their role in an investigation is to fairly and accurately assess the allegations in the charge and then make a finding. If they find that discrimination has occurred, they try to settle the charge. If not successful, the EEOC has the authority to file a lawsuit to protect the rights of individuals and the interests of the public. The EEOC also works to prevent discrimination before it occurs through outreach and education. **Figure 13-2** shows the types of charges filed with the EEOC in 2019.

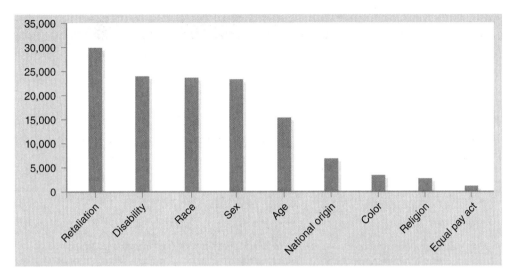

FIGURE 13-2 Type of Charges Filed with Equal Employment Opportunity Commission in 2019*

*Total charges for 2019 was 72,675. Because individuals often file charges claiming more than one type of discrimination, the number of total charges for any given fiscal year will be less than the total number of filed charges.

Data from *"Charge Statistics FY 1997 Through FY 2019,"* U.S. Equal Employment Opportunity Commission 2020. https://www.eeoc.gov/eeoc/statistics/enforcement/charges.cfm

Title VII was further modified and strengthened by the Civil Rights Act of 1991 in an effort to reverse the effects of several U.S. Supreme Court decisions that had the effect of weakening the law. The 1991 legislation also made possible increased financial damages against employers found guilty of discriminatory practices.

You may have seen in a job advertisement that an organization is an affirmative action employer. Some organizations have **affirmative action programs** that recruit and advance qualified minorities, women, persons with disabilities, and covered veterans. Affirmative actions include training programs, outreach efforts, and other positive steps. Affirmative action programs are required of employers who have federal contracts or subcontracts and could also be required by a court as a remedy for past discrimination in the workplace.

Passed in 1990, the **Americans with Disabilities Act (ADA)** affirmed the right of persons with disabilities to equal access to employment, training, services, and facilities available to the public. It defines "disability" as an impairment that substantially limits one or more major life activities (such as seeing or walking), a record of such an impairment, or being regarded as having such an impairment. The ADA covers disabilities such as mental retardation, emotional or mental illness, learning disabilities, and being wheelchair-bound, but not substance abuse or obesity.

In contrast to EEO laws, the ADA not only forbids discrimination but it also requires employers to provide **reasonable accommodation** for disabled individuals who are capable of performing the essential functions of the positions to which they apply. For example, a worktable may be lowered to enable someone to work while seated, a reserved parking spot close to the building made available, the hours of work modified, or job tasks restructured. Many job accommodations cost very little and involve minor changes to a work environment, work schedule, or work-related technologies such as telecommunications devices for the deaf. An accommodation is reasonable as long as it does not impose an undue hardship on an employer, such as a very large expense in a small business.

Amendments passed in 2008 placed new requirements on employers and the courts in deciding whether an individual can be considered sufficiently disabled to receive protection under the ADA. The EEOC is responsible for dealing with complaints filed under the ADA. **Table 13-1** summarizes major EEO laws.

Table 13-1 Summary of Major Equal Employment Opportunity Laws		
Name and Date of Federal Law	**Requirements**	**Covers**
Equal Pay Act of 1963	Requires that men and women performing equal jobs in the same workplace be paid equally.	Virtually all employees.
Title VII, 1964 Civil Rights Act (amended in 1991, 2020 Supreme Court ruling)	Forbids discrimination against someone on the basis of race, color, religion, national origin, or sex. Also applies to gay and transgender workers.	Employers in public and private sectors that have 15 or more employees.
Age Discrimination in Employment Act of 1967	Forbids discrimination against someone who is 40 years of age or older because of age. An amendment to end forced retirement was added in 1986.	Employers with at least 20 employees. Federal government.
Pregnancy Discrimination Act of 1978	An amendment to Title VII that forbids discrimination on the basis of pregnancy, childbirth, or a medical condition related to pregnancy or childbirth.	Employers in public and private sectors that have 15 or more employees.
Americans with Disabilities Act of 1990	Prohibits discrimination against a qualified person with a disability. Requires employers to reasonably accommodate known physical or mental limitations of an otherwise qualified individual with a disability.	Employers in public and private sectors that have more than 15 employees.
Genetic Information Nondiscrimination Act of 2008	Prohibits discrimination on the basis of genetic information.	Employers in public and private sectors that have more than 15 employees.

SEXUAL HARASSMENT

Sexual harassment has been in the headlines for a number of years. Unfortunately, employees in the restaurant industry file more sexual harassment claims than any other industry (Johnson & Madera, 2018). This is not that surprising when you consider that the typical hourly employee is a young woman who reports to a male manager. Because the male manager controls when she works, how many hours she works, and how much money she may make from tips, it creates such a power differential that the woman may feel she can't do anything about being harassed and just puts up with it. If she doesn't want to deal with it, she may look for another job. The turnover rate has been historically high in the restaurant industry.

Customers also engage in sexual harassment and because so many hourly employees rely on tips, they may refrain from complaining. Managers are also likely to be more concerned about an employee sexually harassing another employee than a customer harassing a server. After all, managers are taught that the customer is always right. Managers should exercise sensitivity when balancing complaints about servers or made by servers.

The number of sexual harassment complaints filed with the EEOC and various state agencies continues to increase, as do the numbers of employers and the monetary penalties. In recent years, sexual harassment has been one of the leading causes of legal complaints against employers.

Sexual harassment is a form of sex discrimination under Title VII of the Civil Rights Act of 1964. **Sexual harassment** can be defined as unwelcome sexual advances, requests for sexual favors, and other verbal or physical conduct of a sexual nature when:

- An employment decision (such as being promoted, getting an assignment, or keeping your job) affecting that individual is made because the individual submitted to or rejected the unwelcome conduct; or

- The unwelcome conduct interferes with an individual's work performance or creates an intimidating, hostile, or abusive work environment (Equal Employment Opportunity Commission, 2019).

Certain behaviors, such as conditioning promotions, awards, training or other job benefits upon acceptance of unwelcome actions of a sexual nature, are always wrong. Unwelcome behaviors are considered discriminatory because they treat individuals differently based on their sex.

Unwelcome actions such as the following are inappropriate and, depending on the circumstances, may in and of themselves meet the definition of sexual harassment or contribute to a hostile work environment.

- Sexual pranks, or repeated sexual teasing, jokes, or innuendo, in person or electronic media.
- Verbal abuse of a sexual nature.
- Touching or grabbing of a sexual nature (unwanted).
- Repeatedly standing too close to or brushing up against a person.
- Repeatedly asking a person to socialize during off-duty hours when the person has said no or has indicated he or she is not interested (supervisors in particular should be careful not to pressure their employees to socialize).
- Giving gifts or leaving objects that are sexually suggestive.
- Repeatedly making sexually suggestive gestures.
- Making or posting sexually demeaning or offensive pictures, pornography, calendars, cartoons, or other materials in the workplace.
- Off-duty, unwelcome conduct of a sexual nature that affects the work environment.

A victim of sexual harassment can be a man or a woman. The victim can be of the same sex as the harasser. The harasser may be a supervisor, coworker, or other employee.

Sexual harassment is not limited to the workplace; it is also sexual harassment if it occurs off-premises or at employer-sponsored social events and at private sites if it involves people who have an employment relationship with each other. In addition to involving employees, sexual harassment can involve customers, vendors, and others as either potential perpetrators or victims.

Sexual harassment can result in expensive lawsuits against a foodservice. In addition to monetary losses, if a sexual harassment claim gets a lot of publicity, it will negatively impact the operation. To avoid legal liability and negative publicity, a foodservice needs to do the following.

1. Have a published sexual harassment policy explaining what constitutes sexual harassment and that it will not be tolerated, along with a detailed procedure on reporting and investigating complaints.
2. Train all managers and employees on recognizing and reporting sexual harassment, and how to prevent sexual harassment. An employee who is being sexually harassed by his or her boss must have a way to report the problem that doesn't involve the boss, such as going to someone in Human Resources.
3. Confidentially investigate all complaints and take appropriate actions in a timely manner and protect the victims of sexual harassment as well as the rights of those accused.
4. Train and require managers in customer-service areas, such as dining rooms and bars, to watch for harassing customers and use techniques such as asking the customer to stop and respect the server. If that doesn't work, managers can ask the customer to leave. Managers can also move a server from the table as needed.
5. Create and retain complete and accurate records.

Managers need to be excellent role models and not turn a blind eye to this problem.

Safety and Health in the Workplace

Foodservices have quite a few safety hazards compared with other workplaces, resulting in injuries that may just require first aid to those resulting in an employee who can't return to work for some time. According to AmTrust Financial (2018), a restaurant employee who has a fall that affects the lower back will be out for an average of 23 days. Here are just a few examples of the typical hazards.

- Safety hazards: hot surfaces, slippery floors, sharp blades, steam, flames.
- Chemical hazards: cleaning products, pesticides.
- Biological hazards: bacteria, viruses, molds, insects.
- Other health hazards: heavy lifting, repetitive motions, noise, heat.

Chapter 2 contains a section on how to help foodservice employees stay safe at work.

The **Occupational Safety and Health Administration (OSHA)** is a federal agency (under the Department of Labor) charged with keeping employees safe and healthy at work. The main provision of the **Occupational Safety and Health Act** (1970) is that employers must provide every employee with a safe place to work. In other words, employers must be constantly alert to potential sources of harm in the workplace and remove hazards when possible. Many hazards in a foodservice, such as sharp knives or slippery floors, cannot be removed, so in that case, employees must be trained and monitored for safe practices.

To enforce the Occupational Safety and Health Act, OSHA inspects workplaces and these inspections are not announced in advance. Someone from human resources typically helps the foodservice manager with the inspection. During inspections, OSHA reviews the foodservice's injury and illness records. The inspector will also walk around the premises to do a physical inspection and interview employees. Final findings are discussed with the employer. If violations are found, the employer will be given a reasonable amount of time to make corrections. Inspectors may give citations and also impose fines.

The Occupational Safety and Health Act also asks employees to act in a safe manner as directed by their employers, such as by using personal protective equipment or reading labels of cleaning chemicals, and to report all occupational injuries and illnesses. Employees must receive training about workplace hazards and are allowed to examine safety records. In addition, employees have the right to report unsafe and/or unhealthful working conditions to management and also to file a complaint with OSHA. The rights and responsibilities of workers and employers are listed in **Figure 13-3**.

A business with 10 or more full- or part-time employees must record injuries/illnesses using OSHA Form 300, "Log of Work-Related Injuries and Illnesses." A recordable injury or illness includes any work-related injury or illness that results in loss of consciousness, days away from work, restricted work, or transfer to another job. It also includes any work-related injury or illness requiring medical treatment beyond first aid. Any work-related diagnosed case of cancer, chronic irreversible diseases, fractured or cracked bones or teeth, and punctured eardrums must also be reported (Occupational Safety and Health Administration, 2018).

This information helps employers, employees, and OSHA evaluate the safety of a workplace and implement worker protections to reduce and eliminate hazards. The records must be maintained for at least 5 years, and each February through April, employers must post a summary of the injuries and illnesses recorded the previous year using Form 300A (**Figure 13-4**).

Violence in the Workplace

Workplace violence is violence or the threat of violence against workers. It can occur at or outside the workplace and range from verbal abuse to physical assaults and death. There are no specific OHSA guidelines or standards for workplace violence, but OSHA

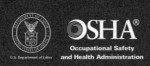

Job Safety and Health
IT'S THE LAW!

All workers have the right to:

- A safe workplace.
- Raise a safety or health concern with your employer or OSHA, or report a work-related injury or illness, without being retaliated against.
- Receive information and training on job hazards, including all hazardous substances in your workplace.
- Request a confidential OSHA inspection of your workplace if you believe there are unsafe or unhealthy conditions. You have the right to have a representative contact OSHA on your behalf.
- Participate (or have your representative participate) in an OSHA inspection and speak in private to the inspector.
- File a complaint with OSHA within 30 days (by phone, online or by mail) if you have been retaliated against for using your rights.
- See any OSHA citations issued to your employer.
- Request copies of your medical records, tests that measure hazards in the workplace, and the workplace injury and illness log.

This poster is available free from OSHA.

Contact OSHA. We can help.

Employers must:

- Provide employees a workplace free from recognized hazards. It is illegal to retaliate against an employee for using any of their rights under the law, including raising a health and safety concern with you or with OSHA, or reporting a work-related injury or illness.
- Comply with all applicable OSHA standards.
- Notify OSHA within 8 hours of a workplace fatality or within 24 hours of any work-related inpatient hospitalization, amputation, or loss of an eye.
- Provide required training to all workers in a language and vocabulary they can understand.
- Prominently display this poster in the workplace.
- Post OSHA citations at or near the place of the alleged violations.

On-Site Consultation services are available to small and medium-sized employers, without citation or penalty, through OSHA-supported consultation programs in every state.

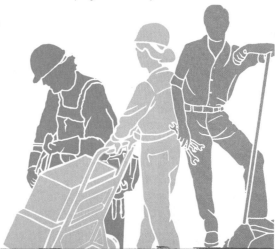

1-800-321-OSHA (6742) • TTY 1-877-889-5627 • www.osha.gov

FIGURE 13-3 Rights and Responsibilities of Workers and Employers Under OSHA

Occupational Safety and Health Administration. Job Safety and Health IT'S THE LAW!. Retrieved from https://www.osha.gov/Publications/poster.html

OSHA's Form 300A (Rev. 01/2004)

Summary of Work-Related Injuries and Illnesses

Year 20____

U.S. Department of Labor
Occupational Safety and Health Administration

Form approved OMB no. 1218-0176

All establishments covered by Part 1904 must complete this Summary page, even if no work-related injuries or illnesses occurred during the year. Remember to review the Log to verify that the entries are complete and accurate before completing this summary.

Using the Log, count the individual entries you made for each category. Then write the totals below, making sure you've added the entries from every page of the Log. If you had no cases, write "0."

Employees, former employees, and their representatives have the right to review the OSHA Form 300 in its entirety. They also have limited access to the OSHA Form 301 or its equivalent. See 29 CFR Part 1904.35, in OSHA's recordkeeping rule, for further details on the access provisions for these forms.

Number of Cases

Total number of deaths	Total number of cases with days away from work	Total number of cases with job transfer or restriction	Total number of other recordable cases
____	____	____	____
(G)	(H)	(I)	(J)

Number of Days

Total number of days away from work	Total number of days of job transfer or restriction
____	____
(K)	(L)

Injury and Illness Types

Total number of . . .
(M)

(1) Injuries ____   (4) Poisonings ____

(2) Skin disorders ____   (5) Hearing loss ____

(3) Respiratory conditions ____   (6) All other illnesses ____

Post this Summary page from February 1 to April 30 of the year following the year covered by the form.

Public reporting burden for this collection of information is estimated to average 58 minutes per response, including time to review the instructions, search and gather the data needed, and complete and review the collection of information. Persons are not required to respond to the collection of information unless it displays a currently valid OMB control number. If you have any comments about these estimates or any other aspects of this data collection, contact: US Department of Labor, OSHA Office of Statistical Analysis, Room N-3644, 200 Constitution Avenue, NW, Washington, DC 20210. Do not send the completed forms to this office.

FIGURE 13-4 OSHA Form 300A

Occupational Safety and Health Administration. OSHA's Form 300A. Summary of Work-Related Injuries and Illnesses. Retrieved from https://www.osha.gov/recordkeeping/new-osha300form1-1-04-FormsOnly.pdf

does require each employer to provide a safe workplace for everyone who works there. The highest-risk areas for nonfatal assaults are retail businesses, such as restaurants, and service organizations, such as hospitals and nursing homes.

Workplace violence may be any of the following types.

1. Someone with no relationship to the business or its employees enters and commits a crime such as robbery or assault.
2. The violence may be worker-on-worker. For example, one employee threatens, harasses, or intimidates a coworker, or becomes physically aggressive toward a coworker.
3. The violence may also be customer-on-worker. Customers can bring violence into foodservices and involve employees.
4. Domestic violence can also find its way into the workplace where the perpetrator shows up at the workplace to carry out acts of violence against someone they know.

The best prevention method is to prioritize a positive and caring work environment by promoting open communication and having ways for complaints and concerns to be expressed in a non-judgmental setting. In addition, employees should be given opportunities to learn new skills and move up the career ladder. When employees exhibit problem behaviors or have performance issues, it is important to maintain consistent and unbiased discipline guided by Human Resources' policies to ensure consistency.

To prevent violence, it is also important for employees to be trained on the following.

- Recognize characteristics of an employee or customer who is more likely to become violent at some point. There is no consistent profile to describe a person who will commit violent acts in the workplace, but violence is often perpetrated by someone who has the following characteristics.
    - Is experiencing family problems, financial instability.
    - Has problems related to drug or alcohol abuse.
    - Has a history of violence or dramatic mood swings.
    - Is a known aggressive personality.
    - Is experiencing certain mental conditions such as depression.
    - Possesses a poor self-image or low self-esteem.
    - Has attendance problems and/or inconsistent work patterns and concentration.
- Alert managers to employees who are having some of the problems listed above. Many larger businesses offer free and confidential counseling programs called **employee assistance programs (EAPs)** for employees with problems such as addiction, family problems, stress, and financial problems. EAP programs are voluntary and offer short-term counseling, referrals, and follow-up services to employees with personal and/or work-related problems. The EAP programs fall under the Human Resources department, but the programs are usually run by an outside company. As appropriate, managers can give an employee the phone number of the EAP. In general, managers can't require the employee to participate as it is a voluntary service. However, managers can require an employee to seek help or counseling as a "condition" of continued employment in some situations, such as failing a drug or alcohol test. Legal counsel is helpful in these situations.
- Watch for warning signs that an employee or customer may become violent and report the concern immediately.
    - Appears to be under the influence of alcohol or drugs.
    - Appears to have been in a fight or shows signs of abuse.
    - Exhibiting mood swings or signs of sleep deprivation.
    - Obvious possession of a weapon.
    - Nervousness or abrupt movements.

- Extreme restlessness, such as pacing and obvious agitation.
- Making threats to others.

Supervisors should speak to the offender immediately and work on de-escalating the situation if the situation is manageable. Though, if the situation is deemed imminently dangerous, the local authority should be called immediately.

- <u>Know the procedures to follow in case of violence and theft</u>, such as getting a manager, calling 911, or pressing a "Panic Button." Safety and security protocols often call for the following, depending on the specific situation.
  - Notify other staff and call security.
  - Stay alert but remain calm.
  - Maintain a safe distance, giving the person plenty of space. Do not turn your back and do not touch the person.
  - Keep obstacles between you and the individual.
  - Be certain you have a way out; avoid dead-end corridors or corners.
  - Listen; do not display anger or defensiveness and do not argue; speak slowly and quietly.
- <u>In the case of an active shooter, the first option is to run away from the shooter, the next option is to hide in an area out of the shooter's view and block entry to the hiding place.</u> Only try to incapacitate the shooter as a last resort. Call 911 when it is safe to do so.

13.2 RECRUIT AND SELECT EMPLOYEES

When a position is open, managers often work to recruit and select a new employee, for example, for a cook's position. A foodservice budget may have four cooks' positions, and each position is either filled or empty. A position is not the same as a job, as each **position** is held by one person and the positions are specific to a given organization. A **job**, such as cook, is a group of tasks and responsibilities that an employee is required to perform.

RECRUITMENT

Recruitment refers to searching for individuals from both inside and outside a business in sufficient numbers and with appropriate qualifications to apply for the positions that need to be filled. In the case of a foodservice with a human resources manager, the recruiting process is typically started with a manager filling out a job requisition form. A **job requisition form** is filled out to request finding an employee for an open position, so it starts the recruiting and hiring process after being signed off by the appropriate managers.

Recruiting applicants from within the foodservice is called **internal recruiting**. For example, in a foodservice found within a hospital, the human resources department will often post open jobs (called job posting) on a central bulletin board or employee newsletter and also on the hospital website. Internal recruiting generates applicants who are well known to the hospital and have a track record. For employees looking for a job with more hours, more pay, different responsibilities, and/or more responsibility, internal recruiting is helpful and also motivational. Some organizations prefer to **promote from within**—meaning promote a current employee to a higher-level position rather than going outside the business to find someone. Filling open positions through internal recruiting also saves time and money. The disadvantages of internal recruiting is the potential for recycling old practices when you might need some fresh ideas.

Most foodservices use both internal and **external recruiting**, meaning recruiting outside of the existing organization. External recruiting is often necessary for entry-level jobs because there are no internal recruits available (unless the job is offering more money, hours, or more desirable shifts). Especially on the management level, external recruiting often brings in candidates with novel ideas from your competitors. The following is a discussion of common external recruitment methods.

1. "Careers" website page of larger foodservices, chain restaurants, and food-service contract companies. If you look at the "Careers" page of a restaurant chain, such as TGI Fridays, you can search and apply for jobs at restaurants in any geographic area. This is a common way that bigger foodservices and food-service contractors get applicants. The advantages of this method are that it is relatively low cost and it shows that the applicants have done some research before applying for a job.

2. "Help Wanted" sign. Something as simple as signs in a foodservice can bring in applicants or refer applicants to a website to apply.

3. Referrals. When someone is looking for a job, they often approach family, friends, and acquaintances for help. If someone works for Sodexo, for example, they may refer a friend to a new job opening in the area. Referrals like this don't cost a thing but can bring in a number of applicants. Formal **employee referral programs**, in which a current employee refers an applicant to the company, are used very successfully by some operators to draw in new employees. In an employee referral program, the employee who makes a successful referral is rewarded with a cash bonus or some other type of incentive. When implementing an employee referral program, it is important to include all employees, ask them to fill out a referral form, require the applicant to undergo and pass the normal selection procedures, and set a period of time for the new employee to work before the other employee receives the reward.

4. Online job boards and job aggregators. Smaller foodservices (that usually don't post jobs on their website) can be successful by posting their jobs onto job boards. You have to pay **job boards**, such as Monster and CareerBuilder, to display your job advertisements. When applicants use a job board, some jobs will allow them to apply directly on the company's website. Other jobs require that the applicant post a resume. Foodservices can then search a job boards' resume database for work experience, education, and skills using key terms to find qualified applicants. Some niche job boards, such as culinaryagent.com, focus on foodservice and culinary jobs and can be more useful. **Job aggregators**, such as Indeed and SimplyHired, gather job postings from job boards and other Internet sites and consolidate them. Applicants then search the listings to find jobs that interest them. There is usually a link to apply directly on the company's website.

5. Print advertisements. With the Internet, the amount of print advertising has decreased significantly. However, local advertising is fairly inexpensive and can be effective. Advertising in a trade, professional, or industry publication, especially for professional jobs, can also be useful.

6. School and college recruiting. If a foodservice is frequently looking for cooks and there are culinary programs in nearby schools and colleges, it makes sense to contact them in order to help their graduates obtain employment. This could be done through internship programs, job fairs, and on-campus interviewing.

7. Employment agencies. Each state has a public agency, often under the Department of Labor, that works with unemployed people to administer unemployment benefits and help them find jobs. The agency may be named a state workforce agency or state employment agency. Foodservices can register job openings with these state agencies for free and each agency maintains a job bank of open jobs, many of which can be accessed online. **Private employment agencies** charge a fee to the employer when they find and place an employee. Private agencies more often place people in white-collar jobs. **Temporary employment agencies** can provide employees who stay for as little as one day or as long as needed. Temporary agencies charge the foodservice by the hour and although the hourly charge is much higher than the foodservice would

be paying, the foodservice neither gives the temporary employee any benefits nor spends any time or money filling a position. The temporary employee is technically employed by the agency and receives a paycheck from the agency. When evaluating temporary agencies, find out how the agency selects and trains employees and if the employees are covered by liability insurance.

Finding foodservice employees can often be quite difficult. To attract more applicants, consider the following.

1. <u>Make sure your website is attractive and complete</u>. Post some videos that show what it is like to work in your foodservice or what employees like about working there. Videos can convey that your foodservice is fun to work at, employees are friendly, the pay is good, and there are opportunities for advancement. Use photos to show happy employees working together (Ganino, 2018; Romeo, 2018).
2. <u>Write engaging job ads</u> with the duties clearly explained, skills needed, and information on the benefits and perks.
3. <u>Participate in job fairs and host an open house event</u>. At a **job fair**, usually one company sponsors the event and sells booths to other companies. The event is advertised to attract candidates. Each company brings recruiters who usually just screen candidates in a fairly brief interview to determine if a full interview at a later date would be beneficial. At an **open house**, a foodservice opens its doors to applicants, who are then interviewed. The open house is advertised with a listing of available jobs in advance.
4. <u>Offer incentives</u> such as flexible schedules, special training classes, help paying off college/culinary school loans, and the like.
5. <u>Use social media</u> to promote opportunities that are available.

SELECTION

After recruiting applicants, the selection process starts. The **selection** process includes the steps from screening the initial applications and resumes through to the point where a candidate best suited for a particular position is offered and accepts the job. The steps vary from business to business, but generally involve screening applications and/or resumes, pre-employment tests and/or work samples, interviews, and finally, background checks and selection of a finalist. The selection process is guided by the job specification (qualifications for a job—including knowledge, skills, and abilities) and job description (responsibilities and tasks of a job), which were discussed in Chapter 12. The qualifications for the job must be **bona fide occupational qualifications**—meaning that they are necessary to perform the duties of the position. The job specification and job description are crucial documents in the selection process as you want the final candidate to be selected fairly and to be able to do the job well once training has been completed.

Diversity gets a lot of attention when it is time to hire employees. **Diversity** is the range of human differences, such as age and ethnicity. Diversity training is important to prevent discrimination and help you select the best candidate. Here are some examples of diversity among applicants.

- Age, ethnicity, and gender (the primary ways we identify differences).
- Culture, religion, national origin, primary language, and accents or dialects.
- Physical attributes (such as obesity), and cognitive abilities.
- Sexual orientation, marital status, and parental status.
- Educational attainment, socioeconomic status, and military service.
- Previous work experience.
- Lifestyle choices such as smoking, hair style, tattoos, and body piercing.

In light of the Equal Employment Opportunity laws, the selection process must be nondiscriminatory and job-related. One way to do that is to apply each step in the selection process in a consistent manner across all applicants. The following are some additional guidelines from the EEOC (Equal Employment Opportunity Commission, 2010).

- Establish neutral and objective criteria to avoid subjective employment decisions based on personal stereotypes or hidden biases.
- Apply the same criteria/standards to everyone applying for the same position from screening to final selection.
- Ensure that selection criteria do not disproportionately exclude certain racial groups unless the criteria are valid predictors of successful job performance and meet the employer's business needs. For example, if educational requirements (such as a high school diploma) disproportionately exclude certain minority or racial groups, these requirements may be illegal if not important for job performance or business needs.
- Employers should ensure that employment tests and other selection procedures are job-related and properly validated for the positions and purposes for which they are used. When applicants take a *valid* selection tool, such as a test, it has been shown that the applicants scoring higher on the test perform better on the job than applicants with lower test scores.
- To ensure that a test or selection procedure remains predictive of success in a job, employers should keep abreast of changes in job requirements and update selecion procedures, including administering tests, accordingly.

Much hiring discrimination comes in the form of unconscious bias (Ruggless, 2016). **Unconscious bias** is a bias that you experience every time you make a snap judgment or assessment of a person or situation. It just happens automatically without really thinking about it. Every recruiter or person involved in hiring has a specific world view and narrow set of personal experiences that affect how they interact with the environment. That world view affects what we look for in a candidate and what each of us might consider a good "fit" for a particular job or position. That world view also provides the unconscious bias toward "people who think and act like me." Ideally, the staff of a foodservice should be as diverse as the communities and population they serve. So, it is recommended that recruiters use tools and tactics to expand the concept of "fit" to include attributes not present in you or in the existing staff, but that could be beneficial in your setting.

If you have ever wondered why you had to fill out an application for a job when you had a perfectly good resume, there are good reasons for that. Resumes give the employer only the information the applicant wants that employer to know. In other words, an applicant may leave things off a resume or color it slightly, or be untruthful. Applications ask for information based on what the employer needs to know. They are legal documents and are often signed off by the applicant as being true. Since the application is standardized, it is easier for a hiring manager to compare applicants in a fair manner. Managers often compare the resume with the applications to establish validity.

Since the majority of applications and resumes are submitted online, businesses use software (called applicant tracking systems) to store each applicant's data in a database. As the applicant moves through the selection process, their information is transferred to another component of the system. Applicant tracking systems allow managers to search and sort through applicants in a number of ways. But first, most software will compare the applications/resumes with the job description and selection criteria. For example, if a cook's position is open, the tracking system will search to see if each applicant has ever had the same job title. It will also search for specific relevant keywords used in the job description such as "prepare," "portion," or "season." An applicant tracking system can identify applications/resumes that lack any keywords. Those applicants may automatically receive a "no thank you" email. The remaining applicants are ranked by how closely they meet the criteria. At this point, a hiring manager can review the applicants and select the best-qualified candidates to go to the next step.

When screening applicants' materials, the hiring manager checks for relevant work history, appropriate skills, and required education. Other factors to consider include the following.

- Was the application completely filled in?
- Is the resume (when used) well written, complete, and free of gaps?
- Does the cover letter seem like the applicant did some research about the company?
- Are there large unexplained lapses between jobs or school attendance?
- What are the reasons for leaving jobs?

Some of these questions can be addressed in an interview.

Employment tests and/or **work samples** may be used during the selection process if they are job-related and applied consistently to all applicants for the same job. Employment tests must be prescreened for possible bias and discrimination. Examples of employment tests, some of which can be administered online, include the following.

- Cognitive ability tests assess mental abilities such as verbal skills, skills working with numbers, and reasoning skills used to find an answer to a problem.
- Physical ability tests measure the ability to, for example, lift 30 pounds.
- Job knowledge tests measure critical knowledge areas needed to perform a job, such as knowledge of basic measurements for anyone involved in preparing recipes and cooking food.
- Job performance tests or work samples ask an applicant to perform a specialized task required in the job, such as use a slicing machine, set a table, or cut vegetables for soup.
- Personality tests assess the degree to which a person has certain traits relevant to job performance such as being conscientious. An integrity test is a specific type of personality test used to assess an applicant's tendency to be honest and dependable.
- Drug testing may be used before or after employment for jobs that, for example, involve safety hazards. Drug testing is controversial and legal advice should be solicited.
- English proficiency tests can be used if proficiency is a bona fide occupational qualification.

Medical exams are often used for physically demanding jobs and for employees working in healthcare foodservices, but, by law, they can only be conducted *after* an employment offer has been made.

Job interviews are frequently used in the selection process. The purpose of a job interview is to determine if an applicant can do the job, wants to do the job, and will fit in with the team. The job interview also informs the applicant more fully about the job, the work environment, and the culture. Supervisors and/or team members may be involved in conducting the interview.

Like any other part of the selection process, discrimination and bias can creep into interviews. According to Cappelli (2019, p. 56), "interviews are where biases most easily show up, because interviewers do usually decide on the fly what to ask of whom and how to interpret the answer." In addition, interviewers like candidates who they consider to be like themselves. If an interviewee went to the same college as you, for example, it is more likely that you will rate this candidate higher than others.

The interviewer's main tool is questions, so it's important to understand the types of questions that can be asked to get a good picture of an applicant and reduce the interviewer's unconscious or selection bias.

- **Closed-ended questions** most often ask for a "yes" or "no" answer, such as "Do you like your present job?"

- **Open-ended questions** require some thought and discussion, such as "How do you feel about working with customers?"
- **Direct questions** can be answered with a specific piece of information, such as "What are you looking for in terms of wages?"
- **Reflective questions** restate what the applicant said in order to get more clarification, such as "Do you mean you left your last job because they did not pay you enough?"
- **Probing questions** seek more information, such as "What was the outcome?" or "What other actions could you take?"
- **Behavioral questions** ask what the applicant has done under certain circumstances in the past, such as "Describe a situation in which you dealt with a customer who was unhappy with his entrée. What actions did you take and what were the results?" An applicant's past behavior is a good guide to future performance.
- **Situational questions** ask what the applicant would do in a hypothetical situation, such as "If your bread supplier was not always providing a fresh product, how would you handle this?"

To learn more about an applicant, the most useful questions are open-ended, reflective, probing, behavioral, and situational. However, at different points in the interview, closed-ended and direct questions are appropriate.

When developing questions, keep EEO considerations in mind. You can't ask questions about age, sex, race, national origin, religion, pregnancy, marital or family status, disabilities, or any other factor that is NOT related to the job. Of course, if a bartender must be 21 years old by state law, it is okay to verify age. If you sell pork barbeque, you would not want to hire someone whose religion forbids pork. So you could ask, "Are you willing to cook and taste test everything on this menu?" Some religions forbid work on the Sabbath or specific holidays, so you can ask, "Are there any days and/or times when you absolutely cannot work?" If an applicant has an obvious disability or has disclosed a disability, you can ask if they will require any changes to the work environment or to the manner that a job is usually performed. Questions about language(s) spoken can only be asked when a certain language is required of the job. An employer can ask if an applicant has the legal right to work in the United States as paperwork is required at the start of employment to verify that.

When writing interview questions, they should be reflective of the job's responsibilities, tasks, and qualifications. Questions should also be clear and concise. Leading questions that convey the correct answers should be avoided. Interviewers should get the applicant to draw from their actual past work experiences to demonstrate job-related competencies, as well as present realistic job scenarios and ask how the applicant would respond.

Because interviews are costly to perform and prone to being subjective and biased, it is crucial that the interview be structured and standardized. During a **structured interview**, the interviewer asks the same set of questions to all applicants. The questions often include behavioral questions as well as situational questions, which tend to have high validity (meaning they are related to job performance). Structured and standardized job-focused interviews are more likely to be objective and not reflect the biases of the interviewer.

The interviewer should always start the interview on time, greet the applicant warmly by name, and introduce themselves by name and title. Start with some small talk on a neutral topic or offer the applicant a beverage as a way to create an informal atmosphere and develop rapport. A seating arrangement that does not put a desk between interviewer and applicant is also conducive to developing rapport. Creating a positive atmosphere helps applicants relax and encourages them to participate fully. At this point, it is a good idea to describe what will occur during the interview along with a brief background on the open position and the nature of the foodservice/business.

The following are the primary areas to be discussed during the heart of the interview.

1. Gather/verify and analyze information about the applicant's knowledge, skills, abilities, work experience, education, and training.
2. Explain the job fully, including responsibilities and tasks, hours of work, overtime requirements, probationary period (if required), wages and benefits, training, performance reviews, and growth opportunities. Make sure the applicant has a copy of the job description and make all job expectations clear. All positive and negative aspects of the job, such as erratic work hours, should be discussed.
3. Gather information to see how well an applicant will fit in with other employees. This is why it is helpful to have coworkers involved in part or all of the interview. Ask a question such as "Tell me about a conflict you had in the past with another employee or manager, and what you did to resolve it." The response: "I never have conflicts" is not an acceptable answer as it is realistic that everyone does, from time to time, have a conflict with someone else.
4. Explain the foodservice's goals, history, and structure.

Table 13-2 lists tips for interviewing.

In wrapping up the interview, the interviewer needs to allow time for the applicant to ask questions. The interviewer may then ask the applicant about their level of interest in the job, and explain the next steps in the process. Always close the interview on a positive note and thank the applicant for their time.

During and/or after an interview, the interviewer needs to take good notes that are professional and based on observable facts. Instead of writing opinions or impressions such as "sarcastic" or "bored," the interviewer should write down job-related facts and direct observations such as "well-groomed and neatly dressed" or "applicant checked his phone multiple times during 30-minute interview."

Once interviews are done and you have selected your top candidates, it is time to do background checks. A **background check** is the process a business uses to verify that an applicant is who they claim to be in terms of, for example, education or employment history. A background check not only helps the employer find out if an

Table 13-2 Tips for Interviewing
• Be nonjudgmental during the entire interview. Do not jump to conclusions. A poor interviewer reaches a decision in the first five minutes.
• Recognize your own personal biases and try not to let them influence you. Be objective. Don't look for clones of yourself.
• Spend most of your time listening attentively. Allow the applicant to do at least 70 to 80% of the talking. Listen to each answer before deciding on the next question. Do not interrupt!
• Use a script with the questions so each interview is equivalent.
• Repeat or paraphrase the applicant's statement to get a better understanding and more information, such as "So you were responsible for the dining room staff in that job?"
• Also, periodically summarize the applicant's statements to clarify points and bring information together.
• Use pauses to allow the applicant to sense that more information is desired.
• Do not use facial expressions to indicate agreement or otherwise telegraph the answer you are seeking.
• Show interest in the applicant but you don't need to show you agree or disagree with their statements.
• Don't be bashful about probing for more information when needed.
• Instead of asking about an applicant's "weaknesses," refer to "areas of improvement."
• Paint a realistic picture of the job. Be honest.
• Always be sincere, respectful, friendly, and treat each applicant in a similar manner.

applicant has not been honest, it also protects the employer from being charged with negligent hiring. The following are guidelines for doing background checks.

- To minimize your liability, ask the applicant in writing to consent to a background check and use that information to make employment decisions.
- Verifying past jobs using references supplied by each applicant is very important. Verifications should include: job start and end dates, job title(s), major job duties, ending salary, and rehire eligibility. If additional job-related information can be obtained, that's fine. Just be aware that many employers will limit the information they give you to lessen their liability.
- If you have three applicants to background check, be consistent in the information you find out about each person.
- Make sure each piece of information you want is job-related.
- Criminal background checks provide information on conviction history, which are important only if they are relevant to the job. For example, it could be important for an applicant who will be handling money. Several states limit employers' use of conviction records to make employment decisions, so getting legal advice is important. It is appropriate to assess the details of each conviction, including how serious it is and how long ago it occurred. Most schools and other facilities where employees care for children, the elderly, and individuals with disabilities, are precluded from hiring any employee with a conviction that may include weapons, violence, domestic violence, physical or sexual abuse, or child abuse or neglect. Prospective employees must pass background checks, such as FBI fingerprint checks or state child abuse registry, before they can start employment in certain jobs.
- Credit checks can be done if an applicant consents; however, some states ban the practice altogether. Some employers do a credit check for employees handling money.
- If the employer thinks they might not hire an applicant because of something in a report compiled by a company the employer used to do the background check, it must give the applicant a copy of the report and a "notice of rights" that explains how to contact the company that made the report. This is because background reports sometimes contain inaccuracies which could cost them job opportunities.
- Employers can't ask for medical information until after offering the job to someone.

Any time you use information obtained through a background check to make an employment decision, you must comply with EEO laws that protect applicants from discrimination based on a person's race, color, religion, sex (including pregnancy, gender identity, and sexual orientation), national origin, age (40 or older), disability or genetic information.

So how do you select the best applicant? In some organizations, each candidate is rated at each step in the process and these ratings are heavily used in the final decision (see **Table 13-3** for an example). In other organizations, candidates are ranked based on objective criteria. Then the candidates are discussed in terms of their abilities, motivation, work ethic, and ability to fit in, and a final selection is made. Records of these ratings should be kept to substantiate that a fair selection process took place.

When a job offer is extended, the salary, amount of paid time off, benefits, start date, and work schedule are discussed, along with any other necessary information such as parking. The candidate is told of any further conditions that must be met, such as a medical examination or drug testing. A candidate is often given time to consider the job offer and get back to the employer by a given date.

The salary offered depends on the candidate's level of experience and the job grade. **Job grades** are groupings of positions that are paid within a similar range of pay. For example, the U.S. federal government has 15 pay grades based on the specific level of work or range of difficulty, responsibility, and qualifications. The higher the grade level,

Table 13-3 Form to Compare Applicants

Comparison of Applicants

Date: _____

Position/Department: _____

Directions: Fill in the Job Qualifications below for this position. Next, rate each applicant using this scale.

1. Does not meet qualification
2. Meets minimum qualification
3. Exceeds qualification

Job Qualifications	Applicant #1	Applicant #2	Applicant #3	Applicant #4
1. Knowledge				
2. Skills & Abilities				
3. Work Experience				
4. Education and Training				

Directions: Rate each applicant below using this scale.

1. Unsatisfactory results
2. Satisfactory results
3. Above average results

	Applicant #1	Applicant #2	Applicant #3	Applicant #4
Pre-employment Testing				
Test 1				
Test 2				
Test 3				
Interview				
Background Checks				
Reference 1				
Reference 2				
Reference 3				
Reference 4				

the higher the pay. There is usually some overlap in terms of pay from one grade to the next. Many factors affect pay, such as the kind of job performed, the industry the job is in, the size and location of the company, how long an employee has been with a company and his/her performance, or whether the employees are unionized.

SPOTLIGHT ON TYPES OF POSITIONS AND OUTSOURCING

Foodservice is a unique industry because the number of customers can vary tremendously from day to day. For example, foodservices close to beaches can be crowded in the summer and close for the winter due to a lack of customers. Weather and the economy also affect the number of customers you have. When the weather is good and people have some extra money in their pocket, they are more likely to eat out. Because of these variations, most foodservices want some staff who have *very* flexible hours.

Each foodservice employee is either employed by the foodservice or another organization. When employed directly by the foodservice, the position may be permanent or temporary. An employee in a **permanent position**, sometimes also called a regular position, can stay in that job until they decide to leave, or the employer asks them to leave or decides the position is no longer needed. An employee in a **temporary position** can stay in that job until a certain date. A temporary employee may be covering an employee on a leave of absence, for example. Sometimes, a temporary employee is brought in to complete a special project. Whether permanent or temporary, each position will fall into one of these categories.

1. **Full-time employee.** The Fair Labor Standards Act does not define the number of hours a full-time employee (or part-time employee) must work. The employer decides the number of hours that must be worked to be full-time (often 35 to 40 hours/week) but some states do define what constitutes full-time or part-time employment. Full-time employees usually receive paid time off (vacation, sick leave, etc.) and benefits such as health insurance.
2. **Part-time employee.** A part-time position requires an employee to work fewer hours/week than a full-time employee. So, if a full-time week is 40 hours, then part-timers work less than that amount—often less than 30 hours/week. However, part-time employees may occasionally work 40 hours in a week and even collect overtime when needed. Part-timers may, or may not, be given paid time off and benefits, but there are some regulations. The Affordable Care Act (ACA) requires employers with 50 or more full-time equivalent employees to offer health insurance to 95% or more of employees who work an average of 30 hours a week. ACA considers an employee who works 30 hours to be full-time. Certain states and jurisdictions also require employers to provide paid sick leave to part-time employees under certain conditions. Casual part-time employees are not normally guaranteed any hours and may only be used to cover sick calls or vacations.
3. **On-call employee.** This employee only works when they are needed, and they may be called into work with little notice. They are not guaranteed any minimum number of hours and most often, they are not given any paid time off or benefits.

Now we will take a look at employees who are *not* employed by the foodservice. **Outsourcing** is when a company hires another company to perform tasks that could be handled in house. For example, a hospital or university may outsource meals to foodservice contract companies. A university may outsource its foodservice because a contractor promises the same or better quality at a lower cost. Here are examples of employees who don't work directly for the foodservice.

1. When a foodservice is outsourced to a foodservice contract company, some or all of the employees are employed by the contract company. For example, in a hospital foodservice run by a contractor, the management team and dietitians may be employed by the contractor while the hourly positions are employed by the hospital. The situation varies depending on the written agreement.
2. As already mentioned, **temporary employment agencies** provide foodservice employees who stay for as little as one day or as long as needed. Temporary agencies charge the foodservice by the hour. The temp foodservice employee is an employee of the temporary agency and receives paychecks (with taxes taken out) from the agency.
3. Becoming more popular in the gig economy characterized by flexible and temporary jobs, foodservices can also use **independent contractors** who are self-employed individuals and may work for more than one client. Using an app such as Pared, foodservice workers (such as cooks) can find short-term jobs in a variety of restaurants in certain areas of the country after a reference check for experience and reliability. As an independent contractor, no taxes are withheld from each paycheck, so independent contractors must pay their own federal and state taxes as well as self-employment tax (which covers Social Security and Medicare taxes).

13.3 TRAIN EMPLOYEES

Training means to instruct and guide the development of a trainee toward acquiring knowledge, skills, attitudes, and behaviors to apply on the job. Most training in the food-service industry is centered on orienting new employees and teaching vital job skills, such as customer service and interpersonal skills, for hourly employees, supervisors, and managers. **Learning** is something trainees do as they respond to training, and learning may happen at the level of knowledge, skills, attitudes, or behaviors. On-the-job coaching by supervisors reinforces the learning acquired in training.

Training has a variety of objectives.

- Introducing new employees to the organization and their jobs.
- Getting new employees up-to-speed and invested in their jobs.
- Helping employees perform their current jobs well.
- Assisting employees to qualify for future job promotions.
- Keeping employees informed of changes within an organization.

Training can also provide opportunities for an employee's personal development.

With a good training program in place, employees can do their jobs more efficiently and be more productive. When employees know their jobs well, managers can spend more time managing and less time dealing with the day-to-day emergencies, such as an accident, often due to poor training or communication. Instead, the food and service quality is more consistent. Costs are also lower, due to less waste, fewer accidents, fewer broken glasses and plates, and so on.

Both employees and guests end up more satisfied due to training. If employees are doing their jobs well, the guests know that, which decreases complaints and also makes them more likely to return. Employees are confident and proud of what they are doing and make fewer mistakes. They are more likely to feel that they are a part of the organization—in other words, loyal—which can translate into lower absenteeism and turnover rates and lower recruiting and training costs. In essence, training gives the employee a dual message: "You are important to this organization, and we care about how you do your job."

Many organizations break down their training programs into different categories, such as the following.

- Onboarding (includes orientation)
- On-the-job training (mostly for new hires or in-house promotions)
- Job-specific skills training (sometimes called **hard skills** or **technical skills**)
- **Soft skills** (refers to interpersonal skills such as communication, collaboration, service recovery, and leadership skills)
- Regulatory and compliance training (educating employees on laws, regulations, and organizational policies that apply to their day-to-day job responsibilities such as anti-harassment training, safety training, or cybersecurity)

Most healthcare foodservices must comply with federal regulations to provide **in-service training**—meaning training while someone is working. Typical in-service training topics include food sanitation, kitchen and fire safety, chemical safety training, ethics, customer service, and modified diets.

ORIENTING AND ONBOARDING NEW EMPLOYEES

Orientation is a specific type of training that usually lasts from a few hours to a few days to introduce a new employee to the workplace and job. If a new employee starts working immediately without any formal orientation, they are likely to feel somewhat confused and uncomfortable. When a manager takes the time to greet new employees and go through orientation procedures, it gives the employee the message that both the employee and the job are important.

Orientation generally has two aspects: an introduction to the organization, department, and position, and a tour and introductions to coworkers. The following topics should be discussed during orientation.

1. Background about the organization and its mission and objectives.
2. Code of conduct including policies regarding dress code, cell phone use, safety procedures, computer use, harassment and discrimination, and behavior that results in disciplinary action.
3. Policies regarding pay, work schedules, paid time off, and benefits.
4. Performance specifics, including job description, performance standards, and how performance is evaluated.
5. Available training, mentoring, and opportunities for advancement.
6. Completion of paperwork for Human Resources (such as benefits or I9 paperwork to make sure an employee is permitted to work in the United States).

The orientation session should be held preferably on the employee's first day of work. The best way to cover the needed information is to use an orientation checklist (**Table 13-4**). Many foodservices have an *Employee Handbook* for employees to take home with much information covered during orientation.

The decision to stay or leave a job, or the perception of a positive or negative work culture, is usually influenced by the orientation. This makes orientation planning and implementation critical to the success of the employee and a positive work environment.

Table 13-4 Orientation Checklist

Orientation Checklist

Introduction to the Restaurant

_____ Welcome the new employee and provide "New Employee Handbook."

_____ Describe restaurant, including history, mission, hours, customer profile, menu.

_____ Show organizational chart.

Pay and Benefits

_____ Review pay periods and when employees are paid.

_____ Explain policy on overtime pay.

_____ Review paid time off (sick time, vacation, etc.) as needed. Explain how to request time off.

_____ Review benefits to which the employee is entitled (as applicable).

Dress Code

_____ Explain dress code (why outside clothes are not permitted) and who furnishes the uniform.

_____ Grooming: Clean, professional appearance, standards on hats, hair, etc.

_____ Additional requirements such as a face mask during a pandemic.

Coming to Work

_____ Describe where to park and approved employee entrances.

_____ Explain how to clock in and out and procedures for missed clock-in or out.

_____ Assign locker and explain its use.

_____ Discuss how to notify supervisor if unable to come to work or if coming in late.

Professional Behavior

_____ Discuss the rules on cell phone use.

_____ Explain the meal and beverage policies, including beverages at the work station.

_____ Review professional behavior guidelines including working in teams.

_____ Explain channels of communication such as meetings and bulletin boards.

_____ Review disciplinary guidelines including limits on lateness/tardiness.

(continues)

Table 13-4 Orientation Checklist (continued)

Security and Safety

_____ Review basic security precautions and procedures (ID badge and codes).

_____ Show what to do in case of fire. Identify pull stations.

_____ Refer employee to review basics of food safety and employee safety in Handbook.

The New Job

_____ Review the job description and performance standards.

_____ Review the daily work schedule including break times.

_____ Review the hours of work and days off, and where schedule is posted.

_____ Explain the probationary period and how and when the employee will be evaluated.

_____ Give examples of why an employee might fail probation.

_____ Explain how training will take place and resources available.

_____ Give tour of restaurant and introduce new employee to other managers and co-workers.

The topics above have been reviewed.

_____

Employee Signature

_____

Date

_____

Supervisor Signature

Just because new employees have gone through orientation does not mean that they are fully functioning in their jobs and integrated with other employees. Orientation is just the first step in the onboarding process. **Onboarding** is a series of events, starting with orientation, that acclimate and engage a new employee to become a contributing member of the team in a reasonable amount of time (such as two to four months, or it could be longer depending on the job). New employees need to build relationships; develop the knowledge, skills, and attitudes to be successful in their jobs; understand company culture, and become familiar with the organization's rules and policies. Once the employee is participating fully in the organization, onboarding is complete.

A written onboarding plan may be used to describe what should be accomplished within certain timeframes, such as the end of the first week and then within 30, 60, and 90 days. The plan also identifies who will be working with the new employee to complete the onboarding process. It is helpful to ask a peer of the new employee (who is a good role model) to help in the process, along with supervisors and managers. As the onboarding process continues, supervisors should give feedback, review progress, and offer encouragement and praise (Little, 2019).

ON-THE-JOB TRAINING

On-the-job training (OJT) refers to how an employee (usually a new employee) is trained to do the various tasks that make up their job. It is commonly used in foodservices. Before conducting on-the-job training, the supervisor should assess the employee's basic skills. Traditionally in OJT, the new employee is placed into the real work situation and trained to do the various parts of the job by an experienced employee or supervisor who uses a technique called tell/show/do/review. In brief, here are the four steps: tell the employee about what he or she is going to learn (such as how to set up a three-compartment sink), show or demonstrate it to the employee, let the employee do it, and then review/coach the new employee's performance. The steps should be modified as needed depending on the new employee's knowledge, abilities, and rate of mastery of new skills.

Some general guidelines for conducting OJT include avoiding training of new job duties at very busy times and making sure the work area is ready. Don't forget to present the big picture so the employee understands how the job contributes to the overall operation and give lots of encouragement and praise. Also, the trainer and trainee should use a checklist (as shown in **Table 13-5**) to keep track of the training, as well as to make use of policy and procedure manuals and training manuals.

Table 13-5 On-the-Job Training Checklist

On-the-Job Training Checklist: Storekeeper

Name of Trainee: _____

Date Starting Training: _____

Name of Trainer: _____

Directions: Write the date in the blank space next to each task when you feel the trainee has mastered the task.

Receiving

_____ Verify items and quantity received against vendor's invoice.

_____ Use barcode scanner.

_____ Spot check quality of incoming goods, including inspecting for damage, spoilage, and correct food temperatures.

_____ Verify pricing.

_____ Make adjustments on the invoice for returns and corrected prices.

_____ Immediately discuss any receiving problems (especially missing items) with chef.

_____ Maintain receiving log.

Storing

_____ Date all incoming food and store in appropriate locations with label face out.

_____ Store frozen and refrigerated food within 30 minutes of delivery.

_____ Rotate stock.

_____ Store raw proteins separately or away from ready-to-eat foods.

_____ Document daily temperature checks of storage areas. Report problems to supervisor.

Recordkeeping

_____ Take physical inventory and record accurately.

_____ Issue stock.

_____ Use inventory and purchasing apps appropriately.

General

_____ Clean storage areas according to cleaning schedule. Clean up spills, etc., immediately.

_____ Follow dress and personal hygiene code.

_____ Come to work on time and ready to work.

_____ Cooperate with other employees.

Upon completion of training, both the employee and trainer sign below to certify that the training has been adequate for the new employee to function in their position.

_____

Employee Signature

_____

Date

_____

Trainer Signature

DEVELOP A TRAINING PROGRAM

Onboarding and on-the-job training are used with new hires. Once an employee is acclimated to the new job and comfortable with performing the job, additional training is often available and may even be required by regulations. Good managers keep an eye on the training needs of their employees. Evidence that additional training is likely needed includes unhappy customers or employees, low productivity, long lines, low sales, high costs, poor product quality, or a high accident rate.

The first step in developing a training program is to complete a **needs assessment**, or determination of what training is needed. You can do a needs assessment at the organizational level, at a department level, or at a job level. The organization may have specific needs, such as concentrating on opening new foodservices. Departments, such as purchasing, also have specific needs. At the job level, job training is always needed for new employees and to refresh and update existing employees.

To help establish specific training needs, managers can use surveys, observations, and other forms of evaluations to identify performance problems. For example, you may look at recent customer satisfaction survey results and see that more customers than usual think they have to wait too long to be served their meals. Before assuming it must be a problem with the servers, you can observe meal service and survey servers, line cooks, expediters, and others. You may discover that the problem is related to work flow (traffic patterns) or equipment issues, in which case training won't help, or perhaps you learn that the servers need more training on the new point-of-sales system in order to get meals out quicker.

Once a training need is identified, an organization may develop its own training programs or use outside companies to develop and/or deliver courses (often through **e-learning** or the use of electronic media). Courses from vendors may be general courses teaching generic skills or a vendor may be asked to develop customized training tailored to the core competencies of the organization (which is going to be more expensive).

A **learning management system (LMS)** is software that organizes, delivers, and manages training programs. The LMS stores and provides learners access to courses and tracks their results. At your college, you likely use a LMS, such as Blackboard or Canvas, to access online courses as well as materials and discussion boards for onsite courses.

Principles of instructional design are used to develop training programs. **Instructional design** describes how a trainer uses learning and instructional theory to develop instructional plans for a specific purpose. For example, to meet regulatory requirements, a trainer will develop a **training unit** for employees that cook on how to keep foods safe to eat. Because keeping foods safe includes a variety of topics, the training unit will include several **training modules** or classes, such as hot preparation and service.

Once the need for a training unit has been identified and its overall training goals have been developed, the instructional designer takes these steps to develop each training module or class.

1. <u>Assess employees' specific needs</u>. Before developing a class, the trainer needs to understand exactly what the employees need to be able to accomplish after the training, as well as the employees' current knowledge and skills. This information will help the trainer develop a relevant training experience.

2. <u>Write learning objectives and how they will be evaluated</u>. A **learning objective** is what you want the employees to do after the training is completed, such as perform a task. Learning objectives should be easy to understand and realistic to accomplish. An example of a learning objective is "Demonstrate how to clean and sanitize his/her work area and equipment according to policy and procedure." Another example is: "Recall minimum internal cooking temperatures for proteins and obtain 90% or higher on a quiz." In both cases, the learning

Table 13-6 Verbs for Learning Objectives (Using Levels of Thinking from Bloom's Taxonomy*)					
					Create
				Evaluate	Develop
			Analyze	Assess	Build
		Apply	Differentiate	Defend	Plan
	Understand	Demonstrate	Interpret	Investigate	Design
Remember	Explain	Estimate	Organize	Monitor	Revise
Define	Compare	Interpret	Compare	Critique	Formulate
Describe	Discuss	Produce	Explain	Appraise	Propose
Recall	Summarize	Solve	Examine	Argue	Establish
Identify	Restate	Execute	Extrapolate	Justify	Assemble
Select	Paraphrase	Implement	Quantify	Review	Modify
List	Organize	Conduct	Contrast	Recommend	Generate
Name		Perform		Prioritize	Construct
State		Complete		Judge	Compose
		Use			

* Data From "A Revision of Bloom's Taxonomy: An Overview," by D.R. Krathwohl, 2002, *Theory Into Practice*, 41(4): 214.

objective includes the quality or level of performance that is required. This way, each objective is measurable, and the trainer can then evaluate whether an employee met each objective.

Trainers use a variety of **evaluation** techniques to see how well trainees recall information, demonstrate skills, exhibit changed attitudes, or improved performance. Sometimes, trainers use a test after training, or they may administer the same test before and after the training to compare results. Other techniques include written assignments, observations, asking questions, simulations, and role playing.

The number of objectives in each lesson varies depending on the lesson length, but normally there are at least two objectives but there could be two or three more. Examples of verbs to use in learning objectives are listed in **Table 13-6**. Table 13-6 is based on Bloom's Taxonomy—a classification of levels of intellectual skills ranging from "remember" to "create" (Krathwohl, 2002).

3. <u>Design the training</u>. Now it's time to focus on the content and **instructional methods** (strategies). In other words, the trainer must make decisions on *what to teach and how to teach it* so employees can accomplish the learning objectives. In terms of what to teach, research shows that a best practice is to break up content into small chunks that people can remember and to limit one session to four to five chunks (Naylor & Briggs, 1963). Employees cannot absorb more than about five chunks of information at one time.

You are no doubt familiar with a variety of instructional methods from attending college courses. Before choosing instructional methods, there are considerations such as the size of the group (from one-on-one training to large groups) or where it will take place—in a classroom, in the kitchen or dining room, or on a computer or other digital device. **Table 13-7** describes some common instructional methods, many of which can take place either in a classroom or in an online environment. Wherever possible, choose an instructional method that involves active learning. **Active learning** is any process by which learners are directly involved in their own learning through, for example, performing a skill, talking, or writing. The more involved an

Table 13-7 Instructional Methods

Presentation Methods (when learners mostly listen or read—these are often supplemented with active learning methods listed next)

- Lecture (often uses PowerPoint slides)
- Reading
- Podcasts
- Video
- Demonstration
- Online self-study

Active Learning Methods (when learners are involved in the learning process, either individually, in pairs, or in groups)

- On-the-job training (tell/show/do/review)
- Practice/skill rehearsal
- Simulation (performing skills—such as ringing up sales—in a situation that looks like the real environment but is really fake)
- Discussion
- Role playing
- Case study
- Games and quizzes
- Question-and-answer sessions

employee is in the training experience, the more likely they will remember and utilize what they learned.

4. <u>Develop all of the materials needed to deliver the training</u>. Resources to support learning may include printed materials, websites, video clips, PowerPoints, podcasts, quizzes, social media, handouts, prework assignments, or case studies.

5. <u>Implement the training</u>. Now it is time to do the training, whether it is classroom-based, computer-based, or on the job. Training should be delivered in an effective and efficient manner to support the employees' mastery of the learning objectives. **Table 13–8** gives tips on facilitating employee learning.

6. <u>Get employee feedback on the training</u>. After any training, the employees should evaluate the training itself using a form such as the one shown in **Table 13-9**. Employee feedback is useful to improve programs.

Table 13-8 Employees Learn Best When...

1. The training environment is informal and resembles the actual work environment.
2. The objectives are clear and very relevant to the employees' job experiences and tasks.
3. Information is presented in fun, interesting, and memorable ways.
4. Written materials are reader-friendly.
5. Employees are participants rather than spectators.
6. The trainer uses a variety of teaching methods.
7. Employees are given opportunities to practice a new skill multiple times over more than one training session.
8. The trainer draws on the experiences of the employees.
9. Employees are treated as responsible adults.
10. The trainer offers lots of feedback and praise.
11. The trainer explains "why."
12. The trainer is enthusiastic, patient, and listens to what the employees have to say.
13. Training is followed up with on-the-job coaching.

Table 13-9 Employee Evaluation of Training

Training Evaluation Form

Title of Training Session: _____

Date: _____ Trainer: _____

Please indicate your level of agreement with each of the following statements.

	Strongly Agree	Agree	Neutral	Disagree	Strongly Disagree
Rate the Course Objectives					
1. The training objectives were clearly defined.	____	____	____	____	____
2. The training objectives provided me with what I needed to learn.	____	____	____	____	____
3. The training taught me what I needed to know and do.	____	____	____	____	____
Rate the Course Delivery					
4. The topics were presented in a logical order.	____	____	____	____	____
5. The topics were relevant to me.	____	____	____	____	____
6. The training was easy to follow and understand.	____	____	____	____	____
7. The distributed materials were helpful.	____	____	____	____	____
8. The length of training was sufficient.	____	____	____	____	____
9. This training will be useful.	____	____	____	____	____
Rate the Trainer					
10. The trainer was knowledgeable about the training topics.	____	____	____	____	____
11. The trainer was well prepared.	____	____	____	____	____
12. Participation and questionswere encouraged.	____	____	____	____	____

Rate Your Overall Reaction

Please write in your answers.

13. Was the training session too long or too short?

14. Was the training worth your time?

15. What were the two most important things you learned from this training?

16. Please add any additional comments.

Table 13–10 gives an example of a training module/class from a training unit on fire safety. A training unit consists of individual modules, or classes, that often act as building blocks. The training unit on fire safety includes a class for kitchen personnel on how to prevent fires, a class for front-of-the-house personnel on how to prevent fires, and a class for all personnel on the steps to take in the event of a fire (seen in Table 13-10).

Table 13-10 Sample Training Module/Class

Training Unit: Fire Safety

Training Module #3: Steps to Take in Case of Fire

Preinstructional Activity: Hand out the restaurant's floor plan to all employees and ask them to work in pairs to locate all fire-related equipment in the restaurant and enter it on the floor plan.

Learning Objective 1: Locate fire alarms, manual activation device for fire suppression system, and fire extinguishers, and explain what each does.

Key Points	Training Methods	Resources & Tools	Time	Feedback/Assessment
1. <u>Fire alarm</u>: Starts alarms to alert occupants to leave, and alerts monitoring company to call fire department. 2. <u>Fire suppression system</u>: Nozzles installed in hood discharge a chemical suppressant designed for grease fires on cooking equipment. Gas and electricity are automatically turned off. Activated by heat/fire or manual switch. 3. <u>Fire extinguishers</u>: Only meant for small fires when an employee has an open evacuation route and environment is not too hot or smoky.	<u>Demonstration/Discussion</u>: - Walk around restaurant and show location of fire alarms, manual activation device for fire suppression, and fire extinguishers. - Ask employees what each piece of equipment does. - Also show employees the <u>automatic sprinkler system</u> and explain how it shoots out water when heat is very high.	Restaurant Safety Manual.	15–20 minutes	Ask employees how many located each piece of equipment correctly. Ask employees how many knew what each piece of equipment does.

Learning Objective 2: Demonstrate the steps to take in case of fire.

Key Points	Training Methods	Resources & Tools	Time	Feedback/Assessment
<u>Steps to take in case of fire</u> (Acronym: LATE) 1. **L**eave fire area immediately and close doors behind you to reduce oxygen for fire to grow. 2. **A**ctivate fire alarm. 3. **T**elephone fire department by calling 911 and give address and location of fire in building. 4. **E**xit (use evacuation plan) and take others with you (closing doors behind you).	<u>Tell/Show/Do/Review</u> - Handout and use Don't Be LATE poster to explain each step. - <u>Explain</u> evacuation plan. - <u>Demonstrate </u>the proper steps for a kitchen fire and *again* for a dining room fire. - <u>Ask small groups of employees to walk through</u> each step of the plan in the kitchen or dining room (depending on where they work). - <u>Review</u> the steps.	Don't be LATE! poster with Evacuation Floorplan.	30–40 minutes	As the employees practice, check their actions.

Learning Objective 3: Use a fire extinguisher.

Key Points	Training Methods	Resources & Tools	Time	Feedback/ Assessment
All employees must know when and how to use a fire extinguisher, and the difference between ABC and K extinguishers. *Only employees who are comfortable using the fire extinguisher will be asked to use it in class or in the event of a fire.* 1. A fire extinguisher should only be used when: - The fire is small. - The area is not too hot or smoky. - You have an evacuation route. - The fire alarm has been pulled. 2. Types of fire extinguishers: - ABC - multipurpose - K-rated – for grease/oil fires **Never use ABC extinguisher or water on fire with grease/oil as it makes fire worse. 3. PASS method: - **Pull the pin while holding the nozzle away from you. - **A**im low at the base of the fire. - **S**queeze the lever slowly and evenly. - **S**weep the nozzle from side to side.	<u>Lecture</u> - Review #1, 2, and 3 in Key Points. <u>Demonstration and Practice</u> - Have local fireman demonstrate PASS. - Ask interested employees to practice with extinguisher with trainer or fireman to supervise.	Local fireman. ABC fire extin-guishers. PASS poster.	15-30 minutes	Feedback from fireman and supervisor on using fire extinguisher.

Closing/Summary: Administer quiz to all employees. Two weeks later, hold fire drill.

13.4 MANAGE EMPLOYEES' PERFORMANCE

"Performance is the value of employees' contributions to the organization over time. And that value needs to be assessed in some way. Decisions about pay and promotions have to be made" (Goler, Gale, & Grant, 2016, p. 91)

Every employee in a foodservice plays a role in how successful that foodservice will be. **Performance management** is the term used to describe how each employee's performance is monitored and assessed to ensure that the employee is contributing appropriately to the foodservice's mission and goals. When an employee starts a job, the job description serves as a guide for performance. Trainers and supervisors help new employees get up to speed through training and coaching, and supervisors

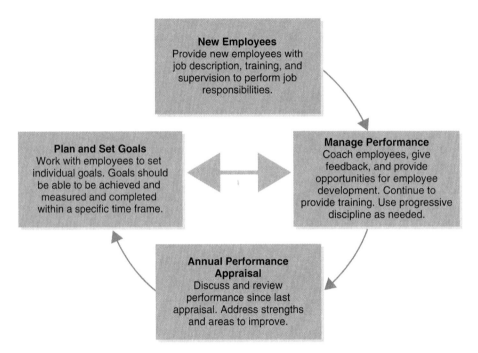

FIGURE 13-5 Performance Management Cycle

continue to observe and evaluate performance after that point. A good supervisor will frequently check in with employees to make sure they understand what is expected of them and why it is important. At the end of probation, an employee often goes through a formal **performance appraisal**, which is then repeated annually. A performance appraisal is a regular review of an employee's job performance and contribution to the organization. Performance goals are often set in a performance appraisal and then reviewed periodically (not just once a year) and at the next performance appraisal. This process is shown in **Figure 13-5**. This section will discuss coaching, annual performance appraisal, and progressive discipline (when performance is suboptimal).

COACHING

Traditionally, coaching has been used by supervisors to give feedback to employees on their performance. **Coaching** was never meant to be a disciplinary action or a training session but simply a way to correct an employee or reinforce an employee for doing something well. As an employee, it is discouraging when your boss seems to focus more on what you are doing wrong than what you are doing right. Over time, the meaning of coaching has changed and today it centers more around collaboration between the supervisor and employee. Good coaches do the following.

1. Give one-on-one performance feedback to an employee, while also asking the employee to be involved in examining and improving their own performance. For example, the coach will ask questions of the employee such as "How do you think you could improve on that?" to encourage the employee to find solutions. The coach should not always give the employee the solution, but rather ask the employee to come up with ideas that might work. Coaches also give praise and encouragement.

2. Provide motivation and guidance to employees who want to move up the career ladder. Coaches can help employees reflect on their goals, strengths, areas of improvement, and options to move to a better job, and then help them develop a plan and challenge them to stay on track.

3. <u>Provide resources to employees</u> who are interested in special training opportunities, new job experiences, taking on new responsibilities, or refer them to people who can act as resources for additional skill development.

Good coaching skills help to engage and retain employees and increase productivity, and are far less costly than formal training. Keep in mind that peer employees can coach each other too.

If coaching employees is so beneficial, why do managers often avoid it? The following are some possible reasons.

- Lack of time. (In most cases, coaching requires only a few minutes.)
- Fear of confronting an employee with a concern about his or her performance. (A mistake—the problem not faced may only get worse, not better.)
- Assumption that the employee already knows they are doing a good job—why bother saying anything? (Your employee would love to hear it anyway.)
- Limited coaching experience. (You can start practicing now.)
- Assumption that the employee will ask questions when appropriate. (Many employees are too shy to ask questions.)

When discussing performance with an employee, do not assume that the employee knows how things are supposed to be done. There are many possible reasons why employees may not be performing up to standards.

- Insufficient training or missed training sessions
- Incomplete on-the-job training
- Inconsistency or lack of enforcement of policies, procedures, and performance standards
- Boredom, lack of growth
- Work volume overload
- Personal problems
- Lack of support or resources to meet employee's needs for equipment and/or materials

Also, ask the employee for their thoughts.

Discuss an employee's performance in private, not with other employees around unless you are giving positive feedback. Supervisors can also schedule regular feedback sessions with employees. Coaching sessions should be documented and kept in the employee's file so that you have records to use for performance appraisals. **Table 13-11** lists additional coaching guidelines.

PERFORMANCE APPRAISALS

Human resources personnel provide guidance about employee evaluation and annual performance appraisals so there is uniformity across the organization. Guidelines typically include the time frames for formal reviews, such as at the end of a probationary period or annual review.

Table 13-11 General Coaching Guidelines

- Actively listen.
- Ask probing questions.
- Provide specific and constructive feedback.
- Be empathetic.
- Act like a personal cheerleader.
- Be confident and consistent.
- Don't be afraid to check on an employee's progress toward a goal.
- As needed, schedule appointments to coach employees.
- Keep each employee's coaching relationship confidential.

Performance appraisals have various roles in foodservice, as they look back over a period of time and also look ahead. They let each employee get an answer to the question "How well am I doing?" as employees get feedback on how they are meeting standards and their performance is discussed. Of course, their performance should be discussed at various points prior to the performance appraisal as part of the coaching process. The appraisal should never be the first time an employee hears about an issue or problem that the supervisor is concerned about. Instead, successes can be recognized and persistent or new performance issues addressed. Opportunities for personal development can also be considered at this time. With supervisory input, employees often set performance goals to achieve within certain timeframes in the future. The performance appraisal often acts as the basis for a possible salary increase or whether an employee may be considered for a promotion. Overall, the performance appraisal improves communication, reminds employees of the foodservice's mission and goals, and helps most employees perform better.

Before a performance appraisal occurs, the supervisor has to complete a performance appraisal form used for the specific job being evaluated. In addition, the employee is often asked to complete a self-evaluation for the supervisor to review before completing their evaluation form. An employee's self-evaluation is often completed using the same performance appraisal form the supervisor will use. In some organizations, the supervisor seeks out information about an employee from other managers, peers of the employee, subordinates of the employee, and/or customers.

There's an expression in the business world that "if you can't measure it, you can't manage it." For performance reviews to work, performance needs to be accurately measured. Therefore, *the performance appraisal form and the supervisor are very important to the success or failure of this process.*

First, let's look at the appraisal form. In order to measure accurately and consistently from employee to employee, the content should include all aspects of the specific job and ask supervisors to evaluate performance based on measurable and observable factors *related to job success.* For an evaluation to be useful, supervisors should ideally compare employee performance with the standards for the job. Supervisors are usually asked to rate employees by utilizing two or more of the following methods.

1. Checklist: Using this method, the supervisor simply checks "yes" or "no" to a series of positive or negative statements, as seen in **Table 13-12**. The checklist usually includes statements about certain job skills as well as workplace behaviors. While a checklist is easy to develop and use, sometimes an employee's skill is neither a "Yes" nor a "No" so the supervisor can't accurately rate the employee. Similary, supervisors may judge various skills subjectively, such as how accurately orders are transcribed.

2. **Graphic rating scale**: The most popular format used to appraise performance is the graphic rating scale (see **Table 13-13**). Graphic rating scales are best used to measure *traits* (psychological or physical characteristics of a person), which is why it is also referred to as a trait rating scale. They are relatively easy to

Table 13-12 Example of a Partial Checklist			
Please select "yes" or "no" for each of these statements.			
Skills	**Yes**	**No**	**Comments**
1. Takes orders accurately.			
2. Able to complete sandwich orders in a timely manner (within standards).			
3. Maintains a clean work station at all times.			
4. Follows portion control guidelines.			

Table 13-13 Examples of Graphic Rating Scale

A.

Performance Dimension	Ratings				
	Poor **1**	**Fair** **2**	**Satisfactory** **3**	**Good** **4**	**Excellent** **5**
Enthusiasm					
Judgment					
Attendance					

B.

Performance Dimension	Ratings				
	Poor **1**	**Fair** **2**	**Satisfactory** **3**	**Good** **4**	**Excellent** **5**
Initiative: Ability to develop useful ideas that are implemented.					
Appearance: Well groomed, neat appearance, meets requirements of uniform/dress policy.					

C.

Job Knowledge				
Important gaps in essential knowledge. Requires frequent super vision.	Occasional lack of knowledge requires supervisor to step in.	Knowledge is adequate to perform job adequately.	Good knowledge of job. Infrequent coaching by supervisor.	Extensive job knowledge allows employee to work independently.
Poor **1**	**Fair** **2**	**Satisfactory** **3**	**Good** **4**	**Excellent** **5**

develop and use, but could have shortcomings. If you used the graphic rating scale shown in Table 13-13A, for example, you may wonder if what you would consider "satisfactory" enthusiasm will be the same as what another supervisor considers the same rating. This can result in inconsistent ratings from employee to employee. In the case of "Attendance," if two absences each month is acceptable, at least there is a standard. When using a graphic rating scale, any traits, such as "creativity," must be truly job-related. The graphic rating scale in Table 13-13B gives a definition of the traits to be measured, and the scale in Table 13-13C gives a description for each rating. Either 13B or 13C take more time to develop but is easier and more accurate to use. Overall, graphic rating scales work best with job-related traits that cannot be otherwise measured, and a definition or anchors should be used. Examples of an employee's conduct should always be given.

3. **Behaviorally anchored rating scale (BARS)**: Instead of trying to rate traits, behaviorally anchored rating scales measure an employee's *behaviors*. BARS combines the graphic rating scale with what is called the **critical incident method**. The critical incidents method is a systematic procedure for identifying behaviors that contribute to the success or failure of employees in a specific

Table 13-14 Example of Behaviorally Anchored Rating Scale

Oral Communication	
Exceeds Acceptable Level of Performance	**7** Expresses ideas in organized and concise fashion.
	6 Actively listens to others. Gives thoughtful responses to questions.
	5 Answers questions directly.
Meets Acceptable Level of Performance	**4** Pays attention when others speak. Clearly enunciates words so others understand.
	3 Gives unclear answers to questions.
Fails to Meet Acceptable Level of Performance	**2** Repeats "you know" or other filler words when speaking. Interrupts others.
	1 Unclear when expressing ideas. Listens poorly. Uses profanity.

situation. Descriptions of actual examples, or incidents, where the employee did something well or poorly are anchored on a numerical scale (**Table 13-14**). The rater considers the anchors, or critical incidents, to help determine how to rate an employee. Although time consuming to set up, BARS is clearly more objective than most graphic rating scales.

4. **Behavior observation scale (BOS)**: The behavior observation scale is a behavior-based measure used to evaluate job performance. The person carrying out the rating uses a five-point scale to gauge the *frequency* with which an employee engages in a behavior described in a critical incident. For example, a supervisor rates how frequently a server anticipates customer concerns by circling "1" for "almost never" to "5" for "almost always."

5. **Management by objectives (MBO)**: Instead of rating an employee's traits or behaviors, management by objectives measures their *results*. Management by objectives is a system that asks all levels of employees to set goals/objectives (with input from supervisors) that contribute to the organization's mission and goals. An example would be "to increase customer satisfaction by 10%." A goal must be specific, objective, and measurable. At the onset, both the employee and supervisor need to agree on the criteria that will be used for measuring if each goal has been reached and the timeframe. The employee then pursues the goals and is evaluated on his/her results at the performance review. MBO is not meant to be used as the sole evaluation technique because it tells little about what a person did to get those results. The person may have done very little to achieve a certain outcome. **Table 13-15** shows some examples of the use of MBO on a performance review form. Developing and using MBO for evaluation is generally quite time-consuming.

6. **Standards-based Method**: Some organizations incorporate standards in their job descriptions, and the *standards* are used in the performance review form. **Table 13-16** gives an example of this format.

7. Narrative Method (Essay): In this method, supervisors must answer questions about employees by writing statements. It requires a lot more time and thought

Table 13-15 Example of MBO Objectives

Objective	% Complete	Results Statement
1. Will pass local health inspection with only one minor deficiency or fewer.		
2. Average customer satisfaction with food will increase from 3 to 4.		
3. Will develop new sanitation class and teach to all kitchen personnel within six months.		

Table 13-16 Example of Performance Standards Used in Server Performance			
Appraisal Performance Standards	**Exceeds Requirements**	**Meets Requirements**	**Needs Improvements**
1. Stocks the service station before each meal using Stocking Guidelines.			
2. Sets tables correctly.			
3. Greets guests cordially within three minutes after being seated.			
4. Explains menu, describes the specials, and accurately answers guests' questions.			

than a simple check yes or no. For example, one question may ask to describe leadership skills used to attain an objective. As you can imagine, this method is more often used with management and executives, not hourly employees.

8. **360-degree performance review**: This type of review uses feedback from coworkers (peer review), supervisors, direct reports, other employees, customers, and vendors (as appropriate). Involving additional people in the appraisal process provides a broader picture of the employee's work performance that is not often considered. Coworkers and others are asked to complete a confidential survey that focuses primarily on discovering strengths, although areas for improvement are also discussed. The survey results are compiled, reviewed, and numeric results are averaged. They are then presented to each employee under review in a constructive way and the information is used to create a personal development plan. This method is more effective when developing employees than when rating employees, although average ratings tend to be quite accurate (Zenger & Folkman, 2012). This type of review can certainly be useful when employees work in teams; however, it is a very time-consuming process. It is also challenging to maintain the confidentiality of the people who contribute feedback.

Each of these formats have their pluses and minuses. The formats chosen will be influenced by available time and money as well as whether traits, objectives, behaviors or actions, compliance with standards, or results are to be evaluated. For example, an appraisal form that uses MBO for measuring results and BARS for measuring behaviors may be appropriate for a number of managers and some hourly employees.

The supervisor has the responsibility of rating an employee's performance and communicating this to the employee. Here are some examples of rating errors that supervisors make.

1. Subjective evaluations: Each supervisor brings to the rating process their own personal values, perceptions, prejudices, stereotypes, and emotions. Supervisors are being subjective when they give higher ratings to employees they like (often employees who they consider to be like themselves—called **similarity error**) or lower ratings to employees they don't like as much. The best advice is to evaluate the performance, not the person.

2. Halo effect: The **halo effect** refers to allowing the rating of one aspect of performance in which an employee excels, such as being cooperative, to positively influence the rating of other factors.

3. Horns effect: The **horns effect** is the opposite of the halo effect and occurs when a poor rating in one aspect of the evaluation negatively influences the rating of other factors.

4. Distributional errors: **Distributional errors** occur when supervisors rate most employees using just one part of a rating scale—specifically the top part, the

middle, or lower part of the scale. For example, supervisors who are too generous with the ratings exhibit **leniency error**. The opposite of leniency error is **severity error**—when everyone is rated below average. Other supervisors rate everyone as average or slightly above average—called the **error of central tendency**. These types of errors can cause problems, such as when you need to fire an employee who has received glowing yearly appraisals.

5. <u>Recency error:</u> **Recency error** occurs when the employee is rated only on his or her most recent performance. Performance review does not begin a month before the appraisal session, but a full year earlier. Recency error frequently occurs because the supervisor has insufficient documentation of employee performance, so that only recent observations are discussed.

Any negative comments should be explained with examples. It is not enough to state that service skills were poor or need improvement. Rather, be specific in terms of the exact task or behavior that must be improved and how to improve it. Training supervisors to perform objective evaluations and to practice making ratings can help avoid these errors.

The performance appraisal interview is a time to help and develop employees, not to punish them. If the appraisal interview is conducted only once a year, it is too late to give praise or remedy problems that were not already discussed during the past year. Since many annual performance appraisals have salary review as a major purpose, be aware that some employees tend not to focus on the evaluation as much as on the increase. **Table 13–17** gives guidelines for preparing and conducting a performance appraisal.

Table 13-17 Guidelines for Preparing and Conducting a Performance Appraisal

<u>Preparing for a Performance Appraisal</u>

1. In advance, explain the performance appraisal instrument and interview process to the employee.
2. If employees are asked to do self-evaluations, ask the employee to complete their form. Self-evaluation is a wonderful way to make the employee more of a doer than a receiver in this process.
3. Set an appropriate time for the interview that is convenient for the employee. Do not do appraisals during the employee's break time.
4. Select a place for the interview that is quiet and informal.
5. Review the employee's file and self-evaluation while filling out the performance appraisal form. Give specific examples on the form, not generalities.

<u>Conducting the Performance Appraisal Interview</u>

1. Establish and maintain a friendly, relaxed, and trusting atmosphere by doing the following.
   • Maintain good eye contact.
   • Don't sit behind a desk.
   • Start with a statement of purpose and agenda.
   • Explain that honesty and feedback are important.
   • Use positive, constructive language instead of negative language; for instance, using "concern" instead of "problem."
   • Actively listen.
   • Be a coach instead of a judge.
2. Start with a discussion of employee strengths and give praise. Don't read directly from the form!
3. Next, identify and ask for the employees to discuss areas that need improvement. Be sure to cite *specific* and concrete examples of less than satisfactory performance. Don't use a "tell-and-sell" approach. Ask the employee to describe any obstacles to better performance. If the employee disagrees with your assessment, listen and be open-minded enough to allow the employee to change your mind.
4. Use a *problem-solving approach* to help them to develop an action plan to improve areas of concern. Make sure this plan has deadlines and is specific, realistic, and measurable.
5. Summarize and conclude on a positive note.
6. Ask the employee to sign the written evaluation form and write down any comments. Make sure the employee gets a copy of the appraisal.

PROGRESSIVE DISCIPLINE

To prevent discipline problems, managers lay out what is expected of new hires, including how and how well to perform job duties (described in the job description and performance standards) and how to conduct themselves (described in the work rules or code of conduct). Indeed, most employees will get their jobs done and cause no problems. However, when an employee breaks a rule, foodservice managers use disciplinary policies and procedures, which should appear in an employee handbook. Typical types of discipline problems and examples include the following.

1. Attendance: Excessive absenteeism or lateness, abuse of paid time off.
2. On-the-job behaviors: Failure to follow sanitation or safety procedures, poor job performance such as undercooked food or incorrect portion sizes, low productivity, sexual harassment of coworker.
3. Dishonesty: Theft of food, beverages, or cash or falsifying information.

Some foodservices categorize disciplinary problems into categories such as minor infractions, major infractions, and causes for immediate discharge. Minor infractions include concerns such as excessive absenteeism or tardiness, violation of cell phone policy, or abuse of break times and meal periods. Major infractions interfere substantially with operations and might include falsifying records, threatening behavior, risking the safety of customers or employees, or refusal to carry out reasonable assignments. Some foodservices also list reasons for immediate firing of an employee, which are usually actions that are illegal (such as theft) or put someone in danger (fighting).

When establishing disciplinary guidelines, most employers use a **progressive discipline** system. Progressive discipline applies corrective measures, such as coaching, in increasing degrees or steps if the behavior continues. In most situations, an employee is given several opportunities to correct the behavior. Progressive discipline approaches rule-breaking as a problem to be solved, not as wrongdoing to be punished. It does not threaten people's self-respect, as punishment does. The overall purpose of progressive discipline is to get the employee to correct behavior *voluntarily*.

The typical progression of disciplinary action starts with an oral counseling and warning, then moves onto a written warning, second written warning, temporary suspension, and termination (**Figure 13-6**). For a minor infraction such as excessive absenteeism (which a company may define as four or more unplanned absences in a month), the first step is usually to start with an oral counseling and warning. A more serious offense, such as falsifying records, might start with a written warning or even a suspension. A **suspension** is when an employee can't go to work for a period of time—often one to three days. Whether or not the employee is paid depends on federal and state wage and hour laws and collective bargaining agreements if there is a union.

Be familiar with your company's policy and procedures on discipline, and make sure employees are also knowledgeable about the process. Disciplinary action should never come as a surprise to an employee. When you are confronted with a disciplinary situation, this series of steps will help you decide what should be done.

1. <u>Collect all of the facts</u>: Keeping an open mind, interview any employees involved and any witnesses. Ask witnesses to write down their version of what happened along with a signature and date. Use these questions as a guide.
   - Did the employee know he was doing something wrong? Were the employee's actions intentional or an accident?

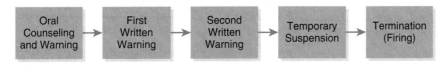

FIGURE 13-6 Steps in Progressive Discipline

- Were there extenuating circumstances such as personal problems?
- How long has the employee worked here and how is their past record (including performance reviews)?
- How serious was the offense? Was anyone injured?
- If you didn't witness the episode, do you have enough evidence to substantiate disciplinary action?

2. <u>Talk to the employee as soon as possible</u>: Explain to the employee what your concern is and ask for their side of the story. Keep an open mind as you listen and ask questions as needed. Every employee has the right to due process, meaning the opportunity to defend himself from any charges.

3. <u>Decide if any action needs to be taken after consulting with your boss and possibly human resources</u>: Any action to be taken must be consistent with past practice and must also be nondiscriminatory. In some organizations, higher levels of disciplinary action (such as suspension or termination) must be reviewed with a representative from human resources to make sure the action is appropriate.

4. <u>Take the action, such as a written warning, and develop an improvement plan with the employee</u>: Many organizations have disciplinary forms that must be filled out, as seen in **Table 13–18**. For the disciplinary meeting, you will likely have another manager or human resources person with you to act as a witness. If the employee is part of a union, the employee will bring a union representative. Explain to the employee the action you are taking and why. Ask the employee to identify some actions he can take so this does not reoccur. Mutually develop an improvement plan including a timeline. Make it clear that you are willing to work with the employee but it remains the employee's responsibility to make the needed changes. Also make it clear what the next step will

---

Table 13-18 Sample Notice of Disciplinary Action

Notice of Disciplinary Action

Employee Name: _____

Department: _____ Position Title: _____

Date and Time of Incident: _____

Type of Incident

_____ Excessive absenteeism/lateness _____ Work quality/quantity

_____ Abuse of break times/meal periods _____ Policy violation: _____

_____ Abuse of cell phone policy _____

_____ Improper uniform _____ Other: _____

_____ Neglect sanitation/safety rules: _____

Description of Incident (include results of investigation and employee comments):

Previous warning(s): _____ Yes _____ No

If yes, give date and type of incident.

Employee Improvement Plan:

Consequences if Improvement Does Not Occur:

_____

Action Taken: _____ Written Warning (Note first or second)

_____ Suspension Date(s): _____

_____ Termination Effective Date: _____

I have discussed the above with the employee.

Date and Time: _____

Supervisor's Signature: _____

_____

Employee Section

Comments: If you disagree with the action taken or anything else, please write here.

Your signature means only that you have been advised of the contents of this warning. It does not signify that you agree with its contents.

_____ _____

Employee's Signature and Date

---

be if the behavior is not corrected. The employee is usually asked to sign any written warnings so the employer has proof that the employee was informed of the contents of the report. From time to time, you will have an employee who refuses to sign the report because they think their signature will signify agreement with the contents of the report. When this happens, explain that the signature means the employee read the document, not that the employee agrees with everything there. If the employee still refuses to sign, have the witness sign that the employee was given the disciplinary action. Each employee should also be given the opportunity to provide a written response to the disciplinary action.

5. <u>Make sure everything is documented (written down)</u>: There are several reasons for keeping good disciplinary records. First, in the event you are ever taken to court, you will need written documentation including the exact nature of the misconduct. Second, the process of writing helps you see the situation more objectively and focus on job-related issues. When documenting, focus on observable, verifiable facts and be nonjudgmental. Don't document opinions or hearsay. Focus on who, what, where, when, and how, as well as the impact of the misconduct. Document accurately and thoroughly, and connect the employee's misconduct to the organization's policies. Mention previous warnings, if there are any. Keep a copy of all documents in the employee's personnel file, including notes on oral warnings. These documents are helpful if the behavior occurs again.

6. <u>Follow-up</u>: Check in with the employee regularly and check for improvement. If the employee's behavior does not meet your expectations, you will need to progress to the next step mentioned in the warning.

Tips for using disciplinary guidelines are given in **Table 13–19.**

Each organization usually has a policy about when disciplinary records can be removed from the employee's file—such as six months for a written warning or 12 months for a final warning (meaning the next step is dismissal). The idea is that if the problem behavior doesn't reoccur within six or 12 months, the employee has learned from the experience.

Table 13-19 Tips for Taking Disciplinary Action

- <u>Be consistent in how you handle disciplinary issues</u>: If you issue a written warning for the second time an employee abuses the cell phone policy, for example, be consistent across all employees. Employees have more respect for a supervisor who is fair and consistent.

- <u>New supervisors should *not* start off being easy about rule enforcement or totally ignore when employees break rules</u>: New supervisors often want employees to like them, but what supervisors really need is for employees to respect them. When new supervisors let employees get away with inappropriate behavior, some employees will test how far they can go before getting into trouble. In the long run, the supervisor will have a real problem getting people to follow rules and meet standards while quality and service suffer.

- <u>Take responsibility for disciplinary action—don't shift the responsibility to your boss or anyone else</u>: Don't tell an employee that your boss or human resources made you take disciplinary action. If you do this, you look like you have little authority or power and employees will not respect you.

- <u>Investigate possible infractions and act as soon as possible after the incident occurs</u>: Waiting too long to take action is not fair to the employee, and inappropriate behavior needs to be corrected as soon as possible.

- <u>Criticize the behavior, not the employee</u>: Be respectful of the employee. Don't let anger or frustration with the employee seep into the tone of your verbal communication or documentation.

- <u>Make sure the employee knows exactly what will happen if misconduct continues</u>.

- <u>Be sure to document the date of the action, name and position of the person issuing the discipline, the level of discipline, a detailed description of the misconduct, specific policy the employee violated, and recent and relevant disciplinary actions taken with the employee</u>: In addition, you should state what will happen if the misconduct occurs again.

The final step in progressive discipline is involuntary **termination**, or firing, of an employee. (Voluntary termination occurs when an employee voluntarily resigns.) Every state in the United States, except for Montana, allows **at-will employment**. At-will employees can be fired at any time and for almost any reason. Likewise, the at-will employee is free to leave the employer at any time and for any reason. Unless an employer gives a clear indication, such as in the Employee Handbook, that it will only fire employees for just cause, it is assumed the employees are at-will employees. At-will employees still cannot be fired for discriminatory reasons or because they have complained about health and safety violations or discrimination in the workplace. At-will employees also cannot be fired for exercising their legal right to, for example, file for worker's compensation or participate in union activities. Some at-will employers do the following to protect their at-will prerogative.

1. Avoid references to "career" employment in recruiting and selecting.
2. Ask new hires to sign at-will statements.
3. Put at-will statements in to the employee handbook that indicate that none of its provisions prevent the company from terminating employees for any reason and at any time.
4. Change "permanent status" to "regular status."
5. Avoid oral and written statements promising any type of job security, such as "As long as you keep doing well, you will have a job working here."

Employers who state they only fire employees for just cause generally have a policy providing causes (such as theft) for being fired and a procedure to follow. Employers must be very careful about how they handle this process. All possible terminations must have input from higher-level managers and human resources personnel. If an investigation needs to be done, the employee should be suspended with pay until the investigation is complete. If firing the employee is justified, some states require the employer to give the employee the final paycheck when they are fired.

Before making a termination decision, you should be able to answer yes to each of these questions.

1. Did the employee know the rule and were they warned about the consequences of violating the rule?
2. Were management's expectations of the employee reasonable? Was the rule reasonable?
3. Did management make a reasonable effort to help the employee resolve the problem before now, and is there proof of such efforts?
4. Was a final warning given to the employee explaining that discharge would result from another rule violation or unsatisfactory performance? Did the employee sign this warning to acknowledge understanding of its terms?
5. In the case of misconduct, did the employee act in willful and deliberate disregard of reasonable employer expectations? Was the situation within their control?
6. Was management's investigation conducted fairly and objectively and did it involve someone other than the employee's direct supervisor?
7. Is dismissal in line with the employee's prior work record and length of service?
8. Did the employee have the opportunity to hear the facts and respond to them in a nonthreatening environment?
9. Has this employee been treated equally with others under similar circumstances?
10. Was the action nondiscriminatory?

In some organizations, there may be an appeal or grievance process that a terminated employee may utilize. This is especially true in union shops where the potential termination may have to be approved by an arbitration panel. If there is one, either the human resources person or the foodservice manager must make sure the employee knows what to do to start that process.

13.5 SCHEDULE EMPLOYEES

Staffing and scheduling are related functions, but they do not have the same meaning. **Staffing** is the process of determining personnel needs, recruiting, and selecting employees. **Scheduling** is the process of assigning an appropriate number of employees to work at specified times and days so that the work of the foodservice is accomplished.

As a manager, it is important to openly and clearly identify schedule needs and expectations during the interview process, since the majority of foodservice positions require work on weekends, holidays, and on both early and late shifts. This should be explained early when screening potential employees. Discussing a candidate's availability and willingness to be flexible during the interview process can prevent the time and monetary loss that will be realized by hiring and training someone who is not a good fit for the position.

The level of staffing an operation requires is tied to a number of factors, such as the type of foodservice (for example, conventional or assembly/serve), number of meals forecasted to be served, and the productivity level desired. The level of staffing also depends on how multiskilled your employees are. If your employees only possess a narrow range of skills, more staffing will be needed. Your menu, the form in which food is purchased, and your production and delivery systems also influence your level of staffing.

Staffing needs are often stated in **full-time equivalents (FTE)**. One FTE is the equivalent of one full-time employee, working 8 hours a day, 40 hours a week (although in some companies this number is a little lower), which works out to be 2,080 hours a year. If you have an eight-hour position that needs to be filled every day of the week, you will need about 1.5 FTEs to fill the position 365 days a year to account for the extra two days every week plus paid time off (vacation, holidays, etc.). For an eight-hour position that needs to be filled five days a week, you will need about 1.1 FTEs.

When talking about labor hours, you need to know the difference between productive hours and nonproductive hours. **Productive hours** are hours when an employee is working. **Nonproductive hours** are hours when an employee is getting paid but is not working on the job. This could include paid time off for sick days, personal days, holidays, or vacation, as examples.

Each functional area of a foodservice often has its own schedule. For example, all food production personnel are often on one schedule while dining room personnel are on a different schedule. The **master schedule** includes schedules for each area within the foodservice. The primary importance of schedules is to control and structure the use of labor hours. Labor hours translate directly to become labor dollars on the cost side of the foodservice's budget.

When creating labor schedules, the manager must first define the work to be completed. This work should match the requirements of the job description to avoid labor disputes. In foodservice operations, the hours of operation and the menu are key drivers in determining how many staff members will be working. Customer demand, meal volumes, and types of service provided are additional factors that impact how many employees are required. The expected volume of customers can vary dramatically between a Friday afternoon and a Sunday morning. If your restaurant sells custom-topped burgers and pizza, the business may be brisk on a Friday or Saturday evening compared with a Sunday late morning. Conversely, if your restaurant is known for its fresh baked pastries, Sunday morning may be one of your highest volume period. The schedule should reflect these high and low volume periods and staffing assignments should be adjusted accordingly.

The manager often creates a scheduling template or master schedule to use throughout the year, which identifies the shifts needed to adequately staff the work. The scheduling template should include each employee's regular days on duty and days off, and also reflect the staffing patterns that support the high and low volume periods of the operation. A master schedule can be revised to include upcoming special events that may require increased or reduced staffing needs as well as to reflect changes to the normally scheduled shifts.

Foodservices also need a mechanism that allows employees to request time off in advance of the schedule writing process. Managers should establish a due date for time-off requests to be submitted to allow sufficient time to incorporate the request into the schedule and ensure appropriate coverage. Managers should establish staffing parameters that set a maximum number of employees who may take the same day(s) off at one time. It is also important to establish rules for using seniority versus a "first come, first served" approach to request for days off and holidays. For the winter holidays or premium vacation weeks, you may rotate who gets off each year. For example, in foodservice operations that never close, such as corrections and healthcare, it is not uncommon to ask each employee to work at least one of the major holidays from November through December (basically Thanksgiving, Christmas, and New Year's Eve) and rotate which day each employee works. So an employee who works Thanksgiving this year will be expected to work Christmas next year, and so on.

Seasonal vacation requests are usually handled differently. For high-demand vacation periods, when multiple employee time-off requests are likely, the manager may establish a practice where the submission due date is one to two months in advance of summer and staff would be asked to enter their desired vacation requests for that period. This will allow the manager adequate time to review and plan for the requests to eliminate short staffing. Again, it is important to establish parameters for the maximum number of employees permitted to have time off during a two-week or other scheduling period. The manager may need to deny a request if multiple employees request the same period off. Working ahead will allow the employees to adjust their plans in advance.

Schedules should be posted at least 14 days in advance and typically reflect the next two-week pay period. This allows staff time to access the schedule for planning purposes. Schedules typically follow a pattern so employees can anticipate when they will be off. Not following a regular schedule or not posting a schedule until late has been abused in segments of the foodservice industry, so Predictive Scheduling legislation has actually been passed in some states and localities. This type of legislation requires employers to give a certain amount of notice to employees about their work schedules. In a tight labor market, where employees can easily find work at the foodservice outlets, it is especially important to be fair and predictable with scheduling.

Computerized scheduling systems, many linked with apps, are now available that provide a more interactive scheduling process. Managers can create an online schedule for staff members to access and view. Some systems allow employees to submit time off requests directly through the system for weeks or months in advance, which then alerts the manager. The system includes the parameters or rules for submitting time off requests and notifies the employee if the request does not meet the schedule parameters. The manager can approve or disapprove the request through the system and include a reply to the employee if the request is denied.

Some systems also allow employees to change shifts with other employees through an email or text process. The employee can anonymously express their desire to give up a shift through a group text to other members of their work team. A coworker can anonymously accept the offer. Their manager is alerted through text or email of this communication and to the identities of the employees who wish to make the change. The system will then alert the manager if there is potential overtime or any additional cost caused by the change. The manager can approve or deny the change before it is incorporated into the schedule.

Schedules should be planned with fairness and take into account the employees' quality of life. In the service industry, happy employees provide and support high-quality customer service. Inconsistent and poorly planned schedules can significantly impact employee morale and engagement. Schedules that equitably distribute labor hours and balance work shifts support productive employees, work/life balance, and a safer work space.

Schedules should not be used as a means to punish or reward employees, although managers have been known to do so. Granting or refusing time off for holidays or vacations should be done in a fair and equitable manner. An employee's work/life quality can be significantly impacted by irregular scheduling. Avoid scheduling an employee from working late to early. If the employee is scheduled to close and work until 10:00 PM, don't schedule them for an opening shift at 6:00 AM the next day. Strive to keep hours of work consistent and balanced. Avoid scheduling staff to work long stretches, such as over five or six consecutive days. This contributes to a higher risk of injury for the employee due to fatigue and creates an unsafe work environment. Young managers are often surprised that employees remember small changes in scheduling and may perceive that schedule changes are based simply on whether or not the manager likes them.

Creating a balanced schedule is not easy. Some seasoned managers consider it an art. The manager is tasked with balancing the needs of the operation, its employees, and controlling budgeted labor hours. The manager, who is familiar with the needs of the employees, their availability to work, and their capabilities within the operation, will have the best chance of success with schedule writing and planning.

To summarize, use these scheduling guidelines.

- Schedules should be patterned. Develop a template or master schedule to use throughout the year for planning purposes.
- Have a staffing plan for regular operational needs and a plan for working short-handed (emergency staffing) that outlines minimum staffing requirements to run the operation.
- Have defined policies in place for schedule posting along with submitting and approving time-off requests.
- Make the schedule as far in advance as possible. In New York City, fast food chains must give employees two weeks' notice.

Table 13-20 Steps to Write a Schedule
1. Know how many positions work each day and know which employees have the skills to work which positions.
2. First, enter regular days off. (This is where a "master schedule" can save time by having regular days off already on the schedule.)
3. Check for any special events (such as catering) scheduled for a particular day that will affect staffing needs.
4. Also check your time-off requests and grant them according to staffing guidelines.
5. Fill in full-time staff first to guarantee they each have the correct number of hours (usually 40).
6. Next, fill in part-time staff according to operational needs and their budgeted number of hours. Review each staff member's total hours to ensure time is distributed equitably.
7. If staff is cross-trained, rotate jobs as needed and practical.
8. Check schedule horizontally and vertically. After you have filled in the schedule, cross-check each day vertically to ensure all positions are covered. You may want to give each daily position a number, then you just need to count them up to make sure you have all positions covered. Check the schedule horizontally to ensure consistency.
9. Have you scheduled someone for a late shift, followed by an early shift, or for six days in a row? Avoid scheduling long stretches. This helps prevent fatigue, job dissatisfaction, and injuries.
10. Total the number of hours for each employee to ensure that guaranteed hours are met but NOT exceeded. Scheduling systems will perform these types of checks for you and provide an alert for scheduled overtime.
11. Don't schedule overtime—unless extenuating circumstances dictate you to do so.
12. Check for cost-effectiveness. Is the lowest pay rate employee who is appropriately trained doing the job? Don't schedule a more highly paid employee to perform a lower classification job. And if a person is in a position that relies on tipping, assure that most of their workday is spent where tips are available as opposed to side work.

- Be completely familiar with schedule rules set within your business such as which day the workweek starts on, rules about consecutive number of days worked that are allowed, or a minimum number of weekends off each month.
- Make your best effort to accommodate employee preferences whenever possible and be practical. Be fair and consistent in scheduling and granting time off.
- Work within your labor budget.
- Make employees aware of the labor budget and the scheduling process. *Labor represents the largest part of your budget, and scheduling can significantly impact the finances of the business.*

Table 13–20 outlines specific steps to take when writing schedules.

13.6 WORK WITH UNIONS

Unions are organizations elected by a group of nonmanagement employees to represent them in bargaining with an employer for wages, hours, and working conditions. Employees often join unions to protect their rights and interests, improve their working conditions and wages/salaries, and give them a voice. There have been unions in the United States since the 1790s.

Most union members in the United States belong to a national or international union, such as the Service Employees International Union, which has foodservice members. Most national unions are affiliated with the American Federation of Labor and Congress of Industrial Organizations (AFL-CIO). The AFL-CIO is not a labor union, but rather a federation of unions that works to advance the interests of its member unions. A **local union** represents employees in a limited geographic area and may include workers, such as foodservice employees, employed by different companies. Most local unions have a charter from a national/international union.

As of 2019, 10.3% of American workers were members of unions. The percentage of workers represented by a union was 11.6% (Bureau of Labor Statistics, 2021). Workers represented by a union include both union members and workers who are not union members but whose jobs are covered by a union contract. Workers who are not union members cannot vote on union business such as election of union officials or ratifying a labor contract. Union membership has declined significantly since the 1950s when over 30% of American workers were union members.

The dealings between unions and management are referred to as **labor relations**. Whereas unions look out for their members in terms of good wages, hours, and working conditions, management is concerned about whether unions will negatively impact profits and productivity. Nowadays, the emphasis in labor relations is for both parties to work together to positively influence costs and output.

Before discussing more about unions, it is important to be familiar with some key terms.

- **Bargaining unit**: The bargaining unit is a group of two or more employees who share common employment conditions and are grouped together and represented by a specific labor union in collective bargaining and other dealings with management.
- **Collective bargaining**: Process in which employees, through their unions, negotiate contracts with their employees to determine pay, benefits, hours, paid time off, safety policies, etc.
- **Collective bargaining agreement (CBA)** or labor contract: During negotiations between the union and the employer, a collective bargaining agreement is hammered out on topics such as pay, benefits, hours of work, and other conditions of employment. The CBA is a legal document for a specific period, such as two years.

By law, all members of a bargaining unit are represented by the union. However, that doesn't mean they are all dues-paying union members. Each union contract includes a section that discusses the extent to which the union can influence new members to join. In a **closed shop**, all members of the bargaining unit must be union members and pay dues. In a **union shop**, a new employee must join the union within a specified period of time after starting employment (such as 30 days). In an **agency shop**, all members of the bargaining unit pay dues, but they are not required to be union members. Under a **dues checkoff provision**, the employer collects dues from union members and nonunion members and then gives the dues to the union. Dues checkoff agreements are legal as long as they are authorized by the employees.

About half of the states have **Right-to-Work laws**, which guarantee that no employee can be required to join a labor union or pay union dues. Therefore, states with Right-to-Work laws *do not allow closed shops, union shops, or agency shops*. The Right-to-Work states are more so in the south and midwestern United States. In 2018, a ruling from the U.S. Supreme Court said that government workers who choose not to join unions are not required to pay dues that pay for collective bargaining.

LABOR LEGISLATION

The **National Labor Relations Act** (also called the Wagner Act) was a significant piece of labor legislation that covered all private-sector employers and nonmanagerial employees not covered by the Railway Labor Act. Up until the National Labor Relations Act was passed in 1935, unions did not get a lot of legal support. That changed after the Great Depression started in 1929. The Wagner Act affirmed the employee's right to organize a union, become a union member, engage in union activities, and go on strike to get better working conditions. If employees chose to be represented by a union, management was required to negotiate with union representatives. It outlawed unfair labor practices by employers such as spying on union meetings, firing pro-union employees, or interfering with the formation of activities of a union.

The National Labor Relations Act also created the **National Labor Relations Board (NLRB)**. The functions of the NLRB include investigation of complaints lodged by unions or employees and oversight of elections in which a union may be selected as the collective bargaining agent for a bargaining unit.

The **Labor-Management Relations Act** (also known as the Taft-Hartley Act of 1947) tried to create a balance between union power and management authority. Unfair labor practices by both unions and management were defined. Unions were not allowed, as examples, to refuse to bargain collectively with the employer, charge excessive initiation fees for new members or dues for existing members, engage in violence when striking, or threaten employees to select a union or support its activities. Management was given more rights during union organizing campaigns, such as discussing the advantages and disadvantages of union membership with employees. States were also given the right to enact laws, the Right-to-Work laws, which allow employees to work in a unionized business without joining the union. Lastly, the U.S. President was given the right to impose an 80-day, cooling-off period to delay a strike if it poses a threat to national safety or health is threatened.

The Taft-Hartley Act also established the Federal Mediation and Conciliation Services, which has two major functions. They are notified of contract expirations and offer to help work on new contracts in order to avoid work stoppages. They also keep lists of available arbitrators. **Mediation** refers to the process by which an impartial third party meets with both sides separately and then suggests compromises or actions that may lead to an agreement. A mediator has no authority to force a party to accept anything. In **arbitration**, a third party conducts hearings to help form the basis of their decisions, which both parties agree in advance will be binding—in other words, both sides must accept the arbitrator's decision.

After union corruption was exposed in the 1950s, the **Landrum-Griffin Act of 1959** was passed. Unions were required to file annual reports with the U.S. Department of Labor on their finances, elections, and other matters. It also established a bill of rights for union members, which required that every union member be given the right to nominate candidates for union office, vote in union elections, participate in union meetings, and review unions' financial records.

HOW TO START (ORGANIZE) A UNION

To organize a union, a series of steps must be taken (**Figure 13-7**). To get things started, union representatives will try to organize one-on-one and group meetings with employees as well as provide literature about the union and its benefits. If a majority of workers want to form a union, they need to get at least 30% of workers in the bargaining unit to sign union authorization cards. A union authorization card is signed by a worker to indicate the worker's desire to be represented in the workplace by the union. Then the National Labor Relations Board will conduct a secret ballot election. During the time before the election, the employer is not allowed to promise or grant benefits to employees, to influence the voting, or to spy on employees. They can discuss the pros and cons of union membership as well as communicate to employees that signing the authorization card doesn't mean they have to vote yes for the union.

If a majority of voters choose the union, the NLRB will certify the union as the representative for the workers. A vote does not need to be taken if the employer agrees to

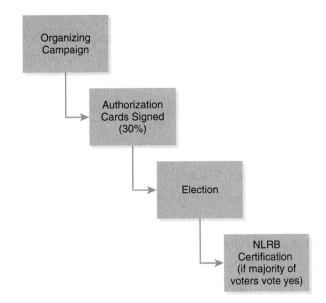

FIGURE 13-7 Unionization Process

let the union represent the workers, which may happen after an employer finds out that a majority of employees signed authorization cards. Once a union has been certified or recognized, the employer is required to meet at reasonable times to bargain in good faith about wages, hours, paid time off, benefits, safety practices, and other topics.

The same process used to certify a union can be used to decertify a union, meaning the union is voted out. However, a union can only be voted out when there is no labor contract in effect.

How to Work Effectively with a Union

If you are working with a union, it is essential to become familiar with the union contract and to oversee how the contract is administered. It is also important to get to know the union stewards and develop a positive working relationship with them. A **union steward** (also called a shop steward or union representative) is a union employee who has been elected as the representative for a group of employees when dealing with management. Union stewards check to make sure the union contract is being administered properly, represent workers in disciplinary and grievance proceedings, and other duties.

A **grievance** is a work-related complaint made by an employee. Often, the grievance is related to dissatisfaction with a disciplinary action, but a grievance may be about any section of the union contract that the employee feels has been violated. The union contract explains how to file a grievance and the series of steps to handle and hopefully resolve the issue. Normally, the first step is for the employee to discuss the concern with the immediate supervisor. An employee may ask the union steward to accompany them to that meeting. If the first step does not produce satisfaction and qualifies as a contract violation, the next step is to put the grievance in writing and submit it to the supervisor's boss. A meeting takes place between all parties and management puts its response in writing. If the problem is still not resolved, the grievance is appealed to the next level of management and additional union officers may be involved. If the problem is not resolved in this step, the union may decide whether or not to use arbitration. Fortunately, most grievances are resolved in the earlier stages.

SUMMARY

13.1 Apply Federal Laws Affecting Human Resources Management

- The Fair Labor Standards Act (FLSA) establishes minimum wage, overtime pay, and youth employment standards. Nonexempt employees (hourly employees) must receive overtime pay for hours worked over 40 per workweek at a rate not less than one and one-half times the regular rate of pay. Exempt employees do not receive overtime pay.
- The Family and Medical Leave Act of 1993 allows eligible employees to take up to 12 weeks of unpaid leave in a 12-month period for birth or care of the employee's child up to 1 year of age, placement of a child for adoption, care of an employee's family member with a serious health condition, or the employee's own health condition involving the inability to perform their job. Upon returning to work, the employee must be returned to their original position or fully equivalent position in terms of pay, benefits, and working conditions.
- Table 13-1 summarizes major Equal Employment Opportunity laws. These laws that make it illegal to discriminate against a job applicant or an employee because of the person's race, color, religion, sex (including pregnancy, gender identity, and sexual orientation), national origin, age (40 or older), disability or genetic information. The laws apply to all types of work situations, including hiring, disciplining, promoting, training, wages, benefits, and harassment. Most employers with at least 15 employees are covered by EEO laws (20 employees in age discrimination cases).
- Sexual harassment is defined as unwelcome sexual advances, requests for sexual favors, and other verbal or physical conduct of a sexual nature when an employment decision is made because the individual submitted to or rejected the unwelcome conduct, or the unwelcome conduct interferes with an individual's work performance or creates an intimidating, hostile, or abusive work environment.
- To avoid legal liability and negative publicity, a foodservice must have a published sexual harassment policy with a detailed procedure on reporting and investigating complaints, train all managers and employees on reporting and preventing sexual harassment, confidentially investigate all complaints and take appropriate actions, and create and retain complete and accurate records.
- The Occupational Safety and Health Act (1970) requires employers to provide every employee with a safe place to work. To enforce this act, the Occupational Safety and Health Administration inspects employers and requires employers to record work-related injuries/illnesses that result in medical treatment beyond first aid, loss of consciousness, days away from work, restricted work, or transfer to another job.
- Employees should be trained on warning signs of workplace violence and know the procedures to follow in case of violence or theft.

13.2 Recruit and Select Employees

- Most foodservices use both internal and external recruiting.
- Common external recruitment methods include posting jobs on the foodservice's website, posting "Help Wanted" signs, asking current employees for referrals, posting jobs on job boards such as Monster or job aggregators such as Indeed, advertising in papers or other publications, recruiting at schools and colleges, and using private employment agencies, temporary employment agencies, or state employment agencies.
- The selection process varies but generally involves screening applications and/or resumes, pre-employment tests and/or work samples, interviews, and finally, background checks and selection of a finalist.
- The selection process is guided by the job specification (qualifications for a job— including knowledge, skills, and abilities) and job description (responsibilities and tasks of a job).
- The selection process must be nondiscriminatory and job-related. One way to do that is to apply each step in the selection process in a consistent manner across all applicants. Also, make sure that selection criteria do not disproportionately exclude certain racial

groups. Employment tests and other selection procedures must be job-related and properly validated for the positions and purposes for which they are used. When applicants take a selection tool that is *valid*, the tool has shown that the applicants scoring higher on the test perform better on the job than applicants with lower test scores.

- Examples of employment tests or work samples include cognitive ability tests, physical ability tests, job knowledge tests, work samples, or drug testing.

- To learn more about an applicant during an interview, the most useful questions are open-ended, reflective, probing, behavioral, and situational. Interview questions should be reflective of the job's responsibilities, tasks, and qualifications.

- Because interviews are costly to perform and prone to being subjective and biased, it is crucial that the interview be structured and standardized. During a structured interview, the interviewer asks the same set of questions to all applicants. Table 13-2 includes tips for interviewing.

- In an interview, you can't ask questions about age, sex, race, national origin, religion, pregnancy, marital or family status, disabilities, or any other factor that is NOT related to the job.

- Once interviews are done and you have selected your top candidates, it's time to do background checks. A background check is the process a business uses to verify that an applicant is who they claim to be in terms of, for example, education or employment history. Applicants need to give permission in writing for a potential employer to do a background check. Employers can't ask for medical information until after offering the job to someone.

- In some organizations, each candidate is rated at each step in the process and these ratings are weighed heavily in the final decision. In other organizations, candidates are ranked based on objective criteria. Then the candidates are discussed in terms of their abilities, motivation, work ethic, and ability to fit in, and a final selection is made.

- Each foodservice employee is either employed by the foodservice or another organization. When employed directly by the foodservice, the position may be permanent (also called regular) or temporary.

Whether permanent or temporary, each employee is either full-time (usually 40 hours, but decided by the employer), part-time, or on-call. Foodservice employees NOT employed by the foodservice itself include foodservice contract company employees (who work for Sodexo, for example), employees from temporary employment agencies, and independent contractors (self-employed).

13.3 Train Employees

- Training introduces new employees to the organization and their jobs, helps employees perform their jobs well, assists employees to qualify for future jobs, and keeps employees informed of changes in an organization. Employees and guests end up more satisfied due to training.

- Training programs often fit into one of these categories: onboarding (includes orientation), on-the-job training, job-specific skills training (technical skills), soft skills, and regulatory or compliance training. Most healthcare foodservices must comply with federal regulations to provide in-service training (training while someone is working).

- Orientation introduces a new employee to the organization and to the job and coworkers. An example of an orientation checklist is in Table 13-4.

- Onboarding is a series of events, starting with orientation, that acclimate and engage a new employee to become a contributing member of the team in a reasonable amount of time. During this process, an employee builds relationships; develops the knowledge, skills, and attitudes to be successful in their jobs; understands company culture, and becomes familiar with the organization's rules and policies.

- Traditionally in on-the-job training, the new employee is placed into the real work situation and trained to do the various parts of the job by an experienced employee or supervisor who uses a technique called tell/show/do/review.

- Once the need for a training unit has been identified and its overall training goals are developed, the instructional designer takes these steps to develop each training module or class: assess employees' specific needs, write learning objectives and how they will be evaluated, design the training—content and instructional methods (preferably active training), develop all of the materials needed to deliver the training, implement the training, and get employee feedback on the training.

- Table 13-8 lists the conditions under which employees learn best.
- Table 13-10 is a sample training module or class.

13.4   Manage Employees' Performance

- Figure 13-5 displays the performance management cycle from orienting and training new employees to coaching and training current employees, and finally to the annual performance appraisal in which the supervisor works with each employee to set individual goals.
- Good coaches do the following: give one-on-one performance feedback to employees, ask employees to be involved in examining and improving performance, provide motivation and guidance to employees who want to move up the career ladder.
- When discussing performance with an employee, do not assume that the employee knows how things are supposed to be done. They may not be performing well because they have missed a training session, are bored, are overwhelmed with work, or lack the necessary equipment.
- Table 13-11 lists general coaching guidelines.
- At performance appraisal time, employees get feedback on how they are meeting standards and their performance is discussed. Successes can be recognized and performance issues can be addressed. Opportunities for personal development can also be considered at this time. With supervisory input, employees often set performance goals to achieve within certain timeframes in the future. The performance appraisal often acts as the basis for a possible salary increase.
- Performance appraisal forms use various methods to rate an employee, such as checklists, graphic rating scales (most popular), behaviorally anchored rating scale, management by objectives, standards-based method, narrative method, and 360-degree performance review. Each format has its pluses and minuses.
- An appraisal form that uses MBO for measuring results and BARS for measuring behaviors may be appropriate for a number of managers and some hourly employees.
- Examples of rating errors that supervisors make include subjective evaluations, halo effect, horns effect, distributional errors (leniency, severity, error of central tendency), and recency error.
- Table 13-17 gives guidelines for preparing and conducting a performance appraisal.
- Typical types of discipline problems include attendance, on-the-job behaviors, and dishonesty.
- Some foodservices categorize disciplinary problems into categories such as minor infractions, major infractions, and causes for immediate discharge.
- Progressive discipline applies corrective measures in increasing degrees or steps if the behavior continues. An employee is usually given several opportunities to correct the behavior.
- The typical progression of disciplinary action starts with an oral counseling and warning, then moves onto a written warning, second written warning, temporary suspension, and termination.
- When confronted with a disciplinary situation, take these steps: collect all of the facts, speak to the employee as soon as possible, decide if any action needs to be taken (you may need to consult with your boss and/or human resources), take the action and develop an improvement plan with the employee, make sure everything is documented, and follow-up. Table 13-18 is a sample disciplinary notice and Table 13-19 gives tips for taking disciplinary action.
- Every state in the United States, except for Montana, allows at-will employment. At-will employees can be fired (terminated) at any time and for almost any reason. Likewise, the at-will employee is free to leave the employer at any time and for any reason. Unless an employer gives a clear indication, such as in the Employee Handbook, that it will only fire employees for just cause, it is assumed the employees are at-will employees. At-will employees still cannot be fired for discriminatory reasons or because they have complained about health and safety violations or discrimination in the workplace.
- Employers who state they only fire employees for just cause generally have a policy

providing causes (such as theft) for being fired and a procedure to follow. Employers must be very careful about how they handle this process. All possible terminations must have input from higher-level managers and human resources personnel. If an investigation needs to be done, the employee should be suspended with pay until the investigation is complete.

13.5 Schedule Employees

- Staffing is the process of determining personnel needs, recruiting, and selecting employees. Scheduling is the process of assigning an appropriate number of employees to work at specified times and days so that the work of the foodservice is accomplished.
- One full-time equivalent is the equivalent of one full-time employee, working 8 hours a day, 40 hours a week (although in some companies, this number is a little lower), which works out to be 2,080 hours a year.
- Productive hours are hours when an employee is working. Nonproductive hours are hours when an employee is getting paid but is not working on the job (such as a sick day).
- The hours of operation and the menu are key drivers in determining how many staff members will be working. Customer demand, meal volumes, and types of service provided are additional factors that impact how many employees are required.
- The manager often creates a scheduling template or master schedule to use throughout the year, which identifies the shifts needed to adequately staff the work. It includes each employee's regular days on duty and days off, and also reflects the staffing patterns that support the high- and low-volume periods of the operation.
- Foodservices need a mechanism that allows employees to request time off in advance of the schedule writing process. Managers should establish a due date for time off requests to be submitted to allow sufficient time to incorporate the request into the schedule and ensure appropriate coverage. Vacation requests may require an earlier due date.
- Schedules should be posted at least two weeks in advance. Also, avoid scheduling an employee from working a closing shift and then an early shift the next day. Consider your employees' quality of life when making schedules.
- Table 13-20 goes through the steps to make a schedule.

13.6 Work with Unions

- Unions are organizations elected by a group of nonmanagement employees to represent them in bargaining (called collective bargaining) with an employer for wages, hours, and working conditions. Most union members in the United States belong to a national or international union. The dealings between unions and management are referred to as labor relations.
- Each union contract includes a section that discusses the extent to which the union can influence new members to join. In a closed shop, all members of the bargaining unit must be union members and pay dues. In a union shop, a new employee must join the union within a specified period of time after starting employment (such as 30 days). In an agency shop, all members of the bargaining unit pay dues, but they are not required to be union members. Under a dues checkoff provision, the employer collects dues from union members and nonunion members and then gives the dues to the union. Dues checkoff agreements are legal as long as they are authorized by the employees.
- About half of the states have Right-to-Work laws, which guarantee that no employee can be required to join a labor union or pay union dues. Therefore, states with Right-to-Work laws *do not allow closed shops, union shops, or agency shops.*
- Up until the National Labor Relations Act was passed in 1935, unions did not get a lot of legal support. This act affirmed an employee's right to organize a union, become a union member, engage in union activities, and go on strike to get better working conditions. If employees chose to be represented by a union, management was required to negotiate with union representatives. The act also created the National Labor Relations Board (NLRB), which oversees elections in which a union may become the collective bargaining agent for a bargaining unit.
- The Labor-Management Relations Act (Taft-Hartley Act of 1947) tried to create a

balance between union power and management authority. Unfair labor practices by both unions and management were defined. States were given the right to enact Right-to-Work laws.

- After union corruption was exposed in the 1950s, the Landrum-Griffin Act of 1959 required unions to file annual reports with the U.S. Department of Labor on their finances, elections, and other matters. It also established the Bill of Rights for Union Members.

- If a majority of workers want to form a union, they need to get at least 30% of workers in the bargaining unit to sign union authorization cards. Then an election will take place and if a majority of voters choose the union, the NLRB will certify the union.

- If you are working with a union, it is essential to become familiar with the union contract and to oversee that it is administered properly. It is also important to get to know the union stewards and develop a positive working relationship with them.

- A grievance is a work-related complaint made by an employee. The union contract explains how an employee may file a grievance and the series of steps (from meeting with the supervisor to others further up the management ladder) to handle the issue. Most grievances are resolved in the early stages.

REVIEW AND DISCUSSION QUESTIONS

1. Discuss the functions of the people who work in the human resources department.
2. How can the human resources department be a competitive advantage for a business?
3. What are five of the rights of American employees in terms of pay and benefits?
4. Briefly describe two EEO laws and the concept of EEO. Which groups are protected by EEO laws in the United States? What are they protected against?
5. What is sexual harassment? How can a foodservice minimize sexual harassment?
6. What is the purpose of the Occupational Safety and Health Act and how is it enforced?
7. Describe different ways in which individuals are recruited to apply for jobs.
8. Explain how the selection process works. Give examples of how this process can be nondiscriminatory and job-related.
9. What are the purposes of the job interview? What is a structured interview?
10. What are the advantages and disadvantages of having on-call employees?
11. What is the difference between orientation and onboarding?
12. When would on-the-job training be useful in a foodservice?
13. Give two examples of active learning methods used to train employees.
14. When is coaching important? Explain how you might coach an employee on improving performance.
15. Describe briefly five methods for doing performance appraisals and when each is used.
16. What is progressive discipline and what are the steps involved? When is progressive discipline required?
17. Explain what at-will employment is. Also explain the purpose of Right-to-Work laws.
18. List three guidelines when developing employee schedules.
19. How does a union organize to get recognition?
20. Describe how having unionized employees affects how a foodservice manager does their job.

SMALL GROUP PROJECT

For the foodservice concept that you created in Chapter 1, develop the following.

1. For one of the job descriptions and specifications that were developed in Chapter 12, write up a list of interview questions that you would use for applicants for this job.

2. Develop a training class, using the format in Table 13-10, on a sanitation topic.

REFERENCES

AmTrust Financial. (2018). *AmTrust financial restaurant risk report*. https://amtrustfinancial.com/getmedia /81e1baeb-df72-445b-9c5b-07a36d33506c/AFS_AmTrust-Restaurant-Statistics-Report_2018_121318.pdf

Bureau of Labor Statistics. (2021). *Union members summary*. https://www.bls.gov/news.release/union2.nr0.htm

Cappelli, P. (2019). Your approach to hiring is all wrong. *Harvard Business Review, 97*(3), 48–58.

Ganino, M. (2018). 4 ways to recruit better restaurant employees. *QSR*. https://www.qsrmagazine.com/mike -ganino-crafting-culture/4-ways-recruit-better -restaurant-employees

Goler, L., Gale, J., & Grant. A. (2016). Let's not kill performance evaluations yet. *Harvard Business Review, 94*(11), 90–94.

Jenks, J. M., & Zevnik, B. (1989). ABCs of job interviewing. *Harvard Business Review*. https://hbr.org/1989/07 /abcs-of-job-interviewing

Krathwohl, D. R. (2002). A revision of Bloom's Taxonomy: An overview. *Theory Into Practice, 41*(4), 212–218.

Little, S. (2019). *What is employee onboarding—and why do you need it? The SHRMBlog*. https://blog.shrm.org/blog /what-is-employee-onboarding-and-why-do-you -need-it

Naylor, J. C., & Briggs, G. E. (1963). Effects of task complexity and task organization on the relative efficiency of part and whole training methods. *Journal of Experimental Psychology, 65*(3), 217–224.

Occupational Safety and Health Administration. (2018). *OSHA injury and illness recordkeeping and reporting requirements*. https://www.osha.gov/recordkeeping /index.html

Romeo, P. (2018). Can't you do better than 'Help Wanted'? *Foodservice Director*. https://www.foodservicedirector.com /workforce/cant-you-do-better-help-wanted

Ruggless, R. (2016). How to tackle unconscious bias in restaurants. *Nation's Restaurant News*. https://www .nrn.com/latest-headlines/how-tackle-unconscious -bias-restaurants

Smith, A. (2018). 13 ways to improve written warnings and manage employees better. *SHRM*. https://www.shrm .org/resourcesandtools/legal-and-compliance /employment-law/pages/ways-to-improve-written -warnings.aspx

U.S. Equal Employment Opportunity Commission. (2019). *Facts about sexual harassment*. https://www.eeoc.gov /eeoc/publications/fs-sex.cfm

U.S. Equal Employment Opportunity Commission. (2010). *Employment tests and selection procedures*. https:// www.eeoc.gov/policy/docs/factemployment_procedures .html

Zenger, J. & Folkman, J. (2012). Getting 360 degree reviews right. *Harvard Business Review*. https://hbr.org /2012/09/getting-360-degree-reviews-right

Managing Quality and Customer Satisfaction

LEARNING OUTCOMES

14.1 Describe approaches to quality.

14.2 Choose appropriate quality tools to support quality management.

14.3 Manage customer satisfaction.

INTRODUCTION

Quality became the fashionable business term of the 1990s, just as the term excellence had dominated much of the 1980s. **Quality** is when a product or service meets or exceeds customer expectations *and* when an organization can provide these products/services in the most cost-efficient manner while complying with regulations and making a profit. Quality is achieved when managers proactively develop specific quality goals or standards and procedures or processes to ensure that they are met or exceeded. Examples of those goals or standards that can be categorized by key performance indicators are shown in **Table 14–1**. **Key performance indicators (KPI)** are measurable values that demonstrate how well an organization is achieving its business goals and objectives. The KPI examples in Table 14–1 are specifically for foodservices.

Quality also involves organizing and leading employees to produce a quality foodservice experience. This process starts with hiring the best employees, training them, and empowering them to reduce time and material waste and make the best decisions to benefit customers. Managers will get better results if they work with employees to build quality into, and remove waste from, products and services.

Managing quality is an example of the management skill of controlling. **Controlling** is a process with three steps.

1. Establish reasonable goals and/or standards for products/services, keeping in mind what your customer expects and also what support employees may need to meet these expectations.
2. Measure and evaluate products and performance against the goal/standards.
3. As needed, rethink and improve processes to meet goals/standards.

© Denis Val/Shutterstock

Table 14-1 Key Performance Indicators	
Category	**Examples**
1. Customer Satisfaction	75% of customers will recommend the foodservice to friends and family. The First-Time Visitor Return Rate will be at least 26% (within a 12-month period).
2. Service	75% of customers rate service as good or better. The kitchen does not run out of a menu item more than once a week.
3. Food Quality	80% of customers rate food as good or better.
4. Sanitation	Mock kitchen inspection results in two of fewer "out of compliance" issues monthly.
5. Revenue	Sales/square foot of $250 or more is maintained.
6. Occupancy	At least 150 covers are served during the dinner period.
7. Financial Management	Maintain liquor costs at 20% of liquor sales or lower. Maintain food cost percentage at 35% or lower.

Goals and/or standards may be set in terms of quantity (such as servers will greet customers within three minutes of being seated), quality (such as temperature and taste of food being served), or cost (such as maintaining food cost percentage at 35% or lower).

This chapter will examine approaches and tools to provide a quality foodservice. The second half of the chapter explores customer satisfaction and what can be done to raise satisfaction scores and improve the customer experience.

14.1 DESCRIBE APPROACHES TO QUALITY

Quality control has been around for many years in the manufacturing industry. Initially, quality control focused on finding defects (or variations from the standard) in a product, service, or outcome (by inspection) and then correcting the problem. Ultimately, finding defects provides information on how to improve inputs or improve processes so that fewer defects occur. Healthcare organizations once preferred the term **quality assurance** to quality control, but quickly advanced to continuous quality improvement (CQI) as hospitals sought to become designated as High Reliability Organizations (HROs). In addition to correcting the processes that produced the errors, both quality control and quality assurance were often responsible for implementing more frequent quality checkpoints or controls so that errors might be caught or prevented.

Within the healthcare field, quality assurance became more than just a reactive process to find where things went wrong. The Centers for Medicare and Medicaid Services (2016) defines quality assurance as: "the specification of standards for quality of service and outcomes, and a process throughout the organization for assuring that care is maintained at acceptable levels in relation to those standards. QA is ongoing, both anticipatory and retrospective in its efforts to identify how the organization is performing." By measuring performance against quality standards, a healthcare organization becomes actively engaged in improving processes (such as producing meals or improving patient outcomes) when needed.

The concepts behind the approaches to quality, to be discussed in this chapter, recognize that both resources (inputs) and activities that are safely carried out (processes) are addressed together to ensure or improve the quality of products and services.

TOTAL QUALITY MANAGEMENT

Quality control was the act of checking and measuring outcomes, but it was not a system that could be applied to any process to improve outcomes. So quality control evolved into **Total Quality Management (TQM)** and Six Sigma. TQM is generally regarded as the beginning of the quality movement and credit for the development of TQM is given to Walter Shewhart, W. Edwards Deming and Joseph Juran. Walter Shewhart developed and used statistical quality control (using statistics and control charts to enhance product control) while working at Western Electric and Bell Telephone Laboratories in the 1920s. He used statistics to reduce variation in manufacturing. Joseph Juran was also trained in these techniques and joined W. Edward Deming in advocating TQM principles in Japan in the 1950s.

In the 1950s, the quality of Japanese products was poor and often joked about. After World War II, Japan was forced to convert its factories that had produced military weapons to ones producing consumer goods. Japan fully embraced TQM. Because they produced high-quality products, Japanese manufacturers dominated U.S. and European consumer markets by the mid 1970s. Examples include Nikon cameras, Toyota cars and trucks, and Sony electronics. After a substantial loss of market share, U.S. and European manufacturers realized that they were very late in adopting quality standards and practices. By the late 1970s, TQM was being taken very more seriously in the United States and being taught in the top MBA programs.

Total quality management is a management philosophy that focuses on responding to customer needs and expectations while continuously examining and improving organizational processes and empowering employees. It advised managers to do the following (Gershon, 2010).

1. Take responsibility for continuous improvement.
2. Focus on work processes to make improvements.
3. Use statistics to measure process performance.
4. Involve employees to identify problems and find solutions.

With TQM, teams of employees are given projects to improve product or service quality. The team may include a leader or facilitator.

The Plan-Do-Check-Act (PDCA) cycle, a basic process improvement model was originally developed by Walter Shewhart and adapted by W. Edwards Deming as the plan-do-study-act (PDSA) cycle. It uses four steps to plan projects and carry out changes. The PDSA cycle doesn't have a beginning and end, so it is normally depicted as a wheel. The cycle is repeated again and again for continuous improvement. The four steps are described in **Table 14-2**. It is especially useful when developing an improved or new design of a process, product, or service.

Another TQM tool was the use of quality circles. **Quality circles** are a group of employees who do similar jobs and meet regularly to identify, analyze, and find and test solutions for quality issues of products or services. The start of quality circles is associated with Japanese management. The basic idea has been adopted and modified by other quality philosophies.

Table 14-2 The Plan-Do-Study-Act Cycle	
1. Plan	Recruit a team. Describe the problem. Analyze possible causes. Develop potential solutions. Complete the statement: "If we do _____, then _____ will happen." Choose the best potential solution and develop an action plan to implement.
2. Do	Carry out the test/change on a small scale. Document what happened including any unexpected findings.
3. Study	Study and analyze the data. Describe the results. Did the plan result in an improvement? By how much/little? Was the action taken worthwhile? Were there unintended side effects? Does the staff understand and support the change?
4. Act	Based on what was learned from the test/change, you can: • Adapt: Modify the changes and repeat the PDSA cycle. • Adopt: Make the change the standard procedure. • Abandon: Change your approach and repeat the PDSA cycle.

CONTINUOUS QUALITY IMPROVEMENT

Continuous quality improvement (CQI) is a systematic approach to measuring, evaluating, and improving products and services. It uses a cyclical process of assessing products or performance, developing and implementing improvement plans, and reassessing results. What makes CQI different is that it involves the *continuous* study and improvement of processes to improve products, services, or outcomes. CQI is not a one-time event—it is a mindset and commitment to collect and use data to improve products and services. CQI is the reason why mobile phones became lighter and thinner and have larger screens and greater capabilities.

KAIZEN

Kaizen is a Japanese philosophy of continuous improvement that involves all employees at all levels. The Kaizen process uses PDCA—Plan Do Check Act—and also a methodology called 5S. The purpose of **5S** is to improve workplace organization and eliminate wasted time looking for needed items or getting ready to work. For example, if the work station for making sandwiches is producing items in a slow manner, these steps can be taken to improve efficiency and decrease waste.

1. Sort: Frequently used items should be easy to reach. Infrequently or unnecessary items can be moved elsewhere.
2. Set in order: Everything in a work station should have a place. A time-and-motion study can help determine the optimal work methods for the employees to eliminate unnecessary motions. Items should be arranged to promote efficient workflow.
3. Shine: To help maintain the order you've created, clean the work station thoroughly and make any physical improvements needed. This affects employee morale and attitude.
4. Standardize: Set standards for a consistently organized work station. Drawings or photos of how it should look will help.
5. Sustain: Initiate controls to keep up the new routines. Make checklists and use them. Update job descriptions. Engage staff with training and positive reinforcement.

SIX SIGMA

In the 1970s, a Japanese company started running a Motorola factory in the United States that made television sets. With groups of employees working on projects and using new quality ideas, the factory greatly decreased costs while also producing televisions with significantly fewer defects. This was the start of Six Sigma.

Six Sigma is a problem-solving quality program that uses a set of methods and tools to reduce errors or variations, lower costs and increase profits, maximize employee job satisfaction as well as customer satisfaction, and earn customer loyalty. Sigma is a statistical measurement that shows how well a process is performing. Higher sigma values mean that there are fewer and fewer defects. At Two Sigma, 95% of products or processes are defect-free. At Six Sigma, there are fewer than 3.5 defects per million products or processes—which is incredibly small. Manufacturers are more likely to adopt Six Sigma than service companies such as retailers, foodservices, and healthcare organizations, but more service companies are receiving training in this discipline.

A key focus of Six Sigma is the use of statistical tools to identify and correct the causes of variations. For example, Six Sigma uses the DMAIC methodology, which relies in part on statistics, as a roadmap for solving problems and improving processes (**Figure 14-1**).

1. <u>Define</u>. Define the opportunity for improvement, the project objectives, and customer needs.

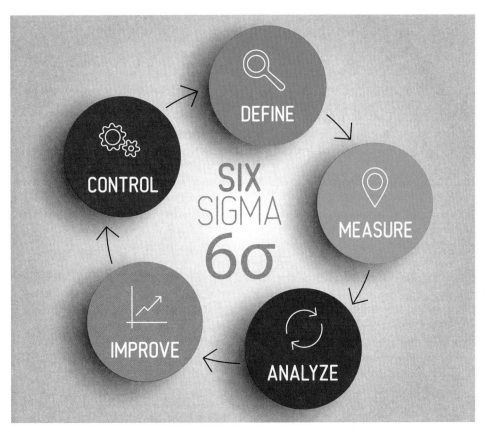

FIGURE 14-1 DMAIC
© Petr Vaclavek/Shutterstock

2. <u>Measure</u>. Once the process/outcome to be improved is identified, the team can map out the process and examine the performance by collecting data and using statistics.
3. <u>Analyze</u>. Analyze the process to identify the root causes. **Root causes** are underlying causes that can be identified and are within management's control to fix. Narrow the pool of root causes to the critical few.
4. <u>Improve</u>. Address the root cause(s) to develop an action plan to improve the process. Implement and verify whether the solutions have improved the process.
5. <u>Control</u>. Establish plans to make sure the improvements are adopted.

DMAIC has been used in restaurants to tackle problems such as order accuracy or order time. For example, Starbucks decreased order time by training baristas to get drink orders and creating a mobile app for ordering.

Six Sigma is different from TQM in that it creates an infrastructure of people in the organization who are trained in Six Sigma methods and can conduct projects and implement improvements. Beginners are Yellow Belts and can advance to the higher level—Master Black Belt.

In practice, Six Sigma is often combined in practice with Lean methods, which is discussed next.

LEAN

Another term that comes up when discussing quality is Lean. Lean is sometimes referred to as the Toyota Production System because it was a foundation for lean manufacturing. **Lean** is a tool used in organizations to streamline manufacturing and production processes by focusing on eliminating waste and smoothing the process flow.

Waste refers to any step or action in a process that is not required for the process to be successfully completed or doesn't add value for the end user. Lean projects emphasize elimination or reduction of anything a customer would not want to pay for. In other words, Lean companies remove any actions that don't add value in the customers' eyes. **Table 14-3** gives examples of potential sources of waste that can be worked on in a lean organization. You can easily recall the eight wastes of lean by using the acronym DOWNTIME.

In a Lean culture, the focus is on teams and employees. Ideally, you want every employee to be a Lean thinker. The Lean organization also tries to bring everyone closer to the processes, so these organizations often eliminate levels of hierarchy.

Lean uses an efficiency tool called **Value Stream Mapping (VSM)** in which a flowchart is developed by a team to document every step in a process. By discussing and agreeing on the process' steps, the team can find what is causing waste, poor flow, and/or errors. The 5S system is also often used in lean organizations. VSM, along with 5S, are excellent tools to create efficiencies and processes that are leaner.

Chick-fil-A has successfully used Lean with employees in some of its units (Reid, 2019). Employees were given training in Lean principles and tools and asked to come up with ideas to decrease waste as long as they didn't sacrifice food safety, people safety, or product quality. Employees came up with many ideas, including a biscuit cutter that cut more than one biscuit out of dough at a time. Employees also recommended a display at the front counter showing the types of dipping sauces available so counter employees would be less likely to have to answer the question "What types of dipping sauces do you have?"

Many organizations are combining the Lean philosophy with Six Sigma. **Lean Six Sigma** brings together the concepts of both waste reduction and quality. Lean Six Sigma is, of course, very customer oriented and relies on capturing the voice of the customer to improve customer satisfaction.

Table 14-3 The Eight Wastes (DOWNTIME)

Waste	Definition	Examples
1. **D**efects	Quality of product or service is not up to standard or produced within acceptable timeframe. Also miscommunication.	Food is overcooked, undercooked, wrong temperature. Service is slow.
2. **O**ver- or under-production	Make too much or too little of products immediately needed.	Excessive amount of leftovers after meals. Menu items are not available.
3. **W**aiting	Waiting for people, materials, or information.	Cooks are waiting for meat order to start lunch preparation.
4. **N**on-utilized talent	Underutilization of team members' skills and creativity.	Employees not fully trained. Employees not actively involved in finding solutions.
5. **T**ransportation	Unnecessary movement of products, equipment, or information.	Sending and resending too many emails. Don't have information when it is needed.
6. **I**nventory excess	Accumulation of inventory or information/data.	Stockpiling food or beverages. Keeping data longer than needed.
7. **M**otion excess	Movements by employees (walking, bending, turning, etc.) that are not of value to the customer.	Line cook makes many unnecessary steps during a shift.
8. **E**xtra-processing/over complicating	Any steps that do not add value to the customer.	Closing procedures for bartender are cumbersome.

ISO 9000

ISO 9000 is a set of quality system standards established by international technical experts from more than 90 countries, as part of the International Organization for Standardization (ISO). There are various ISO standards and ISO 9001 is the model for a quality management system that can be used in large and small organizations to improve efficiency and customer satisfaction. The ISO 9001 standard is the world's most recognized quality management system certification. Companies that achieve ISO 9001 certification benefit from lower costs, higher customer satisfaction, improved efficiency, and new customer opportunities.

ISO 9000 and 9001 are based on these seven Quality Management Principles (QMP).

QMP 1: Customer focus
QMP 2: Leadership
QMP 3: Engagement of People
QMP 4: Process Approach
QMP 5: Improvement
QMP 6: Evidence-Based Decision Making
QMP 7: Relationship Management

Each QMP helps guide performance improvement efforts.

JOINT COMMISSION

The Joint Commission is an independent group in the United States that develops and administers voluntary accreditation programs for hospitals and other healthcare organizations on a fee-for-service basis. Joint Commission standards can help healthcare foodservices measure, evaluate, and improve performance. The standards focus on important patient or resident care and organization functions that are essential to providing safe, high-quality care. The Joint Commission's state-of-the-art standards set performance expectations that are reasonable and achievable.

14.2 CHOOSE APPROPRIATE QUALITY TOOLS TO SUPPORT QUALITY MANAGEMENT

There are a wide variety of quality tools available to use in different situations. This section only looks at some of the most popular and classic tools. They are divided into three sections: cause analysis tools, process analysis tools, and data collection tools.

CAUSE ANALYSIS TOOLS

The following are tools that are used to help determine the reasons why a particular problem has occurred.

- **Root cause analysis.** Root cause analysis is a structured team process used to help identify why and how an unfavorable event occurred so that preventive actions can be taken in the future. The process involves collecting data, charting possible causes, and identifying the most likely root cause(s). Once that is done, a team can design possible solutions, select the best one, and implement and evaluate that solution.
- **Cause-and-effect diagram.** A cause-and-effect diagram (also called a fishbone diagram or Ishikawa diagram after its developer) is helpful for a team to brainstorm possible causes of a problem and sorting those ideas into useful categories. It is an excellent way for visual learners to look at cause and effect. The problem is displayed in a box at the mouth of the fish and possible

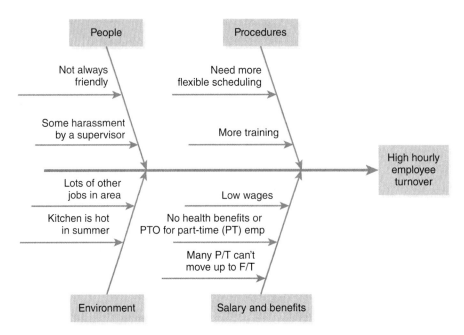

FIGURE 14-2 Cause-and-Effect Diagram

contributors are listed on the fish bones (**Figure 14–2**). Each bone represents a category of possible causes, such as people, procedures, equipment, or policy. The chart is developed through a team effort and displayed so that additions may be made.

- **Pareto chart**. Many years ago, the Italian economist and sociologist Vilfredo Pareto conjectured that 80% of wealth belonged to 20% of the population and later found that his 80-20 split also worked in other situations. Joseph Juran used the Pareto principles to describe how 80% of the variation in a process is caused by approximately 20% of the factors. A Pareto chart shows the factors that contribute to variation in a process as bars, and the bars are arranged with the tallest ones to the left and the shortest to the right. Each bar represents frequency, quantity, cost, or time. For example, **Figure 14–3** is a Pareto chart showing the frequency of common customer complaints. The frequency is listed on the left vertical axis and the percentage on the right vertical axis. The curved line at the top of the chart represents the cumulative total of each problem cause as you progress across the chart. The dotted line that originates from "80%" intersects the cumulative percentage line, showing that 80% of the complaints are caused by two predominant factors. Using a Pareto chart helps a team focus its efforts on the factors that have the most impact.

- **Scatter diagram**. A scatter diagram shows whether there is a relationship between two variables, such as revenue and payroll. The values for one variable are placed on the horizontal axis, and the values for the other variable are on the vertical axis. If the variables are related, the points will fall along a line or curve. If a line seems to form and goes up to the right, there is a positive correlation—meaning that as one variable increases, so does the other. If a line seems to form and goes up to the left, there is a negative correlation—meaning that as the variable on the horizontal axis increases, the other variable decreases. If the points are all over the place, there is no relationship between the two variables. **Figure 14–4** shows a slightly positive correlation between monthly foodservice revenue and payroll—meaning that as revenue increases, so does payroll.

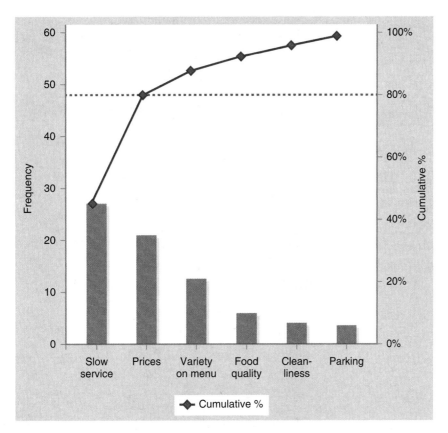

FIGURE 14-3 Pareto Chart: Customer Complaints

PROCESS ANALYSIS TOOLS

Process analysis tools helps managers and employees look more carefully at a process or procedure to troubleshoot issues and make improvements.

- **Flowchart.** Any system can be reduced to a flowchart that indicates the steps in a process and the chronological flow of work. A flowchart (also called a process map) is a graphic representation of an ordered sequence of events,

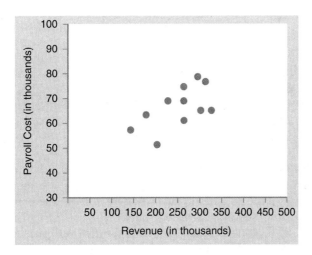

FIGURE 14-4 Scatter Diagram

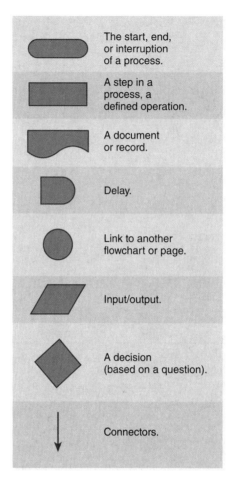

FIGURE 14-5 Flow Chart Symbols

steps, or procedures that take place in a system. Hospital patient traylines and drive-through lines, for example, are all planned using flowcharts. Flowcharts use symbols, each representing a certain kind of function, such as a decision (diamond shape) or processing step (rectangular box). Commonly accepted flowchart symbols are shown in **Figure 14-5**. The symbols are connected with arrows. Flowcharts normally flow from top to bottom or from left to right. A flowchart can be used to develop, document, understand, or analyze a procedure and also to compare present and proposed procedures (**Figure 14-6**). By using a flowchart to lay out a process before it is implemented, it is easier to troubleshoot for mistakes. As a control device, flowcharts can be used to audit a process or workflow and pinpoint concerns such as time delays. A two-dimensional flowchart shows two flowcharts at the same time, such as a trayline making patient trays in the kitchen and trays being delivered to rooms in the hospital. This type of flowchart is called a swim-lane chart because there is a dotted line separating the two flows, which creates something that looks like two swim lanes in a pool.

- **Spaghetti diagram**. A spaghetti diagram traces the path of an item(s) through a process. It measures motions or steps. Lines are used to show the flow of an item, let's say a meal in a fast casual restaurant, from the preparation areas to the service areas (counter, drive-through, pickup). The lines that show the flow of the items look a bit like spaghetti, as seen in **Figure 14-7**. These diagrams are helpful to see possible causes for delay and find ways to accelerate the process.

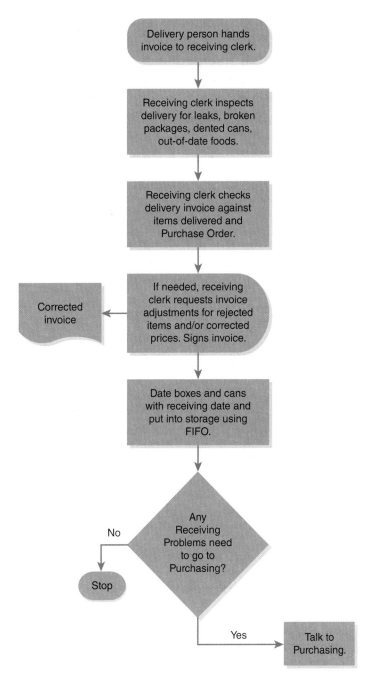

FIGURE 14-6 Receiving Dry Goods Flowchart

- **Failure Mode and Effects Analysis (FMEA).** This technique is used to identify and analyze potential failures within a process. It has been used for many years in the automotive industry as well as other settings. We use FMEA every time we consider the following: What could go wrong and the likelihood of it happening, and if something went wrong, would we know about it in time and how severe would the effects be? If the likelihood of the failure is pretty high and the effects are quite negative, it is time to work on identifying the probable cause(s) of the failure and developing and testing preventive actions to prevent the failure. The Federal Emergency Management Agency actually used FMEA during tabletop drills to pinpoint potential infrastructure failures during floods, earthquakes, fires, and terrorist attacks.

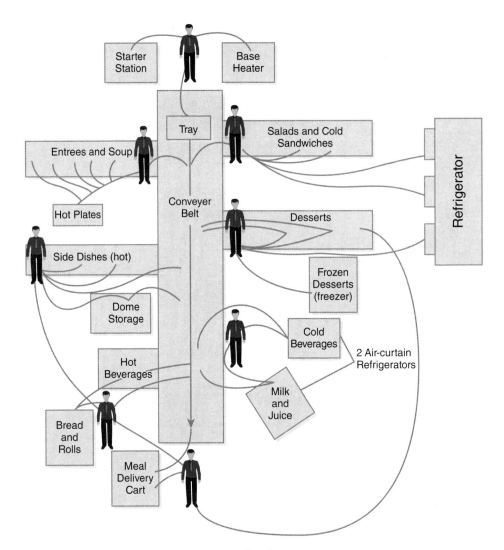

FIGURE 14-7 Spaghetti Diagram: Healthcare Trayline

DATA COLLECTION

This set of tools helps to collect and display collected data.

- **Check sheet.** A check sheet, sometimes called a tally sheet, is designed to collect data in real-time. Check sheets are used to gather how often something of interest happens. For example, a chef keeps a monthly tally sheet that is used when a customer returns a dish to the kitchen. The tally sheet lists common reasons for why a customer returns a dish, such as a hot dish was cold, and the chef checks off the reason. Check sheets may also include a measurement scale divided into intervals that can be checked off. For example, a hospital foodservice uses a Test Tray Assessment form (**Table 14-4**) to collect information on the quality of a patient meal tray sent to an empty patient room. The person evaluating the tray examines the temperature of the hot and cold foods, overall appearance, taste, portion size, and whether the tray contained the correct items. Another type of check sheet is a checklist, which is frequently used in foodservice. A checklist may list supplies to set up a station or steps in a process that has to be completed. For example, closing managers commonly use a checklist of all of the duties, such as cleaning and locking up, that must be done

Table 14-4 Patient Tray Assessment Form

Date: _____   Name of Evaluator: _____

Meal: _____   Floor/Unit: _____

Diet: _____   Travel Time to Room: _____

Directions: Check off whether each item is satisfactory or not. If not satisfactory, please fill in Comments and explain.

	Satisfactory	Not Satisfactory	Comments
Temperature of Hot Foods: Minimum: 140°F (60°C)			
Temperature of Hot Beverages & Soup: Minimum: 150°F (65°C)			
Temperature of Cold Foods: Maximum: 41°F (5°C)			
Appearance			
Taste			
Portion Size			
Correct items on tray			

before the manager can leave. Chapter 13 gives an example of an Orientation Checklist that the supervisor follows and checks off to make sure that the new employee is familiar with certain aspects of the job and workplace.

- **Histogram.** A histogram is a simple graph using bars of different heights to show a frequency distribution of a variable, such as wait time. It is similar to a bar chart but a histogram groups numbers into ranges. For example, **Figure 14-8** shows the wait times for customers to get a table after 6:00 PM on Friday and Saturday nights in a restaurant that does not accept reservations. Each bar corresponds to a different wait time (from 0 to 60 minutes in 10-minute increments) and shows that most customers wait up to 30 minutes to get a table.

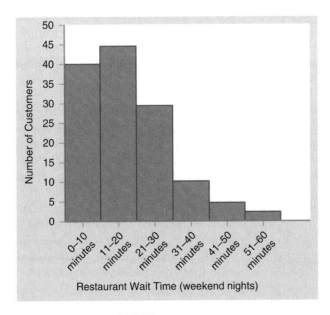

FIGURE 14-8 Histogram: Restaurant Wait Time

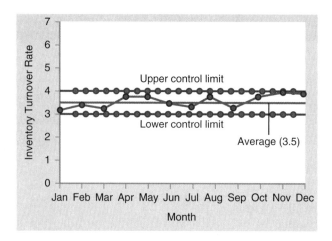

FIGURE 14-9 Control Chart: Inventory Turnover

- **Control chart.** A control chart (also called a Shewhart chart) is a graph that shows data over time, so it demonstrates how a variable or process changes over time. What makes the control chart more valuable is that it includes a central line for the average and two other horizontal lines. These two lines are the upper control limit and the lower control limit. They are chosen so that you can easily see when the data are within acceptable limits. It can help to determine if variations are consistent or desirable. **Figure 14-9** shows a control chart for inventory turnover for one year.
- **Survey.** A survey is used to obtain data from specific groups of people about their behavior, opinions, or knowledge. Customer surveys are common and are discussed later in this chapter.

BENCHMARKING

Any foodservice operation that operates "in a bubble" or without comparison to its competition, is a foodservice that is "at risk." According to the periodical, *Modern Restaurant Management*, 60% of new restaurants fail in the first year, and 80% fail in the first five years. This helps to explain the attractiveness of "franchising" with a restaurant chain with a successful formula for making a profit (Crawford, 2019). But other than being part of a successful chain with feedback from corporate headquarters, a foodservice operator needs to know how they compare with other players in the same market segment. Enter benchmarking. **Benchmarking** is the process of comparing your operation against yourself, a similar operation, or an industry standard.

A benchmark is something that serves as a standard or best practice against which others measure themselves. For an example of benchmarking, consider two managers at separate quick-service restaurants with the same menu and also drive-through service. The managers compare the average number of minutes it takes for a drive-through customer to be served. After a discussion, the manager with the slower drive-through gains some tips on how to serve customers faster. **Internal benchmarking** is when managers compare performance of operations within the *same* organization, such as two Wendy's Unit Managers comparing monthly revenues. Internal benchmarking also includes comparing your own foodservice's performance over time. **External benchmarking** is when a manager compares performance against foodservices *outside* of their organization. Whether internal or external, benchmarking can help you find your strengths and how to maintain them, as well as identify areas in which you can improve and ideas for improvement.

External benchmarking is best between businesses that are comparable in size, volume, and location or setting (urban or rural). Sometimes, benchmarking between the facilities is difficult due to inconsistencies in financial reporting practices. The use of GAAP (Generally Accepted Accounting Practices) is not only important but such an agreement between facilities to count revenue, expenses, and labor in exactly the same fashion, is crucial.

Benchmarking focuses on finding similar operations to share information with and/or finding reputable performance data with which to compare yourself, then using that information to find and implement best practices. To be successful, benchmarking needs to be a continuous process. The following are the four stages in the benchmarking process.

1. <u>What needs to be benchmarked?</u> Your first job is to identify the benchmarking subject. The subject might be a service, a product, or a process. Benchmarking subjects often relate to performance gaps, financial concerns, or unmet customer needs.

2. <u>To whose operation am I going to compare my operation?</u> The answer to this question will depend in large part on what you will be benchmarking. In most cases, pick operations with characteristics (such as size, menu, production system, style of service, type of customers, etc.) as similar to yours as possible. For example, a hospital foodservice director who is a member of the Association for Healthcare Foodservice has access to their Benchmarking Express (TM) program and can benchmark their data (such as costs or productivity) against similar foodservices.

3. <u>How am I going to collect the data?</u> Data from financial reports are often used to examine benchmarks such as food cost percentage or sales per square foot. Most foodservices are already collecting data for benchmarking.

4. <u>What do I do with the collected data and how do I implement changes?</u> You can analyze the data quantitatively or qualitatively. Ultimately, your analysis needs to examine the gap between the aspect of the operation you are studying and the benchmark, or best practice, that you are using. If a gap exists, you can use PDCA, CQI, or DMAIC to make improvements.

As you can see, there is a variety of tools that can be used. What matters is to use the tools most likely to solve the problem and sustain the solution.

14.3 MANAGE CUSTOMER SATISFACTION

You have likely gone out to eat a meal and were quite satisfied with the experience or, at other times, were disappointed and unhappy. In a survey conducted in 2019, the top complaints when eating out included the time it took to be served, prices, quality or taste of the food, rude service, and cleanliness (Fourth, 2019). Since foodservice is a mixture of both products (food and beverages) and service, customers have plenty with which to be happy or unhappy.

BASICS OF CUSTOMER SATISFACTION AND LOYALTY

Table 14-5 lists features of foodservices that can affect how satisfied our customers are. They are broken down into three groups: foods and beverages (the products), employee behaviors (the service), and the physical environment in which the customer experience takes place. The physical environment where the service is produced, delivered, and consumed is known as the **servicescape**, and it can influence customer satisfaction in service businesses (Ryu & Jang, 2008; Bitner, 1992) as well as employee job satisfaction (Parish, Berry, & Lam, 2008).

Table 14-5 Features of Foodservices That May Affect Customer Satisfaction		
Food and Beverages (Product)	**Employee Behaviors (Service)**	**Environment/Atmosphere**
Range of menu choices	Courteous/respectful	Location and parking
Quality of food/beverages (including taste, temperature, freshness, appearance)	Friendly/helpful	Size and layout of dining room
	Competent/reliable service	Attractiveness (colors, furniture, floors, decor, tabletop)
Portion size	Responsive to complaints and requests	Spaciousness
Price	Neat, clean appearance	Temperature/ventilation
Consistency of quality		Acoustics/music/noise
		Lighting
		Cleanliness/neatness
		Employees' appearance
		Interactions among other customers and employees
		Overall ambience

Each customer views and judges the actual meal experience in their own way. For example, two friends go to a new restaurant for dinner. While he thoroughly enjoyed the food, service, and overall experience, she felt the service was a little slow and she didn't like her appetizer. Perhaps her expectations were higher because she had just spoken with someone who couldn't stop raving about the restaurant, and maybe he was just happy to get away from the stress of his job and enjoy some time with an old friend. In any case, they ate at the same restaurant yet had differing experiences.

Customer satisfaction is a psychological concept involving the pleasure of getting what you expected and wanted/needed from an appealing product/service and the *total experience* (not just the service or food). It is highly subjective because each customer has different backgrounds, expectations, values, thoughts, emotions, and previous restaurant experience.

Customer satisfaction is a subjective experience in part because each of us has different expectations. Indeed, your own expectations of meal service in a pizza shop will certainly be different if you were going to a swanky restaurant in the theater district. Your previous foodservice experiences also influence your expectations. According to Goodman (2019), customers have multiple expectations, including that a foodservice will deliver what its brand promises and that the delivery will be consistent from unit to unit (in the case of a multiunit foodservice). Customers also have expectations for speedy, convenient service and frontline employees (such as servers) who will be empathetic and resolve problems quickly.

When we discuss customer satisfaction, we are really looking at how happy the customer is with their **customer experience**. According to Schwager and Mayer (2007), customer experience is "the internal and subjective response customers have to any direct or indirect contact with a company." A direct contact takes place, for example, when the customer is on the foodservice's premises to eat or pick up food. When a customer calls a foodservice to make a reservation or ask a question, that is also a direct contact. Examples of indirect contact include customers viewing the foodservice's website, seeing advertisements, hearing recommendations from friends, or checking online sources (such as Yelp) for reviews.

Customer satisfaction and loyalty are measured in foodservices, hotels, and many other businesses. For example, the **American Customer Satisfaction Index (ACSI)** gathers customer satisfaction data from 46 industries in the United States including some full-service and limited-service restaurant chains such as Denny's and Starbucks. ACSI obtains customer opinions on food quality, service speed, and staff courtesy. Overall customer satisfaction scores for the included full-service and limited-service restaurant chains are often higher than the national ACSI score of 75.7. Industries with low ACSI scores (in the 60s) include Internet service and subscription television providers (American Customer Satisfaction Index, 2020).

In surveys, Ekholm (2018) and Sorofman & McLellan (2014) have shown that more and more retail businesses are mostly or completely competing against the competition working on providing positive customer experiences. *What foodservices want these days are customers who are not just satisfied with their experience, but who have such positive experiences that they become loyal customers who return frequently and recommend the foodservice to others.* For example, a positive experience might be a barista in a coffee shop who addresses a customer by name and remembers what they usually order. Personalized service is one way to improve a customer's service experience.

In general, there is a positive relationship between service quality and customer loyalty (Yadav & Rai, 2019). According to Goodman (2019), loyal customers are "the core of your growth, profits, and reputation." Therefore, providing a positive customer experience to customers is crucial to the success of the business, especially considering that most customers have many choices of where to eat (Maze, 2017).

In any retail business, there are **service failures**—instances when the food, service, or atmosphere did not meet a customer's expectations. Unfortunately, most customers who experience a service failure will not complain, and most simply don't return and worse yet, complain to others. Various surveys, such as the National Customer Rage Survey, have consistently shown the power of negative word-of-mouth reports from unhappy customers, especially given today's opportunities to vent using social media (Arizona State University Center for Services Leadership, 2020; Goodman, 2019). Indeed, angry online reports are quite viral (Berger & Milkman, 2012). Some foodservices, especially chains, have social media teams in-house or use a social media monitoring company to oversee social media, including addressing poor reviews quickly.

Some customers with a complaint would actually say something if they knew where/how to complain and felt they would get a positive outcome. Having employees trained to listen to and resolve complaints (known as **service recovery**) is crucial to keep customers satisfied and loyal (Liat et al., 2017). It is more expensive to find a new customer than to resolve a problem with an existing customer (Goodman, 2019). In other words, keeping your current customers happy is cheaper than finding new customers.

HOW TO IMPROVE THE CUSTOMER EXPERIENCE

In order to give customers an excellent overall experience, there's a great deal more involved than just training employees who work directly with customers. In reality, every part of the organization has a role to play in keeping customers happy (Kandampully et al., 2018; Schneider, 2017; Schwager & Meyer, 2007), including operations, human resources, marketing, information technology, and the physical environment of the foodservice. Managers and supervisors must be excellent role models for providing exceptional customer service experiences as well as recognize employee successes and provide positive coaching. Let's start by discussing operations.

Operations

It all starts with the menu, meaning the foods and beverages served as well as their quality and price. A foodservice can have excellent service, but if the food quality or choices aren't up to your customers' expectations or are overpriced, customers will go elsewhere. In one study, the authors found that food complaints were rated by customers as a more serious failure than complaints about service or atmosphere

(Susskind and Viccari, 2011). Managers, supervisors, and employees can use a number of methods to ensure that meals are high quality.

- Select appropriate menu items based on market research and competitive analysis.
- Purchasing specifications should be developed and used, along with good receiving procedures, to ensure food quality.
- Use photos of plated items to guide production and serving personnel to produce an attractive, consistent product.
- Chefs, cooks, and other personnel should taste products before service.
- Food temperatures should also be tested before service.
- For certain menu items that are prepared and held (such as coffee), there need to be standards about the amount of time each item is held before being discarded.

In addition, production employees need the time, training, tools, and equipment to do their work properly, and the chance to give input on fine tuning production procedures.

Next, the service delivery system must be designed to provide excellent service experiences with an emphasis on *doing things right the first time* and being *consistent* in meeting customer's needs and expectations. Employees should be involved in designing and tweaking the service delivery system. Part of the delivery system should address how to make it easy for customers to complain and for employees to be empowered to solve those problems on first contact using some guidelines and their own judgment and ingenuity. If you use a delivery service as part of your delivery system, it is also important to develop a relationship and require some basic training and standards for delivery partners such as Door Dash, GrubHub, Uber Eats, and Postmates, as they can assist the success or ruin the delivery customer's experience. Some basic customer service techniques are listed in **Table 14-6**.

Human Resources

Service employees with excellent interpersonal skills can help your foodservice attract new customers and retain customers as they shape the customer experience. How service employees interact with customers and meet their needs and wants influence the success of the business.

From the human resources side, it is important to do the following.

- Hire the right employees.
- Provide employees with a living wage that is at least 10% above the median wage in the regional job market (Goodman, 2019).

Table 14-6 Examples of Customer Service Techniques
Promptly greet all customers and use their names if you know them.
Maintain good eye contact with customers and listen intently.
Be prompt and attentive.
Dress appropriately, maintain good body posture, and smile.
Be nonjudgmental about the variety of customers you serve.
Serve and clear food from the diner's left. Serve and clear drinks from the right.
Check with customers frequently to see if there are any concerns and, if so, listen, ask questions, and solve the problem quickly and without drama or argument. End on a positive note.
If any food/beverage is delayed, inform the customers.
Keep your work area clean and neat.

- Provide training, tools, and motivation to ensure job success and advancement to higher-level positions with higher pay.
- Empower employees to turn dissatisfied customers into satisfied loyal customers.
- Provide prompt feedback on performance in a private, nonthreatening atmosphere.
- Motivate employees in part by providing incentives/rewards and recognition from peers and supervisors for quality performance.

Satisfied employees are more likely to deliver better service (Wirtz & Jerger, 2016).

In a study of over 1,400 service employees, Dixon, Ponomareff, Turner, & Delisi (2017) found that managers most often wanted to hire employees who are very empathetic and listen sympathetically to customers. While that makes sense, researchers found that employees categorized as Controllers (not Empathizers) were much better at resolving customer problems, including reducing the effort the customer had to make. Controllers "describe themselves as 'take charge' people who are more interested in building and following a plan than 'going with the flow'.....they're confident decision makers, especially when nobody's in charge, and they're opinionated and vocal" (Dixon et al., 2017, p 113). As you can imagine, controllers want to decide how to help a customer without the need to adhere to strict rules.

Training should include how to establish rapport with diverse groups of customers as well as how to approach complaints, including difficult issues and situations. According to Goodman (2019, p. 228), "the best practice is to provide flexible guidance on the top ten issues and tell employees to use their best judgment for all other situations." Management should make clear how much empowerment is granted to employees to resolve complaints. Training should be ongoing.

Marketing and Information Technology

The marketing of a foodservice influences how customers set their expectations. A foodservice needs to appropriately market its offerings so customers have realistic expectations. Marketing personnel also develop new food promotions and influence policies and procedures, both of which need to involve employee feedback to be successful. Whereas good marketing brings customers in the door, poor food and/or service drives them out.

Technology, such as touchscreens in a foodservice or apps on a smartphone, have been very helpful in making it easier and quicker to order food and also to get it delivered. Having free Wi-Fi for customers or electronic games at the tables for kids are other examples of how technology can enhance excellent customer service. It is important to find the right balance between technology and human interactions. Too much in either direction will make certain customers unhappy. For example, some customers dislike using a computer to order or pay for goods and prefer talking to a person. Social media can be useful to engage individual customers as well as communities of customers.

Physical Environment/Atmosphere

Customers often judge the physical environment more objectively than they judge the food and service. Features of the physical environment should be consistent with the foodservice concept, aesthetically pleasing, and well maintained. The number of customer complaints about the physical environment/atmosphere are generally lower than those about food or service, but customers with these complaints are less likely to return, even if the problem (such as noise) is corrected by the foodservice (Susskind & Viccari, 2011).

The physical facilities also impact employees. In hospital settings, a study showed that employees had more job satisfaction and commitment to their employer when the servicescape was more pleasant and convenient as well as safer (Parish et al., 2008).

HOW TO GATHER CUSTOMER FEEDBACK

When gathering customer feedback, you have to make decisions on what information you want and how to obtain that information. While it is important for a foodservice to get feedback about individual customer experiences, it is equally important to examine and assess a customer's interactions with others in a foodservice—such as managers and other customers, as well as a customer's *overall impression of the foodservice* (Kandampully et al., 2018; Rawson et al., 2013). A customer's overall impression includes all aspects of products, services, and physical environment/atmosphere listed in Table 14-5.

SERVQUAL is an instrument developed by Parasuraman, Berry, and Zeithami (1991) that measures the difference between customer's expectations and perceptions of service quality. SERVQUAL examined service quality from five dimensions: reliability, responsiveness, assurance, empathy, and tangibles. Stevens, Knutson, & Patton (1995) adapted SERVQUAL to develop the DINESERV questionnaire for use in restaurants, which includes 29 questions to measure the same five dimensions of service quality. Respondents are asked to indicate how much they agree or disagree with each statement (from 7 for strongly agree to 1 for strongly disagree). This type of scale is known as a **Likert scale** and is useful for measuring opinions, attitudes, and feelings—constructs that you cannot observe. A Likert scale always has an odd number of responses because the middle choice is "Neither Agree nor Disagree." The following is a sample DINESERV question showing the scale (Stevens et al., 1995).

1. Has personnel who seem well trained, competent, and experienced.

1	2	3	4	5	6	7
Strongly Disagree	Disagree	Some what Disagree	Neither Agree nor Disagree	Somewhat Agree	Strongly Agree	Agree

By today's standards, when customers may only give you three minutes to complete a survey, DINESERV is a bit long. There are certainly many different questions you can ask customers about any aspect of your product, service, or environment, but the longer the survey, the lower the chance that it will be completed. So, it is important to prioritize your questions. Examples of important questions include the following.

1. How likely are you to return to our restaurant/foodservice or request delivery within 30 days? (with a Likert scale from "very likely" to "very unlikely")
2. How likely is it that you will recommend "Foodservice Name" to your friends, colleagues, or family? (with a Likert scale from "very likely" to "very unlikely")
3. Overall, how satisfied were you with your experience today? (with a Likert scale from "very satisfied" to "very dissatisfied")
4. Which of the qualities about the food did you like? (include a list such as taste, texture, portion size, etc.)
5. Was your meal prepared to your satisfaction? (with a Likert scale from "very satisfied" to "very dissatisfied")
6. Which of the qualities about the service did you like? (include a list such as friendly, attentive, prompt, etc.)
7. How would you rate the overall service? (with a Likert scale from "very satisfied" to "very dissatisfied")

Questions 1 and 2 can tell you a lot about your customer loyalty, whereas question 3 looks at overall satisfaction. Questions 4 to 7 ask for feedback on products and service. Depending on the foodservice, you may want to ask what time the customer visited, if a food delivery was on time (in the case of a delivery), and basic customer demographics, such as gender or age.

Closed-ended questions (fixed-alternative) are popular because they require less time for respondents to complete and the results can be quantified easily. **Open-ended questions** allow respondents to answer questions in their own words. In some cases, open-ended questions such as "What would you like us to add to the menu?" may be used. The following are some questions to help you determine whether your questions and responses are effective.

1. Does the question measure something you want feedback on?
2. Will most respondents understand the question as it is intended?
3. Is the question brief, free of bias, and free of double negatives?
4. Is only one question posed?
5. Do most respondents need to answer this question?
6. Does the question provide a list of acceptable responses?
7. Are the response categories both comprehensive and mutually exclusive (the response options don't overlap or conflict)?

Questions and responses should be tested to make sure they are understandable and provide useful data before using them in a formal customer survey.

To gather information from customers and to continually improve customer experiences, there are a number of methods you can use.

1. Customer surveys (online/written) (**Figure 14-10**)
2. Customer interviews (face-to-face, phone)
3. Focus groups/user groups
4. Observations
5. Public postings and reviews on social media

Employees can also provide their impressions of how customers view their experience. Some foodservices hire what is called a **mystery shopper** to eat at the foodservice and report on all aspects of the experience.

Websites with foodservice reviews (such as Yelp or TripAdvisor) are also a great way to read what customers think. In order to make the review sites useful, the business must assure that all of the descriptive information about the restaurant is correct, then it becomes possible to manage the reviews and responses.

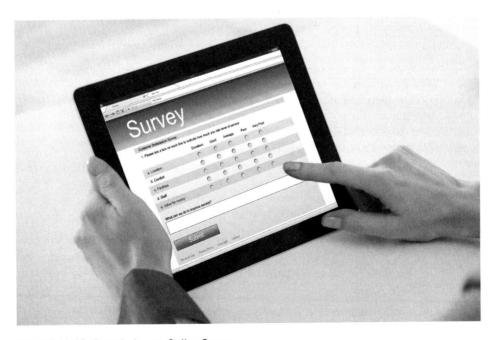

FIGURE 14-10 Completing an Online Survey

© Andrey_Popov/Shutterstock

A popular way to gather customer feedback is to put a link to a survey on a receipt and promise the chance of winning some prize/giveaway/reward by completing the survey. If a survey is delivered on a smart device, you can bundle the survey with the invoice (including the tip), which is another indication of satisfaction. Tracking this information helps to build your customer data base and helps you track successes and failures with each meal served. If you have email addresses, you can also email customers and ask them to complete a survey and thank them for their business.

Texting on a mobile device may be the most common way people communicate today. Asking customers to text reviews using a phone app (in exchange for a free appetizer or beverage) is one of the easiest ways to gather reviews and feedback.

PATIENT SATISFACTION IN HOSPITALS

Patient satisfaction is a very important topic because providers want to provide quality patient experiences and patient care that, in turn, will bring in more patients and provide financial security. Like commercial foodservices, patients do tell others whether they had a good experience at a hospital or not. You can actually compare hospital ratings online at Medicare.gov. For example, you can compare the "patient experience" or "effectiveness of care" at several hospitals in your area.

U.S. hospitals are required to survey a random sample of recently discharged patients using a national standardized survey called the Hospital Consumer Assessment of Healthcare Providers and Systems survey (HCAHPS). The survey includes 29 questions, none addressing food or foodservice directly. Some of the results from this survey are used in the online hospital ratings at Medicare.gov. Hospitals are also allowed to add their own questions. Many of the questions ask how often a patient experienced a critical aspect of hospital care, often related to nursing or physician care, rather than whether they were simply satisfied with their care. Results from this survey allow comparisons between hospitals and are also linked to how much financial reimbursement facilities get from Medicare.

Many hospitals develop their own patient satisfaction surveys to provide additional customized information, or rely on third-party providers, such as Press Ganey Associates or Gallup, to administer and interpret quality patient satisfaction surveys. Press Ganey provides a research-based survey that focuses on multiple aspects of the patient experience, including foodservice.

Questions about food and service generally ask questions about the following.

1. Taste/texture/quality of food
2. Food temperature of hot foods
3. Food temperature of cold foods
4. Appearance of tray
5. Food choices available
6. Meals served in a timely manner (about the same time each day)
7. Whether the meal delivered matches the meal that was ordered (known as **tray accuracy**)
8. Whether the tray included everything, and if not, was it offered
9. Courtesy of employees who serve the food

In addition, patients on a modified diet (such as low sodium) may be asked if someone explained their diet to them so they understood what they were permitted to eat.

To provide excellent service, as well as quality food, hospital foodservices often do the following.

1. Foods are taste tested and temperatures taken in the kitchen according to policy and procedures.
2. Staff are regularly trained and coached on plate presentation guidelines including placement of garnishes.

3. On a regular basis, a **test (or dummy) tray** is sent to an empty patient room, and a manager or Registered Dietitian will test the quality and temperatures of the food, as well as rate the tray appearance and accuracy. Results are communicated to kitchen staff and any problems are reviewed and corrections made.

4. Managers and Registered Dietitians periodically conduct **meal rounds** on patient floors to get patient feedback on food quality and presentation, food temperatures, delivery times, and patients' interactions with dietary staff.

5. Staff who take meal orders and/or deliver patient trays must understand the importance of timeliness and accuracy of food delivery (along with making sure patients have the needed utensils, condiments, and napkins). Trays should be double-checked before leaving the kitchen.

6. Courtesy when delivering meal trays usually includes actions such as knocking at the door before entering, smiling at the patient and making eye contact, introducing yourself and telling the patient why you are there, asking the patient where to place the tray, and making sure the patient can reach everything. Often, a server will deliver about five trays, and then circle back to each patient to see if they have any concerns or need something, such as an extra packet of sugar.

7. Patients who are on modified diets are more likely to be unhappy with the food because they may order menu items that are not allowed on their diet, and then they receive a substitute menu item (that they probably don't like!). It's important to have the Registered Dietitian work closely with these patients to increase meal satisfaction.

The foodservice may also conduct a **plate-waste study** that examines how much food (and which menu item) is left on plates after customers have finished their meals. As trays are returned to the dishroom, some are randomly selected to determine the percentage of uneaten food for one or more specific menu items. If patients show a dislike of a particular item, evaluate whether it should come off the menu.

In a study conducted from 2014 to 2016, Press Ganey Associates and Compass One Healthcare (a contract company) found that patients had low expectations for hospital food. Patients were more likely to give good ratings for food quality as long as their trays were accurate, arrived on time, and delivered in a courteous manner (Press Ganey, 2017). The study also found that patients on modified diets liked to get menus that only show items they are allowed to eat and wanted explanations if an alternate food item had to be served.

SUMMARY

14.1 Describe Approaches to Quality

- Key performance indicators (KPI) are measurable values that demonstrate how well an organization is achieving its business objectives. Examples include measures of customer satisfaction and food quality.

- Quality control has been around for years and focuses on finding defects (or variations from the standard) in a product, service, or outcome and then figuring out why it occurred. Ultimately, finding defects provides information on how to change processes so fewer defects occur in the future.

- Quality control has been replaced with Total Quality Management (TQM) and

Six Sigma. TQM is generally regarded as the beginning of the quality movement. It is a management philosophy that focuses on responding to customer needs and expectations while continually examining and improving organizational processes and empowering employees. It advises managers be responsible for continuous improvement, use statistics to measure process performance, and involve employees to identify problems and find solutions.

- The Plan-Do-Check-Act (PDCA) cycle, a basic process improvement model was originally developed by Walter Shewhart and adapted by W. Edwards Deming as the plan-do-study-act (PDSA) cycle. (Both men helped found TQM.) The cycle (Table 14-2) uses four steps to plan projects and carry out changes. The PDSA cycle doesn't have a beginning and end. The cycle is repeated again and again for continuous improvement.

- Another TQM tool was the use of quality circles.
- Continuous quality improvement (CQI) is a systematic approach to measuring, evaluating, and improving products and services. It uses a cyclical process of assessing products or performance, developing and implementing improvement plans, and reassessing results.
- Kaizen is a Japanese philosophy of continuous improvement that involves all employees at all levels. The Kaizen process uses PDCA—Plan Do Check Act—and also a methodology called 5S. The purpose of 5S is to improve workplace organization and eliminate wasted time looking for needed items or getting ready to work. The steps are Sort, Set in order, Shine, Standardize, and Sustain.
- Six Sigma is a problem-solving quality program that uses a set of methods and tools to reduce errors or variations, lower costs and increase profits, maximize employee job satisfaction as well as customer satisfaction, and earn customer loyalty. Sigma is a statistical measurement that shows how well a process is performing. At Six Sigma, there are fewer than 3.5 defects per million products or processes—which is incredibly small. Manufacturers are more likely to adopt Six Sigma than service companies such as foodservices, but more service companies are trying it out.
- A key focus of Six Sigma is the use of statistical tools to identify and correct the causes of variations. For example, Six Sigma uses the DMAIC methodology, which relies in part on statistics, as a roadmap for solving problems and improving processes. DMAIC stands for define, measure, analyze, improve, and control.
- Six Sigma is different from TQM in that it creates an infrastructure of people in the organization who are trained in Six Sigma methods and can conduct projects and implement improvements.
- Six Sigma is often combined with Lean methods. Lean is sometimes referred to as the Toyota Production System because it was a foundation for lean manufacturing. Lean is a tool used in organizations to streamline manufacturing and production processes by focusing on eliminating waste and smoothing the process flow. Waste refers to any step or action in a process that is not required for the process to be successfully completed. Lean projects emphasize elimination or reduction of anything a customer would not want to pay for. Table 14-3 lists the eight wastes (called Downtime).
- Lean organizations often use value stream mapping, in which a flowchart is developed by a team to document every step in a process, along with the 5S system from Kaizen.
- ISO 9000 is a set of quality system standards established by international technical experts from more than 90 countries, as part of the International Organization for Standardization (ISO). There are various ISO standards and ISO 9001 is the model for a quality management system that can be used in large and small organizations to improve efficiency and customer satisfaction.
- The Joint Commission is an independent group in the United States that develops and administers voluntary accreditation programs for hospitals and other healthcare organizations. Joint Commission standards can help healthcare foodservices measure, evaluate, and improve performance. The standards focus on important patient or resident care and organization functions that are essential to providing safe, high-quality care.

14.2 Choose Appropriate Quality Tools to Support Quality Management

- There are a wide variety of quality tools available to use in different situations. Three categories are discussed—cause analysis tools, process analysis tools, and data collection tools.
- Cause analysis tools include the following.
  - Root cause analysis: Helps identify why and how an unfavorable event occurred so preventive actions can be developed.
  - Cause-and-effect diagram (also called a fishbone diagram or Ishikawa diagram): Helps team brainstorm possible causes of a problem (Figure 14-2).

- Pareto chart: Shows the factors that contribute to variation in a process as bars and the biggest bars are to the left. Each bar represents frequency, quantity, cost, or time. Figure 14-3 shows the frequency of common customer complaints.
- Scatter diagram: Shows whether there is a relationship between two variables, such as revenue and payroll (Figure 14-4).
- Process analysis tools help managers and employees look carefully at a process or procedure to troubleshoot issues and make improvements.
  - Flowchart (also called process map): Is a graphic representation of an ordered sequence of events, steps, or procedures that take place in a system. Figure 14-5 shows common flowchart symbols and Figure 14-6 is an example of a flowchart.
  - Spaghetti diagram: Traces the path of an item through a process. Lines show the flow of an item as shown in Figure 14-7. They are helpful for seeing possible reasons for delays.
  - Failure Mode and Effects Analysis: Is used to identify and analyze potential failures within a process. We use FMEA every time we consider the following: What could go wrong and the likelihood of it happening, and if something went wrong, would we know about it in time and how severe would the effects be. If the likelihood of the failure is pretty high and the effects are quite negative, it is time to work on identifying the probable cause(s) of the failure and developing and testing preventive actions to prevent the failure in the future.
- Here are tools used to collect data.
  - Check sheet: Is designed to collect data in real-time. Check sheets are used to gather how often something of interest happens, such as a dish is returned to the kitchen. Check sheets may also include a measurement scale divided into intervals which can be checked off (Table 14-4). Checklists are another type of check sheet.
  - Histogram: Is a simple graph using bars of different heights to show a frequency distribution of a variable, such as wait time (Figure 14-8). It is similar to a bar chart but a histogram groups numbers into ranges.
  - Control chart: Shows data over time so it demonstrates how a variable or process

changes. What makes the control chart more valuable is that it includes a central line for the average and two other horizontal lines. Called the upper control limit and the lower control limit, they are chosen so that you can easily see when the data are within acceptable limits (Figure 14-9).
- Survey: Is used to obtain data from specific groups of people about their behavior, opinions, or knowledge.
- The process of benchmarking also supports quality management. Benchmarking is the practice of comparing your operation's performance against yourself, similar operations or an industry standard to determine if there are areas for improvement. For example, when managers at two similar quick-service restaurants compare the average number of minutes it takes for a drive-through customer to be served, the manager with the slower drive-through may gain some tips on how to serve customers faster.
- Internal benchmarking is when managers compare performance of operations within the *same* organization. Internal benchmarking also includes comparing your own foodservice's performance over time.
- External benchmarking is when a manager compares performance against foodservices *outside* of his/her organization. Whether internal or external, benchmarking can help you find your strengths and how to maintain them, as well as identify areas where you can improve and ideas for improvement.

14.3 Manage Customer Satisfaction

- Table 14-5 lists features of foodservices that affect customer satisfaction. They include aspects of the food and beverages (product), employee behaviors (service), and the atmosphere/servicescape.
- Customer satisfaction is a psychological concept involving the pleasure of getting what you expected and wanted/needed from an appealing product/service and *total experience* (not just the service or food). It is highly subjective because each customer has different backgrounds, expectations, values, thoughts, and emotions.
- More and more retail businesses are mostly or completely competing against the competition by providing positive customer

experiences. What foodservices want these days are customers who have such positive experiences that they become loyal customers who return frequently and recommend the foodservice to others. According to Goodman (2019), loyal customers are "the core of your growth, profits, and reputation."

- Most customers who experience a service failure will not complain, and most simply do not return and worse yet, complain to others. Some customers with a complaint would actually say something if they knew where/how to complain and felt they would get a positive outcome. Having employees trained in service recovery is crucial to keep customers satisfied and loyal.

- Every part of an organization has a role to play in keeping customers happy including operations, human resources, marketing, information technology, and the physical environment of the foodservice. Managers and supervisors must also be excellent role models for providing exceptional customer service experiences as well as recognize employee successes and provide positive coaching.

- To gather information from customers to improve customer experiences, a foodservice can use customer surveys (online/written), customer interviews, focus groups, observations, public postings/reviews on social media, or a mystery shopper.

- Examples of questions to ask customers are given. Perhaps the most important questions revolve around whether the customer will return to the foodservice or recommend the foodservice to others.

- Common questions asked in hospital foodservice revolve around the quality and temperature of the food, tray appearance, food choices, timeliness and accuracy of the tray, and courtesy of employees who deliver trays. Patients on modified diets are more likely to be unhappy with the food.

- In one study, patients were more likely to give good ratings for food quality as long as their trays were accurate, arrived on time, and were delivered in a courteous manner (Press Ganey, 2017).

REVIEW AND DISCUSSION QUESTIONS

1. What is meant by the term quality? Why is it so important?
2. Is quality management an example of the management function of controlling? Why or why not?
3. Compare TQM with Six Sigma.
4. What does Lean bring to Six Sigma when they are combined? What are Lean's goals?
5. Describe a tool that you can use to help determine the reasons for a problem. Also, describe a tool that helps managers examine a process or procedure to make improvements.
6. What is a control chart?
7. Define benchmarking and give an example of how a foodservice manager might benchmark their operation.
8. What affects whether foodservice customers are satisfied and happy with their purchases and service? List six points and put them into categories.
9. What are service failure and service recovery?
10. What is the big picture in terms of improving the customer experience in restaurants?
11. How do healthcare foodservice managers measure patient satisfaction and what can they do to provide excellent food and service?

SMALL GROUP PROJECT

For the foodservice concept that you created, complete the following.

1. Develop a customer satisfaction online survey for a group of customers who you will serve, and explain how you will summarize and present the data.

REFERENCES

American Customer Satisfaction Index. (2020). *National, sector, and industry results.* https://www.theacsi.org/national-economic-indicator/national-sector-and-industry-results

Arizona State University Center for Services Leadership. (2020). *Customer rage.* https://research.wpcarey.asu.edu/services-leadership/research/research-initiatives/customer-rage/

Berger, J. & Milkman, K. L. (2012). What makes online content viral? *Journal of Marketing Research, 49*(2), 192–205. doi: 10.1509/jmr.10.0353

Bitner, M. J. (1992). Servicescapes: The impact of physical surroundings on customers and employees. *Journal of Marketing, 56*(2), 57–71.

Carrier, N., West, G. E., & Ouellet, D. (2009). Dining experience, foodservices and staffing are associated with quality of life in elderly nursing home residents. *The Journal of Nutrition, Health and Aging, 13*(6), 565–570.

Centers for Medicare and Medicaid Services. (2016). *QAPI description and background.* https://www.cms.gov/Medicare/Provider-Enrollment-and-Certification/QAPI/qapidefinition

Crawford, R. (2019). Restaurant profitability and failure rates: What you need to know. *Modern Restaurant Management.* https://modernrestaurantmanagement.com/restaurant-profitability-and-failure-rates-what-you-need-to-know/

Dixon, M., Ponomareff, L., Turner, S., & Delisi, R. (2017). Kick-ass customer service. *Harvard Business Review, 95*(1), 111–117.

Ekholm, J. (2018). *Why the customer experience matters.* Gartner Blog Network. https://blogs.gartner.com/jessica-ekholm/2018/06/07/customer-experience-matter/

Fourth. (2019). Fourth unveils first annual "Truth about Dining Out" survey results, revealing Americans' eating-out habits, the rise of third-party delivery apps and favorite celebrity chef. https://www.fourth.com/press-room/fourth-unveils-first-annual-truth-about-dining-out-survey-results/

Gershon, M. (2010). Choosing which process improvement methodology to implement. *Journal of Applied Business & Economics, 10*(5), 61–69.

Goodman. J. A. (2019). *Strategic customer service.* Harper Collins Leadership.

Kandampully, J., Zhang, T., & Jaakkola, E. (2018). Customer experience management in hospitality: A literature synthesis, new understanding and research agenda. *International Journal of Contemporary Hospitality Management, 30*(1), 21–56. doi:10.1108/IJCHM-10-2015-0549

Liat, C. B., Mansori, S., Chuan, G. C., & Imrie, B. C. (2017). Hotel service recovery and service quality: Influences of corporate image and generational differences in the relationship between customer satisfaction and loyalty. *Journal of Global Marketing, 30*(1), 42–51.

Maze, J. (2017). Customers not returning despite service: "Intent to return" survey score drops 6.4 percent in April, according to TDn2K. *Nation's Restaurant News, 51*(9), 130–131.

Parasuraman, A., Berry, L. L., & Zeithaml, V. A. (1991). Refinement and reassessment of the SERVQUAL scale. *Journal of Retailing, 67*(4), 420–450.

Parish, J. T., Berry, L. L., & Lam S. Y. (2008). The effect of servicescape on service workers. *Journal of Service Research, 10*(3), 220–238.

Pizam, A., & Ellis, T. (1999). Customer satisfaction and its measurement in hospitality enterprises. *International Journal of Contemporary Hospitality Management, 11*(7), 326–339.

Pizam, A., Shapoval, V., & Ellis, T. (2016). Customer satisfaction and its measurement in hospitality enterprises: A revisit and update. *International Journal of Contemporary Hospitality Management, 28*(1), 2–35.

Press Ganey. (2017). *Food for thought: Maximizing the positive impact food can have on a patient's stay.* [White Paper] Retrieved from https://www.compassonehealthcare.com/files/3015/5958/0020/Compass_One_White_Paper_Rev4_Clean_4.pdf

Rawson, A., Duncan, E., & Jones, C. (2013). The truth about customer experience. *Harvard Business Review, 91*(9), 90–98.

Reid, D.B. (2019). From lean modules to a lean mindset. *Industrial & Systems Engineering at Work, 51*(5), 28–33.

Robbins, S.P., and Coulter, M. (2018). *Management* (14th ed.). New York: Pearson Education Inc.

Ryu, K, & Jang, S. (2008). DINESCAPE: A scale for customers' perception of dining environments. *Journal of Foodservice Business Research, 11*(1), 2–22.

Schneider, B. (2017). How companies can really impact service quality. *People + Strategy, 40*(4), 20–25.

Schwager, A. & Meyer, C. (2007). Understanding customer experience. *Harvard Business Review, 85*(2), 116–126.

Sorofman, J., & McLellan, L. (2014). *Gartner survey finds importance of customer experience on the rise—marketing is on the hook.* Gartner Research. Retrieved from https://www.gartner.com/en/documents/2857722/gartner-survey-finds-importance-of-customer-experience-o

Stevens, P., Knutson, B., & Patton, M. (1995). DINESERV: A tool for measuring service quality in restaurants. *The Cornell Hotel and Restaurant Administration Quarterly, 36*(2), 56–60.

Susskind, A., & Viccari, A. (2011). A look at the relationship between service failures, guest satisfaction, and repeat-patronage intentions of casual dining guests. *Cornell Hospitality Quarterly, 52*(4), 438–444.

Westcott, R.T. (ed.). (2014). *The certified manager of quality/organizational excellence handbook* (4th ed.). ASQ Quality Press.

Wirtz, J. & Jerger, C. (2016). Managing service employees: Literature review, expert opinions, and research directions. *The Service Industries Journal, 36*(15–16), 757–788.

Yadav, M. K., & Rai, A. K. (2019). An assessment of the mediating effect of customer satisfaction on the relationship between service quality and customer loyalty. *The IUP Journal of Marketing Management, 28*(3), 7–23.

Managing Finances

LEARNING OUTCOMES

15.1 Complete and analyze an income statement.

15.2 Complete and analyze a balance sheet.

15.3 Prepare an operating budget and monitor performance.

15.4 Prepare a capital budget.

15.5 Use financial analysis tools.

15.6 Measure productivity.

15.7 Control costs.

INTRODUCTION

When you are at a restaurant and about to pay your bill, have you ever wondered how your money is being used by the restaurant? In other words, if you paid $10 for lunch, how much of that paid for the food and how much paid for the labor? Of course, the restaurant has other operating expenses, so you may wonder if they made a profit on the $10 lunch after paying for food, labor, and other expenses. In almost any business, the bottom line is whether or not the sales dollars cover all of the expenses of doing business plus leave some extra as profit. Noncommercial foodservices, such as an onsite foodservice in a hospital or school, are not usually looking for a profit. Instead, they often look to break even, meaning that they want to bring in just enough revenue to cover their costs. **Figure 15-1** shows how sales in a commercial foodservice are used to pay expenses and provide profit. The two biggest expenses (chunks in the pie) are food/beverage and labor.

Businesses need people to take care of financial matters, such as recordkeeping, accounting, and auditing. **Bookkeepers** have a basic understanding of accounting principles and oversee the recording of the transactions of a business, including revenue, expenses, payment of bills and taxes, and payroll. Bookkeepers maintain the **general ledger**, which is a complete record of all financial transactions. Two important accounts within the general ledger are **accounts payable** (bills for food, etc., that must be paid out) and **accounts receivable** (money that is owed to the business). As you can imagine, records must be up-to-date and accurate so they can be useful for accountants and foodservice managers.

© Denis Val/Shutterstock

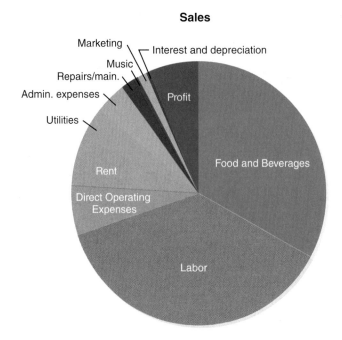

FIGURE 15-1 How Sales Dollars Are Used in a Foodservice

Accounting is the process of recording and summarizing all transactions of the business (which bookkeepers often do) as well as analyzing and verifying the results. Accountants monitor cash flow so you don't run out of cash, prepare important financial statements (such as an income statement or balance sheet) at certain points during the year, and handle tax preparation. A Certified Public Accountant (CPA) is someone who has passed the CPA exam and completed state work experience and education requirements to become licensed. Many accountants in the restaurant industry use the Uniform System of Accounts for Restaurants (USAR) developed by the National Restaurant Association. The USAR is an agreed-upon system of accounting that serves as a set of guidelines for setting up sales categories, expense classifications, income statement, and more. Uniform systems of account also exist for hotels, clubs, and other industries.

Auditing is the evaluation of financial records/statements prepared by accountants. Auditors are CPAs who work outside of the business being audited. After evaluating the financial statements, the auditor gives an opinion of them including whether anything is misstated or there are any irregularities. Auditing's purpose is to ensure the reliability of the financial statements. All public companies must have a CPA firm audit their financial statements before being released to shareholders or the public.

This chapter will introduce you to important financial concepts. Beginning with two financial statements (income statement and balance sheet), the chapter moves on to budgets as well as ways to analyze financial statements, sales, costs, and productivity. The chapter ends with a discussion of what foodservice managers oversee every day— controlling food, labor, and other costs.

15.1 COMPLETE AND ANALYZE AN INCOME STATEMENT

An **income statement** (also called a statement of revenue and expenditures) is a report of revenue and expenses completed for a specific accounting period. An **accounting period** is any specific length of time for which financial records are prepared. The accounting period could be one month, a 28-day period, one quarter of a year (meaning three months), one year, or other period of time that a business decides on. The income statement shows how much revenue came in for a specific period of time for products/services along with the costs and expenses involved in producing them. At the bottom of the income statement, after subtracting all expenses from the revenue, is the **bottom line**: the profit or loss before income taxes are paid.

$$\text{Revenue} - \text{Expenses} = \text{Profit/Loss}$$

This information is crucial in order for owners and managers to understand how the business is doing and make timely business decisions. Many foodservices create income statements every month or 28 days (or more frequently) to keep a close eye on the business. Because a 28-day accounting period makes it easy to compare one period to another, many foodservices prefer that to actual months, which vary in length and in the number of weekends. In one calendar year, there are 12 months or 13 28-day accounting periods.

How to Complete an Income Statement

Income statements are set up like a flight of stairs. On the top step, you have the gross sales (also called revenue or income) for the accounting period (**Table 15–1**). It is called "gross" because expenses have not been deducted from it yet. As you go down, one step at a time, you make a deduction for different expenses, such as food, labor, rent, and so on. At the bottom of the staircase, after deducting all of the expenses, you will see whether the business made money (profit) or lost money (loss). That why the income statement is also called a **profit and loss (P & L) statement**. The following is an explanation of each of the four steps to complete an income statement. Keep in mind that food, beverage, and labor are the three largest expenses in most foodservices.

    Step One. To read the income statement in Table 15-1, let's start by just using the first column, which is in dollars. Sales dollars are recorded for the first quarter of 2021 for food and beverages (meaning alcoholic beverages) in the restaurant and catering. Then these are totaled up and the total is $331,492.

    Step Two. The first deduction from sales is referred to as the **cost of sales** (also called cost of goods sold). The cost of sales is the cost of purchasing the foods and beverages used to generate sales. Food expenses are kept separate from alcoholic beverages so

Table 15-1 Income Statement for Riverside Steaks for the First Three Months of 2021		
Profit and Loss Statement (January 1–March 31, 2021)		
Sales		
Food	$238,183	71.9%
Beverage	76,636	23.1%
Corporate Catering	16,673	5.0%
Total Sales	$331,492	100.0%
Cost of Sales		
Food	$78,157	32.8%
Beverage	17,712	23.1%
Corporate Catering (Food only)	5,335	32.0%
Total Cost of Sales	$101,204	30.5%
Gross Profit	**$230,288**	**69.5%**

(continues)

Table 15-1 Income Statement for Riverside Steaks for the First Three Months of 2021 (continued)		
Controllable Expenses		
Salaries and Wages	$95,323	28.8%
Benefits	19,889	6.0%
Employer-Paid Payroll Taxes/W. Comp	6,630	2.0%
Direct Operating Expenses	19,227	5.8%
Utilities	14,917	4.5%
Administrative Expenses/Fees	12,928	3.9%
Repairs & Maintenance	7,600	2.3%
Music and Entertainment	663	0.2%
Marketing and Advertising	4,040	1.2%
Total Controllable Expenses	*$181,217*	*54.7%*
Controllable Income	**$49,071**	**14.8%**
Noncontrollable Expenses		
Occupancy Costs	$34,807	10.5%
Depreciation	3,961	2.1%
Interest	1,326	0.4%
Total Non-Controllable Expenses	*$43,094*	*13.0%*
Net Income/Net Loss Before Taxes	**$5,977**	**1.8%**

that managers can keep a closer eye on each category. To calculate how much food costs for the period, see **Example 15-1**.

The same formula in Example 15-1 is used to calculate the cost of alcoholic beverages. By adding the value of the inventory at the beginning of a specific period of time to the value of purchases during that period, you have the total value of food or alcoholic beverages available for sale. By subtracting the value of the ending inventory for the period, you now know the *cost of food or alcoholic beverages used during that period*.

So now you have two important numbers: total sales and cost of sales (meaning food and beverage costs). When you subtract the cost of sales from the total sales, you are left with what is called **gross profit**. It is considered "gross" because there are still a number of expenses that haven't been deducted yet. The formula for gross profit is as follows.

Total or Gross Sales − Cost of Sales = Gross Profit
$331,492 − $101,204 = $230,288

EXAMPLE 15-1 HOW TO CALCULATE COST OF SALES

Beginning Inventory + Food Purchased − Ending Inventory = Cost of Sales

Example:

Beginning Inventory − 1/1/2021	$24,000
Purchases for January − March	+ $87,000
Food/Bev. Available for Sale	$111,000
Ending Inventory − 3/31/2021	− $27,508
Cost of Sales	$83,492

Now we need to subtract the remaining expenses (costs) to find out if the business made any money. We are going to do that in *two steps*. First, we are going to deduct the controllable expenses and then the noncontrollable expenses. **Controllable costs**, such as food (which we already deducted), are costs that managers have the power to influence in the short term. Although you can't control every aspect of food costs, you can control them to a large extent. After all, it is the foodservice managers who decide what and how much to purchase and how food is received, stored, and used to reduce theft and waste. While labor is mostly controllable, it also has a noncontrollable element to it. **Noncontrollable costs** are those that managers have little or no control over— such as rent and interest on a loan. Real estate owners determine how much they want to be paid for rent, and banks determine how much interest you pay.

Step Three. We will list and add up the controllable costs first, then subtract them from the gross profit to get what is called the **controllable income** (profit after all controllable costs are removed from sales). As seen in Table 15-1, *controllable costs include the following* (keeping in mind that the cost of food/beverages has already been deducted).

- Salaries/Wages. This is the largest controllable cost in the list. Salaries and wages include all monies paid to employees, including pay for any overtime hours.
- Benefits. Employers often pay a portion of an employee's benefits such as health insurance. Full-timers are more likely than part-timers to receive benefits. The Affordable Care Act (ACA) requires employers with 50 or more full-time equivalent employees to offer health insurance to 95% or more of employees who work an average of 30 hours a week. ACA considers an employee who works 30 hours to be full-time.
- Employer-paid payroll taxes and workers' compensation insurance. Payroll taxes will be discussed later. Employers do pay some payroll taxes for each employee, as well as workers' compensation insurance. **Workers' compensation** programs provide the payment of lost wages, medical treatment, and rehabilitation services to workers suffering from a work-related injury or illness. Most employers purchase coverage for workers' compensation through private insurance companies or they self-fund—meaning they pay out-of-pocket whenever there is a work-related injury or illness.
- Direct operating expenses. These are expenses incurred daily and include cleaning supplies, paper supplies (such as aluminum foil or disposable plates), kitchenware (such as pots), serviceware (such as utensils), laundry, uniforms, exterminating services, and other operating expenses.
- Utilities. These typically include cost of water, electricity, gas, telephone, Internet, and trash removal.
- Administrative Expenses and Fees. Administrative expenses are overhead expenses not directly related to serving food and beverages. Examples of administrative expenses include the cost of supplies such as office supplies, postage, software, and fees paid to accountants or attorneys. This category also includes credit card and debit card processing fees, which are an increasingly significant expense of doing business, as well as the cost of licenses. A business license is required to open any business in the United States. A foodservice license is usually issued by the local or county health department. In order to sell liquor, a liquor license is required.
- Repairs and maintenance costs. Because a foodservice is dependent on heating, ventilation, and air conditioning systems, as well as foodservice equipment, money must be budgeted for repairs and maintenance. In some cases, a foodservice may have a maintenance contract for some equipment, in which case the foodservice pays a set price for repair and sometimes also preventative maintenance for a set period of time. Costs for repairing parking lots and maintaining the grounds must also be budgeted.

- <u>Music and entertainment costs.</u> You can't play copyrighted music (meaning any music by an artist who is signed by a record label) in your foodservice unless you pay the music licensing fees. Using a streaming service, such as Spotify, doesn't mean you paid the licensing fees. Licensing fees are generally paid yearly to one of three companies in the United States—ASCAP, SESAC, or BMI. The amount that must be paid depends on a number of factors, such as the size of the foodservice and how many hours you offer music.
- <u>Marketing and advertising costs.</u> Most foodservices spend money on advertising and other costs involved in promoting the business to current and potential customers. For example, restaurants pay for social media ads, search engine ads, email marketing, and sponsorship of community events (Hale, 2020).

Once the controllable costs are added up, they are then subtracted from the gross profit to get the controllable income.

Gross Profit – Total Controllable Expenses = Controllable Income
$230,288 – $181,217 = $49,071

Step Four. The last step is to subtract the noncontrollable costs from the controllable profit to get your net income (or net loss) before taxes. **Noncontrollable costs** include the following.

- <u>Occupancy costs.</u> Occupancy costs are the costs involved in renting the building or paying a loan if the building is owned. Real estate and property taxes and property insurance are also part of occupancy costs.
- <u>Depreciation.</u> When a business purchases equipment, the expense can be used to reduce income taxes. Depreciation is an accounting method that allocates the cost of a piece of equipment over its life expectancy. For example, if a laptop computer cost $1,600 and has a useful life of four years, you could depreciate for $400/year for four years (assuming it is not worth anything at the end of four years). This is just one method used to calculate depreciation and is called **straight-line depreciation**.

$$\frac{Cost\ of\ asset - Salvage\ value}{Years\ of\ useful\ life} = Annual\ depreciation\ amount$$

$$\frac{\$1600 - \$0}{4} = \$400$$

- <u>Interest.</u> When businesses borrow money from a bank, they have to pay interest on the loan, so interest is another expense.

Once the noncontrollable costs are deducted, you are finally at the bottom line: the net profit or net loss before taxes. (If there is a net loss, the dollar amount will be put in parentheses.) If a business makes a profit, it is likely that income taxes will need to be deducted before you know the real profit.

Controllable Income – Noncontrollable expenses = Net Income/Net Loss Before Taxes
$49,071 – 43,094 = $5,977

Table 15-2 shows a summary of an income statement.

HOW TO ANALYZE AN INCOME STATEMENT

To analyze an income statement, we will use the righthand column in Table 15-1, which features percentages. In the Sales section at the top, Total Sales is divided into three categories: Food, Beverage, and Corporate Catering. The percentages show how much business each category generates: The foodservice is generating 71.9% of sales dollars from food, 23.1% from alcoholic beverages, and 5% from corporate catering (to total 100%). Using the percentages, you can keep track of whether sales are going up

Table 15-2 Summary of the Income Statement
Gross Sales (total sales)
− <u>Cost of Sales (food and beverage cost)</u>
= Gross Profit
− <u>Controllable Expenses (labor cost, direct operating expenses, etc.)</u>
= Controllable Income
− <u>Noncontrollable Expenses</u> (occupancy costs, depreciation, etc.)
= Net Income or Net Loss Before Taxes

or down in these areas over time. That's the beauty of percentages, you can track them over time and also compare them with industry standards.

Under Controllable Expenses and Noncontrollable Expenses, each expense has a percent next to it. That percent was calculated by dividing the expense by the total sales. For example, let's look at salaries and wages.

$$\frac{\$95,323 \ (Salaries \ and \ wages)}{\$331,492 \ (Total \ Sales)} = 28.8\%$$

That means that 28.8% of all the sales dollars are used to pay salaries and wages. If you look at benefits, you will see that the foodservice pays approximately 6% of its sales to pay for employee benefits. Data are available to managers to see whether paying 28.8% of sales for salaries/wages or 6% for benefits is within a normal range for a specific type of foodservice. For some foodservices, these percentages are typical.

When reading an income statement, managers typically analyze the reported data using several yardsticks.

- Previous income statements
- Budgets
- Standards

By looking at prior income statements, managers can watch for trends—such as improvements in sales or increasing food costs. It is also useful to compare the data in income statements to what was planned in yearly budgets. For example, managers can compare their actual sales and expenses to what was planned in the budget. Developing and using budgets are discussed in depth later in this chapter.

To analyze an income statement, managers can compare data in the statement to company standards or industry-wide data that may be used as a goal or standard. Here are some examples.

1. Food cost percentage
2. Beverage cost percentage
3. Cost of sales percentage
4. Labor cost percentage
5. Prime cost percentage
6. Profit margin percentage

In restaurants, food cost percentage is usually close to 33% and labor cost percentage close to 35% (Reynolds & McClusky, 2013), although some restaurants keep food cost and/or labor cost percentages down a bit lower, such as 25%. Food and labor costs run a wide range due to different foodservice concepts, customers, menus, and other considerations. For example, restaurants in expensive cities such as New York City often pay very high rents that have to be offset by higher prices and/or lower payroll and food costs.

A foodservice's **prime cost** is the sum of its food cost and labor expenses. The recommendation for foodservices looking to make a profit is to keep prime cost at about 60 to 70% of sales revenue. If prime cost is 70% of your revenue, this only leaves about 30 cents per dollar for the rest of expenses and profit. Not only does prime cost make up the majority of a foodservice's expenses but it also constitutes the portion of the business that can be manipulated or controlled in order to maximize profit.

Here is how to calculate various percentages.

1. **Food cost percentage** is the proportion of food sales spent on food. The formula for food cost percentage is to divide food cost by food sales. The numbers in the following example are taken from the income statement. Note that you can also calculate a separate food cost percentage for corporate catering.

$$\frac{Food\ cost}{Food\ sales} \times 100 = Food\ cost\ percentage$$

$$\frac{\$78,157}{\$238,183} \times 100 = 32.8\%$$

2. **Beverage cost percentage** is the proportion of beverage sales spent on alcoholic beverages. The formula for beverage cost percentage is to divide beverage costs by beverage sales. So if a foodservice had sales of $10,000 last week, and the beverages cost $2,500, then the beverage cost percentage is 25%. The numbers in the following example come from the income statement.

$$\frac{Beverage\ cost}{Beverage\ sales} \times 100 = Beverage\ percentage$$

$$\frac{\$17,712}{\$76,636} \times 100 = 23.1\%$$

3. **Cost of sales percentage** is the proportion of total sales spent on food and beverages. Using the income statement, you can calculate the **cost of sales percentage** as follows.

$$\frac{Cost\ of\ food/beverage}{Total\ sales} \times 100 = Cost\ of\ sales\ precentage$$

$$\frac{\$101,204}{\$331,492} \times 100 = 30.5\%$$

4. **Labor cost percentage** is the proportion of total sales spent on salaries and wages, employee benefits, and employer-paid payroll taxes/workers' compensation. Using the income statement, you can calculate it as follows. You can also just add up the percentages for salaries and wages, benefits, and employer-paid payroll taxes and workers' compensation (total is 36.8%).

$$\frac{Labor\ cost}{Total\ sales} \times 100 = Labor\ cost\ precentage$$

$$\frac{\$121,842}{\$331,492} \times 100 = 36.8\%$$

5. **Prime cost percentage** is the proportion of total sales spent on food, beverages, and labor. Using the income statement, all you need to do is add up labor cost percentage (36.8%) and the cost of sales percentage (30.5%)—for a total of 67.3%. You can calculate it as follows.

$$\frac{Total\ cost\ of\ sales + labor\ cost}{Total\ sales} \times 100 = Prime\ cost\ percentage$$

$$\frac{\$223,046}{\$331,492} \times 100 = 67.3\%$$

6. **Profit margin percentage** is the proportion of total sales that represents a profit, or it could be a loss, before taxes are paid.

$$\frac{Profit\ before\ taxes}{Total\ sales} \times 100 = Profit\ Margin\ Percentage$$

$$\frac{\$5,977}{\$331,492} \times 100 = 1.8\%$$

The profit shown on this income statement is low—3 to 6.5% would be closer to average (Biery & Sageworks Stats, 2018). To increase profits, a business can decrease expenses while keeping sales the same, increase sales while keeping expenses about the same, or increase revenue and decrease expenses at the same time.

15.2 COMPLETE AND ANALYZE A BALANCE SHEET

Whereas an income statement shows activity for a period of time, such as a month or quarter, the balance sheet gives a snapshot of a company at one point in time. A **balance sheet** provides detailed information about how well a company is doing financially. It is divided into three parts: the company's assets, liabilities, and shareholders' equity. A company's balance sheet is set up like the basic accounting equation shown here.

Total assets = total liability + owner's equity.

On the left side of the balance sheet, companies list their assets. On the right side, they list their liabilities and shareholders' equity (**Table 15-3**). Sometimes balance

Table 15-3 Balance Sheet			
Current Assets		**Current Liabilities**	
Liquid Assets		**Short-term Liabilities**	
Cash in Bank Accounts	$118,612	Accounts Payable	$54,498
Transfer Accts: (PayPal/Venmo)	$5,400	Mortgage Rent or Lease Payments	$11,715
Cash on hand (cashier banks/in safe)	$6,000	Accrued Expenses	$19,378
Accounts Receivable (outstanding)	$84,531	Utilities	$6,931
Inventory	$14,829	Sales Tax	$1,642
Pre-paid expenses	$4,100	Income Taxes	$3,465
Total Liquid Assets	**$233,472**	Payroll	$24,310
Fixed Assets		Benefits (medical, PTO, matching)	$8,167
Real Estate (Buildings/land)	$1,360,000	**Total Short-term Liabilities**	**$130,106**
Major Equipment, furniture/fixtures	$371,044	**Long-term Liabilities**	
Small Equipment: China, flatware.	$52,310	Mortgage (outstanding balance)	$1,143,009
Other Assets (patents, royalties)	$18,921	Long-term Loans	$102,513
Deprecation of Assets	$(24,101)	Other-term Loans (revolving credit)	$7,314
Total Fixed Assets	**$1,778,174**	**Total Long-term Liability**	**$1,252,836**
		Shareholder (Owner) Equity	
		Stock of investments owed back to owners and investors.	$586,104
		Earnings (profit) to be reinvested.	$42,600
		Total Owners Equity	**$628,704**
Total Assets	**$2,011,646**	**Total Liabilities and Equity**	**$2,011,646**

sheets show assets at the top, followed by liabilities, with shareholders' equity at the bottom.

Assets are anything that a company owns that has value. Assets include physical property such as food inventory and money owed from the credit card companies. Cash itself is an asset as well. **Current assets** (also called liquid assets) include cash and other assets that can be converted into cash within one year. **Fixed assets** are the tangible, permanent resources of the business—such as equipment and furniture—and any building or property that the business owns. You can think of fixed assets as those assets needed to operate the business but are not available for sale.

Liabilities are amounts of money that a business owes to others. This can include money borrowed from a bank, rent for use of a building, money owed to food suppliers, payroll owed to its employees, utility bills to be paid, or taxes owed to the government. **Current liabilities** are amounts payable within one year and **long-term liabilities** are amounts payable beyond a year.

Owner's equity (also called **net worth**) is essentially what would be left for the owners from company assets after paying off all liabilities. It is a measure of what has been invested in the business. If the business is a corporation, owner's equity is called **shareholder equity** and represents the value of corporate stock and retained earnings. Retained earnings are earnings used to fund growth or pay off debt. Retained earnings are not paid out as dividends to shareholders. Comparing owner's equity from one accounting period to the next shows how well the owner's investment is doing. If owner's equity is increasing, that is a healthy sign.

In addition to comparing owner's equity, another way to see how the company is doing financially is to calculate the **debt ratio**, the ratio comparing total liabilities with total assets. The debt ratio shows how many assets the company must sell to pay off all of its liabilities. To calculate the debt ratio, just divide the total liabilities by total assets. Here is the formula and an example using the data in Table 15-3.

$$Debt\ Ratio = \frac{Total\ Liabilities}{Total\ Assets}$$

$$0.69 = \frac{\$1,382,942}{\$2,011,646}$$

If the debt ratio is 0.5, it means the company has twice as many assets as liabilities. If the debt ratio is 1.0, the amount of liabilities is equal to the amount of assets, and the business would have to sell all of its assets in order to pay off its liabilities. So the larger the number is, the more debt the company has. Lower ratios, such as 0.3, are considered better debt ratios and make it easier to borrow money. There is risk associated with having too much or too little debt. Borrowing money is a good thing—it is how businesses grow and earn more money. But high levels of debt require a business to generate enough cash to pay it back on time—which can be difficult.

15.3 PREPARE AN OPERATING BUDGET AND MONITOR PERFORMANCE

Budgets are a form of financial planning. Within an organization, top management oversees a **master budget**, that includes three different budgets.

1. Probably the most important type of budget, and the one we think of when we hear "budget," is the **operating budget**. An operating budget includes:
   a. The forecast of revenue (payments for providing meals and/or services)
   b. The forecast of expenses (labor, food, supplies, and other costs)
   c. Profit/loss for a given period (which is basically a minus b.)

The operating budget is often called the annual budget and lasts for 12 months. A **fiscal year** is a period of 12 months that may, or may not, coincide with the calendar year. Each organization decides when the fiscal year starts and ends.

2. A **cash budget** forecasts the organization's cash flow over 12 months. Your checking account is your own cash budget; throughout the year, money is deposited and disbursed or spent. Sometimes, there is very little money in the account, such as after bills are paid, and sometimes there is more money, such as after payments are deposited. A cash budget is helpful to determine if too much or too little cash will be on hand. Too much cash on hand is not desirable because it could be put to better use in an investment. Too little cash causes problems paying suppliers on time and possible credit difficulties.

3. A **capital budget** is money set aside to make major expenditures, such as a new dishmachine or dining-room renovation.

This section will discuss the operating budget.

Before developing a budget, each foodservice must define its accounting period—usually a 12-month period or 13 periods of four weeks each. Each of these accounting periods last for 52 weeks. Using 13 periods of four weeks each means that you can accurately compare performance from period to period because each period has the same number of days. When the accounting period is based on calendar months, the number of days and weekends in each month often differs so comparing performance from month to month is not as accurate.

The operating budget includes information about foodservice costs. Some of the costs, called **fixed costs**, remain the same despite how many meals are being prepared. For example, the amount spent on rent, insurance, or loan payments remain constant (except of course when the rent or insurance go up) regardless of whether sales are high or low. On the other hand, **variable costs** go up or down in response to changes in sales or meals prepared. When more meals are prepared, food and labor costs go up. When fewer meals are made, these costs should decrease.

OBJECTIVES OF OPERATING BUDGETS

Some of the traditional objectives for operating budgets include the following.

*   The budgetary process forces management to carefully examine and prioritize the foodservice's goals and objectives. In a budget, goals and objectives are stated in a quantifiable manner, such as keep food cost under 30%.
*   The budgetary process gives managers an opportunity to review and revise standards of performance, such as labor hours per meal, as well as analyze costs.
*   Once an operating budget is set, it provides a yardstick for measuring department performance. When there is a deviation between the operating budget and actual performance, it is the manager who must determine why and whether standards of performance are being affected.
*   Management uses operational budgets to communicate with and motivate its managers and supervisors to achieve foodservice goals.
*   Checking budgeted figures for sales and expenses against the actual numbers every month allows management to monitor and control costs. A **budget variance** is the difference between the budgeted revenue or expense and the actual amount. In some cases, such as unexpected new sales revenue for one month, you can justify added food and labor expenses because you had increased sales. In other cases, such as higher meat costs than budgeted over three months (with no increase in revenues), you will need to find the cause for the increased costs and make some corrections.

Having budget targets helps managers control costs. Typical budget targets include food cost percentage, labor cost percentage, and prime cost (food cost percentage + labor cost percentage).

Fixed, Flexible, and Zero-Based Budgets

Depending on the budgetary policies of your foodservice, you may prepare a fixed budget, a flexible budget, or a zero-based budget. Fixed and flexible budgets are examples of **incremental budgeting**. With this approach, you use the current budget as a basis for the new budget and add or subtract incremental amounts based on projections, for example, of meals to be prepared or inflation of food or labor costs. Most operating budgets are based on adding a predetermined increment to a budget line.

A **fixed budget** assumes that the volume of business that will be done is known and predictable, and that the costs and revenues will generally stay within projections. Fixed budgets do not provide for wide swings in business volume, either up or down. Most foodservices in healthcare and schools have fixed budgets because they are serving a relatively fixed or static number of customers. Accountants prefer fixed budgets because they can evaluate business performance against variation *consistently* over the life of the budget. It also allows them to schedule how much money (cash) is available to Accounts Payable to cover monthly invoices.

A **flexible budget** adjusts with changes in the volume of sales or activity. With a flexible budget, if sales and revenue go up, allowances are made for higher food and supply purchases and for labor hours to increase as well. A flexible budget adjusts the cost of expenses (on a percentage basis) depending on the level of sales or revenue. For example, a flexible budget may be based on 90, 100, and 110% of the estimated number of meals to be served, so in reality you develop three budgets. Flexible budgets are more useful in situations such as the opening year of a new foodservice when you would expect the sales volume to vary a lot.

Zero-based budgets differ markedly in philosophy and operation from fixed or flexible budgets. Instead of using the current budget as a starting point, the manager begins the process with several blank sheets of paper and a list of the objectives for the foodservice. The manager analyzes the needs and costs of the operation and must *justify all expenses* because the budget starts from zero. Zero-based budgeting is useful to thoroughly review every expense dollar in the budget and build a culture of cost management. It obliges foodservice managers to analyze in depth the objectives, costs, and benefits of each level of expenditure to provide various services. Although zero-based budgeting is a lengthy, time-consuming process, it can reduce costs (Callaghan, Hawke, & Mignerey, 2014).

Revenue and Expense Budgets

The operating budget has two major components: the revenue (sales) budget and the expense budget. The revenue budget includes money coming in from sales. Sales dollars in are often broken down into food (including nonalcoholic beverages) or alcohol sales (if alcoholic drinks are sold). Using a point-of-sale software system, sales can be broken down further by meal/time of day, menu category (such as appetizers, mains, desserts), menu item, and walk-in or drive-thru/takeout/delivery. For the purposes of budgeting, restaurants often project sales for two categories: total food (including nonalcoholic beverages) and alcoholic beverages. Alcoholic beverages are normally separated because they are high in cost and more attractive to steal. Keeping separate records for alcoholic beverages is helpful for *control* purposes.

The revenue (sales) budget is more complicated in many onsite foodservices because they often have more than one revenue center. For example, a university may have revenue coming in from student meal plans, a food court in the Student Union, coffee shops, faculty dining room, catering, vending, and a convenience store. For the purpose of budgeting, each of these represents a separate revenue center and the manager must look at the sales data for each of them to make the sales projection for the following year.

Likewise, hospitals have several revenue centers, such as the main cafeteria (provides meals to employees and often visitors), vending, and catering. If the nursing department requests a catered breakfast, for instance, they have to pay the foodservice department from their budget. In addition, the hospital makes all patient meals. Patient meals are considered a **cost center**, as opposed to a revenue center. This is because the hospital, while it does get some reimbursement for meals from insurance companies, does not credit the foodservice department with that money. The hospital is given a lump sum (mostly from insurance companies) to cover meals, nursing, housekeeping, laundry, etc., for each day a patient is in the hospital. Instead of forecasting revenue for patient meals, the manager will forecast the *number* of patient meals to be served.

The expense budget includes all costs incurred to produce the meals. The two biggest ticket items in the expenses budget are labor and food and beverage. The *labor budget* can be quite complex. In addition to paying wages/salaries, foodservices offering benefits often pay for part or all of the associated costs. Examples of benefits include health insurance, life insurance, uniforms, employee meals, tuition reimbursement, or profit sharing. Lastly, employers pay some payroll taxes. **Payroll taxes** are taxes imposed on employees and employers. For example, as an employee, your employer deducts federal, state, and other taxes from your paycheck. Payroll taxes are usually calculated as a percentage of the wage/salary. *Employers must also pay the following taxes to the federal or state government for each employee and these taxes are **not** taken out of the employee's paycheck.*

- Half of the FICA amount. The **Federal Insurance Contributions Act (FICA)** covers Social Security and Medicare. Half of the required FICA dollars are paid by the employer and the other half by the employee.
- Federal unemployment tax. The **Federal Unemployment Tax Act (FUTA)** requires a small payroll tax that employers pay for each employee.
- State unemployment tax. In almost all states, employers also pay state unemployment taxes and/or other taxes. No state imposes the same tax rate on all employers. The size of the unemployment insurance tax is based on the number of laid-off employees that a company has had and the cost of providing them with unemployment benefits.

Often, the federal and state unemployment taxes are not paid on an employee's full wages/salary. For example, in 2020, the federal unemployment tax is only paid for the first $7,000 of wages/salaries. Likewise, FICA must be paid only up to $142,800 in wages/salary as of 2021. Once that threshold is reached, no more FICA is collected from the employee or the employer.

In the labor budget, predictions are made for the number of hours that each position will work. Those hours are then translated into **full-time equivalents (FTEs)**. An FTE is normally eight hours per day or 40 hours per workweek (depending on how many hours are considered full-time in the business). For instance, if the operation needs three cooks, seven days per week, working eight hours/day, that adds up to 168 hours (3 cooks × 8 hours/day × 7 days/week). If you divide 168 hours by 40 hours/week, every week you will forecast 4.2 FTE for cooking staff.

In most businesses, employees earn **paid time off (PTO)**. This takes the form of vacation days, sick days, holidays, personal days, or other PTOs. These days need to be accounted for in the budget because, as in the example in the last paragraph, you need 4.2 FTE weekly for cooks only when none of the cooks are taking a vacation day or other PTO. Some businesses create a budget that includes a relief factor. The relief factor is a multiplier for each FTE of coverage. The relief factor may be low, such as 1.05 for fast food positions with little paid time off, or high, such as 1.15 for healthcare nutrition

Table 15-4 Sample Labor Budget							
Retirement Community 161—Café Dining Room Labor Budget—Cost Center 1620 Fiscal Year 2021–2022							
Job Title and Job Code	Employee Name	FTE	Annual Hours	Current Hourly Rate	Annual Salary	FICA & Unemploy. Taxes	Total
Café Manager (230)	Jones	1.0	2,080	$30.02	$62,442	$5,219	$67,661
Service Supervisor (226)	Smith	1.0	2,080	$24.75	$51,480	$4,380	$55,860
Café Coordinator (205)	Rodriguez	1.0	2,080	$16.51	$34,341	$3,069	$37,410
Café Coordinator (205)	Lee	1.0	2,080	$16.51	$34,341	$3,069	$37,410
Grill Cook (203)	Abreu	1.0	2,080	$16.06	$33,405	$2,997	$36,402
Sandwich Cook (203)	Harris	1.0	2,080	$16.06	$33,405	$2,997	$36,402
Café Assistant (204)	Figueroa	0.5	1,040	$12.35	$23,400	$2,232	$25,632
Lead Server Café (216)	Franklin	0.5	1,040	$12.15	$12,262	$1,380	$13,642
Lead Server Café (216)	Navarro	0.25	520	$11.00	$5,720	$701	$6,421
Lead Server Café (216)	Betts	0.25	520	$11.00	$5,720	$701	$6,421
Lead Server Café (216)	Patel	0.12	250	$11.00	$2,750	$337	$3,087
15 Servers × 0.233 FTE (208)	Assorted	3.50	7,280	$10.25	$74,620	$9,143	$83,763
Total		11.12	23,130		$373,886	$36,225	$410,111
Additional Paid Hours							
Replacement Time (Relief Factor: 1.1)		1.1	2,300	$15.66	$36,018	$2,755	$38,773
Training Hours		0.15	312	$10.25	$3,198	$245	$3,443
Overtime Hours		0.5	1,040	$18.27	$19,001	$1,454	$20,455
Total		1.65	3,652		$58,217	$4,454	$62,671
Grand Totals		12.87	26,782		$432,103	$40,679	$472,782

departments with generous paid time off. So if the cooking area in a hospital foodservice needs 4.2 FTE weekly, multiply 4.2 by 1.15 to get 4.83 FTE needed to cover the cooking area to include paid time off.

Table 15-4 is a sample labor budget for the main dining room in a retirement community. For each position in the dining room, you can see the FTEs, annual hours, hourly pay rate, and annual salary. Note that a full-time employee works 2,080 hours/year (40 hours × 52 weeks), whereas a half-time employee works 1,040 hours/year. The second to last column lists the FICA and unemployment taxes (federal and state) that the employer pays in addition to the annual salary. At the bottom of the table, you can see the cost of the additional labor hours and costs needed to cover paid time off, training, and overtime hours.

Steps in Planning Budgets

The budget planning process starts well in advance of the start of the new fiscal year. About four to six months into the current fiscal year, it's time to collect and analyze data from the previous two years, including the following.

- Budgets and how they compared with actual revenues/expenses (budget variances)

- Sales revenue
- Food and beverage costs
- Payroll costs
- Direct operating expenses
- Occupancy costs
- Other expenses

These data become the basis of predictions going forward, so it is important to review the historical data and costs. Predictions will be made for revenue, payroll, food, and other expenses on an item–by–item basis.

After collecting and analyzing past data, the following are the steps in planning budgets.

1. <u>Review the foodservice's objectives for the upcoming fiscal year and review your budget targets (such as desired food cost percentage).</u> See **Table 15-5** for some examples of how foodservice objectives can influence budget planning. Managers must analyze the financial feasibility of any new services and also make sure the objectives support the mission and objectives of the parent company or institution (such as a multiunit foodservice operator, school or college, health-care facility, or foodservice contract company).

2. <u>Review factors inside and outside of the foodservice that could affect sales, costs, and/or operations during the next fiscal year.</u> Factors *within* the food-service could include planned renovations, changes in takeout or delivery methods, new software being introduced, change in operating hours, or changes in number of customers to be served. Factors *outside* of the foodser-vice could include new competitors in the area, changes in taxes or occu-pancy costs, changes in the cost of food and beverages, increased benefit costs, or increased wages/salaries. All of these factors will impact your budget. Human resources managers can give advice on changes in labor and benefit costs. Managers who do food and beverage purchasing should gather data on price increases/decreases for the next fiscal year by looking at the Consumer Price Index and the Producer Price Index for food. They should also work with suppliers, prime vendors, and group purchasing organizations to deter-mine if any food products and supplies are expected to change drastically in price or availability. This can occur due to changes in the commodity market, natural and man-made disasters, pandemics, tariffs, or weather/climate effects.

3. <u>Prepare a Budget Worksheet.</u> **Table 15-6** is a budget worksheet for a foodser-vice with a restaurant generating food and alcoholic beverage revenue as well as a small catering business. The data in columns A–C are from the *current* budget year. The remaining columns pertain to the *new* budget year. Because the cur-rent year already has actual revenue and expense data for at least a few months, Column C shows the amount of money you would actually receive/spend for the

Table 15-5 Examples of How Foodservice Objectives Can Impact the Budget	
Examples of Foodservice Objectives	**How They May Impact Budget Planning**
Increase overall customer satisfaction by 10%.	Increase training budget to cover cost of new training programs. Increase labor budget for servers.
Maintain current revenue per worked labor hour.	Keep marketing dollars at same level.
Start new catering program.	Increase food, equipment, labor, and marketing budgets to pull in catering business.
Decrease food cost percentage from 40% to 38%.	Work to decrease food costs.
Increase productivity rate from 3.5 to 3.7 meals per worked hour.	Review position work schedules to determine inefficiencies, then revise work schedules to decrease labor hours.

Table 15-6 Budget Worksheet for FY 2024

	FY 2023 Budget (A)	Percentages (B)	FY 2023 Actual Annualized (C)	Projected % Increase (D)	2024 Budget (E)	Percentages (F)	January 2024 (G)	February 2024 (H)	March 2024 (I)
				3% increase in sales + 2% increase in menu prices					
1. Revenue									
Food	$588,000	81.7%	$605,450	5% total	$617,400	80.9%	$50,000		
Catering (food only)	12,000	1.6	14,100	Goal:20K	20,000	2.6	1,000		
Beverage	120,000	16.7	124,250	5% total	126,000	16.5	10,000		
Total Revenue	720,000	100%	743,800	--------	763,400	100%	61,000		
2. Food Cost				Increase in price					
Proteins	102,900	49%	106,300	3%	109,000	49%	8,700		
Dairy/Eggs	31,500	15	32,600	1%	32,700	15	2,600		
Groceries	18,900	9	20,150	1%	19,600	9	1,600		
Fruits and Vegetables	37,800	18	38,800	2%	39,700	18	3,200		
Baked Goods	10,500	5	10,800	1%	11,000	5	900		
Miscellaneous	8,400	4	8,650	1.5%	8,700	4	750		
Total Food Cost	210,000	100%	217,300	--------	220,700	100%	17,750		
Food Cost %	35.1%	--------	35.1%		34.6%		34.8%		
3. Beverage Cost				Increase in price					
Wine	7,050	28%	7,250	1.5%	7,400	28%	600		
Draft beer	12,850	51	13,600	1.0%	13,400	51	1,000		
Liquor	3,270	13	3,410	1.5%	3,400	13	270		
Bar mix, mixers, etc.	2,030	8	2,050	1.0%	2,100	8	170		
Total Beverage Cost	25,200	100%	26,310	--------	26,300	100%	2,040		
Beverage Cost %	21.0%	--------	21.2%	--------	20.9%	--------	20.4%		
COST OF SALES	235,200 (32.7%)	--------	243,610 (32.8%)	--------	247,000 (32.4%)	--------	19,790 (32.4%)		
GROSS PROFIT	484,800 67.3%		500,190 67.2%		516,400 67.6%		41,210 67.6%		

	FY 2023 Budget (A)	Percentages (B)	FY 2023 Actual Annualized (C)	Projected % Increase (D)	2024 Budget (E)	Percentages (F)	January 2024 (G)	February 2024 (H)	March 2024 (I)
4. Labor Cost									
Salaries/Wages	241,400	91%	245,900	3.0% up	248,600	91%	20,000		
Benefits	8,000	3	8,100	2% up	8,160	3	650		
Employer-Paid Taxes	17,000	6	17,500	3% up	17,510	6	1,400		
Total Labor Cost	266,400	100%	271,500	--------	274,270	100%	22,050		
Labor Cost %	37.0%	--------	36.5%	--------	36.0%	--------	36.1%		
5. Operating Expenses									
Paper supplies	7,600	1.1%	7,950	2% up	7,900	1.0%	650		
Cleaning supplies	15,000	2.1	15,250	2% up	15,300	2.0	1,250		
Uniforms	6,000	0.8	6,400	same	6,000	0.8	500		
Misc. direct expenses	14,000	1.9	14,100	2% up	14,280	1.9	1,150		
Utilities	21,600	3.0	21,000	3% up	22,250	2.9	1,800		
Credit card fees	12,000	1.7	12,200	2% up	12,250	1.6	1,000		
Other Administrative Expenses	14,000	1.9	13,800	2.5% up	14,350	1.9	1,150		
Repairs & Maintenance	16,000	2.2	18,850	2% up	16,320	2.1	1,300		
Music/Entertainment	3,000	0.4	2,900	No change	3,000	0.4	250		
Marketing/Advertising	5,000	0.7	5,500	No change	5,000	0.7	400		
Rent/lease	60,000	8.3	60,000	No change	60,000	7.9	5,000		
Property/Real Estate Tax	7,000	1.0	7,100	Up $400	7,400	1.0	620		
Insurance	5,000	0.7	5,000	Up $300	5,300	0.7	450		
Depreciation	8,000	1.1	8,000	No change	8,000	1.0	670		
Total Operating Exp	194,200	--------	198,050	--------	197,350	--------	16,190		
Income – Expenses =	**24,200** (3.4%)		**30,640** (4.1%)		**44,780** (5.9%)		**2,970** (4.9%)		

entire year based on sales/expenses up to this point in time (that is why it is called "annualized"). Now you can compare that number to the budget for the current year. Column D gives some background on the considerations in deciding on your forecast for 2024. Once you have a budget for 2024, the numbers need to be distributed among the accounting periods for the year.

a. <u>Forecast your sales/revenue.</u> When looking at sales, keep in mind that sales go up when menu prices increase, so increased sales does not always mean that you have more customers. If you intend to raise menu prices, for example so the average check will go up by 2%, you must increase your revenue forecast by 2%. Decreasing menu prices, perhaps due to more local competition, will decrease revenue. You should also compare your sales, average check, and customer counts month-by-month (or accounting periods) for the past two years and look for trends. Perhaps certain periods are slow or you find sales have been increasing overall by an average of 5%. If you decide to increase sales for the next fiscal year by 5%, multiply the current year's budget for revenue by 1.05. For example, let's say you budgeted $700,000 for the current budget year. Just multiply $700,000 by 1.05 to get $735,000. This amount can then be distributed across the 12 months or accounting periods.

Revenue can, therefore, increase because of increased prices or increased sales. When revenue increases because of higher prices, it doesn't mean you need to buy more food or beverages. When revenue increased due to increased sales, you do need to buy more food and/or beverages.

b. <u>Forecast your food and beverage costs.</u> Foodservice industry magazines, such as *Nation's Restaurant News* or *Food Management*, often include information on whether certain food costs will be heading up or down over the next few months or longer. When forecasting your food and beverage costs, you do so by category. For example, in Table 15-6, food is divided into proteins, dairy and eggs, groceries, fruits and vegetables, baked goods, and miscellaneous. If fruit and vegetable prices are expected to go up by 3%, and you anticipate buying a little more because of menu changes, perhaps you may want to increase the budget by 5%. For another item, such as dairy and eggs, perhaps prices are expected to be stable and you don't need to increase the budget.

In addition to increasing costs due to higher food costs, you also have to increase costs due to increased business. For example, in Table 15-6, the budget for bakery goods was $10,500 for 2023. Taking into account a 1% increase in prices and 3% increase in sales, if you multiply $10,500 by 1.04, you get $10,920, which is rounded up to $11,000.

c. <u>Forecast your labor cost.</u> If you have a human resources manager, this person will often provide the forecast for salaries/wages, benefits, and employer-paid taxes. The forecast for salaries/wages has to examine if new positions will be added (in case of growth) or current positions are not filled or removed (in case of downsizing), if current employees will be getting salary/wage increases (often associated with annual employee evaluations), and if starting salaries/wages for new employees will increase. Changes to the minimum wage could change labor costs. Companies that provide benefits can certainly give you information on the costs for the next budget year. Changing benefit providers or hiring more part-time employees without benefits will also change costs. Employer-paid taxes is based completely on the anticipated salaries/wages for the year. Some businesses will also allocate money in the budget specifically for overtime pay.

d. <u>Forecast your operating expenses.</u> For each category, you need to consider how much you need *and* how much the price may change.

e. <u>Check to see if you are hitting your budget targets</u>. Your budget targets might include desired food cost percentage, a cost indicator such as a desired food cost/meal, or a productivity indicator such as meals per labor hour. (Note that when you calculate the food cost percentage in Table 15-6, you must divide the food cost by the total food and catering revenues.) Compare important targets from your current to new budget year, such as food cost percentage, beverage cost percentage, labor cost percentage, gross profit percentage, and the bottom line.

f. <u>The last step is to allocate all line items by month or other accounting period for the next fiscal year</u>. If using 13 four-week accounting periods, it may be tempting to allocate the sales and expenses equally over the periods, but you need to use historical data to judge how busy the business is at different times of year. For example, restaurants tend to be less busy in January after the holidays, but hospitals tend to be quite busy due to the flu season. If using calendar months as the accounting period, you also have to keep in mind the number of weekends and days in each month in order to allocate more accurately.

4. <u>Get opinions and justify the numbers before submitting it</u>. Questions will be asked about why the numbers were chosen. This provides an excellent time to get opinions from budget professionals and to hear how other facilities and departments are handling similar issues and inflation factors. You may need to write up a justification before submission.

5. <u>Implement the budget.</u> Once the budget has been reviewed by the higher ups, you will see which segments of the budget were accepted and which were modified. Plans will soon become reality. This may involve reducing existing staff, hiring new staff, or changing the menu and restructuring purchasing. It may also be time to market and develop new programs and services.

While you might think it is okay to overbudget a little for food, beverage, labor, or expenses, remember that if your costs are higher than your sales, your business will be operating at a loss. *You should carefully compare the "Percentages" columns B and F* (Table 15-6) to see if any line item grew tremendously in the new budget year.

Planning Budgets in Noncommercial Foodservices

Noncommercial foodservices include onsite foodservices that are run by the K–12 school, college, hospital, business, or other organization in which they operate. Noncommercial foodservices are run to provide a needed service: meals and snacks. They are not always tasked with making a profit. Quite a few are run with the goal to simply break even, meaning that enough revenue is brought in to pay for the expenses.

The budgets of noncommercial foodservices often differ from their commercial counterparts in one or two ways: occupancy costs and revenue. Because noncommercial foodservices are housed, for example, within a school or workplace, the foodservice *may not* be charged for occupancy expenses such as rent, utilities, or property taxes. There are also situations when a noncommercial foodservice is charged for and does pay some occupancy costs, such as rent or utilities.

In some noncommercial settings, a number of meals are served for which no revenue is shown on the budget. As mentioned earlier, patient meals in a hospital are considered a cost center because the hospital does not credit the foodservice department with the money it receives from insurance companies in the form of a "room rate." Instead of forecasting revenue for patient meals, the manager will forecast the *number* of patient meals to be served and the food cost per meal or per day. The number of meals to be served is based on the number of patient days that are forecast for the next fiscal year by hospital administration. A **patient day** is when one patient is in the hospital for one day. Most hospitals count up the number of patients in-house at midnight and that number represents the number of patient days for that day. A hospital foodservice knows how many meals they serve per patient day (often about 2.7), so the healthcare manager can project how many patient meals will be prepared for the next year. Note that patients don't always eat three meals a day in the hospital due to meals not being allowed before or after certain tests or surgeries. In other healthcare settings, such as nursing homes or assisted-living facilities, the foodservice director may also provide meals without any revenue for the meals appearing on the budget. In these facilities, foodservice directors often have a target food cost/resident day that is reflected in the budget.

K–12 school foodservice programs do have cash revenue for some of their meals, but school districts participating in National School Lunch (and sometimes Breakfast) Program also receive money from federal and state sources to help pay for meals. **Table 15-7** is an income statement for a school that shows sales revenue along with revenue from the federal and state government. Schools carefully watch their food cost/meal as well as their revenue/meal.

How to Analyze Variances and Decide on Corrective Actions

A **budget variance** is the difference between the actual and budgeted dollars on one of the budget lines (**Table 15-8**). Variances are classified as favorable or unfavorable. A **favorable variance** is one that is preferred—such as higher sales than budgeted,

Table 15-7 Revenue and Expenses for National School Lunch Program at Afton High School for the first quarter, 2022	
Revenue Source	**First Quarter 2022**
Student Lunch Sales	$37,467
Adult Lunch Sales	3,564
Other Food Sales	17,555
Federal Reimbursement (includes USDA supplied foods)	282,211
State	27,799
Miscellaneous	600
Total Revenue	**$369,196**
Expenses	
Salaries and Wages	$109,011
Employee Benefits	44,688
Food Purchases	157,069
Other Supplies	17,891
Operating Expenses - Direct	28,484
Operating Expenses - Indirect	8,122
Total Expenses	**$365,265**
Excess/Deficit	$3,931

food costs or other expenses that come in lower than expected (although it could be due to decreased sales), or more profit than budgeted. Of course, a variance can also be unfavorable. An **unfavorable variance** occurs when a business has lower sales than budgeted, spends more than was budgeted (especially without increased sales), or has lower profits.

Table 15-8 shows an expense report for the month of March for a foodservice with food and beverage sales. The first three columns in the report compare actual sales and expense data for March with what was budgeted for March. The last three

Table 15-8 Expense Report for March for Tom's Smoky BBQ

Current Month			Category	Year-to-Date		
Actual	Budget	Variance, Variance %, **F**avorable or **U**nfavorable		Actual	Budget	Variance, Variance %, **F**avorable or **U**nfavorable
SALES						
$50,500	$52,000	$1,500 (3%) **U**	Food Sales	$148,000	$147,000	$1,000 (1%) **F**
11,800	12,000	200 (2%) **U**	Beverage Sales	$33,500	$33,000	$500 (<1%) **F**
$62,300	$64,000	$1,700 (3%) **U**	*Total Sales*	$181,500	$180,000	$1,500 (1%) **F**
FOOD & BEVERAGE						
$10,800	$9,200	$1,600 (17%) **U**	Proteins	$30,000	$26,000	$4,000 (15%) **U**
2,400	2,500	100 (4%) **F**	Dairy & Eggs	$7,100	$7,000	$100 (1%) **U**
2,500	2,300	200 (9%) **U**	Groceries	$6,600	$6,500	$100 (2%) **U**
4,400	3,800	600 (16%) **U**	Fruits & Vegetables	$12,000	$10,500	$1,500 (14%) **U**
850	900	50 (6%) **F**	Baked Goods	$2,720	$2,500	$200 (8%) **U**
2,700	2,750	50 (2%) **F**	Beverages	$7,400	$7,700	$300 (4%) **F**
$23,650	$21,450	$2,200 (10%) **U**	*Total F & B*	$65,800	$60,200	$5,600 (9%) **U**
LABOR						
$18,100	$18,000	$100 (<1%) **U**	Salaries/Wages	$51,000	$50,400	$600 (1%) **U**
3,000	3,100	100 (3%) **F**	Benefits	$9,700	$9,900	$200 (2%) **F**
1,300	1,280	20 (2%) **U**	Employer Payroll Tax	$3,700	$3,600	$100 (3%) **U**
$22,400	$22,380	$20 (<1%) **U**	*Total Labor*	$64,400	$63,900	$500 (1%) **U**
EXPENSES						
$3,600	$3,800	$200 (5%) **F**	Direct Operating Exp.	$10,600	$10,800	$200 (2%) **F**
$6,000	$6,000	----	Rent	$17,800	$18,000	$200 (1%) **F**
$2,450	$2,500	$50 (2%) **F**	Utilities	$7,150	$7,200	$50 (1%) **F**
$2,500	$2,400	$100 (4%) **U**	Administrative Exp.	$7,200	$7,000	$200 (3%) **U**
$1,800	$1,450	$350 (24%) **U**	Repairs/Maintenance	$4,300	$4,100	$200 (5%) **U**
$125	$125	----	Music	$370	$360	$10 (3%) **U**
$1,000	$800	$200 (25%) **U**	Marketing	$2,200	$2,160	$40 (2%) **U**
$17,475	$17,075	$400 (2%) **U**	*Total Expenses*	$49,620	$49,620	-----
($1,225)	$3,095	$4,320(140%) **U**	**Net Performance**	$1,680	$6,280	$4,600 (73%) **U**

columns compare actual sales and expense data for January through March with what was budgeted for the same time period (called "year-to-date").

The variance in Table 15-8 is calculated by subtracting the budgeted amount from the actual amount. Don't worry whether the number is positive or negative. What matters is if the variance is favorable or unfavorable to the business. This is noted in the chart with the F (favorable) or the U (unfavorable) appearing after the variance. Using the total food and beverage expenses for March in Table 15-8, the **variance percentage** is calculated as follows.

$$\frac{Actual - Budgeted\ Dollars}{Budgeted\ Dollars} \times 100 = Variance\ percentage$$

$$\frac{\$23,650 - \$21,450}{\$21,450} \times 100 = 10\%$$

Since the actual expense was higher than the budget, the variance percentage is unfavorable and the foodservice spent 10% more on food and beverage supplies than was budgeted. This might be acceptable if the sales were also up 10%, but you can see in the table that sales were just a little lower than expected.

When reviewing an expense report, it's helpful to start with the totals—such as total food and beverage costs. In Table 15-8, the totals are all highlighted. You can see pretty quickly if you are significantly over or under in any category. When you look at the variance percentage, focus on the size of the percentage and compare the current month to year-to-date. For example, food and beverage sales were down by 3% in March and up by 1% from budget for year-to-date. Despite the 3% decline in March, which is not huge, sales are just above what was expected for the first three months of the fiscal year. Labor and expenses were pretty much in line with the budget, but the concern that pops out is that food and beverage expenses were up by 9 to 10% both in March and year-to-date. This is where you have to dig into the data to find out what is causing the issue and then develop an action plan to resolve it.

If you have overspent on fruits and vegetables, for example, there are many things to consider.

1. Have there been significant price changes in fruits and vegetables?
2. Are you buying at a competitive price? When were your prices last reviewed?
3. Have there been errors in ordering, receiving, issuing, or inventory valuation?
4. Is there an accounting error due to an invoice charged to fruits and vegetables that really belonged in another category?
5. Has there been significant waste, spoilage, or theft of products?
6. Are customers buying more fruits or vegetables?
7. Have the recipes/menu changed to use more fruits and vegetables?
8. Did the chef start ordering more precut vegetables that are more expensive?
9. Are inventory levels too high? Did the pack size of a fruit or vegetable change so we wound up with more inventory?

A variance in the labor budget may be simpler to solve. The expense report will show whether the overage is in hours worked, dollars paid, or overtime pay. If there are several vacant positions, this can contribute to premium overtime pay. If the business provides benefits like vacation, sick, and holiday pay, look for variations in the amounts of benefit time paid during each pay period. In small operations, the policies should state that no more than one or two people may use vacation or schedule the use of paid time off during the same pay period, as that would exceed the available coverage and could involve paying overtime hours. Overtime hours really hit the labor budget and are to be avoided. Accuracy of hourly employee records should also be checked and compared with the flow of the business' volume cycle.

15.4 PREPARE A CAPITAL BUDGET

Another part of the budget cycle is the **capital budget**, which allocates money for *major* investments, such as equipment or building/renovation projects. The capital budget is separate from the operating budget. Capital equipment includes equipment that is above a stated dollar amount (such as $1,500) and has a useful life of a minimum number of years (such as at least five years). This may or may not include electronic equipment and computers as they tend to become obsolete more quickly. Each organization determines the point at which an equipment purchase is considered capital equipment in terms of dollars and useful life.

Capital equipment is considered an asset of the business and is displayed on the business balance sheet under "Fixed Assets." In accounting, fixed assets are depreciated annually according to their expected useful or productive life cycle. This is why capital equipment is accounted for separately from the operating budget. Most businesses "tag and track" capital equipment until the end of its depreciation (useful life) because used ovens and most other equipment may have some resale market value at that time.

Budgeting for capital expenditures is essential for any business or organization to operate in the long run. Hospitals, for example, set aside a certain amount of money every year for capital expenditures that all departments can apply for. Paperwork is completed and includes information such as details on the piece of equipment, a description of its intended use and benefits, and how soon the investment will pay for itself. Often, the manager must also rank the level of priority for the equipment, such as urgent (needed as soon as possible), essential (perhaps a replacement for worn out equipment), or desirable (needed to improve service or be used to provide a new service).

One of the major responsibilities of a manager is to justify and sell the need for effective and efficient capital equipment purchases to the upper-level managers who allocate this money. You need to make persuasive arguments for new equipment, renovations, or new construction, and to show the negative effects of putting off the project. Whenever possible, demonstrate the value of the capital project to improve the customer experience, improve food safety or employee safety, increase productivity, reduce utility cost, or generate new revenue.

The payback period method is one of the simplest and most frequently used methods for evaluating capital investments. **Payback period** can be defined as the length of time required to earn back the value of an investment from profits or net annual savings. Nonprofit organizations, whose equipment does not generate income, can use labor savings, repair cost savings, utility savings (such as by buying new Energy Star equipment), or food waste savings. In brief, the payback period is the length of time it takes for the cost of an investment to be paid back. When capital investment projects are ranked using this method, the most favorable projects will have the shortest payback periods.

The information required to use this method includes the following.

1. The cost of the investment, meaning the purchase price and all other capital costs required to make the equipment operational (such as installation costs).
2. The net annual savings/earnings (pretaxes).

With this information, you can use the payback period formula as follows.

$$\frac{Cost\ of\ investment}{Net\ annual\ saving/profit} = Payback\ period\ (number\ of\ year)$$

$$\frac{\$8,000}{\$1,500} = 5.3\ years$$

For example, the purchase price of a new Point-of-Sales system is $8,000. It has a useful life of seven years. The estimated net annual savings is $1,500/year. The payback period is a little over five years. Because net annual savings/earnings can vary from year to year, it is more accurate in some cases to simply subtract each year's net savings from the original investment cost until the investment cost is brought down to zero.

A more sophisticated way to evaluate a capital expenditure is called net present value. Before discussing net present value, we need to review several new concepts. A **cash stream** is the term used to describe the series of cash flows to and from the operation. Cash going into an operation is called a cash inflow, cash going out is called a cash outflow. Just as your bank account has a series of cash flows going in (deposits, etc.) and out (debit payments, etc.) of it, so does an investment. Cash outflows related to an investment might include maintenance and supplies. Cash inflows could include operating savings and revenue generated.

To judge the financial feasibility of an investment over its lifetime, the total effect of the cash flows is compared with the original cost of the project. To do this, a common denominator must be used—usually today's dollars. This is because the cost of the investment is expressed in today's dollars (called **present value**), since it is paid for today. The cash flows in each of the future years of the project life are adjusted to represent their value in terms of today's dollars. This process, called **discounting**, allows the future cash flows to be compared with the capital investment cost on an equal basis—today's dollars to today's dollars or apples to apples.

The reason behind comparing today's dollars to today's dollars is that $1.00 today is worth more than $1.00 one or more years from now. This is known as the **time value of money**. If you have $100 in a savings account earning 10% interest, this investment earns $10 of interest after one year, bringing the total investment to $110. Discounting is simply the reverse of compounding interest. In other words, what is $110 one year from now worth to you today at a 10% discount rate? The answer is $100. In order to evaluate a capital investment cost, you need to compare apples to apples, so you need to convert future cash flows to today's dollars.

One last term to define is the cost of capital. The **cost of capital** is the interest rate at which businesses are allowed by banks to borrow money. It is important to keep in mind that at the very least, an investment such as your proposed capital project must earn a return that equals the amount of the loan and the interest paid (or cost of capital).

The concept of net present value is based on the premise that cash going into and out of an investment over time are discounted to the present time at a predetermined rate, usually the cost of capital. The **net present value (NPV)** of a capital investment is the value of the total revenues (over the life of the equipment) discounted to today's dollars, minus the cost of the capital investment. When the net present value is above zero, the capital investment is desirable. When the net present value is below zero, it will be considered a poor investment.

The information you need to calculate net present value includes the following.

1. The cost of the investment, meaning the purchase price and all other capital costs required to make the equipment operational (such as installation costs).
2. The number of years the investment is expected to last.
3. The annual operating savings, cash income, or losses generated as a result of the investment.
4. The depreciation cost (this is considered an expense).
5. The inflation rate for labor costs, benefits, food costs, etc., over the life of the investment.
6. The cost of capital for the facility.
7. Income taxes to be paid on the net cash flow.

The following information is going to be used to determine the net present value of a new dishwasher.

1. The cost is $65,000 including freight, site preparation, and installation costs.
2. The equipment and installation will last 10 years, with $5,000 salvage or trade-in value.
3. The savings resulting from the installation is due to a reduction in labor, about one-third of an FTE. Annual savings of wages and benefits is $12,250, with wages and benefits expected to increase yearly by 3%.
4. Because of the special mechanical system used by the new dishwasher, a factory inspection and one-time parts replacement after five years will be required and cost $3,500.
5. A yearly contract for supplies and maintenance of the machine costs $2,000 (in today's dollars). This contract will increase by 5% every two years.
6. The cost of capital is 9% per year.
7. The investment will depreciate at $6,500/year.

Keep in mind that the actual cost of the investment is the same as its present value because it is stated in today's dollars. Also, any salvage or trade-in value is added to the net cash flow of the last year.

Once you have this information, you can calculate the savings, expenses, and net cash flow for each of the 10 years. In **Table 15-9**, the total expenses (such as $8,500 for Year 1) are subtracted from the savings of $12,250 to get $3,750 net savings before taxes. In the final step, taxes are subtracted from $3,750 and depreciation is added back, to result in a net cash flow of $8,375 for Year 1. Depreciation is deductible as an expense when calculating income tax, but depreciation does not require an outlay of cash year after year. Therefore, in order to convert annual net savings from an investment to a cash flow situation, the depreciation is added back each year.

Now that we know the net cash flow for each of the 10 years, we can convert the annual cash flows to present values, as shown in **Table 15-10**. The discount factor is taken from a Present Value table. If you look under 9% (the cost of capital in this example), for one year, you will find the discount factor is 0.917. At two years, the discount factor is 0.842, and so on.

Table 15-9 Net Cash Flow Over 10 Years										
	Year 1	Year 2	Year 3	Year 4	Year 5	Year 6	Year 7	Year 8	Year 9	Year 10
Savings	12,250	12,600	12,900	13,000	13,400	13,800	14,200	14,600	15,000	15,400
Expense										
Contract	2,000	2,000	2,100	2,100	2,200	2,200	2,300	2,300	2,400	2,400
Overhaul					3,500					
Depreciation	6,500	6,500	6,500	6,500	6,500	6,500	6,500	6,500	6,500	6,500
Total Expenses	8,500	8,500	8,600	8,600	12,200	8,700	8,800	8,800	8,900	8,900
Net Savings Before Taxes	3,750	4,100	4,300	4,400	1,200	5,100	5,400	5,800	6,100	6,500
− Income Tax	1,875	2,050	2,150	2,200	600	2,550	2,700	2,900	3,050	3,250
+ Depreciation	6,500	6,500	6,500	6,500	6,500	6,500	6,500	6,500	6,500	6,500
+ Scrap Value										5,000
Net Cash Flow	8,375	8,550	8,650	8,700	7,100	9,050	9,200	9,400	9,550	14,750

Table 15-10 Converting Net Cash Flow to Present Value			
Year	Net Cash Flow	Discount Factor	Present Value
1	$8,375	0.917	$7,680
2	$8,550	.842	$7,199
3	$8,650	.772	$6,678
4	$8,700	.708	$6,160
5	$7,100	.650	$4,615
6	$9,050	.596	$5,394
7	$9,200	.547	$5,032
8	$9,400	.502	$4,719
9	$9,550	.460	$4,393
10	$14,750	.422	$6,225
		Total Percent Value	$58,095
		Less Initial Investment	$(65,000)
		Net Percent Value	$(6,905)

To calculate the total present value (meaning today's dollars) of the project, you simply multiply the net cash flow for each of the 10 years by the appropriate discount factor, then add up the present value for the 10 years. In this example, the total present value is $58,095. The final steps in calculating net present value is to subtract the cost of the initial investment from the total present value. In this case, the net present value works out to be negative $6,905. In most cases, administration will not look positively on an investment with a net present value less than 0. If it was possible to bring the cost of the investment down to $60,000, the net present value would be a positive $95 and would be viewed more favorably.

The advantages of NPV include that it forecasts cash flows for each year of the project, and then converts them to today's dollars to make a more valid comparison. One disadvantage is that this method does not look at the size of the investment, only its NPV.

15.5 USE FINANCIAL ANALYSIS TOOLS

This section will examine the following financial analysis tools.

1. Comparative and common-size financial statements
2. Break-even analysis
3. Ratio analysis
4. Trend analysis

These tools are useful to interpret financial information to see if costs are too high or low, if the operation is running efficiently, or if operating goals and objectives are being met.

COMPARATIVE AND COMMON SIZE FINANCIAL STATEMENTS

Income statements and balance sheets are important financial statements. There are two ways that you can make these statements even more useful. First, you can compare the results of the two most recent statements by putting them side-by-side, as shown

Table 15-11 Comparative Balance Sheet

Balance Sheet	December 31, 2019 (A)	December 31, 2020 (B)	Change in Value (C)	Change in Percentage (D)
Current assets:				
Cash	$185,250	$192,500	$+7,250	+3.9%
Accounts receivable	5,000	4,500	−500	−10.0%
Inventory	37,500	37,250	−250	−0.7%
Total current assets:	227,750	234,250	+6,500	+2.9%
Fixed assets:				
Equipment	125,000	130,000	+5,000	+4.0%
Furniture and other assets	15,000	14,000	−1,000	−6.7%
Total fixed assets:	140,000	144,000	+4,000	+2.9%
Total assets:	**367,750**	**378,250**	+10,500	+2.9%
Current liabilities				
Accounts payable	162,000	164,000	+2,000	+1.2%
Wages payable	30,000	30,500	+500	+1.7%
Total current liabilities:	192,000	194,500	+2,500	+1.3%
Long-term liabilities				
Long-term debt	20,000	18,000	−2,000	−10.0%
Total long-term liabilities:	20,000	18,000	−2,000	−10.0%
Total liabilities:	**212,000**	**212,500**	+500	+0.3%
Owner's equity	**155,750**	**165,750**	+10,000	+6.4%
Total liabilities & owner's equity	**367,750**	**378,250**	+10,500	+2.9%

in the comparative balance sheet in **Table 15–11**. Column A contains the figures from the December 31, 2019, balance sheet and Column B contains the figures from December 31, 2020. The change in value (Column C) shows how much the balance sheet changed from 2019 to 2020. For example, in 2020, the amount of cash grew by $7,250. The percentage change (Column D) is calculated by dividing the change in value (Column C) by Column A. For example, divide $7,250 by $185,250 to get a 3.9% change. When reviewing a comparative balance sheet, use the percentage column to determine where the biggest changes from year to year took place. In Table 15-11, note that assets went up by almost 3% while liabilities stayed about the same, resulting in increased owner equity. Don't forget that on a balance sheet, the value of the total assets always equals the value of total liabilities plus owners' (or stockholders') equity.

Table 15–12 illustrates a comparative income statement, completed in a similar fashion to the comparative balance sheet. The comparative income statement compares figures from January with figures from February. The final two columns are calculated the same as in the comparative balance sheet.

A second way to make financial statements more useful is to convert them into common-size statements. Common-size statements express each line item on a financial statement as a percentage. For example, in a common-size balance sheet (**Table 15–13**), total assets are given a value of 100% and each type of asset is then expressed as a percentage of that. For example, cash is 50.4% of total assets at the end

Table 15-12 Comparative Income Statement for West Coast Assisted Living Food & Nutrition Services				
Income Statement	**January 2021**	**February 2021**	**Change in Value**	**Change in Percentage**
Revenue				
Residents	$150,000	$135,000	$−15,000	−10.0%
Cafeteria	90,000	82,000	−8,000	−8.9%
Vending	15,000	13,500	−1,500	−10.0%
Nutrition services	5,000	4,500	−500	−10.0%
Total Revenue	280,000	253,000	−27,000	−9.6%
Cost of sales				
Food	95,000	96,000	+1,000	+1.1%
Supplies	7,000	6,500	−500	−7.1%
Other	1,000	1,000	0	0
Total Cost of Sales	103,000	103,500	+500	+0.5%
Gross profit	177,000	149,500	−27,500	−15.5%
Operating expenses				
Salaries and wages	140,000	128,000	−12,000	−8.6%
Payroll taxes and benefits	16,000	14,400	−1,600	−10.0%
Direct operating expenses	8,000	11,000	+3,000	+37.5%
Administrative expenses	8,000	8,000	0	0
Repairs/maintenance	1,000	500	−500	−50.0%
Total operating expenses	173,000	161,900	−11,100	−6.4%
Profit/loss before taxes	4,000	(12,400)	−16,400	−410%

Table 15-13 Common-Size Balance Sheet		
Balance Sheet	**December 31, 2020**	**Percent**
Current assets:		
Cash	$185,250	50.4%
Accounts receivable	5,000	1.4%
Inventory	37,500	10.2%
Total current assets:	227,750	61.9%
Fixed assets:		
Equipment	125,000	34.0%
Furniture and other assets	15,000	4.1%
Total fixed assets:	140,000	38.1%
Total assets:	367,750	100.0%
Current liabilities		
Accounts payable	162,000	44.1%
Wages payable	30,000	8.1%
Total current liabilities:	192,000	52.2%

Long-term liabilities		
Long-term debt	20,000	5.4%
Total long-term liabilities:	20,000	5.4%
Total liabilities:	212,000	57.6%
Owner's equity	155,750	42.4%
Total liabilities & owner's equity	367,750	100%

of December. Total liabilities and owner's equity (together) are also given a value of 100%.

Income statements can also be converted into common-size statements (Table 15-1). When this is done, total revenue is given the value of 100%, and all line items on the income statement are expressed as a percentage of total revenue. For example, in Table 15-1, salaries and wages ($95,323) are 28.8% of total revenue.

BREAK-EVEN AND CVP ANALYSIS

To understand this section, it is important to review some key points. All of the expenses in a foodservice can be classified as either fixed or variable. Fixed costs, which remain constant despite fluctuations in meals served, include occupancy costs, repairs, and other overhead expenses. Food costs are variable costs because they increase or decrease with meal volume. Labor costs include both fixed and variable elements. The following equation shows the relationship between these factors.

$$\text{Fixed costs} + \text{Variable costs} + \text{Profit/loss} = \text{Revenue}$$

The **break-even point** is the point at which the level of sales is equal to a foodservice's combined variable and fixed costs. So, the foodservice is covering its costs but not generating a profit. The following is the formula for the break-even point in sales.

$$\frac{\text{Fixed costs}}{1 - \dfrac{\text{Variable costs}}{\text{Sales}}} = \text{Break} - \text{even point in sales}$$

For example, if a foodservice has monthly sales of $75,000, fixed costs of $15,000, and variable costs of $45,000, you can calculate the break-even point as follows.

$$\frac{\$15,000}{1 - \dfrac{\$45,000}{\$75,000}} = \frac{\$15,000}{1 - 0.6 = 0.4} = \$37,500$$

In the example, the foodservice will generate a profit only after it reaches $37,500 in sales. It is useful to know the break-even point so you have a baseline for the minimum sales needed. When using this formula, the bottom of the fraction is known as the **contribution margin**. The contribution margin is the percent of sales left over after paying for variable expenses (such as food). In this example, the contribution margin is 0.4 or 40%, so for each dollar of sales, 40 cents are available to pay for fixed costs.

Let's say a foodservice doesn't want to just break even. They want to make a profit of at least $13,000. But how much revenue do they need in order to make that profit? This is when you use the **Cost-Volume-Profit formula**—which is the same as the break-even formula except for one addition (profit is added into the formula).

$$\frac{\text{Fixed cost} + \text{Profit desired}}{1 - \dfrac{\text{Variable costs}}{\text{Sales}}} = \text{Target sales revenue}$$

For example, let's say your monthly fixed costs are $25,000 and your variable costs are 40% of revenue. You want to know what level of sales is needed to make $13,000 in profit. So you fill in the equation.

$$\frac{\$25,000 + \$13,000}{1 - 0.4} = \frac{\$38,000}{0.6} = \$63,333$$

So you will need sales of $63,333 to generate $13,000 in profits.

RATIOS

A **ratio** is a comparison of two quantities. For example, food cost percentage is a ratio of food cost to sales. Ratios are only of value when the two numbers being compared are related to each other, such as food cost to food sales. The ratio tells you about the relationship between the numbers. If you compared food cost with beverage sales, the ratio would lack meaning because these numbers are not related.

Ratios can be expressed in various ways.

1. <u>Percentage ratios</u>. Percentages are a ratio in which the second number is 100, so percentage means "per hundred." Food cost percentage is an example. If food cost percentage is 33%, it means that 33 cents out of every $1.00 (or 100 cents) of sales is used to pay for food.

2. <u>Per unit ratios.</u> Average check is an example of a per-unit ratio. When you calculate average check, you are determining how much money each customer spends.

$$\frac{Total\ sales}{Number\ of\ customers\ served} = Average\ check$$

$$\frac{\$1800}{360} = \$5.00$$

Per-unit ratios can be per customer, per employee, per meal period, per patient days, per week, per month, per seat, per productive labor hour, and so on.

3. <u>Common ratio</u>. An example of a common ratio is a ratio of servers to tables, such as 1:5. In other words, each server is in charge of five tables.

Ratio analysis refers to the process of using ratios to analyze how you are doing from a financial or operational perspective. *Financial ratios* can be used to compare or benchmark a business's liquidity, leverage, profitability, or efficiency over time. They often use data from income statements and/or balance sheets. They will be discussed first, followed by a discussion of *operating ratios*.

Ratios are particularly useful when you compare them with previous periods or to other similar operations. A benchmark is something that serves as a standard or best practice against which others measure themselves. **Benchmarking** is the practice of comparing your operation's performance against yourself, similar operations, or an industry standard to determine if there are areas for improvement. For example, when managers at two similar quick-service restaurants compare the average number of minutes it takes for a drive-through customer to be served, the manager with the slower drive-through may gain some tips on how to serve customers faster. **Internal benchmarking** is when managers compare performance of operations within the *same* organization, such as two Wendy's Unit Managers comparing monthly revenues. Internal benchmarking also includes comparing your own foodservice's performance over time. **External benchmarking** is when a manager compares performance against foodservices *outside* of their organization. Whether internal or external, benchmarking can help you find your strengths and how to maintain them, as well as identify areas where you can improve.

Liquidity Ratios

In general terms, **liquidity** looks at the amount of assets a business has that are either in cash form or can be easily sold for cash. Accounting liquidity measures how easily a business can pay bills using their liquid assets. One ratio that measures a business' ability to pay its current bills and short-term liabilities is the **quick ratio** or **acid test ratio**. It is calculated as follows using information from the balance sheet.

$$\frac{Current\ assets - Inventory}{Current\ liabilities} = Quick\ ratio$$

The quick ratio does not include inventory as it is hard to return or sell off perishable foods. The quick ratio is one of the fastest ways to see if a business is liquid enough to pay its bills or creditors. The quick ratio for the balance sheet shown in Table 15-3 is as follows.

$$\frac{\$218,643}{\$130,106} = Quick\ ratio\ of\ 1.68$$

If the ratio is below 1, liquid assets cannot cover short-term obligations. If the ratio gets too high, it indicates that money is sitting idle (in liquid form), and could be worth more if it were reinvested or otherwise used to improve the business' profitability.

Another liquidity ratio, which also measures the ability to pay near-term obligations, is known as the **current ratio**. It is simply the ratio of current assets to current liabilities—current being defined as within one year. A current ratio greater than one indicates that a company can pay its short-term debts using only current assets if need be. It basically indicates how well a business can pay its short-term bills such as for food, beverages, and payroll.

The current ratio for the balance sheet shown in Table 15-3 is as follows.

$$\frac{Current\ assets}{Current\ liabilities} = Current\ ratio$$

$$\frac{\$233,472}{\$130,106} = 1.8$$

This shows that the business has $1.80 of current assets to pay for each $1.00 of current debt. Each operation has to determine the current ratio that best allows them to pay bills without having too much money tied up, which decreases profitability.

Leverage Ratios

Leverage ratios, also called **solvency ratios**, measure a company's ability pay its bills in the long term. The **debt ratio** is an example of a solvency ratio. As already discussed, it is a ratio of total liabilities to total assets. A lower debt ratio likely means the business is more stable. A ratio of 0.5 is considered reasonable.

Profitability Ratios

There are a number of **profitability ratios**. Profitability ratios compare net income before or after taxes to sales, owners' investments or equity, or total assets. They use information from both the balance sheet and income statement to measure management's effectiveness in using the resources available. Profit margin percentage (already mentioned) is also known on **return on sales (ROS)**. ROS measures how efficiently a business turns sales into profits. It is calculated as follows.

$$\frac{Profit\ (net\ income\ before\ taxes)}{Revenue\ or\ sales} \times 100 = Return\ on\ sales\ (percentage)$$

ROS, expressed as a percentage, tells you the percentage of sales remaining after all expenses are paid. Using the income statement in Table 15-1, the ROS is 1.8%, which is on the low side. ROS can vary tremendously depending on the type of foodservice. Restaurants may experience industry averages from 1% to more than 20% depending on market segment and other factors.

$$\frac{\$5,977}{\$331,492} = 1.8\%$$

Other profitability ratios compare net income before or after taxes to owners' investments or equity, or total assets. They use information from both the balance sheet and income statement to measure management's effectiveness in using the resources available. For example, **return on investment (ROI)** is a measure of how well the investment into the business has paid off. There are a number of ways to calculate ROI. This formula is one of them.

$$\frac{Profit\ (net\ income\ before\ taxes)}{Total\ invested\ (owner's\ or\ stockholder\ equity)} \times 100 = Return\ on\ Investment$$

$$\frac{\$63,310}{\$628,704} \times 100 = 10.1\%$$

This ROI formula is also known as return on equity. It shows how well the business is able to turn equity into profits. A 9 to 10% return on equity is average in the restaurant industry.

A final way to look at profitability is to compare profit to your total assets as follows by calculating **Return on Assets**.

$$\frac{Profit\ (net\ income\ before\ taxes)}{Total\ assets} \times 100 = Return\ on\ Assets$$

$$\frac{\$63,310}{\$2,011,646} \times 100 = 3.1\%$$

Return on assets tells you how effectively a business converts the money it invests into net income. In the example, every dollar the business invested in assets generated 3.1 cents of net income. The higher the percentage, the better. The number varies a lot among industries.

Activity Ratios

Activity ratios, also called **efficiency ratios**, tell you how well assets, such as inventory, are being utilized or managed to produce income. **Inventory turnover rate** is an example of an activity ratio. Inventory turnover measures how often a company uses and replaces its inventory during a given period, such as a month or quarter (three consecutive months). If your turnover rate is much lower than the industry average, you are probably overstocked and have some old inventory. For example, if inventory turnover is 1.5 in a school foodservice, that is low when many schools have an inventory turnover of 3 or higher. A low turnover rate may also occur when sales are slower. It is generally desirable to have a higher turnover rate as long as you are not so understocked that you frequently run out of items.

To calculate the inventory turnover rate for a period of time, use the following formula.

$$\frac{Cost\ of\ goods\ sold}{Average\ inventory\ value} = Inventory\ Turnover\ Rate$$

In the prior section, you learned how to calculate cost of goods sold for a period, the top half of the fraction.

To calculate the average inventory value for a period, first add the beginning inventory and the ending inventory, then divide by 2. Following is an example.

Beginning Inventory + Ending Inventory ÷ 2 = Average Inventory

Beginning Inventory (May 1st)		$34,000
Ending Inventory (May 31st)	+	$32,000
		$66,000 ÷ 2 = $33,000

EXAMPLE 15-2 HOW TO CALCULATE INVENTORY TURNOVER

$$\frac{\text{Cost of goods sold}}{\text{Average inventory value for the period}} = \text{Inventory Turnover Rate}$$

Example: $\dfrac{\$99,000}{\$33,000} = 3.0$ *Inventory Turns*

Now you are ready to calculate inventory turnover using the cost of goods sold shown in **Example 15-2** and the average inventory value just computed. Using those numbers, the inventory turnover rate is 3.0 for May.

An inventory turnover rate can also be calculated for alcoholic beverages or one inventory category, such as meats. This is done by dividing the cost of goods sold by the average inventory or ending inventory for those items and can be helpful to locate specific inventory items with low turnover rates.

Inventory turnover is best calculated on a regular basis, such as monthly, and compared over time. It is also a good idea to compare inventory turnover to the industry average and industry standards. For example, an average restaurant inventory turnover rate (across segments) is 4.0 while turnover rates range from 2.5 to 4.0 for foodservices in healthcare or education (Reynolds, 2013, p. 197).

Another example of an activity ratio is the **occupancy rate**. For example, a manager at an assisted-living facility, hotel, or a college dorm needs to know how many rooms are occupied compared with the total number of rooms.

$$\frac{\text{Number of rooms occupied}}{\text{Total number of rooms}} = \text{Occupancy Rate}$$

$$\frac{200}{300} = 67\%$$

As the occupancy rate goes up, you get better utilization of your asset and more income.

A final example of an activity ratio is **seat turnover**. Seat turnover tells you how many times a different customer sat down to eat during a given time period.

$$\frac{\text{Number of guests}}{\text{Number of seats}} = \text{Seat turnover}$$

$$\frac{600 \text{ guests}}{250 \text{ seats}} = 2.4$$

If 600 guests came in for dinner last night, and your dining room has 250 seats, seat turnover would be 2.4—meaning that each seat was used by a little more than two guests during that period.

Operating Ratios

Operating ratios can help you evaluate your ability to generate sales and control costs. It is important for you to choose appropriate operating ratios for your operation. The following are some of the more common operating ratios that utilize sales data.

1. Average check or cover. Average check can be calculated by total revenue or revenue area. For example, a restaurant separates its sales into main dining room, bar, and take-out and delivery. To calculate average check, you must decide which sales you want to capture and also the time period. The time period could be as short as a meal period or as long as a month or year. Keep in mind that average check will differ according to meal period because breakfast

is normally less expensive than lunch, and lunch is less expensive than dinner. The sales and number of customers served must reflect the same time period. In a foodservice such as a cafeteria, you can calculate the average retail transaction in the same manner. In a restaurant, you can use this formula to calculate average check.

$$\frac{Total\ sales}{Number\ of\ customers\ served} = Average\ check$$

$$\frac{\$1,800}{360} = \$5.00$$

2.   Sales per square foot - This ratio is generally calculated using annual sales and total square footage including dining areas, kitchen, storage, rest rooms, etc.

$$\frac{Annual\ sales}{Total\ square\ footage} = Sales/square\ foot$$

$$\frac{\$750,000}{2,750} = \$273/square\ foot$$

According to Bloom Intelligence (2019), if sales/square foot are $250 or higher, a full-service restaurant should be able to create a 5 to 10% profit before taxes (or $300 for a limited-service restaurant).

3.   Sales per seat - This is calculated by dividing the revenue for a certain time period, such as a day or week, by the number of seats available.

$$\frac{Sales\ for\ given\ period}{Number\ of\ seats} = Sales/seat$$

$$\frac{\$100,000}{250} = \$400\ sales/seat\ per\ week$$

4.   Percentage sales by revenue center - The percentage sales of each revenue center is divided by total sales to determine the relative proportion of revenues generated by each revenue center. For example, a university may have revenue coming in from student meal plans, a food court in the Student Union, coffee shops, faculty dining room, catering, vending, and a convenience store. A restaurant may have just two revenue centers: dining room and bar.

$$\frac{Sales\ for\ Revenue\ Center}{Total\ Sales} \times 100 = \%\ sales\ by\ revenue\ center$$

$$\frac{\$100,000}{\$150,000} \times 100 = 67\%$$

Traditional operating ratios also compare costs to sales. Traditional cost-to-sales ratios that were discussed earlier in this chapter include the following.

1.   Food cost percentage.

$$\frac{Food\ cost}{Food\ sales} \times 100 = Food\ cost\ percentage$$

$$\frac{\$78,157}{\$238,183} \times 100 = 32.8\%$$

2.   Beverage cost percentage.

$$\frac{Beverage\ cost}{Beverage\ sales} \times 100 = Beverage\ percent$$

$$\frac{\$17,712}{\$76,636} \times 100 = 23.1\%$$

3. Cost of sales percentage.

$$\frac{Total\ cost\ of\ sales}{Total\ sales} \times 100 = Cost\ of\ sales\ percentage$$

$$\frac{\$101{,}204}{\$331{,}492} \times 100 = 30.5\%$$

4. Labor cost percentage.

$$\frac{Labor\ cost}{Total\ sales} \times 100 = Labor\ cost\ percentage$$

$$\frac{\$121{,}842}{\$331{,}492} \times 100 = 36.8\%$$

5. Prime cost percentage.

$$\frac{Food\ and\ beverage\ cost + Labor\ cost}{Total\ sales} \times 100 = Prime\ cost\ percentage$$

$$\frac{\$223{,}046}{\$331{,}492} \times 100 = 67.3\%$$

6. Profit margin percentage.

$$\frac{Profit\ before\ taxes}{Total\ sales} \times 100 = Profit\ Margin\ Percentage$$

$$\frac{\$5{,}977}{\$314{,}819} \times 100 = 1.8\%$$

Another way of looking at costs involves examining costs *per* meal. Here are some examples. *Keep in mind that you can also calculate these costs per patient/resident day or per student.*

1. Food cost per meal or cover

$$\frac{Food\ cost}{Number\ of\ meals} = Food\ cost/meal$$

$$\frac{\$60{,}000}{20{,}000} = \$3.00/meal$$

2. Supply cost per meal or cover

$$\frac{Supply\ cost}{Number\ of\ meals} = Supply\ cost/meal$$

$$\frac{\$7{,}000}{20{,}000} = \$0.35$$

3. Labor cost per meal or cover

$$\frac{Labor\ cost}{Number\ of\ meals} = Labor\ cost/meal$$

$$\frac{\$70{,}000}{20{,}000} = \$3.50$$

4. Prime cost per meal or cover

$$\frac{Food\ and\ beverage\ cost + Labor\ cost}{Number\ of\ meals} = Prime\ cost/meal$$

$$\frac{\$137{,}000}{20{,}000} = \$6.85$$

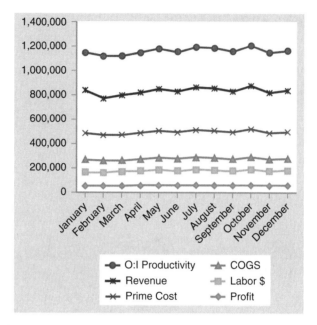

FIGURE 15-2 A Graph is Useful to Analyze Trends

An operating ratio is calculated for a specific length of time. It could be for a meal period, a day, a week, a month, or longer. Be sure that the data used in the ratio are from the same time period.

TREND ANALYSIS

Looking at results, such as cost of sales percentage, over a longer period of time tells you more about the direction or trend in which your business is heading than just looking at a month or two. Trend analysis falls into two categories: internal and external. Internal trend analysis examines data from just your own operation. When you compare data with others outside of your operation, it is external trend analysis.

A graph is very useful for trend analysis. By placing the period of time on the horizontal axis, and the data from various time periods on the vertical axis, you can measure trends in inventory turnover or food cost percentage, for example. **Figure 15-2** shows trends in multiple indicators.

15.6 MEASURE PRODUCTIVITY

Productivity is a measure of efficiency that shows how effectively inputs (such as money and labor) are converted into output (such as meals and revenue). Increasing productivity is one of the best ways to control costs and improve the profitability of a business. The traditional productivity formula is simply a ratio of output to input. The following is an example of a productivity measurement used in foodservices that counts number of meals served, such as K–12 schools. To make this calculation, you need the number of meals produced and productive labor hours from the *same* time period. **Productive labor hours** include only labor hours when employees were on the job—it does not include paid time off hours.

$$Meal\ per\ productive\ labor\ hour = \frac{Number\ of\ meals}{Productive\ labor\ hours}$$

$$18.19 = \frac{41,643}{2,289}$$

Although most productivity formulas used in foodservice utilize just one input (called single factor productivity), multifactor productivity is possible and is calculated by dividing output by a *combination of inputs*. **Table 15–14** lists a variety of productivity ratios in three different categories.

In order to calculate a number of productivity measurements such as meals per labor hour, you must have a single unit of service—a meal. Restaurants often use the term **covers** to indicate the number of meals that were served. If a server has four guests at a table for dinner, it would equal four covers. A hospital foodservice counts the number of meals sent up to the patient floors and the K–12 foodservice counts the number of school lunches served.

However, there are situations in which it is difficult to accurately count meals. For example, many restaurants offer table service as well as take-out service. How will you count the number of covers or meals in a take-out order? In a hospital or business and industry cafeteria, it is also difficult to accurately count meals. When a morning customer buys coffee and a muffin, is that really a meal? Lastly, while a school foodservice

---

Table 15-14 Productivity Ratios

1. Meals or Cover per.......

$$\text{Meals or Covers per paid labor hour} = \frac{\text{Number of covers or meals}}{\text{Number of paid labor hours}}$$

$$\text{Meals or Covers per productive labor hour} = \frac{\text{Number of meals}}{\text{Number of productive labor hours}}$$

$$\text{Meals or Covers per FTE} = \frac{\text{Number of meals}}{\text{Number of fulltime equivalents}}$$

$$\text{Meals per patient day} = \frac{\text{Number of meals}}{\text{Number of patient days}}$$

2. Sales per ...

$$\text{Sales per paid labor hour} = \frac{\text{Sales}}{\text{Number of paid labor hours}}$$

$$\text{Sales per productive labor hour} = \frac{\text{Sales}}{\text{Number of productive labor hours}}$$

$$\text{Sales per FTE} = \frac{\text{Sales}}{\text{Number of fulltime equivalents}}$$

3. Paid or productive labor hours per meal or cover

$$\text{Paid labor hours per meal or cover} = \frac{\text{Number of paid labor hours}}{\text{Number of meals or covers}}$$

$$\text{Example: 0.27 paid hours/meal} = \frac{8,100}{30,000}$$

$$\text{0.27 paid hours} \times \text{60 minutes/hour} = \text{16 minutes}$$

$$\text{Productive labor hours per meal or cover} = \frac{\text{Number of productive labor hours}}{\text{Number of meals or covers}}$$

$$\text{Example: 0.25 paid hours/meal} = \frac{7,500}{30,000}$$

$$\text{0.25 paid hours} \times \text{60 minutes/hour} = \text{15 minutes}$$

counts each lunch meal as "one" meal, what will it do when it sells chips, ice cream, or milk to a child who brought the rest of his lunch from home?

The **meal equivalent** concept was developed to solve this problem. By converting food sales to meal equivalents, you can still determine a per meal cost. For example, in a school lunch program, a la carte and other sales are converted into a lunch meal equivalent by assigning a dollar value to a lunch meal based on the full cost of producing it. So, if a high school had $4,000 of a la carte sales in a week, it would be divided by the full cost of a lunch meal (let's say $4.00) so that à la carte sales are now converted to 1,000 school lunch meals.

The most common method for calculating a meal equivalent is based on sales (but you can also calculate meal equivalents based on cost as just shown). A foodservice with take-out sales or a cafeteria often use **average check** (also called average sale per customer) as a meal equivalent. Average check is an example of a sales-based approach to meal equivalents. It is calculated as follows.

$$Average\ check = \frac{Total\ sales}{Number\ of\ customers\ served}$$

$$\$6.43 = \frac{\$46,400}{7,214}$$

So you can divide take-out or cafeteria sales by $6.43 (average check) to determine the number of equivalent meals served. Using the average check concept assumes that each customer buys a meal. This is not always the case because some customers (especially in a cafeteria) are just getting a beverage or something to go with the lunch they brought from home. To measure an accurate average transaction, calculate it during the busiest meal period when people are most likely to buy a full meal. Another sales-based approach to determining a meal equivalent would be to add up the average selling price of each item in a typical meal.

Some organizations use a cost-based approach to calculating a meal equivalent. In hospitals that serve patient meals and cafeteria customers, you can calculate the average cost of a patient tray by picking the components of the meal (such as 4 ounces chicken, ½ cup rice, ½ cup green vegetable, a roll, beverage, and cake for dessert), costing them out, and adding the costs together. In 2019, the Association for Healthcare Foodservice was using approximately $3.50 as the cost of a standard meal equivalent (AHF, 2019).

In the National School Lunch Program, each student's lunch meal is counted as one meal. If the same foodservice serves breakfast, three breakfast meals are usually counted as two lunch meals (although that could vary depending on the state agency). In addition, three afterschool snacks are counted as one lunch meal. See **Table 15-15** for an example of how meal equivalents are counted in the school lunch program.

Table 15-15 Meal Equivalent Calculations for a National School Lunch Program*			
Categories	**Total Meals or Sales**	**Conversion Factor**	**Meal Equivalents**
Student Lunch	350,000	1	350,000
Adult Lunch	5,000	1	5,000
Student Breakfast	150,000	0.67	100,500
Snacks	15,000	0.33	5,000
Nonprogram Food Sales	$65,000	$3.80/ME	17,105

Total Meal Equivalents: 477,605

* 1 lunch (student or adult) = 1 meal equivalent
  3 breakfasts = 2 lunches
  3 afterschool snacks = 1 lunch
  Nonprogram food sales divided by $3.80 (cost) = Meal equivalents

SPOTLIGHT ON PRODUCTIVITY OF REGISTERED DIETITIAN NUTRITIONISTS (RDNS)

Clinical productivity measures help to determine staffing levels needed for clinical nutrition care in acute and long-term care facilities. Productivity varies depending on the type of facility and patient/resident. Within a hospital, for instance, the time required for patient care can vary between an Intensive Care Unit, a pediatric unit, and a medical floor. Productivity also varies depending on the medical record system being used as well as the amount of time that must be spent in medical rounds or committees.

To understand productivity for RDNs, first you have to collect how much time they spend in direct care and indirect care. *Direct care activities* include time spent seeing inpatients; assessing, planning, and monitoring care for inpatients; medical rounds; and screening patient records to determine which patients need to be visited by a RDN. Whereas direct care activities involve patients and/or their medical records, *indirect care activities* "are those activities required to provide services in that facility but are not directly linked to individuals or groups of patients" (Phillips, 2015, p. 1055). Examples of indirect care activities include staff meetings, research, staff education, travel time to floors, foodservice activities, etc. While RDNs do spend the majority of their time on direct care activities, there is significant variety in how much time is spent in indirect care activities.

Additional data should be collected to calculate the following.

* The average number of patients seen by an RDN per eight-hour day or per hour worked.
* The average number of patients seen per hour spent in direct care.
* The average length of time spent screening.
* The average length of time to complete a comprehensive or a limited assessment.

These data are useful to benchmark a facility's productivity. For more information on productivity benchmarks for RDNs in acute-care hospitals, consult Phillips, Janowski, Brennan, and Leger (2019).

Whichever method is used to determine a meal equivalent, inaccuracies are possible, which can cause problems. For example, when the meal equivalent amount is low, the number of meal equivalents will be inflated, cost per meal will be low, and productivity will appear high. When the meal equivalent amount is high, the number of meal equivalents will be lowered, cost per meal will be high, and productivity will appear low.

There are a number of factors within an organization that influence productivity. According to the Academy of Nutrition and Dietetics (2015), these may include regulatory requirements (such as minimum wage or the Family and Medical Leave Act); the state of the restaurant industry (or healthcare, universities, etc.); technology; the menu and purchasing policies; the kitchen layout and type of production system; and the skills, health, and level of engagement employees bring to work every day. In addition, you need to consider the leadership of the organization and the organization's goals, especially their financial goals.

15.7 CONTROL COSTS

Cost control starts with writing the menu and developing your supply chain or food supplier network. Quick serve and fast food franchisees have very different business models from traditional restaurants or onsite college or healthcare feeding. What they all have in common is the need to pay close attention to the market, inflation, seasonality, and any other changes like shortages or food safety recalls that could affect business costs. Most broad-line food suppliers like Sysco or US Foods have the means to notify customers when there is a significant price change or recall. These suppliers also have search functions for local, seasonal, and sustainably supplied foods.

MENU COST CONTROL

To control menu costs, do the following.

- Make sure that the food cost, selling price, and contribution margin of each menu item is known and tracked.
- Balance high- and low-cost menu items, in order to maintain an average cost that is close to the budgeted cost per meal.
- Assure that ingredients in inventory are used in multiple dishes or recipes.
- Monitor the sales of each menu item and remove or change the price point of poor sellers.
- Take advantage of seasonal food availability and price reductions: For example:
  Summer: Berries, peaches, melons, grapes, green & lima beans, cucumber, cob corn, peppers, tomatoes, zucchini, yellow squash, radishes, Swiss Chard.
  Autumn: Apples, pears, beets, potatoes, broccoli, carrots, Brussels sprouts, eggplant, acorn and butternut squash, and cranberries.
  Winter: Citrus like oranges and grapefruit, cabbage, parsnips, turnips, rutabagas, kale, sweet potatoes and yams.
  Spring: Asparagus, scallions, ramps, fiddlehead ferns, rhubarb, peas, spinach.
- Don't feature seasonally expensive or holiday driven items in high demand such as:
  - Filet mignon or prime rib close to Christmas or New Years.
  - Chicken wings and avocadoes at Super Bowl.
  - Beef or Pork Ribs on holidays such as Memorial, Independence, or Labor Day
- Balance volume discounts with food quality and perishability concerns.

FOOD COST CONTROL

These are some of the best strategies for controlling food and supply cost at the operational level.

Recipes: Provide accurate recipes for each menu item. Match the recipe to the skill level of the staff member preparing it. Some simplification is sometimes needed.

Forecasting: Maintain accurate forecasting records. Check quality of forecast numbers and if production staff are making appropriate amount of food.

Purchasing: Buy from reputable and approved suppliers using group purchasing or competitive bidding to assure the most competitive pricing for all product categories. Use specifications. Buyer needs to be current on market trends and prices.

Receiving: Reject items that are not up to quality standard. Check quantities against purchase order. Keep accurate receiving records.

Inventory: Purchase fresh food Just In Time (JIT) or closest to the date of planned use, whenever possible. Assure inventory rotation and FIFO (first-in, first-out) to maintain food quality, while assuring proper labeling and dating and maintaining ideal storage temperatures.

Issuing: Assure that only authorized receiving and production staff have access to ingredients to prevent theft or product misuse. Use formal requisitions to ensure documentation of the inventory from receiving to consumption.

Value: Assure that recipe ingredients are the best value for the product being produced such as use chuck roast in beef soup, not top sirloin. Use frozen raspberries for a puree rather than fresh berries. Monitor the grade and quality of all of the ingredients.

Portion Control: Assure that over- or underportioning is not occurring. Overportioning is more expensive and is frequently done by staff working for customer tips. Underportioning may reduce customer satisfaction and repeat business will decline. These variances will not only affect perceptions but also cost and nutritional attributes.

Pricing: Review and adjust sales prices on a regular basis.

Control Food Waste: Monitor food waste throughout the entire production process and at the end of the meal. Reward staff for reducing waste or using leftovers in creative ways. Make sure staff receive adequate training on portion control and how to control food waste. Evaluate the cost of precut ingredients against the waste occurring using whole items. Repurpose trimmings.

Supervision: Monitor employee work. Work with others to ensure standards are met. Watch for wasteful practices.

Portion-Control Items and Condiments: Assure that portion-control items (such as condiment and dressing packets, crackers, sugar, sweeteners, and creamers) are available with purchases but not left out to be taken for home use.

Take-out Containers: Use sustainable and natural packaging whenever possible in the smallest possible container. Have staff wrap take-home leftovers in cling wrap or foil.

LABOR COST CONTROL

Compared with food, labor costs are a moving target. When a staff schedule is completed, the manager's intent is to cover all shifts and labor needs for the minimum cost to the business. However, some staff members have their own best interest in mind and attempt to maximize their individual paychecks, which increases the labor cost to the business.

Labor is by far the biggest challenge in the foodservice industry. Foodservice employees are very often young or entry level. They may be simultaneously working other jobs or involved in the gig economy. Foodservice workers in colleges, healthcare, and corrections are more likely to be unionized and have negotiated labor contracts and specific work rules. Each state and some municipalities have different wage and hour laws.

Using the labor budget (hours and FTEs) and master schedule as a guide, do the following.

- Schedule employees to meet the budgeted staffing needs of the foodservice.
- Adjust staffing assignments to anticipate peaks (rush periods) throughout the day.
- Review sales in 30-minute increments and consider adjusting staffing if necessary.
- Stagger clocking in and out times to reflect when and where staff are needed.
- Monitor clocking in and out to prevent staff from getting unapproved overtime pay.
- Hold preshift meetings to make everyone aware of "all" of their assignments and duties as well as inform them about changes.
- Monitor break and meal periods and personal cell phone use.
- Ensure that staff are performing appropriate duties for the assigned rate of pay.
- Cross-train staff so that each skilled position has multiple employees trained to perform the work.
- Schedule production overlap between positions. For example, if three cooks need chopped onions for various recipes, schedule one cook to chop onions for all three. Or if the Sub Station and Salad Bar both need sliced tomatoes, assign to one staff member.
- Monitor and evaluate the work flow daily. Make frequent changes to show staff that attention is being paid to details.
- If an employee is not performing up to expectations, make it obvious that the problem is being addressed. Staff morale and productivity are harmed when unsatisfactory performance is not corrected.

Also, never miss an opportunity to compliment good performance.

Theft Prevention

For foodservice workers, the kitchen and storage areas are an actual (not virtual) Temptation Island. Everything they see at work, they could probably use at home. It is not unusual for employees to make sandwiches at work for their children to take to school the next day. Day after day, the amounts add up. Then, there are the bigger thefts of alcohol, expensive cuts of meat, and more. So, it is not a question of whether or not employees are stealing, but how much. The last thing any business wants is to make it easy. **Table 15-16** lists some general guidelines.

Table 15-16 General Principles of Security and Theft Prevention
1. **Inventory:** Keep the inventory low, check it frequently or maintain a perpetual inventory in the production, inventory, or POS system. Employees know when quantities are not closely monitored.
2. **Receiving:** Secure the receiving area and loading dock. Do not allow chairs or for this to become a hang-out or smoking area for employees. Assure that the receiving staff is inputting each item as it is received and that each item is getting to its proper storage location. Always have receiving monitored by video surveillance. Do not allow staff who place orders to be responsible for receiving as well. If mistakes are made in ordering, the staff member may try to cover the mistakes in the receiving process, and there are cases where staff ordered items for personal use. Maintain strict receiving hours. Rotate receiving duties in order to maintain a business relationship rather than a personal relationship between delivery drivers and receiving staff. Get signatures on invoices and maintain receiving logs. When something critical is missing, "I never saw it come in" is not the best answer to hear from the receiving staff.
3. **Purchasing:** Use group purchasing with prime vendor agreements and broad-line suppliers whenever possible. Try to have contracted or cost-plus pricing (a guaranteed maximum percentage markup), so that there are no surprise price changes. This will allow staff to become familiar with the products and brands being used, so deliveries can be stored and rotated easily. Maintain a purchasing policy that does not allow for frequent substitutions, special purchases, and side deals between the businesses' purchasing agent and the supplier. Take advantage of specials and rebates by requiring a third-party approval.
4. **Purchase order numbers:** Use purchase order numbers and provide copies of orders to the receiving staff. Receive only what is ordered and not what the vendor wants to send or unload. Maintain a separate system for receiving "samples" and trial products.
5. **Order Guide:** Use an Order Guide that contains the product numbers and specifications of each product used for the menu. Use the product numbers. For example, never order "10 loaves of white bread" from a bakery. Loaves can vary from between 10 to 25 slices and also vary by as much as 2 lbs. in weight.
6. **Access:** Do not allow drivers, sales people, or visitors access to the business via the loading dock or by passing the food storage areas. This will help prevent theft as well as decreasing food tampering, sabotage, cross contamination, and prevent sales people from seeing what is being purchased from other vendors. The loading dock should not serve as the employee entrance.
7. **Dumpsters and recycling area**: Monitor these areas closely. Many thefts occur when trash is removed from an operation. Staff will leave packages near the dumpster to be retrieved after work. If the dumpsters are in close proximity to the parking lot, staff can easily take stolen property directly to cars. Make sure all boxes are broken down flat before removal to cardboard recycling. Intact boxes can be used to hide stolen items.
8. **Alarm:** Alarm all entrances and exits that are not meant to be used except in an emergency. If the kitchen is on the first floor or basement level, alarm or lock windows that lead to the outside. Assure that all entrances and exits are alarmed during hours when the business is closed.
9. **Lock up certain items:** Liquor, wine, beer, and expensive food items should be locked in a cage, rack, or a limited access storeroom. Smaller locking racks are available for freezers. Limit access to the keys for these items. Also limit access to expensive spices such as Old Bay Seasoning, Montreal Steak Seasoning, and Middle Eastern Spices, as they come in small containers and are often targets of theft.
10. **ID badge access:** If possible, use ID Badge Access to storerooms so that it is known who was in and out of an area when and where a theft occurred.

11. **Food ordering system with printed tickets:** Use an ordering system where food and drinks are entered into the system before the meals are produced and served. This prevents staff from ordering food that does not get paid for. It also prevents the handing of take-out food to family, friends and coworkers that has not been charged through the cash register.

12. **Linen, aprons, napkins, and uniforms:** Theft can be wrapped in linen and be removed in laundry and uniform bags. Do surprise checks periodically, especially if the same person always carries the linen orders in and out of the business.

13. **Track sales versus inventory:** This can be easy; if a case has 40 hamburgers, check how many were actually charged through the POS system.

14. **Video surveillance:** Maintain on all entrances and exits, and on all self-serve areas where customers access food directly.

15. **Locker and coat areas:** Always maintain an area where staff can safely store belongings. Do not allow outside clothing, purses, shopping bags, or backpacks into areas with food and supply access.

16. **Meal plan sharing:** If a college or business offers a meal plan with "all you care to eat," watch for sharing or for several students trying to eat off of one plan.

CASH HANDLING POLICY

Cash may be the most tempting item of all. And the more a business relies on cash, the more likely someone will figure out how to make some disappear. Cashless systems are improving this but also lend themselves to new types of fraud. Every business with POS systems and cash handling needs a strong cash control policy. See **Table 15–17** for best practices.

Table 15-17 Best Practices for Cash Handling

Vet the cashiers and cash-handling supervisors. Assure that anyone handling cash has had a criminal background check and possibly be Surety Bonded. Employees who are bonded deal with a large amount of cash and the bond provides an insurance policy against theft. Make sure each has been thoroughly trained and has signed off on all of the policies regarding the safeguarding of company assets, keys, security codes, account numbers, deposit and withdrawal slips, and receipts.

Issue each cashier and supervisor with a specific cash bank that provides enough money to provide change to customers at the beginning of a shift or meal service. Set bank amounts for each cashier and supervisor based on cash volume handled. Adjust amounts periodically to prevent service disruptions at the cash register stations. All cashier banks must be verified and reconciled at the beginning and end of each shift.

Standard Operating Procedures (SOPs) must be followed every day and every shift with regard to cash. That includes counting the opening bank and setting up the cash register or POS system. Thieves look for variations to exploit.

Seek 100% Accuracy. Cashiers should always be seeking 100% accuracy at the end of each shift. If a customer says "keep the change," that money should be separated from the deposit. In each transaction, the cashier should be trying to get the payment and the change exactly correct.

"Voids" and "no sales" should be verified by a manager or supervisor. Ideally, voids and no sales should not be accessible to a cashier. Voids are used to take money from customers without completing the transaction in the POS system. This unrecorded money can then be skimmed or removed by the cashier before cashing out for the night. This is why many managers are more suspicious of cashiers whose money is frequently over, than those who periodically run short or under the expected total.

Do not allow cell phones at the registers, as these can be used as calculators and credit card scanners. Do not allow small extraneous objects like paper clips or buttons at the register or in the empty change slot of the cash drawer. These are used as markers or chips to calculate how much untailed money to remove by the end of a shift.

(continues)

Table 15-17 Best Practices for Cash Handling (continued)

Do surprise cashier audits. Ask a cashier to cash out the drawer at an unexpected time. If there is a large overage, the cashier may be stealing from you.

Do frequent cash drops. Businesses, known to have a lot of cash in one location, are frequently the targets of robbery. Many robberies are carried out by disguised employees or friends of employees who know the business's procedures. It is good to have a drop policy and make the policy known. A drop is when, during the course of service, a cashier has more than $800 in their drawer (as an example), and a manager or supervisor counts $500, gives the cashier a receipt for the $500 and places the money in a safe or drop box until the end of the shift. This reduces the possible reward of a robbery, reduces temptation, and helps to keep the cashiers and the business more secure. All staff should be trained on what safety procedures to follow during a robbery.

Separate responsibilities. The cashier who processes customers' orders should not be the employee to count the drawer and reconcile the bank at the end of the shift. Ideally, a manager or supervisor should count the drawer and present the totals to the cashier to verify and sign off on the deposit. The cashier should then double check the change bank for the next shift and initial the verification before placing the bank back in the safe.

Designate a secure and private area for counting money and the day's receipts. This area should be video monitored and staff should not be alone with money during the counting process. Use a cash counting machine to verify all hand counts.

Discrepancies should be rectified during the shift that they occur. Most are very simple. Like being $10 short because a manager took $10 to get the cashier a roll of quarters. The manager gets waylaid by a customer complaint and forgets. Any problems that cannot be solved should be recorded in a discrepancy or error log. Cashiers must understand that frequent mistakes will lead to disciplinary action.

Handle deposits securely. Bank deposits should be made daily to reduce the cash on hand. Staff should never transport money alone and ideally should be accompanied by a security guard. Whether the money is going to an actual bank, to an armored car, to the main hospital cashier, or to the university bursar's office, in the absence of an armed guard, vary the route and the timing of trips to make deposits daily.

All staff must be aware that if they witness or suspect theft, that they must report it immediately, cooperate with any investigation, and keep the investigation confidential. Otherwise, the staff member is subject to disciplinary action up to termination.

Go cashless as soon as possible. It is the future and it is safer. Guests will spend more. Tips will increase. It is less time consuming and safer not having cash to deal with. It is more hygienic. There are transaction fees with credit and debit cards, but there are labor savings at the beginning and at the end of each shift. If your business is located where cash is still king, have customers load cash onto a card at a vending machine.

SUMMARY

15.1   Complete and Analyze an Income Statement

- Businesses need bookkeepers, accountants, and an auditors to take care of financial affairs.
- The income statement (profit and loss statement—Table 15-1) reports revenues and expenses for an accounting period. Revenues minus expenses equals profit or loss.
- To calculate cost of sales, add beginning inventory to food purchased for the period, then subtract the ending inventory.
- The general format for an income statement is as follows.

    Gross Sales (total sales)
    – Cost of Sales (food and beverage cost)
    = Gross Profit
    – Controllable Expenses (labor cost, direct operating expenses, etc.)
    = Controllable Income
    – Noncontrollable Expenses (occupancy costs, depreciation, etc.)
    = Net Income or Net Loss before Taxes

- Labor costs include salaries/wages, portion of employee benefits paid by employer, and employer-paid payroll taxes and workers' compensation insurance.
- Direct operating expenses include cleaning supplies, paper supplies, kitchenware, serviceware, laundry, uniforms, exterminating services, and other expenses.
- Administrative expenses are overhead expenses not directly related to serving food and beverages.
- Noncontrollable costs include occupancy costs (rent or mortgage, real estate and

property taxes, property insurance), depreciation, and interest.

- To analyze an income statement, look at the percentages next to each expense. That percentage was calculated by dividing the expense by the total sales. It is useful to compare the data in income statements with previous periods, to the budget, and to standards such as food cost percentage, cost of sales percentage, labor cost percentage, prime cost percentage, and profit margin percentage. Prime cost percentage is the proportion of total sales spent on food, beverages, and labor. It is recommended to keep prime cost about 60 to 70% of sales.

15.2 Complete and Analyze a Balance Sheet

- Whereas an income statement shows activity for a period of time, such as a month or quarter, the balance sheet gives a snapshot of a company at one point in time. The balance sheet (Table 15-3) is set up as follows: Total assets = total liability + owner's equity.
- Assets are anything a company owns with value, such as cash and inventory (current assets). Fixed assets are the tangible permanent resources such as equipment and furniture.
- Liabilities are amounts of money that a business owes. Current liabilities are payable within one year (such as payroll and utility bills) and long-term liabilities (such as loans) are payable beyond a year.
- Owner's equity (also called net worth) is essentially what would be left for the owners from company assets after paying off all liabilities. It is a measure of what has been invested in the business. If the business is a corporation, owner's equity is called shareholder equity and represents the value of corporate stock and retained earnings.
- Debt ratio compares total liabilities with total assets. If the debt ratio is 0.5, it means the company has twice as many assets as liabilities. Lower ratios are better if the business needs to secure a loan.

15.3 Prepare an Operating Budget and Monitor Performance

- A master budget includes an operating budget (forecast of revenue and expenses), a cash budget, and a capital budget.
- Costs in an operating budget are either fixed (such as rent) or variable (such as food).
- The budget process forces management to examine and prioritize the foodservice's goal and objectives. The budget provides a yardstick for measuring department performance and helps managers control costs.
- Flexible and fixed budgets are two examples of incremental budgeting. Zero-based budgets require a manager to justify all expenses because the budget starts at zero.
- Revenue is often broken down into food and alcohol sales. Many noncommercial foodservices have more than one or two revenue centers. In hospitals, patient meals are considered a cost center.
- The two biggest ticket items in the expenses budget are labor and food and beverage.
- Payroll taxes are imposed on employees and employers. Employers must pay half of the FICA dollars (FICA covers Social Security and Medicare) for each employee as well as federal and state unemployment taxes.
- One full-time equivalent (FTE) is normally eight hours per day or 40 hours per workweek (depending on how many hours are considered full-time in the business).
- The steps to plan a budget are: review the objectives for the upcoming fiscal year and review your budget targets, review factors inside and outside of the foodservices that could affect sales and expenses, prepare a budget worksheet (Table 15-6), get opinions and justify the numbers before submitting the budget, and implement the budget once it has been approved.
- To prepare a budget worksheet, first forecast your sales, then your food and beverage costs and labor. Next comes the operating expenses. Now you can check to see if you are hitting your budget targets such as prime cost percentage. The last step is to allocate all line items by month or other accounting period for the next fiscal year, keeping in mind that sales normally vary throughout the year.
- The budgets of noncommercial foodservices often differ from their commercial counterparts in one or two ways: occupancy costs and revenue. Meals may be served for which no revenue is shown on the budget. Then you need to keep records of the number of meals served.
- A budget variance is the difference between the actual and budgeted dollars on one of the budget lines (Table 15-8). Variances are classified as favorable or unfavorable. Variance percentage is calculated as follows. When looking at variance percentage, focus on the size of the percentage and compare

the current month to year-to-date. You will have to do research to find out what is causing unfavorable variances and then develop an action plan to resolve it.

$$\frac{Actual - Budgeted\ Dollars}{Budgeted\ Dollars} \times 100 = Variance\ Percentage$$

15.4 Prepare a Capital Budget

- A capital budget allocates money for *major* investments, such as equipment or building/renovation projects. Capital equipment is considered an asset. The capital budget is separate from the operating budget.
- Paperwork is completed and includes information such as detailed information on the piece of equipment, a description of its intended use and benefits, and how soon the investment will pay for itself.
- Two methods used to evaluate capital investments include payback period (length of time required to earn back the value of an investment from profits or net annual savings) and net present value. The payback period is calculated by dividing the cost of the investment by the net annual savings or profits. The net present value (NPV) of a capital investment is the value of the total revenues (over the life of the equipment) discounted to today's dollars, minus the cost of the capital investment. When the net present value is above zero, the capital investment is desirable.

15.5 Use Financial Analysis Tools

- Comparative financial statements, such as the income statement or balance sheet, compare the results of the two most recent statements by putting them side-by-side (Table 15-11 and 15-12).
- Common-size statements express each line item as a percentage. In a common-size balance sheet (Table 15-13), total assets are given a value of 100% and each type of asset is then expressed as a percentage of that. Total liabilities and owner's equity (together) are also given a value of 100%. Line items on a common-size income statement are expressed as a percentage of total revenue (Table 15-1).
- The break-even point is the point at which the level of sales is equal to a foodservice's combined variable and fixed costs. So, the foodservice is covering its costs but not

generating a profit. The following is the formula used.

$$\frac{Fixed\ costs}{1 - \dfrac{Variable\ costs}{Sales}} = Break\ even\ point\ in\ sales$$

- The Cost-Volume-Profit formula is the same as the break-even formula except profit is added to fixed costs. This formula can be used to show the level of sales needed to reach a desired profit level.
- A ratio can be expressed as a percentage, a per unit ratio (such as sales/customer), or a common ratio. Financial ratios are used to compare or benchmark a business's liquidity, leverage, profitability, or efficiency over time. They often use data from income statements and/or balance sheets. The following are examples.
  - Liquidity looks at the amount of assets a business has that are either in cash form or can be easily sold for cash. One ratio that measures a business' ability to pay its current bills and short-term liabilities is the quick ratio or acid test ratio. If the ratio is below 1, the liquid asset can't cover short-term obligations. Another liquidity ratio, the current ratio, is simply the ratio of current assets to current liabilities. A current ratio of 1.8 means that the business has $1.80 of current assets to pay for each $1.00 of current debt.
  - Leverage ratios, also called solvency ratios, measure a company's ability to pay its bill in the long term. The debt ratio (already mentioned) is an example of a solvency ratio.
  - Profitability ratios compare net income before or after taxes to sales, owners' investments or equity, or total assets. They use information from both the balance sheet and income statement to measure management's effectiveness in using the resources available. Profit margin percentage (already mentioned) is also known as return on sales (ROS). Other profitability ratios, such as return on investment or return on assets, compare net income before or after taxes to owners' investments or equity, or total assets.
  - Activity ratios, also called efficiency ratios, tell you how well assets are being utilized or managed to produce income.

Examples include inventory turnover rate (cost of goods sold *divided by* average inventory value for period), occupancy rate, and seat turnover.

- Operating ratios can help you evaluate your ability to generate sales and control costs. Examples involving sales include average check or cover, sales per square foot, sales per seat, and percentage sales by revenue center. Examples involving costs include food cost percentage, beverage cost percentage, cost of sales percentage, labor cost percentage, prime cost percentage, and profit margin percentage. Another way of looking at costs involves examining costs per meal, such as food cost per meal, labor cost per meal, or prime cost per meal.

- Internal and external trend analysis of costs and other data tells you about the direction the business is heading.

15.6 Measure Productivity

- Productivity shows how effectively inputs (money, labor) are converted into output (meals, revenue). The traditional productivity formula is simply a ratio of output to input. Table 15-14 lists important productivity ratios such as meals per productive labor hour.

- In order to calculate a number of productivity measurements such as meals per labor hour, you must have a single unit of service—a meal. Because there are situations when it is difficult to accurately count meals, such as a cafeteria, the meal equivalent concept was developed. The most common method for calculating a meal equivalent is based on sales. A cafeteria may use average sale per customer as a meal equivalent. Another sales-based approach to determining a meal equivalent would be to add up the average selling price of each item in a typical meal. Some businesses use a cost-based approach to calculating a meal equivalent. Hospitals, for example, may add up the costs of a typical patient meal and use that total as the meal equivalent.

15.7 Control Costs

- Many ways to control costs are listed in the following categories: menu, food cost, labor cost, theft prevention, and cash handling.

REVIEW AND DISCUSSION QUESTIONS

1. What is the difference between accounting and auditing?
2. What is the purpose and format for an income statement?
3. What is the difference between gross profit and net income/net loss before taxes?
4. Why is it important to compare the current income statement with prior ones as well as the budget and standards?
5. List five important standards used in foodservices and why they are important.
6. What is the purpose and format of a balance sheet?
7. Describe each component of a master budget.
8. Distinguish between fixed costs and variable costs.
9. What are the objectives of operating budgets?
10. Compare how a fixed budget, flexible budget, and zero-based budget are prepared.
11. What is an FTE?
12. List the steps in preparing a budget.
13. How is budgeting for a noncommercial foodservice different from a restaurant?
14. When is a budget variance favorable? When is it unfavorable? Give an example of each.
15. What is a comparative balance sheet or income statement? What is a common-size balance sheet or income statement?
16. How do you calculate break-even point for sales?
17. What is ratio analysis? Why is it done? What types of ratios are commonly computed?
18. Give an example of a profitability ratio and how it is calculated.
19. Give an example of an operating ratio and how it is calculated.
20. Describe trend analysis and why it is useful.
21. Give two examples of productivity ratios and how they are calculated.
22. What is a meal equivalent and why is it used?
23. List important ways to control costs.

SMALL GROUP PROJECT

For the foodservice concept that you created in Chapter 1, develop the following.

1. Develop a one-year operating budget similar to that shown in Table 15-6.

2. Using your budget, calculate the following ratios: food cost percentage, sales of sales percentage, labor cost percentage, and prime cost percentage.

3. Calculate two productivity ratios (your choice).

REFERENCES

Association for Healthcare Foodservice. (2019). *Benchmarking: Compare your facility and explore best practices.* https://ahf.memberclicks.net/benchmarkingexpress

Biery, M. E., & Sageworks Stats. (2018). Restaurants' margins are fatter, but competition is fierce. *Forbes.* https://www.forbes.com/sites/sageworks/2018/01/26/restaurants-margins-are-fatter-but-competition-is-fierce/#e519f7527f9f

Bloom Intelligence. (2019). *Restaurant benchmarks.* http://info.bloomintelligence.com/hubfs/Miscellaneous%20Downloads/Restaurant%20Benchmarks.pdf

Callaghan, S., Hawke, K., & Mignerey, C. (2014*). Five myths (and realities) about zero-basedbudgeting.* https://www.mckinsey.com/business-functions/strategy-and-corporate-finance/our-insights/five-myths-and-realities-about-zero-based-budgeting

Chew, W. B. (1988). No-nonsense guide to measuring productivity. *Harvard Business Review, 66*(1), 110–118.

Dopson, L.R. & Hayes, D.K. (2016). *Food & beverage cost control* (6th ed). John Wiley & Sons, Inc.

Drummond, K. (1997). *Developing and using operating budgets.* American Society for Healthcare Food Service Administrators.

Drummond, K. (1997). *Using meal equivalents and cost allocation methods to prepare performance reports.* American Society for Healthcare Food Service Administrators.

Drummond, K. (1998). *Cafeteria cashiering and menu pricing.* American Society for Healthcare Food Service Administrators.

Drummond, K. (1998). *Capital investment analysis.* American Society for Healthcare Food Service Administrators.

Drummond, K. (1998). *Developing staffing plans and labor cost budgets.* American Society for Healthcare Food Service Administrators.

Drummond, K. (1998). *Financial analysis tools.* American Society for Healthcare Food Service Administrators.

Gregoire, M. B., Theis, M. L. (2015). Practice paper of the Academy of Nutrition and Dietetics: Principles of productivity in food and nutrition services: Applications in the 21st century healthcare reform era. *Journal of the Academy of Nutrition and Dietetics, 115*(7), 1141–1147.

Hale, R. (2020). *How to create your restaurant marketing budget.* https://pos.toasttab.com/blog/on-the-line/restaurant-marketing-budget

Hand, R., Jordan, B., DeHoog, S., Pavlinac, J., Abram. J. K., & Parrott, J. S. (2015). Inpatient staffing needs for registered dietitian nutritionists in 21st century acute care facilities. *Journal of the Academy of Nutrition and Dietetics, 115*(6), 985–1000.

Phillips, W. (2015). Clinical nutrition staffing benchmarks for acute care hospitals. *Journal of the Academy of Nutrition and Dietetics, 115*(7), 1054–1056.

Phillips, W., Janowski, M., Brennan, H., & Leger, G. (2019). Analyzing registered dietitian nutritionist productivity benchmarks for acute care hospitals. *Journal of the Academy of Nutrition and Dietetics, 119*(12), 1985–1991.

Reynolds, D. & McClusky, K. W. (2013). *Foodservice management fundamentals.* John Wiley & Sons, Inc.

© Denis Val/Shutterstock

Marketing and Business Plans

LEARNING OUTCOMES

16.1 Explain the consumer decision-making process and factors that influence it.

16.2 Develop the marketing plan.

16.3 Write a business plan.

INTRODUCTION

According to the American Marketing Association, **marketing** can be defined as follows: "Marketing is the activity and processes for creating, communicating, delivering, and exchanging offerings that have value for customers, clients, partners, and society at large." (AMA, 2017).

The "offerings" mentioned in the definition refer to products or services offered by both for-profit and nonprofit businesses. Products are tangible, while services are intangible—you can't see or touch them. Whether marketing a product or service, marketers want to satisfy consumer wants and needs with products or services they want or need. A consumer's wants and needs are different. For instance, you may go to the drug store because you *need* Advil but end up also buying a magazine there because you *want* to read the cover story. A **want** is a good or service that is desired but not absolutely needed. A **need** is necessary.

Over time, marketing has evolved, resulting in more and more focus on the consumer. At the turn of the 20th century, consumers did not have many purchasing choices and most goods were produced in the region where they lived. Once cars became more common in the 1920s and more roads were built, businesses hired traveling salespeople who greatly increased competition among companies. This era of marketing was known as the "sales era" as businesses increased their selling efforts and worked to sell more product. The "marketing era" started after World War II when many Americans returned from the war effort and started households, which increased the need for products and services. During the war, many businesses had a great deal of scientific and technical innovation that found civilian uses after the war, such as the microwave oven. For the first time, many businesses started to study consumers and decide which products or services they most wanted or needed.

Sales-oriented businesses focus on selling what they make rather than making what the market wants. They are more focused on making a sale than developing a relationship with the consumer. Market-oriented businesses describe themselves as not just selling goods and services but benefits to targeted consumers. Their focus is on customers and becoming aware of their ever-changing needs as well as finding creative ways to satisfy them. Since the marketing era started, it has also progressed from focusing on gaining a larger share of the overall market to retaining customers and developing customer loyalty. Indeed, **relationship marketing** is when a business works to develop long-term connections for the customer that benefit both the customer and the business.

The marketing of a foodservice influences how customers set their expectations. A foodservice needs to appropriately market its products (food) and service so customers have realistic expectations. For marketing to be successful, the business must realize a need to be responsive to the market, have the capacity to respond, and take actionable steps. This chapter will walk you through the basics of marketing, including consumer behavior, the marketing plan, and business plans.

16.1 EXPLAIN THE CONSUMER DECISION-MAKING PROCESS AND FACTORS THAT INFLUENCE IT

Consumers want goods/services that work for them and their individual preferences. If a marketer can connect with a customer's values and interests, while providing for the individual's needs, the customer may become a partner or stakeholder in the product. With luck, frequent communication, and mutually beneficial exchanges, a long-term loyal relationship can develop between the brand and the consumer. If you know people who always buy Ford trucks, Starbucks coffee, Vans or Converse shoes, Ray Ban sunglasses, iPhones, or Levi's Jeans, you have seen this loyalty first hand.

In order to capture consumers' attention and market to them appropriately, you need to understand consumer behavior. According to Solomon (2011, p. 7), **consumer behavior** is the "study of the processes involved when individuals or groups select, purchase, use, or dispose of products, services, ideas, or experiences to satisfy needs and desires." This definition not only looks at how consumers decide whether to make a purchase but it also looks at how marketers influence consumers.

Value plays an important role in purchasing something. **Value** looks at the relationship between the advantages or benefits the buyer gets from a purchase and the sacrifice (i.e., the money spent) that was required. A purchase can provide a wide variety of benefits such as convenience, satisfaction, or relief from hunger. You buy something based on perceived value, in other words, what benefits you expect to get from the purchase. Consumers not only make purchases for the benefits but also for what the purchase means to them in terms of status, reputation, or quality.

According to Lamb, Hair, & McDaniel (2021), there are four different aspects of value.

1. Useful. Will the purchase help save time or effort? Will it make a task easier to complete? Will it increase safety? Will it solve a problem? Will the purchase fill an immediate need (such as food or gas) or a personal need (such as for prestige)?
2. Emotional. Will the purchase be fun and entertaining or provide satisfaction and perhaps happiness? Will the purchase contribute to your health or sense of belonging and make you feel good about yourself? Does the product appeal to your senses or fill a need for something different?
3. Life-changing. Will the purchase provide hope or motivation to do something meaningful and/or different?
4. Social impact. Will the purchase help others, help the environment, or just somehow make the world a better place?

When you purchase something, it often provides more than just one aspect of value. For instance, having dinner out in a nice restaurant provides enjoyment and variety (emotional) as well as fills the need to eat (useful).

Traditionally there are five steps in the consumer purchasing and decision-making process (**Figure 16–1**). A consumer is more likely to go through all of the steps when making an expensive or new type of purchase. Buyers do not take as much time or effort when purchasing low-cost goods or goods that are purchased frequently, such as pasta at the grocery store. In the case of foods, buyers are familiar with at least several brands in a category, and may routinely select one brand. Even if a buyer tries a new brand of, for example, spaghetti sauce, it allows the buyer a chance to evaluate it. For more expensive or unfamiliar purchases, the buyer usually wants to evaluate the product *before* purchase.

The following is a discussion of the consumer decision-making process. A consumer may, of course, skip a step or stop at any point and not make a purchase.

1. <u>Become aware of a want or need</u>. This step is triggered by an internal or (usually) external stimuli that makes the consumer aware that there is a gap between what he or she has and what he or she would like to have. For instance, a parent is about to drive past a favorite pizza restaurant and decides to pick up a hot pizza on the way home from work instead of heating up frozen pizza for dinner. Even though it costs more, it will save time and the family will be happy to eat fresh pizza. Recognizing a want or need can also be caused by a display at a store, a conversation with a friend who made a new purchase, or an advertisement on your video feed or in a magazine. A stimulus can also be sensory through hearing, sight, smell, taste or touch, as in the smell of coffee and cinnamon when you enter a bakery.

2. <u>Gather information and narrow down possibilities</u>. This involves an internal information search (recalling information from previous experiences) and external information search (seeking information from the environment). According to Lamb, Hair, & McDaniel (2021), external information is from a source that is *nonmarketing controlled* (meaning it is not associated with marketers promoting anything) or a source that is *marketing controlled* (meaning marketers are promoting a product). Nonmarketing-controlled sources include speaking with other people who give their evaluations of products they have purchased, unbiased

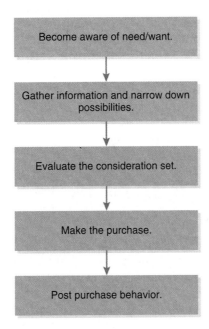

FIGURE 16-1 Consumer Decision-Making Process

sources of information such as *Consumer Reports*, opinion sites such as Yelp or tripadvisor.com, or social media posts made by family or friends. A big source of nonmarketing-controlled information used by many Americans are the reviews and evaluations of products that can be found on Amazon and other websites. Many websites only allow actual users to post reviews to limit any control of marketers.

Marketing-controlled sources of information include advertisements using various media, sales promotions (such as displays, contests, etc.), product packaging, and social media. After gathering information, the consumer has often narrowed down their choices into a list called the buyer's **evoked set** or **consideration set**.

3. Evaluate the consideration set. To evaluate the consideration set, the consumer often decides on some criteria that the purchase should meet. The criteria could include a maximum price or a required attribute. The consumer may also put the possible choices into categories to help make a decision on which product to purchase. The evaluation process is not always objective or rational. Behavioral economists tell us that we do use emotions when making purchasing decisions. They also say that when we are given too many purchase options, it can lead to decision-making paralysis.

4. Make the purchase. If the buyer decides to make this purchase, they must also decide where to buy it and how to pay for it. More expensive items are normally planned purchases that require more time and effort. Less-expensive items are more likely to be unplanned or impulse purchases. Impulse purchases are more likely when products are on sale or the buyer has a coupon.

5. Post-purchase behavior. Post-purchase behavior depends in part on whether the product met the expectations of the buyer and gave satisfaction or dissatisfaction. Expectations tend to rise with the price of the product. If the product did not meet a consumer's expectations, it creates tension, and the consumer may contact the company and write poor reviews on the Internet or social media. Superior customer service can help keep a customer. Marketing works to develop profitable customer relationships, meaning they want satisfied customers who will be loyal to the brand.

The process just described is the traditional straight-line approach. More recently, other models have been developed that describe what is called the **consumer decision journey**. Edelman and Singer (2015) describe how technology has changed this process: "The explosion of digital technologies over the past decade has created 'empowered' consumers so expert in their use of tools and information that they can call the shots, hunting down what they want when they want it and getting it delivered to their doorsteps at a rock-bottom price." (p. 88) **Figure 16-2** gives examples of digital marketing

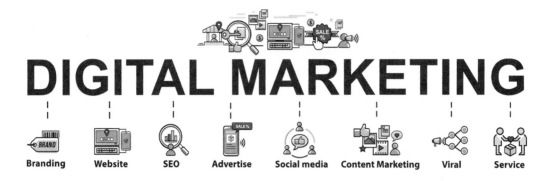

FIGURE 16-2 Digital Marketing

© Buffaloboy/Shutterstock

Streamlining the Decision Journey

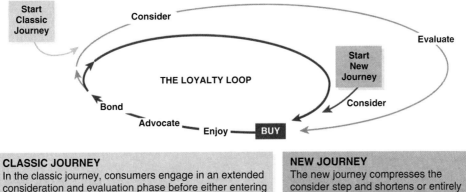

FIGURE 16-3 The Consumer Decision Journey

Reproduced from "Competing on Customer Journeys," by D.C. Edelman and M. Singer, 2015, *Harvard Business Review, 93*(11), p. 89. Reprinted with permission.

technologies (technologies that use an electronic device) and also includes branding and person-to-person service.

As **Figure 16-3** indicates, the consumer, while in the traditional process, may settle on a particular brand and then continues to buy within that brand. This is called the *customer loyalty loop* and illustrates how consumers don't spend as much time considering and evaluating options. When the consumer buys products within the brand and is happy with the purchases, they may advocate for and bond with the brand. Companies that succeed in getting loyal customers work to gather information about customers in order to personalize and customize their purchasing experiences as well as to offer new sources of value (in other words, related products).

Foodservice companies, such as Starbucks, often offer loyalty programs in which consumers receive rewards based on what they spend. Phone apps, such as the Starbucks app, are excellent vehicles for loyalty programs and also encourage customers to place orders for pickup. Loyalty programs are quite popular in foodservice.

There are many factors that influence consumers when making purchase decisions, such as cultural, individual, psychological, and social factors. Cultural factors, including norms, values, and attitudes, likely exert the most influence. Social class also influences what consumers purchase and how marketers communicate. Individual factors include gender, age, self-concept, and lifestyle. Psychological factors look at a consumer's motivation and perception—how consumers select and interpret stimuli such as product design or price. Lastly, social influences are important too. Most consumers regularly ask others for opinions about products, services, or brands. Consumers may use products or services to identify with an opinion leader, a reference group they belong to (such as family) or a group they would like to join (an **aspirational reference group**). Consumers also avoid making certain purchases if it would associate them with a certain lifestyle or group they want to keep away from. For instance, an affluent, middle-aged woman may not want to be seen picking up burgers at a fast food restaurant.

16.2 DEVELOP THE MARKETING PLAN

The **marketing plan** is a document that describes a business' marketing objectives, broad strategies, and specific tactics to achieve the objectives. Developing the marketing plan starts with strategic planning. Strategic planning (discussed in Chapter 12) is a

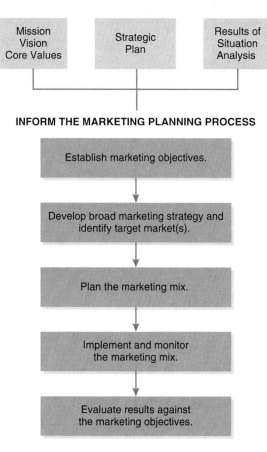

FIGURE 16-4 The Marketing Plan

broad process that looks at the entire business or a part of the business such as marketing. A company's strategic plan should inform the marketing plan (**Figure 16-4**).

START THE MARKETING PLAN

Strategic planning generally starts with a review of the business' mission statement and a situation analysis, both of which will be reviewed here. A **mission** is a broad statement describing what the business does, why the business exists and what purpose it serves for its customers. To expand on their mission statements, many companies nowadays are also listing their **core values** (such as commitment to the local community) or including a **vision** statement that describes their future expectations, including how the organization wants to impact the communities it serves. These statements function as the values the organization wants to project to their internal customers (employees) and external consumers. The mission and vision statements often set the benchmarks for the organization's policies.

An excellent tool for understanding the environment in which a business may launch a new product or service is a **SWOT analysis**, a type of situation analysis in which you identify the strengths and weaknesses *inside your business* and also the opportunities and threats in the *external environment*. Performing a SWOT analysis also helps businesses identify their competitive advantage.

A **competitive advantage** is something unique that is different from and superior to what your competitors offer, such as outstanding value, ambiance, excellence in hospitality and service, or low prices. It is why consumers come to your foodservice and not somewhere else. A competitive advantage generally relies on being competitive on costs (think of fast-food restaurants), product/service differentiation (think of the huge menu at Cheesecake Factory) or serving a niche market (Lamb et al., 2021). A product-service differentiation refers to something offered to consumers that is unique and valuable (other than low prices). Cheesecake Factory is unique because of its many-page menu and also its large portions. A **niche market** is a segment within your target audience that is not being served or not being well served. For instance, fast casual restaurants started out serving a niche market—consumers who wanted someplace to eat that was a notch above fast-food restaurants but didn't require table service.

Whichever competitive advantage a foodservice has, it is important to be able to maintain that advantage in the marketplace. What is called a **sustainable competitive advantage** is one that no competitor can copy (it has nothing to do with being environmentally conscientious, although an organization's sustainable competitive advantage may actually be related to sustainability). If your competitive advantage is that you have low prices (and manage to be profitable), other foodservices can try to imitate that.

In a SWOT analysis, *strengths* look at what your foodservice does well, such as having excellent service or other quality that separates you from your competitors. *Weaknesses* force you to look at what your foodservice lacks or could be doing better, such as lowering food costs or getting help with marketing.

When looking at the external environment, you need to consider the current situation (the state of the industry and your position in it), as well as future changes in the marketplace that could affect you from an economic, competitive, regulatory, or technological perspective. Marketing research is useful to analyze the market and get information about the size and sales potential of various groups of consumers in the area, as well as assess the competition.

Marketing research is the systematic gathering and analysis of data (quantitative and qualitative) related to marketing decisions. Many private marketing companies provide lifestyle and other information about particular consumer markets. For example, NPD Group, Inc. continually collects data for the foodservice industry, such as market share information and consumer purchasing trends. They publish reports on a variety of topics including restaurant delivery and eating patterns in the United States. Marketing companies often use techniques such as survey research, interviews, and focus groups. The Internet is increasingly being used to conduct surveys. **Table 16–1** lists sources of business and marketing data available from the federal government.

In a SWOT analysis, *opportunities* are possible areas for you to do more business, such as underserved markets or increased need for some of your products. Opportunities include any external factors, such as consumers supporting sustainable foods, that could positively impact your foodservice. External *threats*, such as increasing competition,

Table 16-1 Sources of Business and Marketing Data From the Federal Government		
Focus	**Goal**	**Reference**
General business statistics	Find statistics on industries, business conditions	NAICS, USA.gov Statistics, Statistical Abstract of the United States, U.S. Census Bureau
Consumer statistics	Gain information on potential customers, consumer markets	Consumer Credit Data, Consumer Product Safety
Demographics	Segment the population for targeting customers	American FactFinder, Bureau of Labor Statistics
Economic indicators	Know unemployment rates, loans granted, and more	Consumer Price Index, Bureau of Economic Analysis
Employment statistics	Dig deeper into employment trends for your market	Employment and Unemployment Statistics
Income statistics	Pay your employees fair rates based on earnings data	Bureau of Labor Statistics, U.S. Census Bureau

(continues)

Table 16-1 Sources of Business and Marketing Data From the Federal Government (continued)		
Focus	**Goal**	**Reference**
Money and interest rates	Keep money by mastering exchange and interest rates	Daily Interest Rates, Money Statistics via Federal Reserve
Production and sales statistics	Understand demand, costs, and consumer spending	Consumer Spending, Gross Domestic Product (GDP)
Statistics of specific industries	Use a wealth of federal agency data on industries	NAICS, Statistics of U.S. Businesses

Market Research and Competitive Analysis. U.S. Small Business Administration. 2020. https://www.sba.gov/business-guide/plan-your-business/market-research-competitive-analysis.

a shift in consumer behavior, a downturn in the economy, increasing food prices, or new/revised regulations, can disrupt your foodservice. **Table 16–2** gives an example of a SWOT analysis for a self-operated university foodservice.

After the SWOT analysis, the next step is to formulate the marketing plan while keeping in mind the business' mission and strategic plan. The marketing plan includes these steps, although quite often some of these steps are worked on together.

1. Establish marketing objectives.
2. Develop the broad marketing strategy.
3. Formulate an action plan (called the **marketing mix**).
4. Implement and monitor the marketing mix.
5. Evaluate the marketing efforts against the objectives.

Managers should consider marketing objectives that flow from the mission and strategic plan, and also build on strengths, correct weaknesses, exploit external opportunities, and counter threats identified in the SWOT analysis. **Marketing objectives** explain what is to be accomplished through marketing activities and include quantitative measures that are used to confirm if the objective has been accomplished. For example, a marketing objective for a foodservice might be to increase the first-time visitor return rate from 25% to 35% within one year. (The first-time visitor return rate tells you the percentage of first-time customers within the past year who returned again at least once within the same time period.)

The next step is to develop the marketing strategy. This involves determining the broad strategy along with the target market. The **target market** is the specific group of consumers to whom a company plans to market its product/services. A **market** is

Table 16-2 SWOT Analysis for University Foodservice		
Internal Factors	**Strengths** • High satisfaction ratings from students, faculty, and administration in self-operated foodservice. • Cutting-edge menu. • Newly renovated production facilities with extra capacity. • Qualified employees. • Supportive administration.	**Weaknesses** • Retention of quality cooking personnel can be challenging. • Food costs a little higher than desired. • Outdated Point of Sale system.
External Factors	**Opportunities** • More local farms offering organic products. • Local senior meal programs looking for prepared meals.	**Threats** • College-age population/enrollment in decline. • Area colleges being approached by foodservice contract companies. • Increasing threat in food supply of foodborne illness.

any group of people with needs and wants who can purchase something. A **market segment** is a subgroup of people who share one or more characteristics, such as income or age, that may cause them to have similar needs for a product. Each segment responds differently to a marketing offer.

Marketers use characteristics, called **variables**, of individuals (or groups) to divide a market into segments. Markets can be segmented by one variable, such as age, or multiple variables. Marketers often use one or more of these variables.

1. Geography (region of a country or the world, market size, urban vs. rural, climate)
2. Demographics (age, gender, income, education, ethnic background, family situation)
3. Psychographics (values, attitudes, interests, lifestyles, aspirations, personality traits, motivations)
4. Purchasing and spending habits
5. Benefits desired (from a product)
6. Usage-rate (amount of product purchased)

There are also other variables such as social consciousness.

In selecting a target market, a foodservice can treat the entire market as one group of customers (referred to as **mass marketing**) or use market segmentation. **Market segmentation** is a powerful marketing tool that divides a market into distinct groups of buyers with similar variables (such as college-educated women over 65) who likely have similar product needs, as just discussed. A foodservice may decide to focus on one segment or more than one segment (referred to as **multisegment marketing**). In the case of multisegment marketing, the marketing mix (to be discussed) for each target market is often totally different, but they could overlap.

To identify segments, you have to select some of the variables just discussed. The choice of variables is usually determined by the type of product or service. Quite often, some variables from each of these categories are used: geography, demographics, psychographics, and purchasing and spending habits. For example, for a family-friendly restaurant, you may choose a geographic area and some demographic variables, such as age, income, and family situation, as well as purchasing and spending habits. For each segment, the profile should include information about the segment's current size and expected growth, purchase frequency, brand loyalty, and sales potential. For an existing foodservice, you can examine and analyze who your current customers are by doing an audience analysis and using business data and website analytics.

Once you have identified some segments that might be appropriate, you select those you want to target. Many companies will just choose one to three target markets, but it varies depending on the situation. You want each segment to be large enough to justify its own marketing mix and you also want to be able to identify each segment's wants and needs. You also want every customer to be associated with just one segment and be accessible to marketers in some way.

Keeping the target market in mind, the foodservice can now consider some broad strategies to meet its objectives. If your marketing objective is to get more repeat business, and your target audience values convenience, you could make it easier for customers to order take-out with a new phone app and offer curb-side pickup. If the target audience is looking for rewards, the foodservice may consider developing a loyalty program. Each strategy will have a different price tag, so a budget is usually developed at this point.

DEVELOP THE MARKETING MIX

Once you have identified your target market(s) and a broad strategy, it is time to develop your marketing mix. The **marketing mix** is the set of controllable marketing tools that a company uses to produce a desired response from its target market. It is the precise roadmap of the activities that will help achieve the marketing objective. Known as the 4 Ps, it includes: product, price, place, and promotion. However, in retail businesses, we add two more Ps: personnel and presentation. The closer the product or service are targeted using the six Ps to a particular market's unique characteristics, behaviors, and attitudes, the greater the likelihood of getting a positive response.

Before discussing the 6 Ps, we need to discuss the concepts of brand and differentiation. A **brand** is a feature or set of features (such as name, logo, tagline, design, quality, customer experience) that distinguish one product/service from that of the competition. The concept of a brand also includes how these features are perceived by customers. Brands that are well-received by customers can help expand the customer base and increase revenue. **Differentiation** is a marketing strategy to help consumers distinguish your product/service from others. For example, Wendy's makes hamburgers only with meat that has never been frozen. Of course, you can offer distinctive service, serve unique dishes, and have low prices. But, according to MacMillan and McGrath (1997), you can differentiate yourself at any point from when consumers realize they have a want or need. For example, you can differentiate your product/service/customer experience by:

- How consumers find your product (such as Starbucks inside of Target stores).
- How consumers buy your product (such as using a phone app to order).
- How products are delivered (such as by robots).
- How products are paid for (such as using your debit card within the Starbucks app).
- How packaging is disposed of (such as using recyclable materials).

Successful brands connect with the consumer and have a reputation for quality and value. Think of some well-known foodservice brands, such as Dunkin' or Starbucks. If you have a positive connection with either brand, you are probably thinking about a hot coffee beverage in a cup with the logo on it and how you would love to have one right now.

The following is a discussion of each of the 6 Ps.

- <u>Product</u> is the good or service, and also includes, as appropriate, the packaging, brand name, logo, and any guarantee or warranty. The concept of product also includes the value/benefits for the consumer, the nature of the buyer's total experience, and what differentiates this product from others. Having a brand allows a business to distinguish its products from all others and also encourages repeat sales. A foodservice often uses national brands, such as Coca-Cola, and can also develop its own brand, called an **in-house or signature brand**. For example, a foodservice contractor decided to brand its café concept and called it Jazzman's Café. A foodservice can also brand one of its products, such as pizza or coffee. In response to changing food tastes and trends, new products are almost always being considered and some will be test marketed by the larger foodservice companies. New ways to get food to customers, such as the growth of curbside pickup during a pandemic, are frequently studied so as to better serve customers.
- <u>Price</u> is how much is being charged for the product/service. Of all of the Ps, this is the one that can be changed the quickest. In pricing, sellers need to consider the cost of the product and profit to be made, prices of competitors, demand, availability, customer loyalty, and payment methods. To the consumer, the price must indicate a good value for exchange of cash or credit. Price is also important in a foodservice's positioning strategy. Higher prices often indicate higher quality and reinforce the image of a more expensive foodservice such as found in fine dining. Lower prices are often more appropriate for a product when it is first introduced as a way to reach more people. To protect against sales slumps, foodservices offer lower prices in the form of deals and special promotions,

such as $5 footlong hoagies or 2 for 1 pizzas, to increase orders. Some restaurants are experimenting with dynamic pricing, which means prices are adjusted based on customer demand—such as higher prices during the weekend and lower prices during the workweek. Dynamic pricing works better when you don't have a printed menu, so it is more useful when customers order on a delivery platform such as GrubHub.

- <u>Place</u> includes everywhere that the seller makes the product or service available to the market. This includes retail stores, websites, phone apps, and placement on social media. Picking the best location for a foodservice, such as a restaurant, includes a lot of considerations, such as if the location is visible and convenient for customers, traffic flow, parking availability, zoning regulations, cost, and safety and security. Ghost kitchens don't have a storefront or dining room but only have a kitchen space (possibly shared) to produce meals for delivery. Pop-up shops use a current foodservice for short periods of time. A part of this P is also physical distribution—which involves getting the product/service to where it is needed in good condition. With the increase in food delivery to homes, getting the food there so it tastes and looks great can be a real challenge. Some pizza parlors limit delivery to within just a few miles of the store or limit how many orders are taken for delivery at one time to improve its quality.

- **Promotion** includes communications by marketers that mainly *inform*, *remind*, and/or *persuade* potential buyers to purchase something. Promotion is also used to simply *connect* to the target market. Your market research can help you determine the communication channels and activities that will best reach your target segment and build your brand's reputation. **Table 16-3** list different forms of promotion, including advertising, public relations, sales promotion, personal selling, and social media and content marketing. You can inform, remind, and persuade consumers through paid ads, video marketing (including using influencers), Facebook, newspaper, publicity, direct mail, infomercials, outdoor billboards and graphics on buildings, sponsorship of events or public radio programs, and word of mouth. For many foodservices, effective methods of generating immediate sales are personal selling (suggestive selling) and sales promotion. These are also the ideal methods for interacting with customers, getting feedback and suggestions, and performing service recovery and generating good will. Table 16-3 lists different forms of promotion.

Table 16-3 Forms of Promotion

1. **Advertising** (any form of *paid* presentation or promotion of an idea, product, or service where the brand or sponsor is clearly identified). Advertising is a one-way communication targeted at the target audience(s). Traditional advertising is found in newspapers, magazines, and television. Nowadays, more advertising money is being used on digital advertising, meaning advertising on the Internet and social media sites. While the cost of advertising is high, it does communicate to a lot of people so the cost per contact is low.

2. **Public relations** (the act of promoting a product or service by building good relationships with the public and potential consumers). People working in public relations communicate information about a company, product or service to various media, such as in a cooking column that appears online or in a newspaper or magazine. Public relations specialists generate positive publicity for their clients and the products and services they sell. What makes public relations different is that they persuade audiences via *unpaid* methods. They do so by writing for the web, writing pitches about a product that is sent to journalists and others, creating special events, and writing and distributing press releases. A **press release** is a brief news story with contact information that is sent to targeted members of the media. The purpose of the press release is to make an announcement (such as a new product or a foodservice sponsoring a local 10K run), provide information, and hope the news will be picked up and distributed. Public relations employees also control a brand's image on social media and work to dispel unfavorable reviews, rumors, and stories that negatively affect the brand.

(continues)

Table 16-3 Forms of Promotion (continued)

3. **Sales promotion** (incentives to stimulate sales of a product or service). These are usually short term such as free samples, coupons, contests, or rebates. They also include point-of-purchase displays. Sales promotions complement advertising.

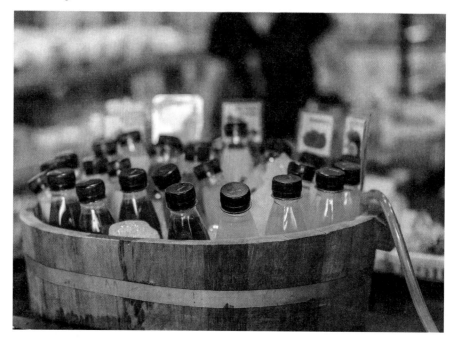

Example of a Point-of-Purchase Display

© John and Penny/Shutterstock

4. **Personal selling** (when a person with great interpersonal skills and trained in sales techniques, demonstrates the product, gives samples, or simply delivers information). Personal selling builds relationships with consumers and increases the perceived value of a product or service. While personal selling works better face-to-face, it can also be done on the phone or Internet.

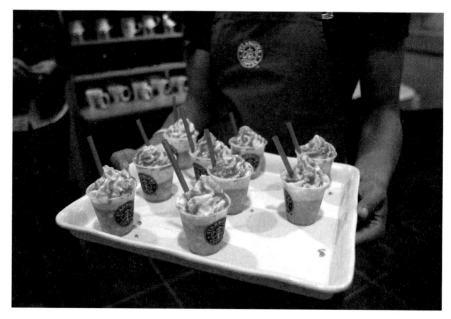

Example of Personal Selling

© Rblfmr/Shutterstock

5. Social media and content marketing. **Content marketing** is a type of marketing that involves the creation and distribution of materials (such as blogs and videos) intended to attract a specific audience and stimulate interest and purchases. This requires the foodservice or brand to develop positive promotional content, such as in written and video formats, and then use digital marketing, search engine optimization, and social media to attract customers to the business's website or social media channel. **Search engine optimization** is the practice of optimizing a website so it will appear toward the top of searches by search engines. Content marketing generates positive buzz about the brand and encourages conversations in the media, such as Twitter posts. Social media such as Facebook, YouTube, TikTok, Periscope, Reddit, and Tumblr are used to distribute videos, photos, and/or posts. Podcasts can be used and distributed on social networks (Facebook, Pinterest, LinkedIn, Instagram, and Snapchat). Consumers can speak directly with other consumers and the company on social media. In this manner, marketers are using social media as important parts of marketing campaigns. As global competition for the attention of consumers intensifies, controlling what shoppers see on digital media is becoming more vital to marketers.

- <u>Personnel</u> Service employees with excellent interpersonal skills can help your foodservice attract new customers and retain customers as they shape the customer experience. How service employees interact with customers and meet their needs and wants influence the success of the business. Service employees can not only help provide an excellent service experience but can also use suggestive selling to increase sales.
- <u>Presentation</u> Atmosphere is the most important element of a foodservice's presentation. Any part of a foodservice that influences the way guests experience dining will contribute positively or negatively to the restaurant's atmosphere. This can include the physical layout, tabletop appearance, furnishings, lighting, music, employee appearance, and how the food is presented.

SPOTLIGHT ON PROMOTIONS IN ONSITE FOODSERVICES

Onsite cafeterias found in businesses, schools, colleges, hospitals, and other healthcare organizations have somewhat captive customers. Sure, a high school student could bring lunch from home and a business employee can eat lunch out. To maintain interest and excitement in the cafeteria, foodservice managers like to have a long menu cycle and they also like to develop and implement a wide variety of promotions. The following are some examples.

- Feature daily Chef's specials that bundle an entrée with one side to add variety and offer value.
- Highlight sustainable options such as organic or locally sourced foods as well as healthy alternatives.
- Make Grab-and-Go foods easy to pick up, such as by using mobile kiosks.
- Every month, have a special events day where the main meals have a theme. The theme could be related to a holiday (such as Valentine's Day), a sports event (such as Opening Day for a local team), a cuisine from anywhere in the world, or national food holidays such as National Pancake Day. You can get some ideas for special promotions from your food distributors as well as theme day materials and foods.
- Ask customers to bring in their favorite recipes for the chef to make and possibly add to the menu.
- Offer combos such as half sandwich or wrap and a small soup.
- Develop a loyalty program in which customers build up points through number of visits, amount spent, or items purchased (such as cups of coffee).
- Offer discounts off of whole meals or offer buy one, get one free.
- Offer coupons, such as for a free cup of coffee.

When planning a special promotion, it is important to gauge whether a sufficient number of your customers are interested and if the idea is consistent with the organization's mission. If the idea looks like a good one, plan well in advance and speak to a variety of people. The cost of any promotion needs to be compared with its benefits so you don't wreck your budget. Design a written plan, including objectives, that includes all details and exactly how the plan will be executed. Review the plan with employees. After the promotion, evaluate the results against the objectives.

As businesses attempt to connect with consumers and form lasting and financially beneficial relationships, they will need to market themselves in ways that give customers faith, trust, and confidence in the products and the brand behind the products. There are several ways to accomplish this.

- <u>Corporate social responsibility</u>. A business should be depended upon to do what is right, fair, and responsible. That includes delivery of promised services, honoring warranties, protecting consumer's private information, protecting the environment, and preventing foodborne illness or food recalls. The business should not violate wage and hour laws, abuse exempt staff, or allow discrimination or sexual harassment. In other words, they should play by the rules and treat all stakeholders with care and respect. Not all businesses engage in corporate social responsibility because "profit is king" may still be the philosophy at the boardroom or investor level.
- <u>Cause marketing</u>. Cause marketing refers to marketing programs by for-profit brands based on a social or charitable cause. It can also involve a collaborative effort between a for-profit company and a non-profit for mutual benefit. Many businesses gain customer faith and repeat business by marketing causes and even other brands. *Newman's Own* foods promote "all profits to charity." Ben & Jerry's Ice Cream pledged money to activist organizations, including the Women's March, from the sales of a limited-edition ice cream. At the local level, small businesses such as restaurants support youth sports, volunteer fire departments, and food banks.
- **Green marketing**. Green marketing indicates that a business is doing all that it can to improve the environment and minimize damage caused by its production and business practices. These practices include using more organic products, using less water and more Energy Star Appliances, buying nontoxic cleaning products, and supporting animal rights. Green marketers tout sustainability, which is not only attractive to young consumers, but 4 out of 10 Americans claim to be dedicated to purchasing green products. (Lamb, Hair, & McDaniel, 2021) **Greenwashing** is a term used to describe corporations who give the impression of being environmentally conscious whether or not the company is really being environmentally friendly.
- **Social marketing**. Social marketing creates programs designed to influence human behavior on a large scale, such as making environmentally sound food choices.

IMPLEMENT AND EVALUATE THE MARKETING PLAN

Once the marketing plan is developed, it needs to be turned into a series of specific actions and steps. Someone will need to determine who is going to be involved, what they will do, and when they will do it. The marketing plan may call for involving other parties such as a public relations firm or an advertising department. It is important that employees are involved in developing the marketing plan so that they buy into the work that needs to be done. It is important to gain everyone's acceptance of the plan.

Once the plan is implemented, it is time to monitor how the implementation went and start to evaluate marketing results. To evaluate any marketing plan, you can go back to the objectives and measure how well the plan succeeded. Some common ways to evaluate the success of marketing efforts include the following.

- Sales: How many products did you sell? What were your projected and actual sales?
- Profit: How much profit did you make?
- Website: Did the website and Facebook traffic go up? How many requested additional information? How many became leads? How many became new customers?

It is also helpful to review how close to budget the project was.

16.3 WRITE A BUSINESS PLAN

Planning a new business or doing a renovation of an existing facility *begins* with formulating the details of the project into a written plan known as a **business plan** or **prospectus**. The business plan explains why the project is important (the rationale) and the goals of the project, such as serving new customers and being profitable. A business plan describes the business in detail and is used to seek and secure approvals and/or loans. It includes the following sections.

1. **Company Overview**. This section includes a description of the business including its mission and vision. This section also includes information about the company's key products or services, its customers, major business goals and objectives, the size and organization of the business, backgrounds of key members of the team, and the company's history and profitability (as applicable). State whether you have or intend to incorporate your business, form a partnership, or form a limited liability company. (In a corporation or limited liability company, your personal assets won't be at risk in case of lawsuits or bankruptcy.) Explain the competitive advantages that make the business a success. In the case of an existing business that is planning an expansion or renovation, the goal and objectives of the project should be explained.

2. **Industry Analysis**. The industry, such as fast casual restaurants, needs to be described, including whether this segment is growing, mature, or (hopefully not) declining. Barriers to entry are noted as well as the typical customer profile and an analysis of the competition (who are the major competitors and what are their products' pricing, benefits, and positioning).

3. **Operating Plan**. This section includes details about the location of the business; the menu; how much total space is needed and how the space will be allocated to each function; business operations including who will manage it, when it will be open, and how foods will be purchased, produced, and served; who the customers will be and how many will be served; the labor needed and salaries/wages; how regulatory requirements will be met; and how the operation will be unique.

4. **Marketing Analysis and Plan**. The market analysis includes detailed information on your target market (including demographics such as age and level of education) and an analysis of who are the competing businesses in the area. Competitive research will show what other businesses are doing and what their strengths are. The marketing plan starts with marketing objectives and describes what is unique about your business. The marketing plan explains how you will attract and keep customers using your product or service including pricing and customer benefits. The marketing plan also discusses how the company will promote and distribute the product/service to prospective customers (such as home delivery, etc.).

5. **Financial Feasibility Study**. The financial feasibility study examines the start-up costs for a new business or the renovation/expansion costs for an existing business. For a new business, you have to develop a projected **profit and loss statement** in which you project your sales and expenses (food, beverage, labor, lease, etc.) for a period of time, such as four or five years. By projecting sales and expenses, you can estimate your net profit/loss. A cash-flow statement is also useful as you need to forecast how money will flow in and out of your business so that you don't run out of money during the start-up phase. For a renovation, the costs of the project must be fully laid out and justified through, for example, increased sales or cost savings. The financial plan will need to show how the business can pay for building or renovation costs and succeed financially over time.

6. **Funding Request**. If you're asking for funding, this is where to outline how much you will need and the length of time your request will cover. Give a detailed description of how you'll use the money, such as to buy equipment,

inventory, and pay salaries and specific bills until revenue increases. If your business is already established, include financial statements such as income statements, balance sheets, and cash flow statements for the last three to five years.

The emphasis for a business plan should be on the financial justification. For example, will a kitchen renovation result in increased sales that will justify the expense, and how quickly will the renovation costs be paid off?

A business plan usually starts with an executive summary and ends with an appendix. The executive summary is best written after completing the business plan. It is basically a summary of each section. Supporting documents can be put in the appendix, and may include resumes, detailed marketing analysis, examples of marketing pieces, blueprints, equipment documentation, credit histories and other financial documents, and product photos.

SUMMARY

16.1 Explain the Consumer Decision-Making Process and Factors that Influence It

- Whether marketing a product or service, marketers want to satisfy consumer wants and needs with appropriate products and services.
- Sales-oriented businesses focus on selling what they make rather than making what the market wants. Market-oriented businesses describe themselves as selling not only goods and services but also benefits to targeted consumers.
- Value looks at the relationship between the advantages or benefits the buyer gets from a purchase and the sacrifice (i.e., the money spent) that was required. Value has four aspects: will it be useful, will it fill emotional needs, will it change your life, or will it have a social impact?
- The consumer decision-making process includes five steps: become aware of a want or need, gather information and narrow down possibilities, evaluate the consideration set, make the purchase, and post-purchase behavior.
- Figure 16-3 shows the more recent consumer decision journey, which includes a loyalty loop.
- Many factors influence consumers when making purchase decisions: cultural (norms, values, attitudes, social class), individual (gender, age, self-concept, lifestyle), psychological (motivation, perception), and social (influences such as friends, family, and aspirational reference groups).

16.2 Develop the Marketing Plan

- The marketing plan is a document that describes a business's marketing objectives, broad strategies, and specific tactics to achieve the objectives. Developing the marketing plan starts with strategic planning. Strategic planning is a broad process that looks at the entire business, or a part of the business such as marketing.
- The business's mission, vision, core values, and strategic plan all inform the marketing planning process.
- An excellent tool for understanding the environment in which a business may launch a new product or service is a SWOT analysis, a type of situation analysis in which you identify the strengths and weaknesses inside your business and also the opportunities and threats in the external environment. Performing a SWOT analysis also helps businesses identify their competitive advantage.
- The marketing plan includes these steps, although quite often some of these steps are worked on together.
  - Establish marketing objectives.
  - Develop broad marketing strategy and identify target market(s).
  - Formulate the action plan (marketing mix).
  - Implement and monitor the marketing mix.
  - Evaluate the marketing efforts against the objective.
- Market segmentation divides the market into distinct groups of buyers with similar variables who likely have similar product needs.

- Marketers often use geographic, demographic, and psychographic variables to segment the market, along with examining purchasing habits and amount of product purchased (usage-rate).
- You want each target market to be large enough to justify its own marketing mix and you also want to be able to identify each segment's wants and needs. You also want every customer to be associated with just one segment and be accessible to marketers in some way.
- The marketing mix is the set of controllable marketing tools that a company uses to produce a desired response from its target market. It is the precise roadmap of the activities that will help achieve the marketing objective. Known as the 4 Ps, it includes: product, price, place, and promotion. However, in retail businesses, we add two more Ps: personnel and presentation. The closer the product or service is targeted using the 6 Ps to a particular market's unique characteristics, behaviors, and attitudes, the greater the likelihood of getting a positive response.
- Promotion includes communications by marketers that mainly *inform*, *remind*, and/or *persuade* potential buyers to purchase something. Your market research can help you determine the communication channels and activities that will best reach your target segment and build your brand's reputation. Table 16-3 lists different forms of promotion, including advertising, public relations (always using unpaid methods), sales promotion (such as samples, coupons, rebates, point of purchase displays), personal selling, and social media and content marketing.

- Differentiation is a marketing strategy to help consumers distinguish your product/service from others.
- To help market yourself in ways that give customers trust and confidence in your products, consider corporate social responsibility, cause marketing, and green marketing.
- Once the marketing plan is developed, it needs to be turned into a series of specific actions and steps. Employees should be involved in the planning and implementation.
- Once the plan is implemented, it is time to monitor how the implementation went and start to evaluate marketing results. To evaluate any marketing plan, you can go back to the objectives and measure how well the plan succeeded.

16.3 Write a Business Plan

- Planning a new business or doing a renovation of an existing facility *begins* with formulating the details of the project into a written plan known as a business plan or prospectus. The business plan explains why the project is important (the rationale) and the goals of the project, such as serving new customers and being profitable.
- The sections of a business plan include the following.
  - Executive summary.
  - Company overview.
  - Industry analysis.
  - Operating plan
  - Marketing analysis and plan.
  - Financial feasibility study.
  - Funding request.
  - Appendices.

REVIEW AND DISCUSSION QUESTIONS

1. Explain what marketing is. What's the difference between marketing and sales?
2. Discuss the concept of value.
3. Describe the five steps in the traditional consumer decision-making process. How has this process recently changed?
4. What factors inform the marketing planning process?
5. Briefly explain the steps in the marketing planning process.
6. How is mass marketing different from marketing to a specific segment?
7. Give five examples of variables used to segment markets.
8. Give the purpose of the marketing mix and describe the 6 Ps.
9. Contrast advertising and public relations.
10. What is content marketing?
11. How can you evaluate whether a marketing program was successful?
12. Describe the purpose of a business plan and its six major components.

SMALL GROUP PROJECT

For the foodservice concept that you created, complete the following.

1. Develop and write up a theme day event involving your menu that is consistent with your concept and customers.

2. Include your menu. Describe each menu item, including its portion size and how it will be cooked and served.

3. Describe three low-budget ways to market your promotion to inform and attract customers.

REFERENCES

American Marketing Association (AMA). (2017). *Definitions of marketing*. Retrieved from https://www.ama.org/the-definition-of-marketing-what-is-marketing/

Armstrong, G., & Kotler, P. (2020). *Marketing: An introduction* (14th ed). Pearson.

Bojanic, D., & Reid, R. (2016). *Hospitality marketing management* (6th ed). John Wiley & Sons, Inc.

Deiss, R. & Henneberry, R. (2021). *Digital marketing for dummies* (2nd ed). John Wiley & Sons, Inc.

Edelman, D. C., & Singer, M. (2015). Competing on customer journeys. *Harvard Business Review, 93*(11), 88–100.

Gingerella, B. (2019). 4 dining event ideas for December. *Foodservice Director.* https://www.foodservicedirector.com/operations/4-dining-event-ideas-december

Jennings, L. (2016). Dunkin' Donuts promotion aims to steal thunder from Starbucks loyalty shift. *Nation's Restaurant News.* https://www.nrn.com/advertising/dunkin-donuts-promotion-aims-steal-thunder-starbucks-loyalty-shift

Kotler, P., Bowen, J. T., Makens, J., & Baloglu, S. (2017). *Marketing for hospitality and tourism* (7th ed). Pearson.

Lamb, C. W., Hair, J. F., & McDaniel, C. (2021). *MKTG 13*. Cengage Publishing.

MacMillan, I., & McGrath, R. G. (1997.) Discovering new points of differentiation. *Harvard Business Review, 75*(4), 133–140.

Solomon, M.R. (2017). *Consumer behavior: Buying, having, and being* (12th ed.). Pearson.

© Denis Val/Shutterstock

Being an Effective Leader

LEARNING OUTCOMES

17.1 Explain and classify theories of leadership.

17.2 Discuss the delegation process.

17.3 Manage change.

17.4 Describe guidelines for negotiating.

INTRODUCTION

As mentioned earlier, leading is one of the four management functions along with planning, organizing, and controlling. **Leading** is a process by which managers use motivation and other skills to guide and influence the actions of others to accomplish the business's goals and objectives. When managers motivate subordinates, influence how teams are working, or actively listen to concerns from a group of employees, they are leading. While a first-line production manager spends time motivating their employees in the kitchen to ensure a smooth operation, top managers are spending more time creating a vision, inspiring others, setting long-term goals, and managing change.

A leader is a person whom people follow voluntarily. You don't have to be a born leader, you don't have to be magnetic or charismatic; you just have to get people to work for you voluntarily, willingly, to the best of their ability. In theory, you have authority over your people because you have been given **formal authority** by the organization. As the boss, you have the power to control hiring, firing, raises, rewards, and so on. In reality, your authority is anything but absolute. Real authority is given by your subordinates and you have to earn the right to lead them. It is possible for you to be the **formal leader** of your group but have someone else who is the **informal leader** actually calling the shots.

As you get more leadership experience, you will develop your own leadership style. **Leadership style** encompasses the traits, skills, and behaviors that leaders and managers use when they interact with subordinates. In this chapter, you will read about a number of leadership styles and how our views of effective leadership styles have changed over the past 100 years. Neck, Houghton, and Murray (2020, p. 338) give a more contemporary view of leadership style here.

"Despite numerous debates regarding the nature of leadership, there is a general view that today's leaders are most likely to be critical thinkers who lead from a position of influence rather than power, and who use their decision-making, motivational, and communication skills to inspire others with their vision in order to generate results. Researchers have discovered that effective leadership can produce astonishing results."

This chapter will begin with a look at theories of leadership from the 1920s to now. Several leadership/management skills will also be discussed including how to delegate tasks, manage change, and negotiate.

17.1 EXPLAIN AND CLASSIFY THEORIES OF LEADERSHIP

Leadership theories try to explain the keys to effective leadership, such as a leader's traits or behaviors or relationships with followers. When discussing leadership, we will refer to a leader's subordinates as followers. **Followers** are obviously in lower positions on the organizational chart and have less power and authority than the leaders. The concept of **followership** refers to individuals' capacity to work with leaders. In addition, when we use the term leader, keep in mind that this person is a manager, although they will often be in the top management ranks.

TRAIT THEORIES

Early leadership theories compared various personal characteristics or traits, such as intelligence or sociability, of leaders and nonleaders to determine if certain traits predicted effective leadership. Additional examples of traits include height, physical appearance, fluency of speech, or perseverance. Notice that some of these traits are truly physical traits (height), personality traits (perseverance), while others are more like knowledge, skills, and abilities (fluency of speech). Research into the trait theory of leadership was done mostly between the 1920s and the 1930s. At that time, it was thought that leaders were born, not made. Today, we realize that both are possible. You are born with some natural leadership abilities, such as being persuasive, but you can also learn and develop leadership skills. Leadership is a popular training topic in organizations as well as in colleges and universities.

Research into traits did not result in a list of traits that *all* leaders possessed and the researchers found no consistent relationship between traits and a leader's effectiveness. More recent studies have shown that there are some traits that are important for effective leadership although not all are required for success (**Table 17-1**). Within the foodservice industry, the Elliot Group has identified these traits as very important for leaders: trustworthiness, flexibility, life-long learner, visionary, and drive (Ray, 2019). You will notice some overlap between the traits in Table 17-1 and those identified by the Elliot Group.

Table 17-1 Traits Associated with Leadership
1. Drive/ambitious
2. Desire to lead
3. Honesty/integrity
4. Self-confidence
5. Intelligence/cognitive abilities
6. Knowledge of the field
7. Outgoing.

Data from "Personality and leadership: A Qualitative and Quantitative Review," by A.T. Judge, J.E. Bono, R. Illies, R. & M.W. Gerhardt, 2002, *Journal of Applied Psychology*,. *87*(4): 765–780. "Leadership: Do traits matter?" by S.A. Kirkpatrick & E.A. Locke, 1991, *Academy of Management Executive, 5*(2): 48–60. "Trait-based perspectives of leadership," by S. J. Zaccaro, 2007, *American Psychologist, 62*(1): 6–16.

BEHAVIORAL THEORIES

Rather than focusing on traits, researchers started to look at what effective leaders actually do. Leadership research in the 1940s and 1950s examined leaders' behaviors as they interacted with work groups and individuals, and how their overall behavior influenced performance. Researchers looked for behaviors that were hallmarks of effective leaders. First, we will look at studies completed at several universities.

Researchers at the University of Iowa identified three leadership styles.

- **Authoritarian leaders** make almost all of the decisions and directed subordinates on exactly what to do. Subordinates were expected to carry out all directions while working under close supervision. Employee behavior is closely controlled through rules, rewards, and punishments.
- **Democratic leaders** guide and coach employees to do their jobs, as well as encourage them to participate in decision making.
- **Laissez-faire leaders** give complete freedom to the employees/group to complete tasks and the leader does not give any feedback.

Each style can be useful in different situations. For example, authoritarian leadership is appropriate in an emergency, such as a fire, when you need to make sure everyone gets to safety quickly. Democratic leaders work well when they have capable, motivated employees who like to be involved in decision making. Laissez-faire leadership may work when individuals or teams need the independence to do their work how they see best and take ownership.

These studies brought to light a central issue in leadership theory. To get high levels of performance and achieve goals, should a leader pay more attention to getting work done (such as the authoritarian leader) or focus more on the employees (found in the democratic leader) or try to do both?

Researchers at Ohio State University wanted to identify behaviors of successful leaders, so they asked leaders to complete questionnaires. Based on the results, they identified two dimensions of leader behavior that accounted for most of the leaders' behaviors.

- *Structuring* – These behaviors focus on defining roles so that goals are reached, setting clear procedures and standards, establishing formal lines of communication, giving directions, and setting deadlines.
- *Consideration* – These behaviors focus on developing positive interpersonal relationships with employees involving support, trust, and friendship, and being considerate of employees' well-being and satisfaction.

Each leader's structuring and consideration behaviors exist independently, so each leader would fit into one of the following categories or styles.

1. High Structuring and High Consideration
2. High Structuring and Low Consideration
3. Low Structuring and High Consideration
4. Low Structuring and Low Consideration

In many (but not all) situations, leaders who ranked high in both structuring and consideration had subordinates with high satisfaction and high levels of performance.

The two dimensions identified at Ohio State are similar to those in the next set of studies. At the University of Michigan, researchers described these styles of leadership behavior based on questionnaires completed by leaders.

- *Production-oriented* leaders emphasize work methods and directing work.
- *Employee-oriented* leaders emphasize interpersonal relationships and taking a personal interest in the needs of employees.

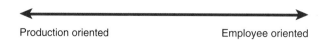

Production oriented   Employee oriented

FIGURE 17-1 University of Michigan One-Dimensional Leadership Style

Although these are analogous to structuring and consideration, one big difference is that the Michigan researchers considered these two styles to be at opposite ends of the same continuum, so a leader was either more employee oriented or more production oriented—not both (**Figure 17-1**). The conclusion of the Michigan studies was that being more employee-oriented and exerting a general rather than close level of supervision yielded better results.

Blake and Mouton (1985) devised the Managerial Grid (**Figure 17-2**), which shows the possible combinations of leadership with regard to concern for people (employees) and concern for production, the same dimensions identified by others. However, their model is different because they ranked a leader's use of each of these behaviors on a scale from 1(low) to 9 (high). For example, a leader with a low concern for production and a high concern for people puts a lot more time into having satisfying relationships than directing work. Each style noted in Figure 17-2 has its own characteristics and

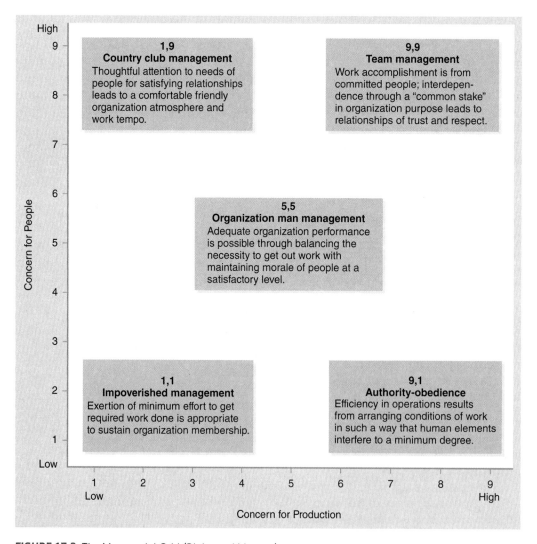

FIGURE 17-2 The Managerial Grid (Blake and Mouton)

Reproduced from Mouton, J., & Blake, R. (1985). *The Managerial Grid III: the key to leadership excellence.* Gulf Publishing Company. Reprinted with permission.

limitations. Of course, the researchers advocated a 9, 9 team leader orientation high in concern for both people and production for an organization to be successful. Although Blake and Mouton encouraged the 9, 9 orientation, research did not always support that it was effective (Nystrom, 1978).

Up to this point, researchers were trying to figure out which traits or behaviors would predict which leaders were successful, and which style works best in all situations. Since there was not any one style of leadership that fits all situations, researchers started to explore which leadership styles worked best in different situations.

CONTINGENCY MODELS OF LEADERSHIP

Contingency models of leadership not only take into account traits and behaviors but also the situation or context in which a leader is working. How effective a leader will be depends on the interaction between what the leader is like (traits), what he or she does (behavior), and the situation. Given the variety of situations in which a leader functions, it is no surprise that what makes a leader successful in one situation may lead to poor results when the circumstances and people change. Contingency theories gained prominence in the late 1960s and 1970s.

Fiedler Contingency Leadership Model

Introduced in 1967, Fiedler's contingency model was the first to specify how situational factors interact with leader traits and behavior to influence leadership effectiveness (Fiedler, 1967). Fiedler's model describes two leader styles, relationship-oriented and task-oriented, and the kinds of situations in which each style is most successful. An important aspect of Fiedler's model is that the work group and situation affect the extent to which a leader's traits and behaviors will be effective.

Using this model, a person's leadership style, either task-motivated or relationship-motivated, is identified using a scale Fiedler developed. Fiedler believed that leadership style is relatively fixed so a leader was more oriented toward either tasks or relationships, not both.

Next, you look at three situational variables to determine how favorable or unfavorable the situation is.

1. Leader-follower relations. This is the level of confidence and trust followers have in their leader. The situation is more favorable when the leader has more influence.
2. Task structure. The task structure varies between being very clear and well-defined to vague and unstructured. The situation is more favorable when the leader provides a well-defined task.
3. Leader's position power. The more power a leader has to direct followers and provide rewards, promotions, etc., the more favorable the situation.

The more influence and control the leader has over the situation, the more favorable the situation is.

Using these three variables, Fiedler identified eight different situations that were either favorable or unfavorable for the leader (**Figure 17-3**). He determined that task-oriented leaders performed better in either very favorable or very unfavorable situations (seen in situations 1, 2, 3, and 8); whereas relationship-oriented leaders performed better in moderately favorable situations (seen in situations 4–7).

The Fiedler contingency model has been criticized (Mitchell et al., 2017), but there is much research evidence to support the model (Peters et al., 1985; Schriesheim et al., 1994). One of its biggest shortcomings is that the leadership style is fixed. So, if you are a task-oriented leader, and you are in a situation in which being relationship-oriented would be more suitable, either you change the situation to fit your leadership style, or you bring in another leader—neither of which are good alternatives. Much future research will state that the leader needs to change their style.

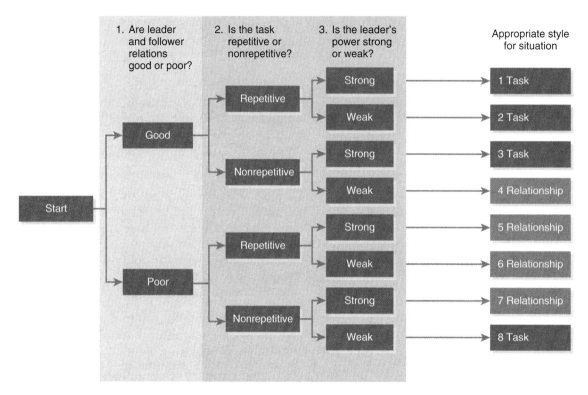

FIGURE 17-3 Contingency Leadership Model – A Decision Tree

Reproduced with permission from Lussier, R. N. (2017). Management fundamentals: Concepts, applications, and skill development. Sage Publications.

Path-Goal Model (House)

The **path–goal model** can best be thought of as a process in which leaders select specific behaviors that are best suited to the followers' needs and the working environment so that they can guide and support followers to perform well and meet goals that are compatible with the organization (House, 1971). Robert House developed this model. The term "path goal" refers to the job leaders have to perform to give followers a clear path, without barriers, to goal achievement.

House identified the following leadership styles that motivate followers.

1. <u>Directive style</u>. The leader lets followers know what is expected of them and provides instructions on how to perform tasks including standards and a timeline for completion. This style is most useful when followers have low abilities and do not mind, or even want, close supervision.

2. <u>Supportive style</u>. The supportive leader is friendly and pays attention to followers' needs. It is a more appropriate style to use when employees are capable and motivated, the task is simple, or when employees need a little guidance.

3. <u>Participative style</u>. Using this style, the leader asks for employee feedback and input to make decisions. It works well when employees want to be involved and the task is complex.

4. <u>Achievement-oriented</u>. Using this style, a leader works to motivate followers to set tough goals and perform at their highest level. This leader provides both directive and support behaviors.

In contrast to Fiedler, House believed that leaders are flexible and can utilize different styles.

The optimal leadership style depends on two sets of situational factors: subordinate and environmental (**Figure 17-4**). Subordinate situational factors include the degree to

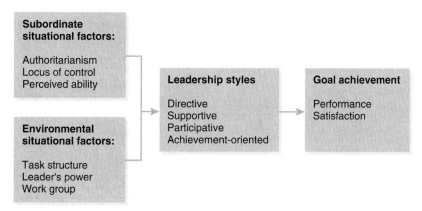

Note: The situational factors determine the leadership style which affects goal achievement.

FIGURE 17-4 Path-Goal Model

Note: The situational factors determine the leadership style, which affects goal achievement.

Data from "A Path-Goal Theory of Leadership Effectiveness," by R. House, 1971, *Administrative Science Quarterly, 16*(3): 321–338.

which they want to be told what to do (authoritarianism), their locus of control (how much they believe they control their successes and failures), and their perceived ability to perform their job (ability). Environmental situational factors include the repetitiveness of the job (task structure), the leader's power (formal authority), and the extent to which coworkers contribute to job satisfaction (work group).

The model suggests that leaders should adjust their style to make up for shortcomings in the subordinate or the work setting. Also, the leader should not try to provide something that is already being provided for in the environment or is not appropriate for a subordinate. For example, a participative style, rather than a directive style, is suitable for a subordinate who has an internal locus of control and tends to be more achievement oriented.

Hersey and Blanchard's Situational Leadership Theory

Using Hersey and Blanchard's Situational Leadership® model, there are two dimensions of leadership behavior: task (directive) and relationship (supportive) behaviors (Hersey & Blanchard, 1969; Hersey & Blanchard, 1977). Task behaviors are used to get work done, such as telling an employee what to do and how to do it. Relationship behaviors would include listening and encouraging. High or low levels of these two dimensions can form the basis for four leadership styles (**Figure 17-5**).

What makes this theory different is that the leader chooses which style will work best by considering the readiness levels of the followers. The authors describe the followers' readiness as their ability (competence) and willingness (commitment) to perform the task. The emphasis on choosing a style that works with the followers is important because it acknowledges that the followers are crucial in getting work done.

The following are descriptions of each leadership style.

1. Telling style. When followers are low in readiness, a leader needs to use this directive approach to give explicit directions and closely supervise. This style works best when the completion of the task is of the utmost importance and the followers are not as skilled or eager as the leader would like them to be.

2. Selling style. When followers have the willingness to do a job but lack some ability, the leader needs to be both directive and supportive. Using the selling (also called coaching) style, the leader explains what needs to be done and why it is important, while selling their ideas to the followers in a persuasive manner.

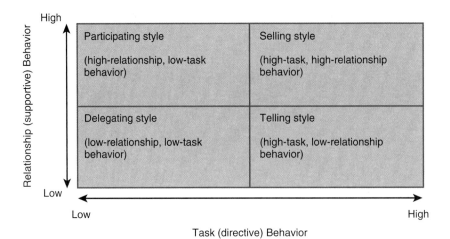

FIGURE 17-5 Hersey-Blanchard Situational Leadership Theory

Data from P. Hersey and K. H. Blanchard, (1977). Management of Organization Behavior: Utilizing Human Resources, Prentice Hall Inc.

3. <u>Participating style</u>. When followers have the ability to do a job but lack the confidence or simply need a little guidance, the leader does not need to be very directive but does need to be very supportive. This style emphasizes sharing of ideas and decision-making between the leader and followers.

4. <u>Delegating style</u>. When followers are both competent and motivated, the leader can use a low-task and low relationship style. Leaders can delegate tasks to employees and monitor progress.

As employees become more capable and willing to perform, the leader decreases supervision as well as supportive behaviors. Despite its popularity, research does not generally support the theory (Graeff, 1997).

CONTEMPORARY LEADERSHIP

Up to this point, leadership theories have looked at traits, then behaviors, then the situation the leader was in. Contemporary leadership theories build on past research to explain how effective leaders interact and build relationships with followers as well as motivate and support them. Contemporary theories show different ways that leaders use their influence and power.

Leader-Member Exchange Theory

Leader-member exchange (LMX) theory does not focus on the specific characteristics of an effective organizational leader. Instead, it focuses on the nature and quality of the exchanges and relationship between a leader and *each* follower. Before LMX theory, researchers looked more at how leaders acted toward all of their followers as a group. Successful LMX leaders develop high-quality relationships with each follower, including high levels of mutual trust and respect, which boosts a follower's job satisfaction, productivity, and performance toward organizational goals (Bauer & Erdogan, 2016). A central premise of this theory is that leadership is more effective when leaders have a positive relationship with each follower.

Early LMX research found that leaders often have two groups of followers: an in-group and an out-group. If this is starting to sound like cliques from high school, you have the right idea. The leader considers in-group members to be competent, trustworthy, and motivated, and gives them more time, information, better assignments, and rewards such as higher performance ratings. In-group members are more likely to be given opportunities to grow and are also more likely to engage in organizational citizenship behaviors. **Organizational citizenship behaviors** are when someone takes an action that goes beyond the call of duty.

Out-group members, on the other hand, receive less respect, trust, and support, and are often seen as less competent and motivated as in-group members. As expected, out-group members get easier tasks to complete, less communication and rewards, and fewer opportunities for advancement. They are also less satisfied with their jobs.

So why do in-groups and out-groups exist? One possibility is that due to limited time and energy, it can be difficult for leaders to establish quality exchange relationships with all followers (Anand et al., 2016). In addition, in-group members may be particularly competent. Research shows that in-group members are often similar in many ways to the leader, such as in gender, personality, or demographics (Liden et al., 1993).

Of course, when a leader has an in-group and an out-group, the differences between the groups (such as in status and rewards) will create tension and conflict. When members from each group work together on a team, there will be less group cohesiveness and more conflict. Because leaders need to bring out the best in everyone, they must listen to and support all of their followers for the organization to be successful.

Later research focused more on how LMX theory was related to goal achievement and organizational effectiveness. In order for an organization to be successful, a leader must listen to and support all of his or her followers. Research has shown that quality leader-member exchanges and relationships are consistently related to member job satisfaction, job performance, and organizational commitment (Gerstner and Day, 1997). When leaders and followers interact well and enjoy positive relationships, all parties accomplish more and the organization thrives.

Transactional and Transformational Leadership

A **transactional leader** is one who leads primarily by using social exchanges with followers along with exchanging rewards (or in some cases punishments) for completion of certain tasks/goals. This type of leader sets goals for followers and motivates them mostly by using rewards and punishments. The transactional leader works within the organizational culture to maintain the status quo.

While the transactional leader is more likely to be a first-line manager or in middle management, transformational leaders are usually in the top management ranks. **Transformational leaders** (**Figure 17-6**) inspire followers to look at problems in new ways while inspiring and motivating them to work together toward a shared vision and (often) extraordinary goals. A transformational leader is:

- Inspiring
- Energetic and enthusiastic
- Inclusive
- Collaborative
- Emotionally intelligent
- Team oriented
- Empowering
- Innovative
- Respected and respectful

Transformational leaders are quite capable of changing an organization's culture and developing a new vision and goals in large part by their ability to overcome resistance to change, asking followers to question established views (including the leader's views), and by making followers understand their vital roles in making the vision a reality. Transformational leaders are also excellent listeners and truly support employee growth and development.

Research has shown that groups led by transformational leaders have higher levels of performance and employee satisfaction than groups led by other types of leaders (Dvir

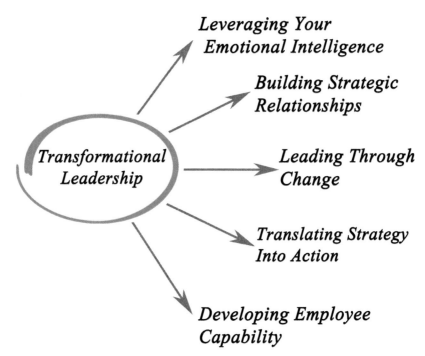

FIGURE 17-6 Transformational Leadership

© Arka38/Shutterstock

et al., 2002; Robbins and Coulter, 2018). In a study conducted in restaurants, Mostafa (2019) found that transformational leadership affects social relationships in a way that enhances customer-oriented behaviors.

Transactional and transformational leaders are not opposites. It is likely that many transformational leaders started out as transactional leaders using more of a "telling" style. Over time, some transactional leaders adopt more of a "selling" style, become more innovative and inspiring, and evolve into transformational leaders.

Charismatic and Visionary Leadership

Charisma can be defined as someone's compelling ability to attract and influence other people. A **charismatic leader** is an enthusiastic, energetic, and confident individual who uses their personality and actions to motivate and inspire high levels of performance, trust, and commitment. Much of their strong influence derives from the fact that they are skilled communicators and can articulate an engaging vision. They also reach followers on a deep, emotional level. By supporting followers, they also inspire confidence.

According to Conger and Kanungo (1998), charismatic leaders tend to have these characteristics.

1. They have a strategic vision that is frequently presented to followers in an inspiring way.
2. They will take risks to achieve that vision.
3. They are sensitive to their followers' needs.
4. They assess the environment for growth possibilities.
5. They may choose unconventional behavior at times in part to build trust and commitment in followers.

While research supports the positive effect of charismatic leaders on performance (LePine, Zhang, Crawford, & Rich, 2016), other research shows that while a moderate level of charisma is appropriate, having too much charisma is not helpful and makes the leader less effective (Vergauwe et al., 2017).

Although charismatic leaders are very skilled at presenting their organizational vision, it doesn't mean that they are also visionary leaders. Likewise, visionary leaders are not necessarily charismatic. There are certainly examples in the business world of leaders who are both charismatic and visionary, such as Steve Jobs of Apple who was very charismatic and also envisioned years ago how we would be using computers and mobile phones today.

Visionary leaders create and communicate an energizing vision of the future that provides direction for strategic planning and goal setting as well as taps into the enthusiasm and emotions of their followers. For example, Ron Shaich pioneered the fast-casual segment of foodservices when he started Panera Bread. He envisioned a foodservice that provided more upscale food, service, and decor than fast-food restaurants yet still used counter service for speed. Panera has been very successful financially and the company has been a leader in developing clean, healthy menus and using technology. Visionary leaders also work to *create* new opportunities in the market and *prevent* threats in the environment rather than just preparing for them.

Authentic and Servant Leaders

Authentic leaders are genuine; they don't try to imitate someone else. Because they are open, honest, and genuine, they are trusted by their followers. Authentic leaders are guided by their sense of ethics and lead by example. Building honest, meaningful relationships with followers is important along with involving them in making decisions and empowering them to take actions. Authentic leaders are sensitive to the needs of their followers.

With **servant leadership**, leaders share power with the employees and *serve the employees* and often the community. Servant leaders place their employees' needs ahead of their self-interest. By doing so, the servant leader moves beyond transactional leadership and helps align the employee's sense of purpose with the organization's mission. Servant leaders empower and develop employees as well as provide a powerful role model for prioritizing the needs of others.

At Zingerman's, which started as a Jewish delicatessen in Ann Arbor, Michigan, the founders embraced servant leadership from its start in 1982. Effective servant leaders have six responsibilities (Zingerman's, 2016).

1. Provide an inspiring and strategically sound vision.
2. Give great service to the staff.
3. Manage in an ethical manner.
4. Be an active listener and teacher.
5. Help staff succeed.
6. Say thanks to let people know they made a difference.

In addition to serving employees, they also support the local community. From its original business, Zingerman's now runs a number of foodservices and other businesses.

In a study involving nurses, *authentic leadership* was associated with higher levels of job satisfaction and self-reported higher performance (Wong & Laschinger, 2013). Likewise, research in a restaurant chain showed that *servant leadership* was positively related to restaurant performance, employee job performance, and customer service (Liden, Wayne, Liao, & Meuser, 2014).

TRENDS AND FUTURE ISSUES IN LEADERSHIP

The concept of **distributed leadership** (**Figure 17-7**) comes from the world of education and is being discussed more in business settings. With distributed leadership, leadership responsibility is distributed throughout the organization. In other words, power

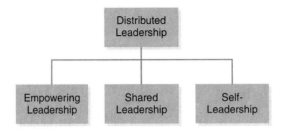

FIGURE 17-7 Distributed Leadership

is shared. There are different ways to distribute power, from empowering employees to act independently to shared leadership to self-leadership. Shared leadership is when the leader shares responsibility with teams or other groups or even individuals to achieve goals. Self-leadership is the ability to lead yourself to achieve your goals while also working toward organizational goals. Self-leadership involves having a sense of who you are and where you are going. Daniel Goleman, the psychologist who first discussed the concept of emotional intelligence, feels that top-notch leaders are different because they have superior self-leadership.

There are a number of issues that will affect leadership now and in the future. For example, as business becomes more globalized, **cross-cultural leadership** will become more important. Note that most of the theories discussed in this chapter were developed in the United States and don't cross over to all countries and cultures. Another issue is the fact that the percentage of American women in leadership positions lags substantially behind men and this is especially true for women of color. Organizations need to work on reducing both gender and racial inequality in the workplace to enable more capable individuals to move up the career ladder. Increased technology has also changed leadership and will continue to do so.

17.2 DISCUSS THE DELEGATION PROCESS

Delegation is when a manager asks a subordinate to accomplish an objective or task (that is not already in the employee's job description) and also gives the responsibility and often some authority to make certain decisions and/or use resources to do so. **Authority** is the right of a manager to direct others at work, to make decisions, and to use resources. Authority is not the same as power. **Power** is the ability to influence others' behavior. **Responsibility** refers to the obligation of the employee to perform the task. When responsibility to complete a task is delegated (assigned) to someone, so is accountability. **Accountability** means answering to your boss for the results. For example, if the executive chef delegates preparing a catered luncheon to a line cook, the line cook is accountable to get the job done, but the executive chef is ultimately accountable as well.

Delegation is actually a form of participative management that gives the manager more time to do his or her own work and the subordinate an opportunity to build knowledge, skills, confidence, and job satisfaction. A measure of a manger's effectiveness lies in the ability to get work done through other people. By delegating, a manager has more time for important managerial activities such as planning or organizing. As a manager, you can, therefore, improve your efficiency and achieve more by delegating. When you delegate appropriately, you are also assessing, training, and developing employees. Employees become more self-reliant, skilled, versatile, and promotable. In brief, delegation improves the performance of both the manager and the employee.

WHY MANAGERS DON'T LIKE TO DELEGATE

Despite the benefits, managers can state many reasons for *not* delegating, such as the following.

- I can do the job faster. I can do the job better.
- My employees won't get the job done right.
- My employees don't have the time.
- If I ask someone to do this job and the person messes up, it could be costly and I'm still responsible anyway.
- My employees don't have as much clout as I do to get things done around here.
- My employees don't know enough about my job to do any of it, and that's just the way it is.

Underneath the countless excuses for not delegating lie some managerial attitudes that often need redirection. Managers who do not want to delegate may be insecure and do not want to delegate due to a fear that the employee will either do a better job or a poor one for which the manager will be responsible. Other managers won't delegate because they consider themselves indispensable to the operation and do not want to share their authority with anyone. Some managers simply don't have any trust or confidence in their employees to complete a delegated assignment, or they are perfectionists who feel only they can do the job right. Managers who are not well organized often don't delegate because they never get to the first steps of organizing a task to be delegated. This type of manager is likely to spend the day reacting to problems, often called fighting fires, rather than delegating.

In order to get a good start at delegating, a manager needs to do the following.

- Consider which subordinates could take on additional responsibilities.
- Realize that giving an employee additional authority will not lessen the manager's power and will actually improve the manager's performance if delegating is successful.
- Let others makes mistakes, as long as they are not major.
- Be willing to invest time in monitoring and developing employees.

Managers also need to be receptive to listening to ideas from subordinates that may initially seem to be far-fetched but may actually be worth trying out.

STEPS IN DELEGATION

Delegation actually comprises four steps: preparation, the delegation discussion, monitoring, and evaluation. To prepare, a manager needs to develop a delegation plan, including objectives and a timeline, and decide which subordinate would be most appropriate. A manager's job can be divided into three categories: work that only a manager can perform, work that that can be delegated right away, and work that can be delegated as soon as someone is trained to do it. Only the manager should perform certain tasks, such as discipline, counseling, performance evaluations, complex activities, handling sensitive situations, or dealing with circumstances that require the manager's unique knowledge or abilities. Tasks that can be delegated are those where the manager does not need to be directly involved, such as routine activities, technical matters, fact-finding, or attendance at certain meetings.

Once an appropriate task or activity has been chosen, the manager needs to set objectives so the employee knows exactly what results are expected. A deadline also needs to be set, along with checkpoints along the way where the manager and employee will discuss progress toward the objectives as well as any problems that may occur. Checkpoints could be set weekly, for example, and completed via email, phone call, or detailed report. The level of authority and autonomy given to the employee must be based on a realistic appraisal of their capabilities. The employee needs to know exactly what authority they have while completing this assignment. For example, is the employee expected to make recommendations to the manager and then help decide the next step or is the employee being given the responsibility to carry out a complete task without preapproval? If the employee is given the authority to use restricted resources, the manager needs to give the employee access to them.

When selecting someone to accept a delegated task, look for an employee who has both the ability and the time to perform the task. Although there are situations when it is appropriate to delegate to a team of employees, it is easier in some ways to delegate to a single employee. By giving a task over to one person, the manager has more control and this lessens any confusion. There is a tendency to delegate to the same employee or group of employees because they can be relied on to do a job well; as a result, they are often overburdened with work and may resent the added pressure when others have time to spare. Delegated tasks should be distributed as evenly as possible among capable employees who want the challenge. Also, don't just delegate jobs that are undesirable. Delegate whenever possible in order to give employees interesting, challenging work.

Now that you have a plan and a capable, willing employee, it's time to have the delegation discussion. This discussion should include all details such as the objectives, the amount of authority and resources available, the controls such as progress reports and deadlines, and how results will be evaluated and recognized. Effective delegation does not mean telling someone what to do, but rather mutually discussing and agreeing on what is to be accomplished and how it is to be monitored and evaluated. Frequently, employees are asked to do certain functions but can't get them done because they were not given enough authority. It is crucial to delegate enough authority in order to get the job accomplished but not so much that it could be abused.

Once a task is delegated, it needs to be monitored to evaluate progress and give any needed feedback. All parties need to agree on the degree of monitoring and the deadline dates during the delegation discussion. An assignment can be tightly or loosely monitored, depending on the task, the employee, and the desired results. Tight controls not only reduce the chance of confusion or error but also reduce the authority of the employee. Loose controls allow the employee more initiative and creativity. Whether controls are tight or loose, it is important to follow up on schedule, show the employee that this project is important, and give support as needed.

While monitoring, the manager may find that progress is poor or even nonexistent, in which case they need to find out why. If the employee doesn't have the time or ability to get the job done, perhaps the job should be assigned to someone else. If the employee is sincerely trying to get something accomplished but needs more guidance or training, the manager needs to provide that. The best option is to give some help in hopes of getting things moving in the right direction. Under some circumstances; however, it is necessary to reassign the task, which in many cases could have been avoided if the most appropriate employee had been chosen initially to do the job.

The last step is to assess the completed task by comparing it with the results agreed upon at the beginning of this process and to hold the employee accountable for the results. Of course, an honest discussion with the employee is important to improve understanding. Recognize and reward the good work accomplished. Emphasize what the employee learned from their mistakes to keep up motivation to take on future assignments. Any criticisms should be stated in a constructive manner.

SPOTLIGHT ON REVERSE DELEGATION

Here's a common situation. A manager delegates a task to an employee. They discuss and agree on a plan of action. After a week or two, the employee confronts the boss and says, "We've got a problem." The worker explains many reasons why they cannot complete the task. In essence, the employee is dumping the assignment back onto the boss. This is referred to as **reverse delegation**. The employee may be doing this because they lack confidence, do not really know enough to do the job, are afraid of making a mistake and being criticized for it, or simply realized later on that they did not want to take on the added responsibility.

What should the boss do? The manager should listen and discuss the dilemma but make it perfectly clear that the task is still the employee's responsibility to complete. To encourage the employee to think through their own problems, the manager can ask questions such as "What do you recommend?" and have an informed discussion that hopefully results in some positive action by the employee.

If a manager takes back incomplete work, it gives the message to the employees that they will not be held responsible for their actions or inactions. It also fosters employee dependence on managers to solve all of the problems. Of course, sometimes it is just that a manager made a poor choice of which employee to complete a task. The best way to handle reverse delegation can be summed up by this statement: "Don't bring me problems, bring me solutions."

17.3 MANAGE CHANGE

Change within a foodservice organization is a given. In order to keep up with conditions both outside and inside the business and be competitive, change is essential. An important component of business success is having an organizational culture that values change and innovation. Innovations in the foodservice industry, such as a new cooking technology, help give an operation an advantage or uniqueness, but only if the employees can handle change.

THE CHANGE PROCESS

People pass through four phases when they are faced with change: fear/denial, anger/resistance, exploration or resignation, and commitment (**Figure 17-8**). It is an ongoing process and can reverse at any point. How quickly and easily certain employees go through this process depends on their readiness for change, evaluation of the benefits and efforts it will require, and ability to adapt.

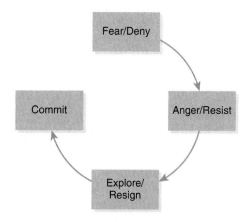

FIGURE 17-8 The Change Process

Fear and denial are often the first reaction to an announcement of change, particularly when the change is unexpected or unexplained. Employees may have a fear of the unknown (such as when a new manager takes over), losing the routine and having to do something differently (such as when a new menu is implemented), or of possible incompetence (such as being asked to use a new computer system). When employees first hear of changes, they often like to think that it won't affect them. In other words, they deny that change is coming.

The second phase sees anger and resistance to change. Once the employee has gotten over the denial and admitted that they will be involved in this change, they often resist the change. In many kitchens and dining rooms, employees will tell managers that "we've always done things this way" and they are not interested in changing now.

In the third phase, employees explore the change further and/or resign themselves to it. By now, some employees start to realize that the changes are here to stay and there doesn't seem to be any going back to the old ways. Resistance decreases; however, this should not be interpreted universally as acceptance because some people intend only grudging compliance. During this stage, these individuals often do no more than what they absolutely must—frequently while looking for other employment. Other individuals, meanwhile, actively explore the nature of the change and experience a transition to the final stage of the change process.

In the fourth and final phase, employees start to commit themselves to the change. As time goes on, the change becomes more routine. Employees will naturally move to this stage at different times. This phase is marked by a lack of complaining or longing about the old ways. Employees become able to identify with and refocus their efforts on the new set of expectations.

WHY EMPLOYEES RESIST CHANGE

There are many reasons why employees resist change.

1. <u>Fear of the unknown/uncertainty</u>. For most people starting a new job, the first few days or weeks can be nerve-wracking because everything is new. The same thing happens when employees are confronted with a change in their workplace and job. They wonder whether they will be able to successfully adjust to the changes and whether there will be some loss—such as a pay cut, a less flexible schedule, switch to another department resulting in a loss of social relationships, or even loss of status or loss of a job.

2. <u>Self-interest or group interest</u>. What is in the best interest of the organization is not always in the best interest of every employee and work team. We will naturally resist changes in our routine that take us out of our comfort zone such as a change in work assignment or schedules or splitting up a work team that gets along really well into new teams. We will also resist changes when we feel we will be worse off after the change is made, especially when others appear to benefit from the change.

3. <u>Anxiety about learning new skills</u>. As happens frequently in any industry, new skills, such as computer and software knowledge, have to be learned. Some employees will be truly afraid that they won't be able to learn a new skill and be proficient at it. Many will also fear looking stupid if they don't pick things up quickly.

4. <u>Lack of trust in superiors</u>. If employees lack the faith to think that superiors will make the right changes, they will likely not be supportive.

5. <u>Not being consulted</u>. When employees are involved in deciding on how changes will be implemented, they are less likely to resist. Having changes just dropped on employees without any involvement (and often little advance notice) just decreases job satisfaction and increases resistance.

6. <u>Poor communication/lack of clarity</u>. When change is being considered or is definitely happening, how the change is introduced and explained will help

determine how much resistance there will be. If the need for change is discussed early and a good argument for change is given, employees will be more likely to get on board. At this point, you will need to start showing the benefits for the employees.

7. Inadequate rewards. Some employees will resist if they feel they will have to put in more effort to make the changes without any type of reward. Management should consider the issue of reward early in the process.

LEADING CHANGE

To increase success, it is best to organize the change process into three stages: creating a climate for change, engaging employees while transitioning into the change, and sustaining change (Kotter, 1996). Only necessary and useful changes should be made in an organization, and change should be by gradual evolution, not sudden revolution.

Creating a Climate for Change

This stage occurs after there has been a realization that some type of change needs to occur and before an actual change is implemented. The key in this stage is to build support for the change via honest communication and involvement of employees to create a clear vision of change. The following are some guidelines.

1. Create an awareness for the need to change. Discuss with employees the need for, and reasons behind, the change, as well as how important it is to them and the organization.
2. Communicate the vision for change—well in advance of the implementation date—with the expectation that it will succeed and will improve a situation.
3. Ask employees to participate in the decisions about how the change will be made. Having a team approach stimulates employees to discuss, make suggestions, and think positively about the change, discourages resistance, and encourages employee commitment to the change rather than mere compliance.
4. Gain the support of key people who have influence in the areas likely to be affected.
5. Acknowledge both the benefits—such as improved customer service or procedures that require less time—and short-term difficulties involved in making the change.
6. Help employees see how the proposed change will affect them, both directly and indirectly. Create a win-win situation.
7. Allow employees to express their feelings about the change.
8. Make sure there is some kind of reward available for employees involved in the change, such as recognition from management or training in new skills. The question from employees, "What's in it for me?" needs to be addressed ahead of time.

During this phase, frequent meetings of employee groups are essential to good planning and communication. A final plan should be drawn up that describes who does what, when, where, and how. This plan should be communicated in training sessions and visibly posted. Adequate training is crucial to the next stage.

Engaging Employees During the Transition

During this stage, the operation continues to serve guests and operate normally, while at the same time, change is introduced into one or more areas that could potentially disrupt normal activities. To maneuver successfully through this phase, follow these guidelines.

1. Keep employees fully informed of everything going on, through periodic progress reports that should also communicate the vision.
2. Continue to ask employees for advice and help.

3. Enable the employees to reach a series of short-term goals to provide encouragement as the overall change starts to take place.
4. Managers should be very visible in leading the change effort and very supportive of the employees' efforts. Let them know how important their work is and how much it is appreciated. Use rewards.
5. Remove as many barriers as possible so employees are not frustrated.
6. Continue to remind the employees of the need for change and its benefits.
7. Constantly monitor and evaluate how well the implementation is working.

During this stage, resistance is often still felt. Use **Table 17-2** for methods to deal with it.

Sustaining Change

At this point, the change has been implemented, but there are certainly still bugs to be worked out. New procedures written out on paper don't always survive the test of being used day-in and day-out. The original plan most likely needs to be modified in places. Managers often make the mistake of declaring the overall effort a success too early. It is appropriate to evaluate the change by answering several questions such as the following.

- Did the change solve the problem it was meant to?
- What did the change fail to accomplish and why?
- Are the benefits of this change still worth the costs involved?
- How has this change affected the employees involved?

Table 17-2 Methods for Dealing with Resistance to Change

Exhibit I
Methods for dealing with resistance to change

Approach	Commonly used in situations	Advantages	Drawbacks
Education + communication	Where there is a lack of information or inaccurate information and analysis.	Once persuaded, people will often help with the implementation of the change.	Can be very time consuming if lots of people are involved.
Participation + involvement	Where the initiators do not have all the information they need to design the change, and where others have considerable power to resist.	People who participate will be committed to implementing change, and any relevant information they have will be integrated into the change plan.	Can be very time consuming if participators design an inappropriate change.
Facilitation + support	Where people are resisting because of adjustment problems.	No other approach works as well with adjustment problems.	Can be time consuming, expensive, and still fail.
Negotiation + agreement	Where someone or some group will clearly lose out in a change, and where that group has considerable power to resist.	Sometimes is a relatively easy way to avoid major resistance.	Can be too expensive in many cases if it alerts others to negotiate for compliance.
Manipulation + co-optation	Where other tactics will not work or are too expensive.	It can be relatively quick and inexpensive solution to resistance problems.	Can lead to future problems if people feel manipulated.
Explicit + implicit coercion	Where speed is essential, and the change initiators possess considerable power.	It is speedy and can overcome any kind of resistance.	Can be risky if it leaves people angry with the initiators.

Reproduced from "Choosing Strategies for Change," by J.P. Kotter & L.A. Schlesinger, 2008, *Harvard Business Review, 86*(7–8): p. 135. Reproduced with permission.

Another question to ask is whether the employees were adequately involved and rewarded.

In addition, do not let up. Hold onto the new ways of behaving and make sure employees don't shift back to old habits. Be persistent with instituting the changes until they are sustained. Change is an ongoing process that needs to be integrated into the organizational culture.

ORGANIZATION DEVELOPMENT

Organization development (OD) is a contemporary process that uses social and behavioral sciences to increase organizational effectiveness and assist the change process in both individuals and the organization. A central theme of OD is to create and manage change so that individuals can develop and organizations perform better. Organization development is usually led by someone in the human resources department. The **change agent** is the person in charge of overseeing an organizational change effort. Specific methods used in OD to implement changes are called **organizational development interventions**. Examples include training and development, team building, developing and collecting survey feedback, job design, direct feedback, and force-field analysis. Using **force-field analysis**, a group brainstorms all the forces that foster change and forces that diminish the chances of change—then diagrams each force, including its strength. The group members can then develop ways to increase the driving forces and decrease the diminishing forces to make the change a reality.

17.4 DESCRIBE GUIDELINES FOR NEGOTIATING

Negotiation is a type of discussion in which two parties are trying to reach an agreement that both parties find acceptable (**Figure 17-9**). Negotiations occur frequently in the workplace. For example, employees may need to negotiate work schedules, salaries, or project deadlines. **Table 17-3** gives tips on what you should do before and during negotiations.

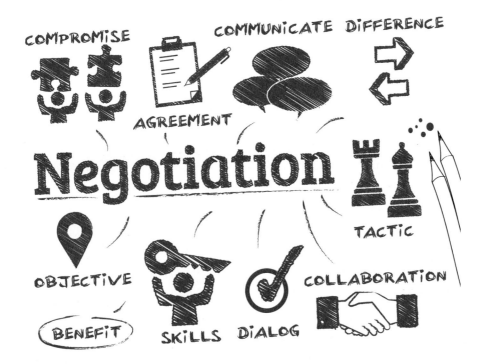

FIGURE 17-9 Negotiation

© Trueffelpix/Shutterstock

Table 17-3 Tips for Negotiating

Before Negotiations

- Know your strengths and weaknesses as a negotiator, as well as the strengths and weaknesses of the other party.
- Think about the situation from the other party's perspective. You probably know what you want but try to anticipate what the other person will want too. Try to understand their needs and concerns and think about how you can address them.
- Unbundle the items to be negotiated. Break it down into its parts. Identify objectives for each of the items, including an optimum goal, target goal, and minimum goal. The optimum goal is where you start bargaining and it represents the best deal you can get. The target goal is set lower but is still acceptable. The minimum goal is just that—the minimum you will accept.
- Determine which items are most important to you and which are less important. You may need to use the less-important items as leverage to get what you rank as most important.
- Find evidence that will help support any of your positions.
- Have a back-up plan—called the **best alternative to a negotiated agreement** (Ury et al., 1992). The best alternative to a negotiated agreement (BATNA) is the course of action if negotiations do not work out and no agreement can be reached. Ask yourself: "What will I do if I don't reach an agreement?"
- Think about different ways the meeting could proceed, potential objections you will face, and all possible outcomes. Consider ways to move the meeting toward a positive outcome.
- Plan to negotiate at a good time for both parties to avoid a sense of urgency or stress.

During Negotiations

- Build trust by being honest and considerate.
- Establish rapport early by finding areas on which you both agree. Bring up items where you are pretty sure the other party can say "yes." Agreement also helps build trust.
- Actively listen and pay attention to all of the nonverbal messages.
- Don't talk too much. By listening more than you talk, you will learn more about the other party.
- Be confident, but not overconfident.
- Describe your needs in a concise, clear manner, and explain how your proposal is beneficial to all parties. Persuade others to support your point of view.
- Focus on the negotiation issues, not the people or personalities you are negotiating with.
- Present your arguments logically. Bring materials to support your position. Referring to some fair standard other than your opinion is helpful.
- Ask open-ended questions such as "What is your biggest concern with...?" Find out more about the needs and concerns of the other party.
- Paraphrase others' statements to clarify issues and correct misinterpretations. Clarify issues and analyze the nature of the disagreement before exploring solutions.
- Work together to find workable and creative solutions.
- Remain calm and cool. Refrain from getting irritated or angry.
- Don't take "no" personally.
- Try not to think of winning the negotiation. Instead, work toward a win-win solution.

SUMMARY

17.1   Explain and Classify Theories of Leadership

- Leadership style encompasses the traits, skills, and behaviors that leaders and managers use when they interact with subordinates.
- Early research (1920s and 1930s) into traits did not result in a list that all leaders possess and there was no consistent relationship between traits and a leader's effectiveness. Later research did find some traits to be important, but not essential, including honesty, drive, and cognitive abilities.

- The next set of research (1940s and 1950s) focused on behaviors.
  - Researchers at the University of Iowa identified three leadership styles: authoritarian, democratic, and laissez-faire.
  - Researchers at Ohio State University identified two dimensions of leader behavior: structuring and consideration. These behaviors exist independently and a leader may be high or low in either dimension. In many (but not all) situations, leaders who

ranked high in both structuring and consideration had subordinates with high satisfaction and high levels of performance.

- University of Michigan researchers felt that leaders were either more production oriented or more employee oriented (not both).
- Blake and Mouton's Managerial Grid (Figure 17-2) shows possible combinations of leadership with regard to concern for people and concern for production.

- Contingency models of leadership take into account not only traits and behaviors but also the situation or context in which a leader is working. How effective a leader will be depends on the interaction between what the leader is like (traits), what he or she does (behavior), and the situation.

  - Fiedler's Contingency Leadership model describes two leader styles, relationship-oriented and task-oriented. He determined that task-oriented leaders performed better in either very favorable or very unfavorable situations (seen in situations 1, 2, 3, and 8 in Figure 17-3); whereas relationship-oriented leaders performed better in moderately favorable situations (seen in situations 4–7).
  - House's Path-Goal Model (Figure 17-4) shows a process in which leaders select specific behaviors (directive, supportive, participative, or achievement-oriented) that are best suited to the followers' needs and the working environment so that they can guide and support followers to perform well and meet organizational goals.
  - Using Hersey and Blanchard's Situational Leadership® model, there are two dimensions of leadership behavior: task (directive) and relationship (supportive) behaviors. Depending on the follower's readiness (ability and willingness), a leader can choose a telling style, selling style, participating style, or delegating style (Figure 17-5).

- Contemporary leadership theories build on past research to explain how effective leaders interact and build relationships with followers as well as motivate and support them.

  - Leader-member exchange (LMX) theory focuses on the nature and quality of the exchanges and relationship between a leader and *each* follower. Research has shown that quality leader-member

exchanges and relationships are consistently related to member job satisfaction, job performance, and organizational commitment.

- A transactional leader is one who leads primarily by using social exchanges with followers along with exchanging rewards (or in some cases punishments) for completion of certain tasks/goals. The transactional leader works within the organizational culture to maintain the status quo.

- While the transactional leader is more likely to be a first-line manager or in middle management, transformational leaders are usually in the top management ranks. Transformational leaders (Figure 17-6) inspire followers to look at problems in new ways while inspiring and motivating them to work together toward a shared vision and (often) extraordinary goals.

- A charismatic leader is an enthusiastic, energetic, and confident individual who uses their personality and actions to motivate and inspire high levels of performance, trust, and commitment. Much of their strong influence derives from the fact that they are skilled communicators and can articulate an engaging vision.

- Authentic leaders are genuine; they don't try to imitate someone else. Because they are open, honest, and genuine, they are trusted by their followers. Authentic leaders are guided by their sense of ethics and lead by example.

- Servant leaders share power with the employees and *serve the employees* and often the community. Servant leaders place their employees' needs ahead of their self-interest. By doing so, the servant leader moves beyond transactional leadership and helps align the employee's sense of purpose with the organization's mission.

- Trends and future issues in leadership include distributed leadership (Figure 17-7), cross-cultural leadership, and the reduction of gender and racial inequality.

17.2 Discuss the Delegation Process

- Although managers are often wary of delegating tasks, it can give the manager more time to do their own work and the subordinate an opportunity to build knowledge, skills, confidence, and job satisfaction.

A measure of a manager's effectiveness lies in the ability to get work done through other people.

- Delegation actually comprises four steps: preparation, the delegation discussion, monitoring, and evaluation. To prepare, a manager needs to develop a delegation plan, including objectives, a timeline, and checkpoints, and decide which subordinate would be most appropriate.
- The delegation discussion should include all details such as the objectives, the amount of authority and resources available, the controls such as progress reports and deadlines, and how results will be evaluated and recognized. Effective delegation does not mean telling someone what to do, but rather mutually discussing and agreeing on what is to be accomplished and how it is to be monitored and evaluated.
- Once a task is delegated, it needs to be monitored to evaluate progress and give any needed feedback.
- The last step is to assess the completed task by comparing it with the results agreed upon at the beginning of this process, and hold the employee accountable for the results. Of course, an honest discussion with the employee is important to improve understanding.
- Reverse delegation is when an employee tries to dump the assignment back onto the boss.

17.3   Manage Change

- Figure 17-8 shows the change process (fear/deny, anger/resist, explore/resign, commit).
- There are many reasons why employees resist change such as fear of unknown, uncertainty, self-interest, anxiety about learning new skills, lack of trust in superiors, poor communication, not being consulted, or inadequate rewards.
- Tips are given for creating a climate for change, engaging employees while transitioning into the change, and sustaining change.
- Table 17-2 explains methods for dealing with resistance to change.
- Organization development (OD) is a contemporary process that uses social and behavioral sciences to increase organizational effectiveness and assist the change process in both individuals and the organization. A central theme of OD is to create and manage change so that individuals can develop and organizations perform better. Organization development is usually led by someone in the human resources department.

17.4   Describe Guidelines for Negotiating

- Negotiation is a type of discussion in which two parties are trying to reach an agreement that both parties find acceptable.
- Table 17-3 gives tips for what to do before and during negotiations.

REVIEW AND DISCUSSION QUESTIONS

1. What did trait theories, behavioral theories, and contingency models of leadership say about leadership?
2. Do you think managers use a contingency approach to be effective leaders? Explain why or why not.
3. What is the premise of leader-member exchange theory?
4. Differentiate between a transactional leader and a transformational leader.
5. Can a leader be both charismatic and visionary? Explain.
6. Why is trust between a leader and followers so important? Give two examples of how a leader builds trust.
7. How can a leader distribute leadership throughout the organization?
8. Why can it be hard for a manager to delegate?
9. Give three tips on how to successfully delegate a task or project.
10. Why do employees fear change?
11. Why do people in organizations resist change? Name three ways a manager can reduce resistance to change.
12. What are four things you can do to be an effective negotiator?

SMALL GROUP PROJECT

For the foodservice concept that you created in Chapter 1, develop the following.

1. Assume you have a managerial role in your foodservice. Describe your role and where it exists in the organizational chart. Describe two tasks you might be able to delegate to a capable employee and the procedure you would follow to do so.

2. As the Production Manager, you make changes to the menu every year in the spring and in the fall to take advantage of seasonal fruits and vegetables. The cooks do not always like menu changes as they have to change some of their routines and it takes some time to figure out how popular the new items will be. Describe five specific ways you could create a climate for change so that the cooks were less upset about changing the menu.

REFERENCES

Anand, S., Vidyarthi, P. R., & Park, H. S. (2016). LMX differentiation: Understanding relational leadership at individual and group levels. In T. N. Bauer & B. Erdogan (Eds.), *The Oxford Handbook of Leader-Member Exchange* (pp. 263–291). Oxford University Press.

Anthony, S. D., & Schwartz, E. I. (2017). What the best transformational leaders do. *Harvard Business Review.* https://hbr.org/2017/05/what-the-best-transformational -leaders-do

Bauer, T. N., & Erdogan, B. (Eds.). (2016). *The Oxford Handbook of Leader-Member Exchange.* Oxford University Press.

Blake, R.R., & Mouton, J.S. (1985). *The Managerial Grid III: The key to leadership excellence.* Gulf Publishing.

Conger, J. A., & Kanungo, R. N. (1998). *Charismatic leadership in organizations.* Sage.

Dvir, T., Eden, D., Avolio, B. J., & Shamir, B. (2002). Impact of transactional leadership on follower development and performance: A field experiment. *Academy of Management Journal, 45*(4), 735–744. doi: 10.2307 /3069307

Fiedler, F. E. (1967). *A theory of leadership effectiveness.* McGraw-Hill.

Fiedler, F. E., & Chemers, M. M. (1974). *Leadership and effective management.* Scott, Foresman and Company.

Gerstner, C. R., & Day, D. V. (1997). Meta-analytic review of leader—member exchange theory: Correlates and construct issues. *Journal of Applied Psychology, 82*(6), 827–844. doi: 10.1037/0021-9010.82.6.827

Graeff, C. L. (1997). Evolution of situational leadership theory: A critical review. *The Leadership Quarterly, 8*(2), 153–170. doi: 10.1016/S1048-9843(97)90014-X

Harvard Business Review. (2011). *HBR's 10 must reads on leadership.* Boston: Harvard Business School Publishing.

Hersey, P., & Blanchard, K. H. (1969). Life cycle theory of leadership. *Training & Development Journal, 23*(5), 26–34.

Hersey, P., & Blanchard, K. H. (1977). *Management of organization behavior: Utilizing human resources* (3rd ed.). Prentice Hall, Inc.

House, R. J. (1971). A path-goal theory of leader effectiveness. *Administrative Science Quarterly, 16*(3), 321–339. doi: 10.2307/2391905

Judge, T. A., Bono, J. E., Illies, R., & Gerhardt, M. W. (2002). Personality and leadership: A qualitative and quantitative review. *Journal of Applied Psychology, 87*(4), 765–780. doi: 10.1037/0021-9010.87.4.765

Kirkpatrick, S. A., & Locke, E. A. (1991). Leadership: Do traits matter? *Academy of Management Perspectives, 5*(2), 48–60. doi: 10.105465/ame.1991.4274679

Kotter, J.P. (1996). *Leading change.* Harvard Business School Press.

Kotter, J. P., & Schlesinger, L. A. (2008). Choosing Strategies for change. *Harvard Business Review, 86*(7–8), 130–138.

LePine, M. A., Zhang, Y., Crawford, E. R., & Rich, B. L. (2016). Turning their path to gain: Charismatic leader influence on follower stress appraisal and job performance. *Academy of Management Journal, 59*(3), 1036–1059.

Liden, R. C., Wayne, S. J., Liao, C., & Meuser, J. D. (2014). Servant leadership and serving culture: Influence on individual and unit performance. *Academy of Management Journal, 57*(5), 1434–1452. doi:10.5465 /amj.2013.0034

Liden, R. C., Wayne, S. J., & Stilwell, D. (1993). A longitudinal study on the early development of leader-member exchanges. *Journal of Applied Psychology, 78*(4), 662–674. doi: 10.1037/0021-9010.78.4.662

Lussier, R.N. (2019). *Management fundamentals: Concepts, applications, and skill development* (8th ed.). Sage Publications, Inc.

Mitchell, T. R., Biglan, A., Oncken, G. R., & Fiedler, F. E. (2017). The contingency model: Criticism and suggestions. *The Academy of Management Journal, 13*(3), 253–267. doi: 10.5465/254963

Mostafa, A. M. S. (2019). Transformational leadership and restaurant employees customer-oriented behaviours: The mediating role of organizational social capital and work engagement. *International Journal of Contemporary Hospitality Management, 31*(3), 1166–1182. doi 10.1108 /IJCHM-02-2018-0123

Neck, C.P., Houghton, J.D., & Murray, E.L. (2020). *Organizational behavior: A skill-building approach.* Sage.

Nystrom, P. C. (1978). Managers and the hi-hi leader myth. *Academy of Management Journal, 21*(2), 325–331. doi: 10.2307/255767

Peters, L. H., Hartke, D. D., & Pohlmann, J. T. (1985). Fiedler's Contingency Theory of Leadership: An application of the meta-analysis procedures of Schmidt and Hunter. *Psychological Bulletin, 97*(2), 274–285. doi: 10.1037/0033-2909.97.2.274

Ray, J. (2019). 5 traits all effective leaders have. *Nation's Restaurant News.* https://www.nrn.com/workforce/5-traits-all-effective-leaders-have

Robbins, S. P., & Coulter, M. (2018). *Management* (14th ed.). Pearson Education Inc.

Schriesheim, C. A., Tepper, B. J., & Tetrault, L. A. (1994). Least preferred co-worker score, situational control, and leadership effectiveness: A meta-analysis of contingency model performance predictions. *Journal of Applied Psychology, 79*(4), 561–573. doi: 10.1037/0021-9010.79.4.561

Torben, R. (2011.) Top 12 reasons why people resist change. https://www.torbenrick.eu/blog/change-management/12-reasons-why-people-resist-change/

Ury, W.L., Fisher, R., & Patton, B. (1992). *Getting to yes: Negotiating agreement without giving in* (2nd ed). HMH Books.

Vergauwe, J., Wille, B., Hofmans, J., Kaiser, R. B., & De Fruyt, F. (2017). Too much charisma can make leaders look less effective. *Harvard Business Review.* https://hbr.org/2017/09/too-much-charisma-can-make-leaders-look-less-effective

Wong, C. A., & Laschinger, H. K. S. (2013). Authentic leadership, performance, and job satisfaction: The mediating role of empowerment. *Journal of Advanced Nursing, 69*(4), 947–959. doi: 10.1111/j.1365-2648.2012.06089.x

Zaccaro, S. J. (2007). Trait-based perspectives of leadership. *American Psychologist, 62*(1), 6–16. doi: 10.1037/0003-066X.62.1.6

Zingerman's. (2016). The 6 responsibilities of a Zingerman's servant leader. https://drive.google.com/file/d/0B1tNMeL_C8YYVm1obDRoTnNBTnM/view

GLOSSARY

A

ABC inventory method   A classification of each inventory item into one of three categories based on their dollar value and usage so managers pay more attention to higher-value items.

accent lighting   Lighting that is used to add interest, such as by accenting artwork. A form of direct lighting.

accountability   Being responsible to your supervisor for your actions and performance.

accounting   The process of recording and summarizing all transactions of the business as well as analyzing and verifying the results.

accounting period   Any specific length of time for which accounting functions are performed and analyzed, such as a fiscal year.

accounts payable   In a business, a bill that must be paid to suppliers and others.

accounts receivable   In a business, money that is owed to the business.

acquisition   When one company buys all or part of another.

active learning   Any process by which learners are directly involved in their own learning.

active listening   Being engaged and attentive to what the speaker is saying, including nonverbal messages.

activity ratios   Ratios that tell you how well assets are being utilized or managed to produce income. Also called efficiency ratios.

adaptive strategies   Strategies that a business uses when reacting to changes in the business environment.

administrative management theory   A management theory that put an emphasis on design of an organization and how well it is managed.

adulterated foods   Foods that are harmful to health; prepared, packed or held under unsanitary conditions; or contain filth or part of a diseased animal.

advertising   Any form of *paid* presentation or promotion of an idea, product, or service where the brand or sponsor is clearly identified.

affirmative action programs   Programs in businesses that recruit and advance qualified minorities, women, persons with disabilities, and covered veterans. Include training programs, outreach efforts, and other positive steps.

aflatoxin   A group of toxins produced by molds found on crops such as peanuts and tree nuts.

Age Discrimination in Employment Act   Prohibits discrimination in employment decisions against employees 40 years of age and older.

agency shop   With unions, when all members of the bargaining unit pay dues, but they are not required to be union members.

air gap   An interruption in the drain pipe from a sink to prevent sewage from flowing into the sink.

à la carte   A type of menu in which each individual item has its own price.

© Denis Val/Shutterstock

American cheese   A cheese made by blending one or more natural cheeses (often cheddar is included) with texture- and flavor-altering ingredients. Less expensive than natural cheese.

American Customer Satisfaction Index (ACSI)   A source of customer satisfaction data from 46 industries in the U.S.

American-style service   Service where food is arranged on plates in the kitchen and then placed in front of each guest.

Americans with Disabilities Act (ADA)   A federal law that prohibits discrimination against individuals with disabilities in all areas of public life, including jobs, schools, transportation, and all public and private places that are open to the general public.

AP (as purchased) quantity   The weight or volume of an item exactly as it was purchased.

aquaculture   Breeding, raising, and harvesting fish and shellfish. Farming in water.

arbitration   When a third party conducts hearings to help form the basis of his or her decisions, which both parties agree in advance will be binding.

aspirational reference group   A reference group that a consumer would like to belong to.

assembler   In a pod, the person who collects the hot and cold food items for each tray and checks the food for quality and accuracy of the diet order.

assembly   In foodservice, putting components of a meal together on plates/trays to be served.

assembly-serve operation   A foodservice where meals are prepared and most of the items are made from convenience foods.

assets   Anything that a company owns that has value.

assisted-living facilities   Facilities that provide residents with housing, food, housekeeping, and daily assistance with tasks such as dressing and bathing. Often also provide laundry services, recreational and religious activities, and part-time nursing help.

attitudes   A learned tendency to evaluate people, situations, etc., in a positive or negative manner.

at-will employment   When employees can be fired at any time and for almost any reason.

auditing   The evaluation of financial records and statements prepared by accountants.

authentic leaders   Leaders who are open, honest, and genuine. Trusted by their followers.

authoritarian leaders   Leaders who make almost all of the decisions and direct subordinates closely.

authority   Right of a manager to direct others at work, make decisions, and use resources.

automated guided vehicles   Robotic vehicles often used for delivery of items.

automatic slicers   A piece of foodservice equipment that slices meats, cheeses, vegetables, and more. Can slice items without an operator.

average check   Average sale per customer.

B

background check   The process a business uses to verify that an applicant is who they claim to be in terms of, for example, education or employment history.

back-to-back arrangement   When two rows of foodservice equipment are laid out back-to-back, often with a hood overhead. Rows are parallel.

bacteria   One-celled organisms that are invisible to the eye, some of which are in food and can cause illness.

bain-marie   A piece of foodservice equipment that consists of a hot water bath used in the hot production area to keep soups, sauces, etc., warm.

baking   Cooking foods by surrounding them with heated dry air. Same as roasting but applies to baking breads, cakes, etc.

balance sheet   A document that provides detailed information about how well a company is doing financially. Includes the company's assets, liabilities, and shareholders' equity.

banquet service   Service where guests are all seated at tables and served preset menu items at the same time.

barcodes   A label with vertical lines, spaces, and numbers that tell you information about the item. Machine readable.

bargaining unit   A group of two or more employees who share common employment conditions and are grouped together and represented by a specific labor union in collective bargaining and other dealings with management.

base   A piece of equipment placed underneath a plate to keep the plate hot or cold.

batch cooking   Cooking small quantities as needed during meal service.

behaviorally anchored rating scale (BARS)   A performance appraisal technique that measures an employee's behaviors. Combines the graphic rating scale with anchors or critical incidents for each rating.

behavior observation scale   A behavior-based measure used to evaluate job performance. The person carrying out the rating uses a five-point scale to gauge the frequency with which an employee engages in a behavior.

benchmarking   The practice of comparing your operation's performance against yourself, similar operations, or an industry standard to determine if there are areas for improvement.

best alternative to a negotiated agreement   The course of action if negotiations don't work out.

beverage cost percentage   Cost of alcoholic beverages divided by alcoholic beverage sales.

beverageware   Everything that holds a beverage, such as cocktail glasses.

big data   Complex data sets that can be used to recognize patterns and business opportunities.

blast chiller   A piece of equipment that reduces the temperature of hot food quickly.

blueprints   An architectural/construction drawing of how a building or renovation will be constructed.

boiling   Cooking a food in a liquid that is bubbling rapidly.

bona fide occupational qualifications   Job qualification that is necessary to perform the duties of the position.

bone china   Strongest china you can buy. Lightweight with thin, delicate edges.

bookkeepers   Individuals with a basic understanding of accounting principles and who oversee the recording of the transactions of a business.

bottom line   The profit or loss noted at the bottom of the income statement before income taxes are paid.

bottom-line purchasing   In purchasing, awarding an order to whomever has the lowest bottom line or overall price.

braising   A cooking method with two steps: searing or browning the food (usually meat) in a small amount of oil or its own fat (to seal the outer layer and maintain moisture inside) and then adding liquid and simmering until done.

brand   A feature or set of features that distinguish one product/service from that of the competition.

break-even analysis   A tool to determine at which point your business or new product/service will start to be profitable.

break-even point   The point at which the level of sales is equal to a foodservice's combined variable and fixed costs.

bridge method   A series of steps to use to convert from one type of measurement to another.

brix   Measurement of the sugar content of a watery solution such as the packing medium in canned fruit.

broadline distributors   In foodservice, companies that sell a wide variety of food and nonfood supplies, including some foodservice equipment.

broiler   A piece of cooking equipment that cooks with heat above the food.

broiling   Cooking with radiant heat from above.

broken case   A case that is not full.

broker   An agent that represents food processors or manufacturers. Supplies product samples to foodservices and places orders to a distributor. Does not maintain their own inventory, but makes a commission on sales.

budget variance   The difference between budgeted revenue or expense and the actual amount.

buffalo chopper   A piece of food preparation equipment that uses an S-shaped blade and rotating bowl to turn large pieces of vegetables into small pieces and to chop meats finely.

buffet   Service in which customers serve themselves (some staff may help with certain items) from chafing dishes, refrigerated food wells, platters, etc.

bureaucracy   A type of organization characterized by a hierarchy with a clear chain of command and division of labor, along with formal rules and job performance judged by productivity. Also called mechanistic organization.

business plan   A document that describes a new project or business in detail and is used to seek and secure approvals and/or loans. Also called a prospectus.

butter chip   A slice of butter on a small square of moisture-proof material and a paper on top. Continental butter chips are completely covered in foil.

bypass line   A cafeteria layout that separates different counters so customers can bypass certain stations.

C

cage-free eggs   Eggs laid by hens that are able to roam up and down in indoor houses, and have access to fresh food and water. Not required to have access to the outdoors.

can-cutting test   When a buyer (and others) evaluate different brands and qualities of a canned product, such as canned pears.

capital budget   A budget of money set aside to make major expenditures.

carbon steel   A material used to make pots and pans. Must be cleaned and seasoned. Heats fast and evenly.

carrier   A person who carries a pathogen but has no symptoms.

cart   An open cart with shelves used to collect and transport items in a foodservice.

cash-and-carry distributors   In foodservice, a company, such as Restaurant Depot, Costco, or Gordon Foodservice Store, that sells to smaller foodservices.

cash budget   A budget that forecasts a business' cash flow over 12 months.

cash stream   The series of cash flows to and from a business.

cast iron   A heavy, durable material used to make pots and pans.

cause-and-effect diagram   A diagram (also called a fishbone diagram or Ishikawa diagram after its developer) that is helpful for a team to brainstorm possible causes of a problem and sorting those ideas into useful categories.

cell pack   A style of packaging when each item in the carton is protected from damage.

central distribution centers   For multi-unit operations, a building with supplies and trucks that deliver to the individual units.

centralized ingredient room   A room where employees measure and weigh the ingredients for each recipe that cooks will be preparing.

centralized meal assembly   When meal assembly takes place in one central location.

centralized purchasing   When purchasing within an organization is conducted by a purchasing department (not individual departments).

centralized service   Service in which trays are assembled in the main kitchen and then transported to the patient's rooms or dining rooms for service.

chain of command   Line of authority from the top of an organization down to lowest position.

chain restaurant   Restaurant with multiple units in one city, a region, or across U.S.

change agent   The person in charge of overseeing an organizational change effort.

char-broiler   A piece of cooking equipment with flames that come from below the grill. Similar to outdoor barbecue grill at home.

charismatic leader   An enthusiastic, energetic, and confident individual who uses their personality and actions to motivate and inspire high levels of performance, trust, and commitment.

check sheet   A sheet designed to collect data in real time. Also called a tally sheet.

cheese melters   A piece of cooking equipment that does not cook foods—it only melts cheese, toasts bread, or browns the top of a casserole.

ciguatoxin   A toxin found in fin fish that is not destroyed through cooking and can cause nervous system symptoms.

clamshell griddle   A griddle that speeds cooking by applying heat to both sides of the product.

close-ended questions   Questions that are answered by selecting from a limited number of response options.

closed shop   With unions, when all members of the bargaining unit must be union members and pay dues.

coaching   When supervisors give feedback to employees on how they are doing and also collaborate with employees to improve performance.

collective bargaining   Process in which employees, through their unions, negotiate contracts with their employees to determine pay, benefits, hours, paid time off, safety policies, etc.

collective bargaining agreement   Labor contract between a union and management.

color rendering index   A measure of how well an artificial light shows natural colors compared with daylight or incandescent light.

combination steamer oven   A convection oven with a steamer that can be used for: convection heat, pressureless steam, or a combination of both.

command group   A group made of a manager and the employees they supervise. Also known as a functional command group.

commercial blender   A blender that is more heavy-duty than home versions.

commercial food processor   A piece of food preparation equipment that can cut foods in many different ways.

commercial foodservices   Foodservices that operate to provide meals and make a profit, such as restaurants.

commissary   A central production kitchen that produces meals for delivery off-site such as to airplanes and school lunch rooms.

commissary operation   A foodservice that prepares food in a central kitchen and then transports it to external satellite kitchens where the meals are served. Foods may be distributed in bulk, pre-portioned, or pre-plated—hot, cold, or frozen.

communication   Act of transmitting information, ideas, and meaning through various channels.

communication channel   Means in which a message is transmitted—such as oral, written, electronic, or nonverbal.

compact fluorescent lamps (CFLs)   Ideal lightbulbs to save energy and money as they are about three times more efficient than incandescent bulbs, last for years, and don't emit heat.

compensation   The process of creating and maintaining an internal wage and salary structure and ensuring that this structure is administered fairly and consistently.

competitive advantage Something unique that is different from and better than what your competitors offer.

competitive strategies Strategies used to beat the competition.

compost Organic material that can be added to soil to help plants grow.

conceptual skills Skills that help managers better understand complex and abstract situations so as to analyze a problem and develop a creative solution.

conduction When heat is transferred from something hot to something touching it that is cooler.

consensus When all members of a group support, to some degree, a decision or action.

Consolidated Omnibus Budget Reconciliation Act Federal regulation that gives workers and their families who lose their health benefits the right to choose to continue group health benefits provided by their group health plan for limited periods of time under certain circumstances such as voluntary or involuntary job loss.

consumer behavior The study of how consumers select, purchase, and use products and services.

consumer decision journey The steps involved when a consumer is deciding what to purchase.

content marketing A type of marketing that involves the creation and distribution of materials (such as blogs and videos) intended to attract and educate a specific audience and stimulate interest and purchases.

continental butter chips Small pieces of butter completely covered in foil.

contingency theory A theory that each organization needs to manage and organize itself differently depending on its external environment and technology.

continuing care retirement community (CCRC) Facility that offers assisted living and/or skilled nursing care along with independent living for elderly adults.

continuous-feed food processor A piece of food preparation equipment that is more heavy duty than batch bowl processors and is excellent when you have large quantities of food that need to be chopped, diced, sliced, and more.

continuous quality improvement (CQI) A systematic approach to measuring, evaluating, and improving products and services. Uses a cyclical process of assessing products or performance, developing and implementing improvement plans, and reassessing results.

contribution margin The amount of money left over when you subtract the food cost from the selling price of a menu item.

control chart A graph that shows data over time, so it demonstrates how a variable or process changes over time.

controllable costs Costs, such as food, that managers have the power to influence in the short term.

controllable income Profit after all controllable costs are removed from sales.

controlling A function of management that involves monitoring employees' performance, products being made, and services being delivered, as well as keeping an eye on food costs, sales, and other important indicators.

controls Methods to influence how something is managed or done.

convection When heat is spread by moving air, steam, liquid, or hot fat.

convection microwaves A microwave oven that adds forced hot air to help brown or crisp food surfaces.

convection ovens A type of oven that uses radiant heat and forced air to cook foods. Cooks quicker than a nonconvection oven.

conventional operation A foodservice where meals are prepared and served and most of the menu items are cooked from scratch.

conveyor ovens Ovens with a wire conveyor that carries foods through a space where the hot air hits the food from all angles. Used for pizza, calzones, hamburgers, and more.

conveyor-type dishwasher Large dishwashing machine used in foodservices that move full racks of dishes from the wash to rinse to sanitizing rinse cycle.

cook chill system   A system of producing food that involves these steps: cook, chill for a period of time, then reheat and serve.

cook freeze system   A system of producing food in which food is cooked then frozen rapidly using a blast chiller or blast freezer. Foods are then usually thawed before reheating.

core values   The essence of a company's identity, principles, and beliefs.

cost-benefit analysis   A way to compare the costs and benefits of an alternative, where both are expressed in dollars.

cost center   A department or part of an organization that does not generate revenue and incurs costs.

cost of capital   The interest rate at which businesses are allowed by banks to borrow money.

cost of goods sold   The cost to purchase the foods and beverages purchased to generate sales. Also called cost of sales.

cost of sales percentage   The total cost of foods and beverages divided by total sales.

cost-plus pricing   Pricing based on the cost of the product plus a fixed markup.

cost-plus percentage pricing   Pricing based on the cost of the product plus an additional percentage.

Cost-Volume-Profit formula   A formula used to determine the needed sales level to cover costs and provide a given profit.

counter service   Serving customers at a counter.

covers   In restaurants, the number of meals served.

coving   Flooring material found at the base of walls to keep the juncture of the wall and floor clean.

credit memo   A document that shows the amount of money that does not need to be paid on an invoice due to items being rejected, returned, etc.

critical control points (CCPs)   Any point, step, or procedure in which a food safety hazard can be prevented, eliminated, or reduced to an acceptable level.

critical incident method   A procedure to identify behaviors that contribute to the success or failure of employees in a specific situation.

cross contamination   The transfer of harmful bacteria from uncooked foods, people, and equipment/surfaces to ready-to-eat foods and cooked foods.

cross-cultural leadership   The process of leading followers representing many cultures.

cross-functional team   A team of employees from different functional areas (departments) of the company who work on a common project/goal.

crystal glass   A type of glass that is not as sparkly as lead crystal but its appearance is favored over glass.

current assets   Assets such as cash or other assets that can be converted into cash within one year. Also called liquid assets.

current liabilities   In a business, amounts of money that must be paid within a year.

current ratio   The ratio of current assets of a business to its current liabilities.

customer experience   How customers respond to any direct or indirect contact with a company.

customer satisfaction   A psychological concept involving the pleasure of getting what you expected and wanted/needed from an appealing product/service and *total experience* (not just the service or food).

cycle menu   A menu that changes daily for a certain length of time, such as one week. Commonly used in many onsite foodservices.

D

data   Unorganized facts and numbers.

date label gun   A tool designed to print a date on a sticker that is then put on a box or product. Used by receiving so each can or item is marked with the date it was received.

debt ratio   A ratio comparing total liabilities to total assets of a business.

decentralized meal assembly   A system in which food is transported in bulk from the production area to a location(s) closer to the point of service where the meals will be assembled/served.

decentralized service   Service in which food is moved in bulk from a main or central kitchen to a galley or satellite kitchen where meals are assembled and served.

decibels   A measurement of the intensity of sound.

decision-making process   A process that involves selecting a course of action to: solve a problem (such as decrease labor costs), take advantage of an opportunity (such as expand a business), or simply make a management decision (such as set long-term goals).

decision tree   In problem-solving, a diagram of the possible outcomes for different actions that could be taken.

deck oven   A standard oven with several shallow oven spaces. Food is placed directly on the metal, ceramic, or cementitious floor or deck of the oven. Used in bakeries and pizzerias.

deep-fat frying   In cooking, to immerse a food in hot fat, where it tends to cook evenly and quickly.

deglaze   In cooking, to swirl a liquid in a pan to dissolve cooked particles of food remaining on the bottom of the pan.

delegation   When a manager asks a subordinate to accomplish an objective or task (that is not already in the employee's job description) and also gives the responsibility and often some authority to make certain decisions and/or use resources to do so.

demand-controlled kitchen ventilation (DCKV)   A kitchen ventilation system that saves energy by adjusting the quantity of kitchen hood exhaust and incoming outdoor air to reflect the amount of cooking taking place under the hood.

democratic leaders   Leaders who guide and coach employees to do their jobs, as well as encourage them to participate in decision making.

departmentalization   The process of grouping related activities together to form departments, such as cold food production.

design   Developing a new or renovated foodservice space starting with creating a concept until the building/renovation is completed.

diet order   In a healthcare facility, the order for which foods someone can and can't eat, such as a low-sodium or regular diet.

differentiation   A marketing strategy to help consumers distinguish your product/ service from others.

differentiation strategy   A strategy that requires a business to create products or services that are unique and valued by customers.

digital instant-read thermometer   A thermometer with a stainless-steel stem and a digital readout that takes approximately 15 seconds to measure temperature.

dinnerware   Plates, bowls, and dishes.

directional plan   A flexible plan that spells out general guidelines. Also called an options-based plan.

direct issues   Received items that do not go into storage, but instead go directly to production (such as bread).

direct lighting   Lighting used to put light in a specific area.

disaster   When the activities of a community or region are seriously disrupted by natural hazards or other event that causes widespread harm and losses.

discounting   Estimating the present value of a future payment(s) that will be received at a later time.

distributed leadership   When leadership responsibility is distributed or shared.

distribution   In foodservices, the process of getting food from where it was produced to where the customer will be served.

distributional errors   When evaluators rate most employees using just one part of a rating scale—specifically the top part, the middle, or lower part of the scale.

distributor   A company that supplies goods to businesses such as restaurants and healthcare facilities.

diversity   The range of human differences, such as age and ethnicity.

docking station   A specialized piece of equipment that can rethermalize food trays, and, at the same time, keep cold foods cold.

door-type dishwasher   A dishwasher that accommodates one rack full of dishes.

drained weight   The weight of a can's content once the liquid is completely drained.

dry-heat cooking methods   Cooking that transfers heat without the use of water or steam. Relies on hot air, hot fat, hot metal, or radiation.

dry sauté   A low-fat cooking method of browning foods in little or no fat.

dry stores   A storage area for foods that don't require refrigeration or freezing.

dues checkoff provision   With unions, when the employer collects dues from union members and non-union members and gives the dues to the union.

dynamic equilibrium   Steady state.

E

effective managers   Managers who choose appropriate goals and activities to make a business successful.

efficient managers   Managers who get the most output of goods or services from the smallest amount of inputs.

egg products   Eggs that are removed from their shells and processed to produce whole eggs, egg yolk, or egg whites in refrigerated, frozen, or dried forms. Must be pasteurized.

e-learning   Learning through electronic media and technologies.

80-20 principle   When applied to time management, the idea that 80% of the results comes from 20% of the actions taken.

electric heat strips   Contains one or more rows of heating elements inside a metal or ceramic cover that radiates the heat.

electric induction cooktops   A burner that produces a magnetic field so that only the cookware gets hot.

electronic communication   Messages that use electronic media such as emails, texts, Skype, Facebook, or Twitter.

elevation   A view looking sideways at an object, such as a drawing of how the front of a restaurant will look.

emergencies   Similar to disasters but occur on a much smaller scale.

emotional intelligence   Your self-awareness and self-management, but also your ability to sense how others are feeling and handle the emotions of others.

employee assistance programs   Programs offered by some employers that give free and confidential counseling and help for employees with addictions, family problems, stress, or financial problems.

employee development   Initiatives of both the employer and an employee in which the employee gains more education, skills and abilities, job experiences, and relationships (such as a mentor) to move up the career ladder.

employee referral programs   A program in which a current employee refers an applicant to the company and receives a reward if the applicant is hired.

employee relations   Creating a positive work environment for employees.

employment tests   Tests used to help determine the best qualified candidate for a job. May include cognitive ability tests, physical ability tests, job knowledge tests, or drug testing, depending on the job.

English service   Service in which the server holds a large dish of food and serves each guest individually, starting with the host.

environment   The conditions or surroundings in which a person, business, or system operates.

EP (edible portion) quantity   The weight or volume of an item after all inedible or nonservable parts are trimmed off.

Equal employment opportunity (EEO)   A concept that people should be treated equally in employment matters. EEO laws make it illegal to discriminate against a job applicant or an employee because of the person's race, color, religion, sex (including pregnancy, gender identity, and sexual orientation), national origin, age (40 or older), disability, or genetic information.

Equal Employment Opportunity Commission (EEOC)   An agency of the Department of Justice that enforces most of the EEO laws. Has the authority to investigate charges of discrimination against employers after an employee files a complaint.

Equal Pay Act of 1963   Federal regulation that requires covered employers to provide equal pay for men and women who are performing the same (equal) work.

equity theory   A motivational theory based on the concept of fairness and how the employee perceives their outputs/inputs compared with others. When inequities occur, employees are less motivated.

error of central tendency   When evaluators evaluate everyone as average or slightly above average.

evaluation   In training, the process used to see how well trainees recall information, demonstrate skills, have changed attitudes, or improved performance.

evoked set   The narrowed-down set of choices a consumer puts together after evaluating a variety of products. Also called consideration set.

exempt employees   Employees such as many executive, administrative, and professional employees who meet special legal requirements, such as being compensated on a salary basis at a rate not less than $684 per week (as of 2020), so they are not entitled to overtime pay. Also called salaried employees.

expectancy theory   A motivational theory that states that motivation to behave in a certain way is a function of expectancy, instrumentality, and valence.

external benchmarking   When a manager compares performance with foodservices *outside* of their organization.

external recruiting   When a company recruits applicants from outside of the company.

extrinsic motivation   When you do something to get a reward that is external to the work itself.

F

facilitate   To guide (not direct).

Failure Mode and Effects Analysis (FMEA)   A technique used to identify and analyze potential failures within a process.

Fair Labor Standards Act (FLSA)   Federal regulation that establishes minimum wage, overtime pay, and youth employment standards.

Family and Medical Leave Act   Federal regulation that makes it possible for an eligible employee (one who has been employed for at least one year and has worked for at least 1,250 hours) to take up to 12 weeks of *unpaid* leave in a 12-month period for certain specified reasons (such as childbirth) without loss of employment.

family-style service   Service in which large serving platters and bowls of food are placed on the guests' table, and they are passed around the table for diners to serve themselves.

farm-raised seafood   Seafood that is raised using aquaculture.

favorable variance   A variance that is preferred, such as higher sales than budgeted or lower food costs.

Federal Unemployment Tax Act (FUTA)   A federal regulation that requires a small payroll tax that employers pay for each employee that helps pay unemployment benefits.

Federal Insurance Contributions Act (FICA)   A federal regulation requiring employers and employees to pay Social Security and Medicare taxes.

feedback   In a system, when outputs are examined to see how well the system is functioning.

feedback   In communication, asking for clarification or verification of a message.

filtering   The withholding of information because the sender thinks the information is either not needed or the receiver doesn't want to receive it.

first-in, first-out (FIFO) method   A method of stock rotation in which foods are shelved based upon use–by or expiration dates, so older foods are used first.

first-line manager   Managers who supervise hourly employees. Also called supervisor.

fiscal year   A period of 12 months.

fixed assets   Tangible permanent resources of a business.

fixed budget   A budget that assumes the volume of business that will be done is known and predictable, and that the costs and revenues will generally stay within projections.

fixed costs   Costs in a budget that remain the same despite the level of sales or number of meals prepared.

flexible budget   A budget that adjusts with changes in the volume of sales.

5S   A methodology used in Kaizen to improve workplace or work-station organization and eliminate wasted time looking for needed items or getting ready to work.

flash freezing   Freezing food rapidly to prevent the formation of ice crystals.

flats   Packaging used for certain fruits and vegetables that only contain one layer of product.

flavor   An attribute of a food that includes its taste, aroma, feel in the mouth, texture, and temperature.

flight-type dishwasher   A dishwasher used only in high-volume foodservices that does not use racks, but instead dishes are moved through the cycles on a moving belt.

flowchart   A graphic representation of an ordered sequence of events, steps, or procedures that take place in a system.

fluid ounces   A measure of volume.

fluorescent tubes   Lighting that is durable and spreads light over a large area. Often used in foodservice kitchens.

focused differentiation or focused low-cost strategies   Strategies that develop low-cost or unique products for a specific regional or niche market.

followers   Subordinates of a leader.

followership   Individuals' capacity to work with leaders.

food cost percentage   Cost of food divided by total sales. Often falls between 25 and 35%.

food pulpers   A type of foodservice equipment that is used to collect and dispose of food scraps.

food safety management system   A comprehensive use of practices, such as standard operating procedures, training, and pest control, that a foodservice can use to ensure food safety.

foodservice consultant   Individuals who provide expertise and experience for foodservices when such expertise is not available in house. Often, they are members of the Foodservice Consultants Society International.

foodservice contract company   A profit-making company that may be hired to provide meals for clients such as healthcare facilities, schools, colleges and universities, correctional facilities, or other organizations that need meals.

foodborne illness   A wide spectrum of illnesses resulting from eating food contaminated in one of these ways: biological contamination such as bacteria, chemical contamination such as cleaning products, or physical contamination.

foodservice subsidy   In onsite foodservices, the amount of money that an organization spends to cover the foodservice costs that are not covered by prices/income.

food specification   A written, detailed description for each food purchased including size, color, quality requirements, packaging information, and other relevant information.

food terrorism   When food is deliberately made unsafe and causes injury or death and/or disrupts stability.

food waste   Food that is produced to eat but is never consumed.

foot-candles   A measurement of light intensity. The illuminance on a one square foot surface from a light source.

forecast   In foodservice, a prediction of how much of each menu item will be needed for a specific time period or meal.

force-field analysis   A brainstorming method in which the group lists all of the forces that foster change and forces that diminish change—then diagrams each force, including its strength.

forged knives   A type of knife created from one solid piece of metal. Better quality than stamped knives.

formal authority   The right to give directions to subordinates because of your position in the organizational chart.

formal communication   Communication among people that takes place based on lines of authority set up in an organizational chart.

formal leader   The leader as officially designated within the group or organization.

formal groups   A group with designated members and specific functions, such as hot food production. Created via formal authority.

formal purchasing   A purchasing process that uses competitive proposals or bids.

franchisee   The person/company granted the rights to run a unit of a multi-unit retail operation, such as Dunkin', and pays fees and royalties.

franchise restaurant   A chain restaurant run by a third-party operator who has the rights to use the chain's name, design, and system of operation in exchange for fees/royalties, marketing, and advising.

franchisor   A multiunit operator that sells the right to open stores using its brand.

free-range eggs   Eggs produced by hens that are able to roam in indoor houses with continuous access to the outdoors and food and water.

freeriding   In a group, when a member puts in less effort than when working alone. Also known as social loafing.

French service   Service distinguished by some food being prepared (sometimes just partially prepared) and served table-side such as carved prime rib, Caesar salad, or a flambé dish such as crêpes Suzette or steak Diane.

freshwater fish   Fish that live all or most of their lives in streams, rivers, ponds, lakes, and reservoirs.

fryers   A piece of cooking equipment that holds oils and cooks foods such as French fries.

functional structure   When organizational structure is based on creating departments that each have their own functions.

full-line distributors   In foodservice, companies that sell a wide variety of food and nonfood supplies.

full-time employee   An employee who typically works 35 to 40 hours/week. The number of hours needed may be decided by the business or the state.

full-time equivalents (FTE)   One FTE is the equivalent of one full-time employee who works eight hours a day, 40 hours a week (although in some companies this number is a little lower), which is 2,080 hours a year.

fungi   Organisms that feed on organic matter, including molds, yeast, and mushrooms. Can spoil food.

G

galley (satellite) kitchen   A kitchen that receives mostly prepared foods from another location and then meals are assembled and served.

Gantt chart   A bar chart that depicts the tasks that must be completed for a project to be finished.

general ledger   A complete record of all financial transactions for a business.

Genetically Modified Organisms (GMO)   Common term used by consumers to describe foods that have been created through genetic engineering.

ghost kitchens   Foodservices that only have a kitchen space to produce meals and meals are delivered. Also called virtual kitchens.

goals   Desired outcomes.

goal setting theory   (Locke) A motivational theory that says that working toward a clear goal is a major source of motivation

grading   A process in which foods are graded on quality. Not required by regulations, completed voluntarily by food processors/manufacturers.

gram   Unit of weight in the metric system.

grapevine   Informal communication within an organization, sometimes called the rumor mill.

graphic rating scale   A popular format used to complete performance appraisals. Lists the traits each employee should have and then each is rated on a numbered scale.

grass-fed cattle   Cattle that are only fed grass, forage, hay, or silage so they grow at a slower pace and are normally slaughtered up to 12 months later than grain-fed cattle.

green marketing   A marketing approach in which a business shows all it is doing to improve the environment and minimize damage caused by its production and business practices.

greenwashing   When corporations give the impression of being environmentally conscious whether or not the company is really being environmentally friendly.

griddle   Polished, flat cooking surfaces used to cook pancakes, eggs, hamburgers, and other foods.

griddling   Cooking foods such as pancakes on a solid, flat griddle.

grievance   A work-related complaint made by an employee.

grilling   Cooking with a heat source under the food.

gross profit   The amount of money left over after subtracting food cost from sales.

group cohesiveness   Group members who actively work together, participate, and recognize member contributions.

group dynamics   The study of how group/team members interact with each other. Also called group process.

group purchasing   When an organization purchases items along with other organizations to increase buying volume and decrease prices paid.

group purchasing organization   An entity that puts together the purchasing volume for various members (such as hospital foodservices in a metropolitan area) so that member needs are met and the higher purchasing volume helps get lower prices than if each member purchased individually.

group roles   How a group member is expected to perform because of their position in the group.

groupthink   When group members agree on a course of action that they know is not optimal instead of expressing doubts or disagreeing with the consensus. This can happen when some group members feel a need to conform.

growth strategies   Steps to grow a business.

H

halal Meat prepared according to Muslim law.

halo effect When an evaluator allows the rating of one aspect of performance in which an employee excels, such as being cooperative, to positively influence the rating of other factors.

Hawthorne effect The experience in which performance of the employees is influenced by the people they are working with—including fellow employees, groups, and managers. Employees performed better when they felt managers cared about their workplace and gave them a chance to be heard.

Hazard Analysis Critical Control Point (HACCP) system A prevention-based food safety system.

heat lamps Lamps using infrared bulbs that can keep plated food warm before service.

Hierarchy of Needs Theory (Maslow) Theory that states that people are motivated by five types of needs: physiological, safety, social or belonging, esteem needs, and self-actualization.

high carbon stainless steel A material used to make a knife blade with excellent durability and edge retention.

histogram A simple graph using bars of different heights to show a frequency distribution of a variable, such as wait time.

homogenized A process in which the fat in milk is divided into tiny pieces that are then evenly dispersed throughout the milk.

horizontal (lateral) communication When information flows among people at about the same level in an organization.

horns effect When an evaluator allows a poor rating in one aspect of the evaluation to negatively influence the rating of other factors.

hot holding cabinet A piece of foodservice equipment that holds sheet pans and steam table pans and keeps prepared foods hot.

hourly employees Employees who are paid by the hour and are entitled to overtime pay if working over 40 hours in a week.

human or interpersonal skills Skills that look at how well someone relates to and understands other people. Also called soft skills.

human resource management The department in a company that oversees hiring, employee development, compensation, safety and health, and employee and labor relations.

human resource planning A process in which human resource professionals analyze the present labor supply, forecast how many employees with specific knowledge and skills will be needed in the future, and consistently maintain a skilled workforce that avoids employee shortages or surpluses.

I

immersion blenders Stick blenders that go directly into a pot of food to blend, puree, or emulsify.

incandescent bulb A traditional light bulb that tends to capture color better than fluorescent lighting but is not energy efficient and does not last very long.

income statement A report of revenue and expenses completed for a business for a specific accounting period. Also called a profit and loss (P & L) statement.

incremental budgeting When the current budget is used as the basis for the new budget and the manager adds or subtracts incremental amounts based on projections.

independent contractors Self-employed individuals who may work for more than one client.

independent manufacturers' representative A manufacturer's salesperson who represents a number of product lines from more than one manufacturer.

independent restaurant A restaurant that is not part of a multiunit or chain. Often a single restaurant with an owner who is engaged in daily operations.

indirect lighting Lighting that is pointed upward and mostly washes the ceiling and upper walls with light instead of aiming at a certain spot.

individually quick frozen (IQF) A process in which foods are frozen separately so they are less likely to stick together.

informal communication Communication between people independent of their organizational relationship, level of authority, or job functions.

informal groups Groups in an organization that form for social reasons or because members have common interests.

informal leader An individual with influence in an organization but who does not hold any position of formal authority over others who follow their lead.

informal purchasing A procedure to purchase foods in which the buyer requests and evaluates prices from suppliers, then places the order, receives the shipment, and reviews and approves the invoice.

information Data that have been organized and can be used to make decisions.

infrared thermometers Thermometers that measure surface temperatures (not internal temperatures).

ingredient room A space usually in the dry goods storeroom area where personnel weigh and measure the ingredients for each recipe, which is then given to the cooks or other personnel responsible for preparation.

in-house or signature brand When a foodservice develops its own brand.

inputs What goes into or operated on by a system.

in-service training Training given to employees during the course of their employment.

inspection For foods, a physical inspection to assure that the food is wholesome and safe to eat.

instant read thermometer (bimetal thermometer) A thermometer with a stainless steel stem and a dial or digital readout that takes approximately 15 to 20 seconds to measure temperature.

instructional design A process that a trainer uses to develop instructional plans using learning and instructional theory.

instructional methods Teaching strategies.

integration The need to coordinate efforts throughout the organization to create a smooth workflow and meet goals.

intermediate-term plan A plan that is longer than short term but less than long-term.

internal benchmarking When you compare performance of operations within the *same* organization.

internal recruiting When a company recruits applicants from within the company. Also called promote from within.

intrinsic motivation When you do something because it is internally satisfying and you enjoy it, such as feeling competent at work.

inventory The amount of foods, beverages, and supplies that are on hand.

inventory turnover rate A measurement of how often a company uses and replaces its inventory during a given period.

Invitation for Bid Request for prices for a one-time purchase or prices over a period of time. Used when purchasing items that any vendor could provide.

invoice A list of items purchased with the prices charged and total due.

invoice receiving When the receiving clerk uses the supplier's invoice to check the name/description and quantity of each item delivered.

ISO 9000 A set of quality system standards established by international technical experts from more than 90 countries, as part of the International Organization for Standardization.

J

jargon   Special words or expressions used in a profession or group.

job   A group of tasks and responsibilities that an employee is required to perform.

job aggregators   Websites that gather job posting from job boards and other Internet sites and consolidate them.

job analysis   Examining an existing job to get a picture of what exactly is involved, including tasks or work activities, responsibilities, work conditions, interactions with others, equipment used, supervision needed, and qualifications.

job boards   Websites that list open positions (usually for a fee) and often accept job applications.

job description   A document listing the responsibilities and tasks of a job.

job design   The process of identifying tasks and responsibilities to form a complete job.

job enlargement   A process that widens the scope of a job by asking an employee to perform a greater number of tasks. Also called horizontal loading.

job enrichment   When an employee is given more freedom, control, and/or responsibility over their work to make the job more challenging, rewarding, or interesting. Also called vertical loading.

job expansion   The process of making jobs less specialized. Accomplished through job enlargement, job enrichment, or job rotation.

job fair   An event where employers take booths in a location for a specific time period during which they screen and recruit new employees.

job grades   Groupings of positions that are paid within a similar range of pay.

job requisition form   A form that requests finding an employee for an open position. Starts the recruiting and hiring process after being signed off by the appropriate managers.

job rotation   When employees do different jobs on a rotating schedule.

job satisfaction   Your attitude toward your job, meaning the degree to which you feel positive or negative.

job simplification   Reducing the number of tasks that each employee performs to improve overall efficiency.

job specification   Minimum qualifications for a job.

just-in-time purchasing   When a buyer purchases goods so that they're delivered just as they're needed to meet customer demand.

K

Kaizen   A Japanese philosophy of continuous improvement that involves all employees at all levels.

key performance indicators   Measurable values that demonstrate how well an organization is achieving its business goals and objectives.

kickback   An amount of money or other item of value given to someone illegally as a reward for giving someone else some business or help.

kilogram   A unit of weight in the metric system.

Kosher   For food, satisfying the requirements of Jewish law.

L

labor cost percentage   Cost of labor divided by total sales. Often runs close to 35% but varies a lot.

Labor-Management Relations Act   Legislation that tried to create a balance between union power and management authority. Defined unfair labor practices by unions and management.

labor relations The dealings between unions and management.

laissez-faire leaders Leaders who give complete freedom to the employees/group to complete tasks and the leader does not give any feedback.

Landrum-Griffin Act of 1959 A labor law that required unions to file annual reports with the U.S. Department of Labor and also established a bill of rights for union members.

lateral relationships Positions that are on the same horizontal line, or similar level, in a hierarchy (organizational chart).

layout The process of arranging the actual physical facilities, such as where the walls will be and the equipment.

layout pack Packaging for bacon in which it is laid out on oven paper so it can be put on a sheet pan and put right into the oven.

lead crystal A material used to make some glassware. Because of concerns about lead safety, lead-free crystal is preferred.

leader-member exchange (LMX) theory A contemporary leadership theory that focuses on the nature and quality of the exchanges and relationship between a leader and *each* follower.

leadership style Encompasses the traits, skills, and behaviors that leaders and managers use when they interact with subordinates.

leading A management function that involves using motivation and other skills to guide and influence the actions of others to accomplish the business' goals and objectives.

lead time The time between when an order is placed and when it is delivered.

Lean A tool used in organizations to streamline manufacturing and production processes by focusing on eliminating waste and smoothing the process flow.

Lean Six Sigma Brings together the concepts of quality and waste reduction. Very customer-oriented.

Learning Acquiring new knowledge, attitudes, behaviors, skills, and values.

learning management system (LMS) Software that organizes, delivers, and manages training programs.

learning objective In training, what you want employees to do after training is completed.

LED (light-emitting diode) bulbs Produce light approximately 90% more efficiently than incandescent light bulbs and last a long time.

leniency error When an evaluator is too generous with his/her ratings.

leverage ratios Ratios that measure a company's ability to pay its bills in the long term. Also called solvency ratios.

liabilities Amounts of money that a business owes to others.

liaison A person who establishes and maintains communication between two or more parties.

Life Safety Code A document that provides guidance on building construction, renovation, and operational features to minimize the effects of fires, smoke, and panic.

Likert scale Usually a five- or seven-point scale used to measure a respondent's agreement with given statements. Can be used to measure customer satisfaction.

line authority The authority to direct subordinates to perform job duties as shown in the chain of command in the organizational chart.

line-item purchasing Choosing who to purchase from by awarding whoever has the lowest price for each item on the list. Results in ordering from multiple vendors. Also called cherry picking.

linguistic style A person's characteristic speaking pattern.

liquidity The amount of assets a business has that are either in cash form or can be easily sold for cash.

liter Unit of volume in metric system. A liter contains 1,000 milliliters.

local union   A union that represents employees in a limited geographic area.

long-term liabilities   In a business, amounts that are payable beyond a year.

long-term plan   A plan that covers from three to 10 years.

long-term skilled nursing facilities   In-patient facility used by older adults who need daily medical assistance.

low-cost strategy   A strategy that focuses on driving costs lower than rivals so products can be sold at lower prices and more customers will be attracted.

L-shape arrangement   When foodservice equipment is laid out so it makes an L shape.

lugs   Packaging used for certain fruits and vegetables that contain two layers of product.

lumen   Measure of light output.

M

maintenance roles   In a group, behaviors that strengthen and maintain the group or team.

make-or-buy analysis   A comparison of whether to purchase foods that have been processed to some degree or prepare from scratch. Examines costs, quality, and labor/skills/equipment required for preparation.

makeup air   In ventilation systems, outside air that is brought inside a building.

management   Overseeing and coordinating the work activities of others so jobs are completed according to standards and in an efficient manner in order to achieve goals.

management by objectives (MBO)   A system that measures an employee's results after goals and objectives are set and results are measured.

management theory   A collection of ideas explaining how a manager should act, such as how to motivate employees or implement plans that help accomplish the organization's objectives.

manager   A person whose job is to oversee and coordinate the work activities of others to ensure that organizational goals and objects are being achieved efficiently and effectively.

manual slicers   A piece of foodservice equipment that slices meats, cheeses, vegetables, and more. The operator must move the carriage holding the item past the rotating blade to slice.

marbling   Fat that is found distributed throughout meat.

market   Any group of people with needs and wants who can purchase something.

market form   For a food product, the temperature of the food, its shape (whole or cut up), and whether it is raw or cooked.

market segment   A subgroup of people who share one or more characteristics, such as income or age, that may cause them to have similar needs for a product.

marketing   The activities involved in creating, communicating, and delivering goods and services that have value for consumers and other parties.

marketing mix   The set of controllable marketing tools that a company uses to produce a desired response from its target market. Includes the 6 Ps: product, price, place, promotion, personnel, presentation.

marketing objectives   Objectives that discuss what is to be accomplished through marketing activities.

marketing plan   A document that describes a business' marketing objectives, broad strategies, and specific tactics to achieve the objectives.

market pricing   The current price on the market. Used for items with prices that fluctuate frequently such as produce.

marketing research   The systematic gathering and analysis of data (quantitative and qualitative) related to marketing decisions.

market segmentation   A marketing tool that divides a market into distinct groups of buyers with similar variables (such as college-educated women over 65) who likely have similar product needs.

markup   The difference between the selling price and the actual cost of an item.

mass marketing   Treating the entire market as one group of customers.

master budget   In a business, the operating budget, the cash budget, and the capital budget.

master cleaning schedule   A schedule that includes what should be cleaned and when, as well as who is responsible and who checks that the work is done properly.

master maintenance schedule   A list of the preventive maintenance required for each piece of foodservice equipment and how often it needs to occur.

master schedule   The schedule for all functional areas of a business.

materials handling   The movement, protection, storage, and control of products as they move through the foodservice.

material safety data sheet (MSDS)   A safety document that contains data about a hazardous substance, including chemical safety and how to use the product safety, to the end user.

maximizing   An approach to making decisions in which managers spend a lot of time evaluating different options.

meal equivalent   A tool used to convert all meals and cash sales to a standard unit - a meal.

meal pattern   The menu categories that will be used for a meal and the number of choices to be offered in each menu category.

meal rounds   In healthcare, when a manager checks on patients to get their feedback on food quality and presentation, food temperatures, delivery times, and patients' interactions with dietary staff.

mechanistic organization   A type of organization characterized by a hierarchy with a clear chain of command and division of labor, along with formal rules and job performance judged by productivity. Also called bureaucracy.

mediation   Process by which an impartial third party meets with both sides separately and then suggests compromises or actions that may lead to an agreement.

melamine   A material used to make dinnerware that is lightweight and doesn't break easily.

menu engineering   An analysis of menu items based on each one's popularity and contribution margin, then determining which items to improve or remove from the menu.

merchandising   The process of presenting products for sales in ways that influence a shopper's purchasing decision.

merger   When two companies form one company.

micro-markets   Small self-service retail stores offering foods and snacks in workplaces, colleges, healthcare facilities, and other locations.

microorganisms   Very small, living organisms such as bacteria and viruses.

milliliters   Unit of volume in metric system.

misbranded foods   A food whose label information contains false or misleading information or omits required information.

mise en place   A classical French cooking term that refers to all the preparation and organization of ingredients that must be done *before* a recipe is made.

mission statement   A broad statement describing what the business does, why the business exists, and what purpose it serves for its customers.

modified diet   A diet that has been adjusted with regards to its nutrient content or texture.

moist-heat cooking methods   Cooking that involves water, a water-based liquid, or steam as the vehicle of heat transfer.

molds   Fungi that are made of many cells and can sometimes be seen—such as mold on bread. Some molds cause illness.

motivation   A force inside us, such as needs, that energizes us to engage in persistent goal-directed behavior. Not a trait.

moving average   A forecasting method.

multisegment marketing   In marketing, focusing on more than one segment.

mycotoxins   A poisonous substance made by a few molds that also may cause allergic reactions.

mystery shopper   A shopper who is hired by the store they visit to report on all aspects of the customer experience.

N

National Labor Relations Act   Legislation that affirmed an employee's right to organize a union, become a union member, engage in union activities, and go on strike to get better working conditions.

National Labor Relations Board (NLRB)   Federal board that investigates complaints lodged by unions or employees and oversees elections in which a union may be selected as the collective bargaining agent for a bargaining unit.

National Shellfish Sanitation Program (NSSP)   A federal and state cooperative program recognized by the FDA to oversee shellfish safety from the quality of the water in the areas they grow to their processing and shipping.

need   In marketing, something that is necessary for consumers.

needs assessment   In training, identifying employees' current level of competency to create meaningful training programs focused on what employees really need.

negative reinforcement   When someone is rewarded for desired behavior by having something unpleasant removed.

negotiation   A type of discussion in which two parties are trying to reach an agreement that both parties find acceptable

net present value (NPV)   For a capital investment, the value of the total revenues (over the life of the equipment) discounted to today's dollars, minus the cost of the capital investment.

niche market   A segment within your target audience that is not being served or not being well served.

noise   In communication, anything that hinders the communication process.

noncommercial foodservices   Onsite foodservices whose primary role is to provide meals (generally not to make a profit). Run by the business, school, college, hospital, or other organization in which they operate.

noncontrollable costs   Costs that managers have little or no control over, such as rent.

nonexempt employees   (hourly employees) Employees who are paid by the hour for the hours they work. Must receive overtime pay for hours worked over 40 per workweek at a rate not less than one and one-half times the regular rate of pay.

nonproductive hours   Hours when an employee is getting paid but is not working on the job.

nonprogrammed decisions   Decisions that deal with unique or unusual situations that need to be addressed because they could have major consequences. The situations are usually nonrepetitive and more complex, and information is more likely to be ambiguous or incomplete. Often made by higher-level managers.

nonselective menu   A menu that does not offer any choices. Also called a preselective menu.

nonverbal communication   Transfer of information using mostly body language (facial expressions, gestures, posture) and no words.

norms   In groups, guidelines or ground rules of how group members will behave.

norovirus   A highly contagious virus that causes vomiting, stomach pain, and diarrhea.

O

objectives Statements that describe how and when goals are to be accomplished.

occupancy rate The percent of total rooms/units/beds that are being used.

occupancy sensors Motion detectors that can turn lights on.

Occupational Safety and Health Act A law that requires employers to provide every employee with a safe place to work.

Occupational Safety and Health Administration A federal agency charged with keeping employees safe and healthy at work.

onboarding A series of events, starting with orientation, that acclimate and engage a new employee to become a contributing member of the team in a reasonable amount of time.

on-call employee An employee who only works when they are called in.

onsite foodservices Foodservices that provide meals and snacks for people at work, at school, at university, in a healthcare facility, childcare center, correctional facility, or other organization.

on-the-job training (OJT) A hands-on method used to train new employees to do the various tasks that make up their job.

open house When a business opens its doors to job seekers to inquire about open positions.

open-door policy When a manager encourages employees to come discuss matters of concern to them.

open-ended questions Questions in which the respondent answers in their own words.

open storerooms Storage areas that employees can all access.

open system A system that is open to the external environment.

open well In a steam table, a well that has an exposed heat source at the bottom, and you can use dry or moist heat (with a spillage pan) to keep foods warm.

operating budget A budget that includes a forecast of revenues, expenses, and profit/loss for a given period.

operating ratios Ratios that help managers evaluate their ability to generate sales or control costs.

operational planning Setting short-range objectives and strategies to improve the ability of each subsystem (such as production or service) to perform its activities while supporting the overall strategic plan.

operations The steps in which a business' products or services are produced. In foodservices, the steps or processes from planning menus to cooking and serving foods and cleaning up.

oral communication Messages of words that are spoken.

organic U.S. Department of Agriculture certified organic foods are grown and processed according to federal guidelines addressing factors such as pest and weed control and animal raising practics.

organic beef Beef from cattle that are raised in living conditions accommodating their natural behaviors (like the ability to graze on pasture), are fed 100% organic feed and forage, and do not receive antibiotics or hormones.

organic eggs Eggs laid by hens raised on organic feed and with access to the outdoors.

organic milk Milk that comes from cows that must have outdoor access year-round, be able to graze on grass for a certain number of days each year, and do not receive hormones or antibiotics.

organic organization Organizations with fewer management levels, decentralized authority, more broadly defined jobs, and a loose organizational structure.

organizational behavior (OB) The study of how people act and behave in the organizational setting.

organizational chart A graphic display of an organization's hierarchy and departments.

organizational citizenship behaviors When an employee takes an action that goes beyond the call of duty.

organizational culture   Encompasses the values, practices, and expectations that guide the actions of managers and employees in an organization or business.

organizational design   The process of creating the formal arrangement of jobs and positions within the organization so it runs efficiently and effectively.

organizational development   A contemporary process that uses social and behavioral sciences to increase organizational effectiveness and assist the change process in both individuals and the organization.

organizational development (OD) interventions   Specific methods used to implement changes.

organizational structure   The formal arrangement of jobs and positions within an organization, including reporting relationships, that will help the people in the organization achieve its mission and goals.

organizing   A function of management that involves structuring and coordinating the work of a business into tasks, jobs, and departments to accomplish the business' goals and objectives.

orientation   A specific type of training to introduce a new employee to the workplace and job.

outputs   The products/services made by a system.

overrun   In ice cream production, the amount of air that is worked into the ice cream.

outsourcing   When a business hires another company to perform tasks that could be handled in house.

owner's equity   What would be left for the owners of a business from assets after paying all liabilities. Also called net worth.

P

packers' brands   In foodservice, private label foods carried by large national distributors.

padding   In foodservice, when someone increases the number of forecasted portions to be made by production personnel in order to avoid running out.

paddle   A beater used in a mixer to do most mixing.

paid time off   When an employee gets paid when not at work, such as a paid vacation day.

pan-broiling   A cooking method similar to griddling, except it is done in a sauté pan or skillet. As fat accumulates, it is poured off.

pan-frying   To cook foods in a moderate amount of fat in a pan over a moderate heat.

pandemic   An event in which a disease spreads across several countries and affects many individuals.

panini press   A two-sided piece of cooking equipment that cooks paninis.

pantry or garde manger   An area in the kitchen where cold foods are prepared.

parasites   Organisms that can be transmitted to humans by consumption of contaminated food and water. Can cause physical harm because they live in a host organism and get food from or at the expense of the host.

parallel arrangement   When foodservice equipment is laid out in two or more straight parallel lines.

Pareto chart   A chart that shows the factors that contribute to variation in a process. Based on the Pareto principle that 80% of the variation in a process is caused by about 20% of the factors.

part-time employee   An employee who works fewer hours/week than a full-time employee, such as less than 30 hours/week.

par value   In inventory, the amount of a product that is needed to meet production requirements for one order period plus a small amount of safety stock. The maximum amount of a food to keep on hand.

pass-through refrigerators　A foodservice refrigerator with doors on two opposite sides so an employee can load foods on one side and another employee can grab foods from the opposite side.

pass window　In a foodservice, a window from the kitchen into the dining area where finished plates are passed to servers.

path-goal model　A leadership theory/model developed by House. The best leadership style is when leades select specific behaviors that are best suited to the followers' needs and the working environment.

pathogens　Micro-organisms that cause disease.

patient day　In healthcare, when one patient is in the hospital at the hour at which the hospital does their daily patient count.

payback period　Length of time required to earn back the value of an investment from profits or net annual savings.

payroll taxes　Taxes imposed on employees and employers.

percentage forecasting　A method of forecasting.

performance appraisal　A formal evaluation of how an employee is performing. Usually completed at the end of a probationary period as well as yearly.

performance management　How each employee's performance is monitored and assessed to ensure that the employee is contributing appropriately to the business' mission and goals. Includes annual performance appraisal.

performance standards　How well parts of a job must be completed.

permanent position　A position that is not temporary. Also called a regular position.

perpetual inventory　When inventory records are maintained so that every time receiving accepts deliveries, the amounts for every item are immediately entered into the inventory records, and likewise issued items are removed from inventory. Ensures that the number of each item in stock is accurately reflected in the records in real time.

personal protective equipment (PPE)　Using equipment, such as face masks, to prevent spreading disease.

personal selling　When a person with good interpersonal skills and sales techniques demonstrates a product, gives samples or simply delivers information.

physical inventory　When every item in inventory is counted up and entered into an inventory management system.

plancha　A griddle that gets very hot very fast and is used for browning, sealing, caramelizing, or blackening foods, and is ideal for getting a flavorful crust.

planetary mixers　A mixer in which the beater moves around the bowl, which is stationary, during operation.

planning　A management function that involves identifying and selecting appropriate goals (a desired outcome such as increased sales) and choosing strategies (a course of action) to achieve them.

planning team　Group of individuals who work together to plan a new facility or renovate an existing one.

plate-waste study　When a foodservice manager looks at how much food and which menu items are not being eaten.

plus/delta evaluation　An evaluation tool that collects data on what is going well and what needs to be improved.

poaching　To cook a food submerged in liquid at a temperature of 160° to 185° F (71° to 85°C).

pods　A smaller and more efficient type of trayline used in healthcare facilities.

point of origin　For food, the place where the food came from, such as a Maine lobster.

point of service　Where the customer is served/given the food.

policy　A guideline(s) for making decisions that is expressed in fairly broad terms.

porcelain china (china)   Dinnerware made of a fine-particle clay fired at high temperatures. Results in dinnerware that is very durable and nonporous.

portion control   Serving standard portion sizes agreed upon by the foodservice.

position   A specific instance of a job—such as four Cook positions. Cook is a job and there are four positions for cooks.

positive reinforcement   When a behavior has pleasant consequences, such as a reward.

positive risk   When you invest time or money in new programs, equipment, personnel, or systems that could result in the long-term saving of money (decreased costs) or gaining a competitive edge over your competition (increased revenue).

pot wash machines   Machines specifically built to wash and sanitize pots and pans. May be front or side loading.

power   The ability to influence others' behavior.

Pregnancy Discrimination Act of 1978   A law that forbids job discrimination on the basis of pregnancy, childbirth, or a medical condition related to pregnancy or childbirth.

present value   When the cost of something is expressed in today's dollars.

press release   A brief news story with contact information that is sent to targeted members of the media.

pressure fryers   A lidded fryer that uses pressure to cook faster and make food extra crispy.

preventive maintenance   Service that is regularly performed on a piece of equipment to increase its lifespan and lessen the chance of it failing to work.

primal cuts   The sections of meat that are the first to be separated from the carcass of an animal during the butchering process.

prime cost percentage   Sum of food and beverage cost percentage and labor cost percentage.

prime cost   In foodservice, the costs for food/beverages and labor.

prime vendor contract   In foodservice, special pricing that a distributor offers to foodservices for the items they frequently buy over a specific period of time.

private employment agencies   Companies that will find and place an employee for an employer. Fees are charged to the employer.

probability   The likelihood that an event will occur.

problem solving   The process of identifying a problem and considering and taking corrective action.

problem-solving team   A team that may function either as a team or group to discuss and come up with solutions for a problem.

procedures   Step-by-step descriptions of actions required to carry out the policy.

process analysis tools   A set of tools that help managers and employees look more carefully at a process or procedure to troubleshoot issues and make improvements.

procurement   The process of finding suppliers for goods a company needs and purchasing those goods and services.

product flow   The flow of food from receiving to plated meals.

production areas   Locations in a foodservice kitchen where hot food and cold food are prepared.

production meeting   Meetings held by production managers or chef managers before meals are made to give special directions, handle missing ingredients, etc.

production schedule   Documents that communicate to employees which menu items need to be prepared and how many, along with pertinent instructions.

productive hours   Hours when an employee is working.

productivity   A measure of efficiency that shows how effectively inputs (such as money, and labor) are converted into output (such as meals and revenue).

profitability ratios Ratios that compare net income before or after taxes to sales, owners' investments or equity, or total assets. Use information from both the balance sheet and income statement to measure management's effectiveness in using the resources available.

profit margin percentage Proportion of total sales that represents a profit.

pro forma income statement A statement that projects sales and expenses for a business for a period of time.

programmed decisions Decisions that are concerned with relatively routine problems (often repetitive) and are often made by lower-level managers.

programs A set of activities to fulfill an objective during a specific period of time.

progressive discipline Discipline in the workplace that applies corrective measures in increasing degrees or steps if the undesirable behavior continues.

promote from within When managers try to fill vacant positions with individuals who already work at the business.

promotion Communications by marketers to inform, remind, and/or persuade potential buyers to purchase something.

psychology of menu design How the physical menu design can influence what customers order.

public relations The act of promoting a product or service by building good relationships with the public and potential consumers.

punch list List of items and tasks that need to be completed or fixed before a construction project can be considered finished.

purchase order A sales agreement stating the items to be purchased, pricing, credit terms, and delivery date.

purchase requisition A document listing items that need to be purchased.

purchasing In a foodservice, determining what, how much, and when to purchase food and supplies, who to order from, and then receiving and paying for the goods. The purchasing agent is always trying to get good value for the money spent and to have adequate supplies on hand.

Q

quality When a product or service meets or exceeds customer expectations *and* when an organization can provide these products/services in the most cost-efficient manner while complying with regulations and making a profit.

quality assurance Standards for the quality of service and outcomes, and the process to maintain those standards. An ongoing process that looks back and also forward.

quality circles A group of employees who do similar jobs and meet regularly to identify, analyze, and find and test solutions for quality issues of products or services.

quality control Finding defects in a product, service, or outcome and then correcting the problem.

quick ratio A ratio that measure a business' ability to pay its current bills and short-term liabilities. Also called acid test ratio.

R

racks Foodservice equipment on wheels designed to hold sheet pans and/or steam table pans.

radiation The transfer of heat through energy waves from a source to the food.

range A widely used piece of cooking equipment that has burners on top and oven underneath.

rapid cook ovens   An oven using newer technologies to cook foods, such as heated sandwiches, quickly.

ratio   A comparison of two quantities.

reach-in refrigerators   A foodservice refrigerator that you reach into to put foods away or get an item you need.

ready-prepared operation   A foodservice where most menu items are prepared and then either chilled or frozen for later use.

real authority   The authority a manager is given by subordinates.

reasonable accommodation   Any change to a job, the work environment, or the way things are usually done that allows an individual with a disability to apply for a job, perform job functions, or enjoy equal access to benefits available to other individuals in the workplace.

receiving   The duties associated with checking in delivered items to make sure the items are exactly what was ordered and the quality of the items meets specifications.

receiving log   A document that a receiver uses to note the date and time of each delivery, along with the name of the supplier, invoice number, purchase order number, and description of goods received.

recency error   When the evaluator rated employees only on his or her most recent performance.

recruitment   Searching for individuals from both inside and outside a business in sufficient numbers and with appropriate qualifications to apply for the positions that need to be filled.

reduced-oxygen packaging   Packaging of food in which a reduced-oxygen level in the sealed food package results in extended shelf life and improved quality retention.

reinforcement theory   (Skinner) A motivational theory that says how people behave depends on the consequences—whether they were rewarded, ignored, or punished.

relationship marketing   When a business works to develop long-term connections for the customer that benefit both the customer and the business.

renewal strategy   A strategy that is used when a company has declining performance. Often involves cutting costs and restructuring operations.

Request for Proposal (RFP)   A request to bid on providing goods and/or services. Outlines the bidding process, contract terms, and criteria to be used to pick the winning vendor.

resources   Inputs into a system such as employees and money.

responsibility   The obligation each employee, at any level, has to carry out certain activities or tasks or see that someone else has done so.

restaurant concept   Everything about a restaurant that affects your customer's image of the restaurant, such as the atmosphere, customers, location, food.

residential care facilities   Provide accommodations for elderly residents who need some help and support with daily care. Often referred to as assisted-living facilities or personal-care homes.

return air   Air returning to the heating, ventilation, and air conditioning system from inside a room.

return on assets   A measure of how effectively a business converts the money it invests into net income.

return on investment (ROI)   A measure of how well the investment into a business has paid off.

return on sales   A measure of how efficiently a business turns sales into profits. Also called profit margin percentage.

reverse delegation   When an employee tries to dump an assignment back onto his/her supervisor.

Right-to-Work laws   Laws that guarantee that no employee can be required to join a labor union or pay union dues.

risk   The probability that the predicted outcomes of a course of action will occur, and it varies on a continuum from certainty to uncertainty. The possibility of injury, damage, or loss.

risk management   A process in which potentially risky events are managed proactively to minimize outcomes such as injuries, damages, or loss.

roasting   Cooking with heated dry air.

roll-in refrigerators   A foodservice refrigerator designed to roll a rack into. Has no shelves.

room service programs   Service for hospital patients in which they order meals using a menu in their room and then the meal is delivered within 30 to 45 minutes.

root causes   Underlying reasons that explain why a problem exists.

root-cause analysis   A structured team process used to help identify why and how an unfavorable event occurred so that preventive actions can be taken in the future.

rules   A prescribed guide for conduct.

runner   In healthcare foodservice, the person who takes the food carts up to the patient rooms. In restaurants, the person who brings plated meals from the kitchen to the table.

S

safety stock   A small amount of inventory used to meet higher-than-expected customer demand.

salamander   A small broiler that is often mounted above the range.

salaried employees   Employees that are not paid by the hour and instead earn a yearly salary. In most cases, they are not able to collect overtime pay.

sales mix   Proportion of total sales that each menu item generates.

sales promotion   Incentives to stimulate sales of a product or service.

saltwater fish   Fish that live all of most of their lives in an ocean.

satellite kitchen   A kitchen that is not the main kitchen for a foodservice but is used to assemble and/or serve meals. Also called a galley kitchen.

satisficing   A decision-making style in which a manager works fast and looks for an acceptable decision, which is not necessarily the optimum decision.

sautéing   Cooking food quickly in a small amount of fat over high heat.

scatter diagram   A diagram that shows whether there is a relationship between two variables, such as revenue and payroll.

scheduling   The process of assigning an appropriate number of employees to work at specified times and days so that the work of a business is accomplished.

schematic drawing   A floor plan showing where walls, doors, windows, equipment, and tables are placed in a foodservice.

scientific management school   A group of researchers in the early twentieth century who worked on finding efficient ways for workers to perform tasks to increase worker efficiency.

scramble (scatter) system   A cafeteria set up so customers can walk to a variety of stations to make food and beverage choices. Also called hollow square cafeteria.

Scombroid poisoning   A foodborne illness after eating certain fish that weren't properly refrigerated.

Seafood Inspection Program   A voluntary, fee-for-service program that inspects and grades seafood (fresh and frozen). Overseen by NOAA Fisheries.

sealed bid   A document handed in by the vendor in response to an Invitation for Bid. Placed in a sealed envelope that won't be opened until the given date and time.

sealed well   In a steam table, a well that has the heat source underneath so you can add water into the well to provide moist heat.

search engine optimization   The practice of optimizing a website so it appears toward the top of searches by search engines.

seat turnover   A ratio that tells how many times a different customer sat down to eat during a given time period.

section   A drawing of a space in which the structure looks as though it has been sliced in half vertically.

segment   Part of an overall market with distinguishing characteristics.

selection   A process that moves from screening job applicants to making the final choice.

selective menu   A menu that offers at least two choices in each menu category.

self-managed work teams   A work team that is given the responsibility and authority to do what is needed to produce an output with little or no supervision.

self-operated foodservice   An onsite foodservice that is run and operated by the organization in which it operates, *not* by a foodservice contract company.

self-oriented roles   In a group, selfish behaviors that disrupt the group.

self-service   A style of service in which each customer serves themselves. Common at buffets, for example.

semi-selective menu   A menu that offers at least two choices in some categories, while other categories have only one choice.

servant leadership   Leaders who share power with the employees and *serve the employees* and often the community.

service   How the food is given/presented to the guest.

service failures   Instances when the food, service, or atmosphere did not meet a customer's expectations.

service recovery   How employees resolve customer complaints.

servicescape   The physical environment where the service is produced, delivered, and consumed.

severity error   When evaluators rate everyone's performance below average.

sexual harassment   Unwelcome sexual advances, requests for sexual favors, and other verbal or physical conduct of a sexual nature when an employment decision affecting an individual is made because the individual submitted to or rejected the unwelcome conduct, or the unwelcome conduct interferes with an individual's work performance or creates an intimidating, hostile, or abusive work environment

shareholder equity   The value of corporate stock and retained earnings for a corporation.

shellfish   An aquatic animal with a shell, such as lobsters.

shellfish poisoning   A foodborne illness caused when shellfish feed on algae that produce toxins.

shingle pack   Packaging for bacon in which it is layered.

short-term plan   A plan that covers one year or fewer.

shrinkage   The loss of products due to damage, waste, spoilage, and theft.

similarity error   When an evaluator's rating is biased toward employees whom they perceive to be similar to themselves.

simmering   Cooking a food in a liquid that is bubbling gently at a temperature of about 185° to 200° F (85° to 94°C).

single-use plan   A plan that is used just once to address a unique situation and achieve a particular goal.

single-use (or disposable) temperature indicators   A sensor that changes color when it reaches a certain temperature and can only be used once.

single-use (or event) menu   A menu designed and used for only one meal or occasion. Often used in catering.

Six Sigma   A problem-solving quality program that uses a set of methods and tools to reduce errors or variations, lower costs and increase profits, maximize employee job satisfaction as well as customer satisfaction, and earn customer loyalty.

skilled nursing facilities In-patient facility used by older adults who need daily medical assistance.

slab-pack A style of packaging in which items are placed into a carton without any packaging materials.

slicers A piece of foodservice equipment that slices meats, cheeses, vegetables, and more. Either manual or automatic.

smallwares Pots, pans, knives, and other hand tools, measuring tools, and utensils used for a variety of kitchen duties.

Smoke-roasting A cooking method and way to flavor foods. Also called pan-smoking.

social marketing Programs designed to influence human behavior on a large scale, such as making environmentally sound food choices.

Social Security Act of 1935 Established Social Security and unemployment insurance.

soft skills Includes non-technical skills such as people skills, problem solving, and teamwork.

source reduction To eliminate waste before it is created.

sous vide When raw food is vacuum packaged in an impermeable bag, cooked in the bag, rapidly chilled, and refrigerated for later use. Uses reduced oxygen packaging.

spaghetti diagram A diagram that traces the path of an item(s) through a process.

span of control The number of subordinates a manager has. Also called span of management.

specials Menu items that rotate and appear seasonally or weekly or for just one meal or day.

specialty distributors In foodservice, distributors who handle only one category or good, such as dairy or fountain beverages.

specification A detailed description of food or equipment used when purchasing.

specific plans Plans that clearly define objectives and don't allow any flexibility or room for interpretation.

spiral mixer A mixer in which the beater is stationary and the bowl revolves around it.

spoken menu system In healthcare foodservice, when patients give their meal orders directly to a foodservice employee in their rooms. The same employee returns later with the meals.

stability strategy A strategy that involves either slow growth or staying the same.

staff authority When an individual or department has responsibility to advise, assist, or support others in an organization but no formal authority.

staffing The process of determining personnel needs, recruiting, and selecting employees.

stamped knife A knife that is thinner and less expensive than forged knives.

standardized recipe A recipe that has been tested and adapted for use in a specific kitchen location so any cook in that kitchen can follow the written instructions to produce the same quantity and quality of food every time.

standards of fill Federal requirements that explain how much food must be in a container (such as a can or box) so the container appears well filled and the buyer is not deceived.

standards of identity Federal requirements that define the nature of a specific food in terms of types of ingredients the food must contain and/or how it is made in order to use a name such as fruit jam.

standards of quality Federal minimum requirements for the quality of certain food products.

standing committees A task force that is more permanent in nature and members may rotate.

standing orders   An order in which the delivery person takes a quick inventory of items, such as number of bread loaves, and stocks up to an agreed-upon par level.

standing plan   A plan that is used frequently and provides a set of procedures to use in a recurring or repetitive situation.

static menu   A menu that, in general, stays the same but is often updated once or twice a year. Also called a restaurant-style menu.

station   A designated area in a kitchen where a certain part of production takes place.

status   In groups, a perceived ranking relative to other group members.

steamers   A piece of cooking equipment in which steam circulates in a closed cavity and cooks food. Many steamers use pressure or convection to speed up the cooking process.

steaming   To cook a food with steam.

steam-jacketed kettles   A kettle heated by steam that is pumped into a space between the inner and outer walls of the kettle. Come in a wide variety of sizes.

steam table   A piece of foodservice equipment that uses steam to keep cooked foods warm.

stir-fry   Cooking bite-size foods over high heat in a small amount of oil.

stockouts   When the inventory level of an item is zero.

stock requisition   A form used to request items in inventory.

stoneware   A material used to make dinnerware. Heavy in weight and thick in appearance.

straight line arrangement   When foodservice equipment is laid out in a straight line.

straight line depreciation   A method to calculate depreciation (the process of expensing an asset over its useful life).

strategic planning   Establishing the overall mission, goals, and long-range objectives and strategies for the business.

strategies   Courses of action to achieve goals and get a business to where it needs to be.

structured interview   An interview in which the interviewer asks the same set of questions to all applicants.

style of service   How food is given/presented to the guest.

SWOT analysis   A tool to help identify the strengths and weaknesses inside your business and also the opportunities and threats in the external environment.

subsystem   A system within a system.

suppliers   Companies that sell food, beverages, and equipment to foodservice operations. Also called vendors.

supply air   Air going into a room from the heating, ventilation, and air conditioning system.

supply chain   A system of suppliers, transportation companies, and buyers who interact to get products to consumers in an efficient manner. Also called distribution channel.

supply chain management   Efforts to ensure that the supply chain runs efficiently and effectively.

suprasystem   A large system that integrates smaller systems.

survey   A research method usually involving questions used to collect information from a specific group or groups of individuals.

suspension   A disciplinary action taken in the workplace in which the employees can't go to work for a period of time.

sustainable competitive advantage   A competitive advantage that no competitor can copy.

system   A set of interrelated parts that work together for a purpose.

systems theory   A theory based on the principle that the parts of a system are best understood in the context of the relationships with each other and other systems.

T

table d'hôte menu   A menu that offers a complete meal for a fixed price.

table service   A style of service in which customers are seated and a server takes their order and serves their food and beverages.

take-out service   Any purchased food that is not eaten on premises. Can be ordered in many different ways.

target market   The specific group of consumers to whom a company plans to market its product/services.

task group   A group that includes members from different departments to work on a specific objective. Sometimes called a task force.

task roles   In a group, behaviors that help accomplish the group's objectives.

taste   Sensations perceived by the taste buds on the tongue, including sweet, salty, sour, bitter, and umami.

technical skills   The job-specific knowledge, methods, and techniques needed to perform tasks. Also called hard skills.

temperature danger zone   The temperature at which bacteria grow rapidly, between 41°F and 135°F (5°C and 57°C).

temporary employment agencies   Companies that provide an employer with employees who stay for as little as one day or as long as needed.

temporary position   A position that exists for just a period of time.

termination   Firing an employee from a job.

test tray   In healthcare, when a food tray is sent to an empty bed so that a manager can evaluate the quality of the meal and the speed at which it was delivered. Also called dummy tray.

texture (of food)   How a food feels in your mouth—such as crispy, crunchy, juicy, or lumpy.

Theory X managers   Managers who feel that the average employee is lazy and needs to be closely supervised.

Theory Y managers   Managers who feel that employees are not inherently lazy and will contribute to the organization when trusted and empowered.

thermistor thermometer   A thermometer that measures temperature with a resistor. Takes temperature within 10 seconds and uses digital display. Can measure temperatures of thin foods.

thermocouple thermometers   A thermometer that uses a thermocouple to measure temperatures. Measures quickly and uses a digital display.

360-degree performance review   A technique to do a performance appraisal that utilizes feedback from coworkers (peer review), supervisors, direct reports, other employees, customers, and vendors (as appropriate).

three-needs theory   (McClelland) A motivational theory that identifies three needs that are learned: need for achievement, affiliation, and power.

tilt skillet   A piece of cooking equipment that looks like a large griddle or frying pan. Very versatile piece.

Time and Temperature Control for Safety (TCS) foods   Foods such as meat, poultry, and seafood that require time and temperature controls to prevent the growth of bacteria.

time management   Techniques to use your time more effectively so you accomplish more and get better results.

time value of money   Money in the present is worth more than an equal amount in the future.

Title VII of the Civil Rights Act of 1964   As amended by the Equal Employment Opportunity Act of 1972, Title VII prohibits discrimination because of race, color, religion, sex, or national origin in employment decisions. Helps ensure that decisions, such as hiring, firing, promotion, and compensation, are made on job-related criteria.

top management team   A team made up of the president and other top executives who develop the mission, goals, and strategy for the organization.

total quality management   A management philosophy that focuses on responding to customer needs and expectations while continuously examining and improving organizational processes and empowering employees.

toxin   A poisonous substance.

traditional trayline system   In healthcare, a system in which a patient's tray is assembled one item at a time using the patient's menu with food choices indicated.

training   Instruct and guide the development of a trainee toward acquiring knowledge, skills, attitudes, and behaviors to apply on the job.

training module   A training class.

training unit   A series of training classes.

transactional leader   A leader who leads primarily by using social exchanges with followers along with exchanging rewards (or in some cases punishments) for completion of certain tasks/goals.

transformation   The process of inputs being turned into outputs in a system.

transformational leaders   Leaders who inspire followers to look at problems in new ways while inspiring and motivating them to work together toward a shared vision and (often) extraordinary goals.

tray accuracy   Whether a meal tray contains all the appropriate foods and other items.

tray service   A style of service used mostly in healthcare where meals are assembled on trays and the trays are transported to the patient's bedside.

trim   The weight or volume of food that is removed, such as potato peels, and not used.

Truth in Menu laws   Laws that require menu items to be presented honestly and accurately on the menu with regard to factors such as the weight of a piece of meat or its point of origin.

two-factor theory   (Herzberg) A motivational theory that separated factors that increase motivation, referred to as satisfiers or motivators, from those whose absence leads to job dissatisfaction, such as salary.

U

unconscious bias   A bias that you experience when you make a snap judgment or assessment of a person or situation.

unfavorable variance   A variance that is not desirable, such as when a business has lower sales than budgeted.

Uniform Commercial Code (UCC)   State laws that govern all commercial transactions including purchasing and the obligations of a buyer to its employer. Also covers product warranties.

union shop   With unions, when a new employee must join the union within a specified period of time after starting employment.

union steward   A union employee elected as the representative for a group of employees when dealing with management.

unity of command   When each position in an organization reports to just one person.

V

value   The relationship between the advantages or benefits the buyer gets from a purchase and the sacrifice that was required.

Value Stream Mapping   A tool used by Lean practitioners in which a flowchart is developed by a team to document every step in a process that will help identify waste and poor flow.

variable costs Cost in a budget that goes up or down in response to changes in sales or meals prepared.

variables In marketing, characteristics of individuals or groups that help divide the market into segments.

variance percentage The variance divided by the budgeted dollars and expressed as a percentage.

variety In fruits and vegetables, different types such as Honeycrisp apples (red and sweet) or Granny Smith apples (green and a little sour).

ventless hood A ventilation hood that doesn't require fans or ductwork because it uses two or more levels of filters to remove grease and other contaminants from the air.

verbal communication Messages composed of words that are either spoken or written.

vertical communication Communication that goes up or down the organization's chain of command.

vertical cutter mixer A piece of food preparation equipment that can be used to puree, chop, or mix.

viruses A micro-organism that is smaller than a bacterium and invades living cells and then uses them to grow and reproduce.

virtual kitchen A foodservice that is just a kitchen. All food is prepared and then delivered to customers. Also called a ghost kitchen.

visionary leaders Leaders who create and communicate an energizing vision of the future that provides direction for strategic planning and goal setting as well as taps into the enthusiasm and emotions of their followers.

vision statement An organizational statement describing their future expectations and achievements, including how the organization wants to impact the communities or areas it serves.

W

wait service A style of service in which servers take food orders from diners at tables and serve food and beverages.

walk-in refrigerators A large refrigerator made for foodservices that you walk into and contains shelving.

want In marketing, a good or service that is desired but not absolutely needed.

waste In a lean organization, any step or action in a process that is not required for the process to be successfully completed or doesn't add value for the end user.

white space In page design, the blank space surrounding and in between the content/graphics.

wild-caught seafood Seafood caught from a lake, ocean, river, or other natural habitat.

workers' compensation State-regulated programs that provide the payment of lost wages, medical treatment, and rehabilitation services to workers suffering from a work-related injury or illness.

work flow The flow of employees doing their jobs.

work groups Three or more people (often more) who come together to achieve a specific goal(s). Includes a clear leader/manager who usually has decision-making authority.

work specialization Dividing work activities into separate jobs. Also called division of labor.

work teams A specialized type of group in which members work intensely with each other to complete an entire process. Leadership is often shared among the members.

wok range Gas-fired rings that heat round or cone-shaped pots. Used in Chinese, Vietnamese, and Thai cooking.

work samples Tangible examples of an applicant's work, such as a baked good or a marketing piece.

write-ins   Alternate items written onto a patient's menu to replace something on the menu.

written communication   Messages that include writing such as reports and memos.

Y

yield percent   Percent of a food that is edible.

Z

zero-based budgets   A budget that does not look at prior budgets and the manager must analyze needs and costs of the operation to *justify all expenses* because the budget starts from zero.

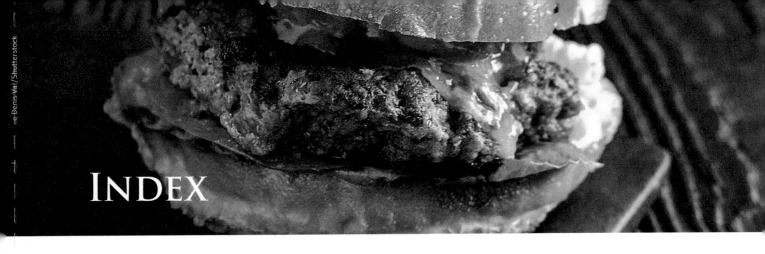

INDEX

Note: Page numbers followed by f or t represent figures or tables respectively.

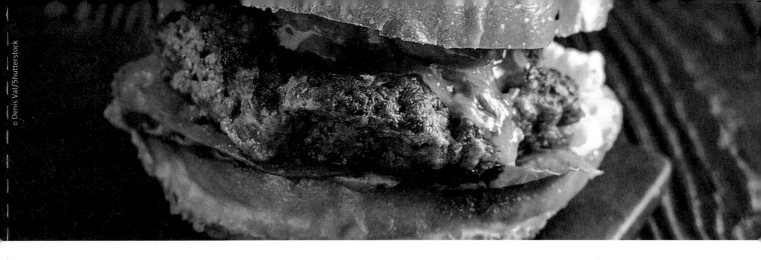

APPLICATIONS FOR CHAPTER 1

LEARNING OBJECTIVE 1.1 DESCRIBE COMMERCIAL AND NONCOMMERCIAL FOODSERVICE SEGMENTS

1. Give an example of each of the following types of foodservices and explain why your example is correct.

   A. Commercial foodservice:

   _____

   _____

   B. Noncommercial foodservice:

   _____

   _____

   C. Onsite foodservice:

   _____

   _____

   D. Foodservice contract company:

   _____

   _____

2. When is an onsite foodservice commercial? When is an onsite foodservice noncommercial?

   _____

   _____

   _____

   _____

   _____

3. In which foodservice segment would you possibly want to work? Explain why.

_____

_____

_____

_____

_____

4. You work in the franchise office at Dunkin' Donuts. What qualifications do you look for in potential franchisees? List four. Briefly explain the application process for potential franchisees.

_____

_____

_____

_____

_____

_____

_____

_____

_____

_____

5. Pick a professional organization in **Table 1-2** that you may want to join in the future. Look at their website online and list at least four benefits of membership.

_____

_____

_____

_____

_____

LEARNING OBJECTIVE 1.2 DISCUSS THE PROS AND CONS OF SELF-OPERATED AND CONTRACTED FOODSERVICES

6. Is the foodservice at your college/university commercial or noncommercial? Explain your answer.

7. Find an article on foodservice contract companies using one of these foodservice industry magazines: *Foodservice Director* or *Food Management*. Write a paragraph to summarize the article.

8. Go to the website of a foodservice contractor and go through their job postings. Find a job you might like to apply for, either now or after you finish your education. Now consider that a similar job is also available, but you would be working directly for the organization/institution. Which job would you prefer and why?

LEARNING OBJECTIVE 1.3 APPLY SYSTEMS THEORY TO A FOODSERVICE ORGANIZATION

9. In your own words, describe the process from inputs to outputs of a foodservice system in one paragraph.

_____

_____

_____

_____

_____

_____

_____

_____

10. Find an article in a foodservice magazine that discusses how something in the *environment* affects foodservices. Summarize the discussion.

_____

_____

_____

_____

_____

_____

_____

_____

11. The chef in the restaurant where you work is making changes to how a number of menu items will be garnished. Name four subsystems that could be affected and why.

_____

_____

_____

_____

_____

_____

_____

LEARNING OBJECTIVE 1.4 CONTRAST TYPES OF FOODSERVICE OPERATIONS

12. Make a table that summarizes the advantages and disadvantages for each type of foodservice operation. You can only state two advantages and two disadvantages for each—so state the most important.

_____

_____

_____

_____

_____

_____

_____

_____

_____

_____

_____

13. Describe a foodservice segment that would likely benefit from having a conventional operation. Justify your answer. Do the same with the remaining types of operations.

A. Conventional:

_____

_____

_____

_____

B. Ready-Prepared:

_____

_____

_____

_____

C. Assembly/Serve:

_____

_____

_____

_____

D. Commissary:

_____

_____

_____

_____

14. The flow of food in a conventional operation is depicted in this diagram. Draw a similar type of diagram to show how a commissary and also a ready-prepared foodservice operate. You can use additional steps/boxes as needed.

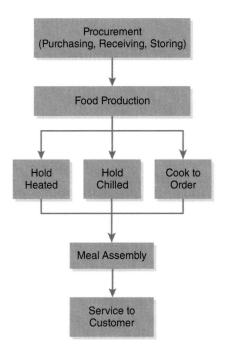

A. Commissary

_____

_____

_____

_____

_____

_____

_____

_____

_____

_____

B. Ready-Prepared

_____

_____

_____

_____

_____

_____

_____

_____

LEARNING OBJECTIVE 1.5 DISCUSS FOODSERVICE TRENDS

15. Using restaurant industry magazines (such as _Restaurant Business_ or _Nation's Restaurant News_), find two additional trends affecting restaurants that were not directly discussed in the text and discuss them briefly.

_____

_____

_____

_____

_____

_____

_____

_____

_____

16. Do restaurant trends affect onsite foodservices and if so, why? Explain your answer.

_____

_____

_____

_____

_____

_____

_____

_____

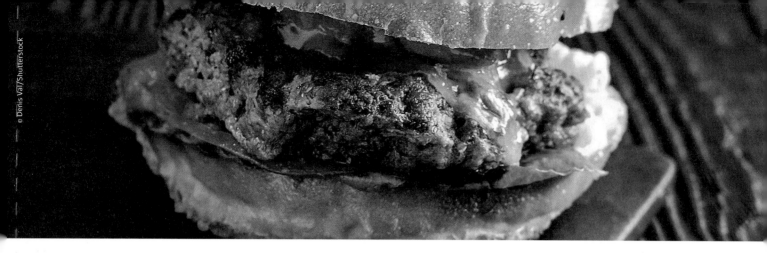

© Denis Val/Shutterstock

APPLICATIONS FOR CHAPTER 2

LEARNING OBJECTIVE 2.1 DISCUSS CAUSES AND PREVENTION OF FOODBORNE ILLNESS

1. Circle each food below if it is a TCS food or if it contains TCS ingredients.

bread	raw chicken breast	cut onions
egg salad	boiled potatoes	head of lettuce
alfalfa sprouts	cooked fish	cut melon
uncooked quinoa	rice pudding	cooked beans
blue cheese	fried rice	scrambled eggs
cooked sausage	cold cereal	sliced lettuce with tomato
fresh broccoli	fish taco	coffee latte

2. The causes of foodborne illness are listed here. Answer the question for each.

Causative factors	How can you **prevent** foodborne illness caused by this factor?
Bacteria	

Causative factors	How can you <u>prevent</u> foodborne illness caused by this factor?
Viruses	_____ _____ _____ _____ _____ _____ _____ _____
Parasites	_____ _____ _____ _____ _____ _____ _____ _____
Fungi (mold and yeast)	_____ _____ _____ _____ _____ _____ _____ _____

Seafood and Plant Toxins	
	_____
	_____
	_____
	_____
	_____
	_____
	_____

3. One of the restaurant managers did a sanitation inspection. The results showed the following situations encountered by the manager. Describe what problem each situation could cause, which type of pathogen(s) could be involved, and how to prevent the problem.

   A. The grill cook was cooking hamburgers, and some of the burgers were undercooked.

   _____

   _____

   _____

   B. Apples were being placed directly from the box (in which they were delivered) into the food processor.

   _____

   _____

   _____

   C. An employee using the restroom did not wash her hands.

   _____

   _____

   _____

   D. A can of open nuts in the bakery contained mold.

   _____

   _____

   _____

E. An employee was mixing tuna salad with his hands and no gloves.

_____

_____

_____

F. In the refrigerator, raw chicken was on a rack above cooked meat.

_____

_____

_____

G. The eggs being served were soft and runny.

_____

_____

_____

H. Cooked lasagna was held on the steam table well below the required temperature for 5 hours.

_____

_____

_____

I. The tap water being used was noticeably cloudy.

_____

_____

_____

J. Fresh tuna and baked potatoes wrapped in foil were left unrefrigerated on a cook's table for a lengthy period of time.

_____

_____

_____

LEARNING OBJECTIVE 2.2 DESCRIBE SAFE PERSONAL HYGIENE PRACTICES

4. As an assistant manager, you have been asked to have a brief meeting with production employees to review why employees should not report to work if they have recently experienced vomiting, diarrhea, or jaundice. List the major points you will discuss at this meeting.

    _____

    _____

    _____

    _____

    _____

    _____

    _____

    _____

5. The Employee Handbook states each of the following dress code requirements. Explain *why* each one is important.

    A. Clothes and aprons are clean and in good condition.

    _____

    _____

    B. Shoes must be closed-toe, low-heeled, and have skid-resistant soles.

    _____

    _____

    C. The only jewelry allowed is one plain ring.

    _____

    _____

    D. Nail polish and/or fake fingernails are not allowed.

    _____

    _____

    E. Any cuts, wounds, or boils must be covered in a waterproof bandage.

    _____

    _____

LEARNING OBJECTIVE 2.3 APPLY FOOD SAFETY PRINCIPLES

6. Which type of thermometer should be chosen in each of these situations?

   A. A cook is grilling a steak and wants to know if it has reached the desired temperature.

   _____

   B. The chef is testing food temperatures and wants a digital thermometer that is not too expensive.

   _____

   C. The grill cook needs to test the surface temperature of a griddle.

   _____

   D. A supervisor needs the most inexpensive food thermometer to test the temperature of foods on a steam table.

   _____

   E. The receiving clerk wants to measure surface temperatures of incoming refrigerated foods.

   _____

7. Go to the website (www.cooper-atkins.com) of Cooper Atkins, a manufacturer of thermometers, and browse the bimetal, digital, thermocouple, and infrared thermometers. Compare the temperature range and accuracy of a bimetal to a thermocouple thermometer.

   _____

   _____

   _____

   _____

8. While doing an inspection of the receiving and storage areas, the purchasing manager had the following concerns. How would you correct each situation and why?

   A. When milk is delivered, temperatures were not taken.

   _____

   _____

   B. Shellfish are delivered without shellfish identification tags.

   _____

   _____

   C. Canned goods that were received only two days ago show rust on the cans.

   _____

   _____

D. Cereals and rice are put into storage before eggs and poultry.

_____

_____

E. Cases of soft drinks that were just delivered were placed on top of soft drinks that were already in stock.

_____

_____

F. Someone put aluminum foil on a refrigerator shelf.

_____

_____

G. The thermometer in the walk-in refrigerator is at the back of the unit.

_____

_____

H. Food is stored on the floor of the dry goods storeroom.

_____

_____

I. Cut leafy greens and tomatoes are being stored at 45°F (7°C).

_____

_____

9. How often do cooks and food preparation workers have to clean and sanitize their work areas and equipment? How are table surfaces cleaned and sanitized?

_____

_____

_____

_____

_____

_____

_____

10. Following are the steps to clean and sanitize a mixer. Number them in the correct order.

    _____ Wash the stationary parts with a cleaning solution with detergent and appropriate tool, such as a cloth towel or brush. Rinse with clean water.

    _____ Disassemble the equipment.

    _____ Allow all surfaces to air-dry.

    _____ Unplug the equipment.

    _____ Wash, rinse, sanitize the removable parts in a three-compartment sink or run them through a dishwasher if appropriate.

    _____ Sanitize the food-contact surfaces of the stationary parts with a sanitizing solution.

11. Some foodservices are allowed to serve raw or undercooked TCS items. Identify which foodservices can do this, and what they must do to be in compliance.

_____

_____

_____

_____

_____

12. The following is part of a Production Sheet that tells the cooks how much to make of each menu item. Fill in the appropriate minimum internal cooking temperatures in the last column.

Menu Item	Recipe Number	Minimum Internal Cooking Temperature
Prime Rib	59	
Chicken Milano	75	
Stuffed Turkey Breast	101	
Meat Lasagna	164	
Roast Pork	216	
Sirloin Steak	99	
Grilled Salmon	123	
Elk Burger	188	
Mac & Cheese	377	
Broccoli	404	
Rice	510	

13. Develop a PowerPoint slide that shows what a cook should do when hot food is not served right away.

14. Fill in the blanks.

When foods are not served immediately, you must hold hot foods at an internal temperature of (a)_____ or higher and cold foods at an internal temperature of (b) _____ or lower. Temperatures must be checked at least every (c) _____ hours, and if a hot food is below (d) _____ at that time, you have to throw it out. However, if you check the temperature every two hours and find that a hot food is below (e) _____, you can reheat it up to (f)_____ and put it back into the hot-holding unit.

15. Develop a PowerPoint slide showing how to use a three-compartment sink.

Learning Objective 2.4 Manage Food Safety

16. List and describe five components of a food safety management system.

_____

_____

_____

_____

_____

_____

_____

_____

_____

_____

_____

17. Put the following HACCP steps in order.

_____ Establish control procedures and critical limits.

_____ Verify that the system works.

_____ Establish monitoring procedures.

_____ Determine critical control points.

_____ Establish documentation procedures.

_____ Conduct a hazard analysis.

_____ Establish corrective actions to be taken.

18. Using the following recipe, determine the critical control points and how to control and monitor each critical control point to prevent the introduction of hazards.

Fruit Salad Recipe Ingredients:	Steps:
4 cantaloupes 4 honeydew melons 8 pounds strawberries, washed and drained 15 kiwi, peeled and sliced 6 oranges, juiced	1. Wash the melons. Cut the melons into ¾-inch cubes. 2. Remove stems from strawberries and cut into halves or quarters. 3. Combine fruit with orange juice and toss gently.

_____

_____

_____

_____

_____

_____

_____

_____

_____

_____

_____

_____

Learning Objective 2.5 Explain How to Have a Successful Sanitation Inspection

19. Read "What to Expect When You're Inspected: A Guide for Food Service Operators" by the New York City Health Department at https://www1.nyc.gov/assets/doh/downloads/pdf/rii/blue-book.pdf. Write a paragraph describing what you learned.

_____

_____

_____

_____

_____

_____

_____

_____

_____

_____

_____

_____

LEARNING OBJECTIVE 2.6 MAINTAIN AN ACCIDENT-FREE WORKPLACE

20. You are training new employees about kitchen safety. Develop a set of flash cards with the following questions and put the answers on the other side.

   a. Why are you more likely to cut yourself with a dull knife?
   b. Why do cooks put a damp towel under the cutting board?
   c. Why shouldn't you put a dirty knife into the sink?
   d. How do you store knives so they are secure and won't cut someone?
   e. Why is it a bad idea to use a spatula when the mixer is mixing?
   f. Why is it a bad idea to use a wet potholder?
   g. Why should you keep pot handles turned in from the edge of the range?
   h. Why should you put foods into the fryer slowly?
   i. Why should you not turn your back on hot fat in a pan?
   j. What happens if you throw water on a grease or electrical fire?
   k. Why shouldn't you stand on a chair to reach something?
   l. Why do you need to unplug equipment before cleaning?
   m. Why do you have to lift with your legs?
   n. Why are carbon dioxide and nitrogen tanks locked down or chained to something?

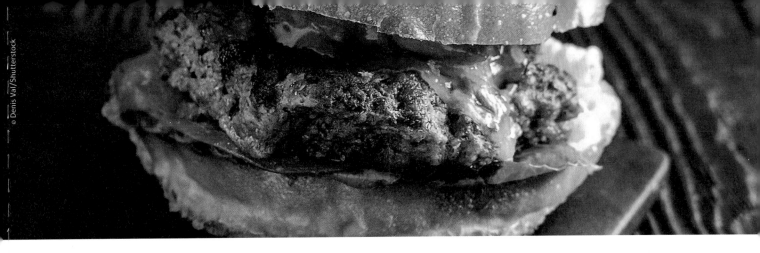

APPLICATIONS FOR CHAPTER 3

LEARNING OBJECTIVE 3.1 IDENTIFY TYPE OF MENU

1. Name the three ways in which menus may vary.

   _____

   _____

   _____

   _____

   _____

   _____

2. Compare à la carte menus to table d'hôte menus.

   _____

   _____

3. Which type of menu is usually used by each of the following businesses? Each question may have more than one answer.

   a. A restaurant?

   _____

   _____

   b. A university?

   _____

   _____

   c. A caterer?

   _____

   _____

© Denis Val/Shutterstock

    d. A foodservice for employees of a pharmaceutical company?

_____

_____

4. Name one type of healthcare facility likely to use nonselective menus and why.

_____

_____

LEARNING OBJECTIVE 3.2 PLAN MENUS

5. You are one of the managers at a new Italian restaurant that is opening in a few days. Discuss four problems you could encounter (from the customer's and manager's point of view) if the menu is not well planned out.

_____

_____

_____

_____

_____

_____

_____

_____

6. Using the following information, calculate the food cost percentage and labor cost percentage for March.

March sales: $38,004.00   Food and beverage cost: $12,161   Labor cost: $13,330

    a. Food cost percentage:

_____

_____

_____

    b. Labor cost percentage:

_____

_____

_____

7. Name three instances when a restaurant/foodservice's menu falls under governmental regulations and briefly discuss the requirements.

a.

_____

_____

_____

_____

b.

_____

_____

_____

_____

c.

_____

_____

_____

_____

8. What is the target market for a restaurant you like? Name the restaurant and briefly explain your answer.

_____

_____

_____

_____

_____

9. Why are each of these meals *not* very appealing?

a. Macaroni and cheese, buttered carrots, mashed potatoes with cheddar cheese

_____

_____

b. Beef stew, mashed potatoes, butternut squash

_____

_____

c. Grilled chicken, grilled vegetables, grilled potatoes

_____

_____

d. Tomato soup, ravioli with tomato sauce, lettuce and tomato salad

_____

_____

e. Chicken nuggets, tater tots, onion rings

_____

_____

10. Find a restaurant menu on the Internet that exemplifies sustainability. Write down the website address and give three reasons why the menu is sustainable.

_____

_____

_____

_____

_____

_____

11. Put the following _steps for planning menus_ into the proper order.

_____ Plan the appetizers.

_____ Plan breakfast.

_____ Plan desserts for lunch and dinner.

_____ Plan lunch entrées.

_____ Plan side dishes for lunch and dinner.

_____ Plan dinner entrées.

_____ Plan beverages and condiments for all meals and bread(s) for lunch and dinner.

12. The following menu is for a university in New Jersey with a diverse student body, mostly 18 to 24 years old. The menu includes lunch and dinner meals for

five days. At each of these meals, a full salad bar (with rotating items) and grill/sauté station are available. At lunch, a sandwich bar is set up. Evaluate the university menu using these criteria.

A. The menu should reflect the food habits and preferences and sociocultural backgrounds of the customers.

B. The menu should offer variety without too much repetition.

C. The menu should offer visually appealing meals with different textures, colors, shapes, sizes, and cooking methods.

LUNCH	Monday	Tuesday	Wednesday	Thursday	Friday
Soup of the Day	-White Bean & Tomato Soup	-Chicken Corn Chowder	-Black Bean Soup	-French Onion Soup	-Manhattan Clam Chowder
Entrée	-Mongolian Beef	-BBQ Pork Loin	-General Tso's Chicken	-Jerk Chicken with Pineapple Mango Salsa	-Texas Flank Steak
Sides	-Brown Rice Pilaf -Mongolian Vegetables	-BBQ Baked Beans -Stewed Corn, Tomatoes, and Okra	-Chinese Broccoli -Steamed Jasmine Rice	-Coconut Basmati Rice -Fried Plantains	-Sautéed Green Beans -Spanish Rice
Salads	Salad Bar	Salad Bar	Salad Bar	Salad Bar	Salad Bar
Grill/Sauté Special	-Philly Cheesesteak Sandwich	-Korean BBQ Beef	-Vegetarian BBQ	-Sweet and Sour Chicken Stir-Fry	-Grilled Teriyaki Chicken Sandwich
Sandwiches	Sandwich Station	Sandwich Station	Sandwich Station	Sandwich Station	Sandwich Station
DINNER					
Soup of the Day	-White Bean & Tomato Soup	-Chicken Corn Chowder	-Black Bean Soup	-French Onion Soup	-Manhattan Clam Chowder
Entrée	-Beef Fajitas	-Corn Meal-Crusted Catfish -Manicotti	-Meat Lasagna -Roasted Pork Loin w/Apple Chutney	-BBQ Pork Ribs -Collard Greens with Ham	-Cheese Ravioli -Pepper Steak Lo Mein
Sides	-Rice Pilaf -Sautéed Broccoli	-Baked Sweet Potatoes -Macaroni & Cheese	-Garlic Mashed Potatoes -Sautéed Broccoli Rabe	-BBQ Baked Beans -Collard Greens	-Asian Stir-Fried Vegetables -Steamed Jasmine Rice
Salads	Salad Bar	Salad Bar	Salad Bar	Salad Bar	Salad Bar
Grill/Sauté Special	-BBQ Ribs	-Chicken Breast Sliders	-Beef and Broccoli Stir-Fry	-Steak Quesadilla	-Sausage and Pepper Sub
Specialty Bar	Taco Bar	--------	Ramen Noodle Bar	------	Pasta Bar

_____

_____

_____

_____

_____

_____

_____

_____

_____

_____

_____

_____

_____

_____

13. Write a one-week (Monday–Friday) lunch menu for an elementary school including portion sizes. The menu should feature kid-friendly foods that are tasty and economical. The National School Lunch Meal Pattern for Grade K–5 requires the following.

- Milk: 1 cup daily, 5 cups/week
  - Only fat-free or low-fat allowed.
  - Must offer at least two choices daily.
- Meat or Meat Alternates: 8 - 10 oz. weekly (1 oz. daily minimum)
  - One ounce cooked, skinless, unbreaded portion of beef, poultry, or fish = 1 ounce.
  - One-half cup of yogurt = 1 ounce of meat/meat alternate.
  - Two tablespoons of nut butter = 1 ounce of meat/meat alternate.
  - One-quarter cup of drained beans/peas = 1 ounce of meat/meat alternate.
- Vegetables: ¾ cup/day minimum + Fruits: ½ cup/day minimum
  - Each week, must include ½ cup dark green vegetable, ¾ cup red/orange vegetable, ½ cup legumes, ½ cup starchy vegetable, and ½ cup any type of vegetable.
  - One cup of leafy greens counts as ½ cup of vegetables.
- Grains: 8 to 9 oz./week
  - Half the grains offered must be whole grains.

Monday	Tuesday	Wednesday	Thursday	Friday

LEARNING OBJECTIVE 3.3 DESIGN A PRINTED MENU

14. Explain the concept of "truth in menu."

   _____

   _____

   _____

15. Write menu descriptions for the following four appetizers.
   Oysters on the Half Shell:

   _____

   Shrimp Cocktail:

   _____

   Cheese Plate:

   _____

   Nachos:

   _____

16. Design a printed menu for the following menu items and create a restaurant name. Highlight the Filet Mignon and Crab Cakes as they bring in the most money.

   Appetizers: Oysters on the Half Shell ($7.50), Shrimp Cocktail ($7.50), Cheese Plate ($9.50), Nachos ($6.00)

   Soup & Salad: French onion soup ($7), Soup of the Day ($7), garden greens ($7), Margarita Salad ($8.50), early spring salad ($7), Iceberg wedge salad ($7)

   Entrées: Grass-fed Filet Mignon with creamed spinach and baked potato ($28), barbecue beef meatloaf with baked beans and coleslaw ($20), roasted half chicken with scalloped potatoes and carrots ($22), braised lamb shank with roasted mushrooms and mashed potatoes ($25), grass-fed burger on brioche bun with fries ($14.50), baked salmon with roasted beets and orange salsa ($26), crab cakes with sweet potato wedges and slaw ($26)

   Desserts: Tiramisu ($7), red velvet ice cream cake ($8), cheesecake ($7), brownie sundae ($7), ice cream ($6)

LEARNING OBJECTIVE 3.4 SET MENU PRICES

17. You spend $20 for dinner. The restaurant maintains its food cost percentage at 33% and its labor cost percentage at 35%. How much of your $20 went toward paying for food? How much of your $20 went toward labor?

   _____

   _____

   _____

   _____

18. Calculate possible selling prices for the following entrées using the three methods in the chart. Finally, recommend selling prices for each entrée in the final column.
Desired Food Cost Percentage: 33%
Desired Prime Cost Percentage: 65%
Contribution Margin for Entrées: $9.25

Entrées	Food Cost	Labor Cost	Food Cost Percentage Method	Prime Cost Method	Contribution Margin Method	Recommended Selling Prices
Grilled Steak	$8.26	$6.55				
Half Roast Chicken	$4.40	$5.60				
Fish of the Day	$5.24	$6.00				
Pork Chops	$5.89	$6.15				
Hot Turkey Sandwich	$3.05	$5.60				
Cheeseburger	$3.25	$3.87				

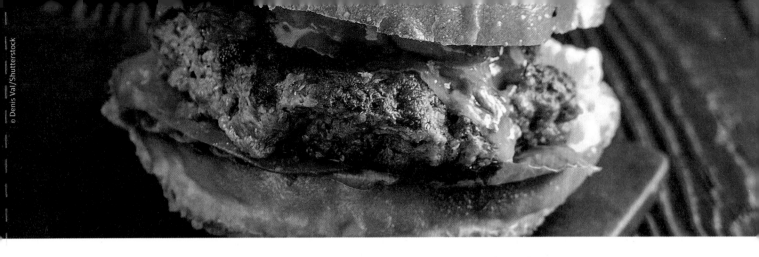

APPLICATIONS FOR CHAPTER 4

4.1 EXPLAIN HOW TO SELECT FOODSERVICE EQUIPMENT

1. Why is stainless steel used in much cooking equipment (such as ovens) and aluminum used in many pots and pans?

_____

_____

_____

_____

_____

_____

2. How is NSF certification different from UL certification?

_____

_____

_____

3. As a restaurant manager, you are discussing a possible purchase of a new ice machine with a manufacturer's sales representative from Scotsman, a major brand. You also plan to speak with an independent manufacturers' representative who represents another major brand, Manitowoc, as well as check out ice machines on the Internet. What are the pros and cons of using each of these methods to help make a purchasing decision?

_____

_____

_____

_____

_____

_____

4.2 CHOOSE AN APPROPRIATE POWER SOURCE

4. Describe four considerations when deciding on whether to use gas, electric, or steam.

_____

_____

_____

_____

_____

_____

5. Equipment using which power source(s) generally must have an exhaust hood overhead?

_____

_____

4.3 DESCRIBE FEATURES OF COMMON KITCHEN EQUIPMENT

6. As the chef, you need to roast four top sirloin roasts, averaging about six pounds each. Which oven would you rather use: a range oven, a full-size convection oven, or a full-size combi-oven? As part of your research, look at specification sheets for each type of oven to compare the interior size of the oven itself. Explain why the oven you choose is the best choice to produce a quality product.

_____

_____

_____

_____

_____

_____

_____

_____

7. Match each piece of equipment with the food items it cooks well. A food item may be matched with more than one piece of equipment.

    _____ Conveyor oven   A. Toasted sandwich

    _____ Microwave oven   B. Soup

    _____ Combi-oven   C. Beef roast

    _____ Steam jacketed kettle   D. Lots of bread and rolls

    _____ Griddle   E. Pizza

    _____ Cook-and-hold oven   F. Oven-fried chicken

    _____ Rack oven   G. Vegetables

    _____ Convection oven   H. Sirloin steak

    _____ Rapid cook oven   I. Pancakes

    _____ Char-broiler

8. What is the difference between a char-broiler, regular broiler, salamander, and cheese melter? Which one does not cook food?

_____

_____

_____

_____

_____

_____

_____

9. Develop a list of "Dos and Don'ts" that will be posted next to the slicer to remind employees of safety issues.

_____

_____

_____

_____

_____

_____

_____

10.   As a salad preparation worker, you need 20 pounds of sliced carrots for a recipe. Which tool would you use and why?

_____

_____

_____

_____

11.   In the bakery, you need to do the following. Which attachment would you use?

A. Make frosting.

_____

B. Make a muffin batter.

_____

C. Make pizza dough.

_____

D. Make whipped cream.

_____

12.   Enter the name of the smallware into the blank that matches the description given.

A. _____ A shallow, rectangular pan used in the kitchen and bakery.

B. _____ A stainless steel pan used to hold foods in a steam table or cook foods in a steamer.

C. _____ A shallow and often slope-sided pan used for sautéing, frying, browning, and making egg dishes.

D. _____ A large, straight-sided pot that is taller than a saucepot and is used to make soups.

E. _____ A small knife used to trim and cut fruits and vegetables.

F. _____ A type of spatula used to turn food during cooking.

G. _____ With straight or slanted sides and a handle, this piece of equipment is the workhorse of rangetop cooking.

H. _____ A knife, often 10 inches long, used for heavy-duty cutting, chopping, and more.

I. _____ A knife used to slice breads and cakes.

J. _____ A handheld bowl with small holes or mesh used to drain liquid.

K. _____ A hand tool used to beat and whip.

4.4   DESCRIBE CONSIDERATIONS TO SELECT DINNERWARE, BEVERAGEWARE, AND FLATWARE

13.   Find an appropriate dinner plate and flatware for each of these types of foodservices using a website for restaurant equipment. Describe their key qualities (such as 18/0 stainless steel flatware in a simple pattern) and explain what makes each choice appropriate.

A. Bistro

_____

_____

_____

_____

_____

_____

B. Fine-dining restaurant

_____

_____

_____

_____

_____

_____

C. Restaurant serving mostly families with children

_____

_____

_____

_____

_____

_____

4.5 WRITE EQUIPMENT SPECIFICATIONS

14. Using the one-week menu found in Chapter 3 (Table 3-1), list two pieces of equipment (you must include an oven) that are needed to prepare this menu. Use the guidelines in the textbook to write up a specification for each piece of equipment, keeping in mind the following:

   A. Each meal is served to 300 residents daily.
   B. The budget allows for low- to mid-priced equipment.
   C. Equipment that is multi-functional is a plus.
   D. Key considerations also include energy and maintenance costs as well as employee safety and ease of cleaning.

   _____

   _____

   _____

   _____

   _____

   _____

   _____

   _____

   _____

   _____

   _____

   _____

   _____

   _____

   _____

   _____

   _____

   _____

   _____

4.6   DEVELOP AN EQUIPMENT MAINTENANCE PROGRAM

15.   Using the website, www.webstaurantstore.com, find a gas combi-oven made by Alto-Shaam. For almost every piece of equipment on this website, the manufacturer's spec sheet and the Manual are available (on the right-hand side further down the equipment page). Look into the Manual and write down below two items that should be inspected monthly and two items to be inspected yearly.

_____

_____

_____

_____

_____

_____

_____

_____

_____

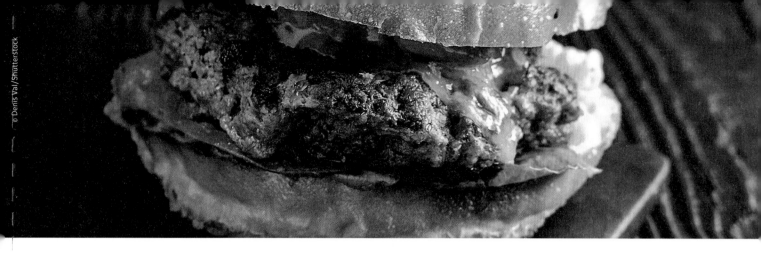

APPLICATIONS FOR CHAPTER 5

5.1 DEVELOP A BUSINESS PLAN AND ORGANIZE THE PLANNING TEAM

1. Distinguish between design and layout.

2. Which part(s) of the business plan would include each of these statements?

   A. The typical customer is a male or female of about 25 to 35 years old, who is a college graduate with an income of $50,000 or more.

   B. The restaurant will be open for lunch and dinner six days a week with Mondays off.

   C. Sales for the first six months are forecasted to be $320,000.

   D. The goal of the kitchen renovation is to provide a more varied menu to our clientele and increase their satisfaction.

E. Fast-casual pizza restaurants are becoming very popular.

_____

_____

F. In addition to local advertising, the restaurant will also participate in popular town events such as Restaurant Week.

_____

_____

G. We should increase sales enough to completely pay for renovation costs within 18 months.

_____

_____

3.   Which member(s) of the planning team will:

A. Design the heating, ventilation, and air conditioning system?

_____

_____

B. Choose possible tables and chairs for the dining area?

_____

_____

C. Do all the final drawings (blueprints)?

_____

_____

D. Help you select an appropriate range and fryer?

_____

_____

E. Build or renovate the new space?

_____

_____

F. Design the plumbing system?

_____

_____

G. Recommend colors and window coverings in the dining room?

_____

_____

H. Help you select energy-efficient equipment?

_____

_____

I. Recommend how to lay out the equipment in the hot food production area?

_____

_____

4. List four examples of codes or regulations that the planning team may consult during the design and layout phase.

_____

_____

_____

_____

_____

_____

5.2 Design The Environment

5. Why do most foodservice kitchens need an independent makeup air supply?

_____

_____

_____

6. Why must hood filters be cleaned regularly?

_____

_____

7. Name three considerations when choosing lighting for a hot food production area. Also recommend a specific light bulb or tube including lighting intensity and color temperature.

_____

_____

_____

_____

_____

_____

_____

_____

8. Name three ways to lessen the noise in the kitchen.

_____

_____

_____

_____

_____

_____

9. Find a restaurant that is LEED certified and describe two ways in which the design is sustainable.

_____

_____

_____

_____

_____

5.3   PLAN THE FLOW OF FOOD AND WORK

10. This box represents the outer walls of a foodservice that includes a loading dock/receiving area, two walk-in refrigerators, one walk-in freezer, a dry goods storage room, hot food production area, cold food production area, and a room for washing dishes and pots. Designate on the drawing where each of these areas will be located, drawing walls and doors as needed. Also draw doors in the outer walls that open into the dining area.

Trace the product flow from delivery to the dining area as well as the flow of dirty dishes and pots and pans to the dishwashing/pot-washing areas. How would you rate product flow and overall work flow?

[blank boxed area]

5.4   LAY OUT A FOODSERVICE

11.   Visit a foodservice that offers cafeteria service, such as a dining hall at your college or university. Make a drawing below of the serving areas showing the approximate location of each station. Label each station and also show how people flow into and out of the cafeteria from the kitchen and dining area.

12. Prepare a schematic drawing for a kitchen with a hot food production area and cold food production. The production areas supply hot and cold foods that are placed on steam tables and other heating/cooling equipment in serving areas close to the kitchen. Using ¼-inch scale graphing paper, draw a 24 feet x 22 feet kitchen (each ¼-inch represents 1 foot). Within this space, use the following templates found in **Figure 5-17:** range with griddle and broiler, stacked convection ovens, floor-model charbroiler, convection steam cooker, countertop steam kettle (12 gallons), tilting skillet, two roll-in refrigerators, and table with double sink and drainboards. You will also need cook's tables. Make sure all gas equipment is under a ventilation hood. Use a dashed line to designate where the hood will be.

5.5   EXPLAIN THE PROCESS FROM BLUEPRINTS TO INSPECTION

13. Explain the difference between an RFP and IFB.

_____

_____

_____

_____

14. Google "RFP school district cafeteria renovation remodel" and find an actual RFP from a school district requesting bids to remodel a cafeteria. Explain briefly the selection process that will be used by the school district and how long the project will take.

_____

_____

_____

_____

_____

_____

_____

_____

_____

_____

_____

_____

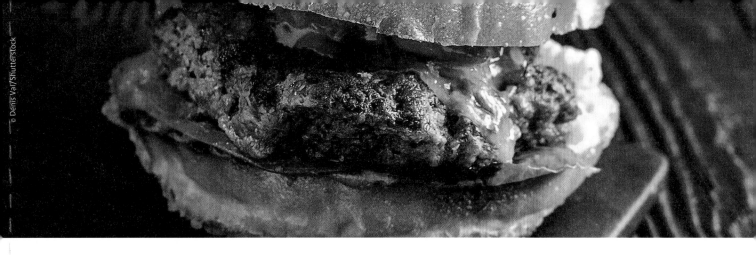

APPLICATIONS FOR CHAPTER 6

LEARNING OBJECTIVE 6.1 MEASURE INGREDIENTS ACCURATELY

1. 1 cup = _____ tablespoons

2. 4 pints = _____ quarts

3. 6 quarts = _____ gallons

4. 2 quarts = _____ fluid ounces

5. 1¼ pounds = _____ ounces

6. 1 kilogram = _____ grams

7. 1 fluid ounce = _____ milliliters

8. ¾ cup = _____ tablespoons

9. ½ cup = _____ teaspoons

10. ¾ cup = _____ fluid ounces

11. 12 oz. = _____ pound

12. Represent this amount in pounds using decimals: 12 lbs. 9 oz.

_____

LEARNING OBJECTIVE 6.2 CONVERT UNITS OF MEASURE

13. Convert 20 tablespoons to cups.

_____

_____

14. Convert 54 ounces to pounds.

_____

_____

15. You need to serve 175 servings of lemonade (portion size is 12 fl. oz.). How many gallons should you make?

_____

_____

16. Convert 3¼ cups of all-purpose flour to ounces (1 cup = 4.3 oz.).

_____

_____

17. Convert 24 tablespoons of walnuts to pounds (1 pound = 4 cups).

_____

_____

18. You have a container of cinnamon that weighs 1 pound 2 ounces. How many tablespoons can you measure from the container? Use Appendix D to find information on cinnamon.

_____

_____

LEARNING OBJECTIVE 6.3 USE YIELD PERCENT AND CALCULATE AP OR EP QUANTITY

19. If Romaine lettuce has a 75% yield, what percent of the Romaine lettuce is trim?

_____

20. A cook has 50 pounds of fresh whole potatoes that need to be peeled and quartered. How many pounds of potatoes will they yield?

_____

_____

21. You have three pounds of fresh oranges. After peeling and removing the membranes from each section, you have 1.6 pounds. What is the yield percent?

_____

22. A cook is putting 77 pounds of whole chickens (broiler-fryer size) into the oven to roast. How many pounds of chicken (including skin) will it yield?

_____

_____

23. A recipe calls for 10 pounds of sliced eggplant. How many pounds do you need to order?

_____

_____

24. You will be serving 120 people a 3-ounce portion of fresh pineapple chunks. How many pounds of pineapple do you need to order? If a case of fresh pineapple weighs approximately 26 pounds, how many cases will you order?

_____

_____

LEARNING OBJECTIVE 6.4 DEVELOP A STANDARDIZED RECIPE AND ADJUST RECIPE YIELD

25. The following are the ingredients for cornbread. The recipe makes 16 servings and you want the recipe to yield 60 servings (enough for one full-size sheet pan). Calculate how much of each ingredient will be needed.

Yield: 16 Servings	Yield: 60 Servings
¼ cup olive oil	
1 cup all-purpose flour	
1 cup cornmeal	
1½ teaspoons baking powder	
½ teaspoon baking soda	
¼ teaspoon salt	
¾ cup unsweetened almond milk	
1 teaspoon lemon juice	
½ cup chickpea brine	
⅔ cup sugar	

LEARNING OBJECTIVE 6.5 CALCULATE COST OF A RECIPE AND PORTION

Directions: Use Appendix D to calculate the AP costs per unit for #26–#33.

26. A 25-pound bag of salt costs $36.50.

   a. AP cost per pound

   _____

   _____

   b. AP cost per cup

   _____

   _____

   c. AP cost per tablespoon

   _____

   _____

27. Iceberg lettuce is packed 24 heads to a case and one case costs $14.50.

   a.   AP cost per head

   _____

   _____

   b.   AP cost per pound

   _____

   _____

28. A case of jam contains 12 jars and each jar contains 8 ounces. The case cost $37.99.

   a.   AP cost per jar

   _____

   _____

   b.   AP cost per ounce

   _____

   _____

   c.   AP cost per tablespoon (1 tablespoon weighs 0.6 ounces)

   _____

   _____

29. A case of frozen carrots includes 12 - two-pound boxes and costs $37.50.

   a.   AP cost per box

   _____

   _____

   b.   AP cost per pound

   _____

   _____

   c.   AP cost per 3-ounce serving

   _____

   _____

30. A container of three pounds of grated mozzarella costs $15.67.

   a.   AP cost per pound

   _____

   _____

b. AP cost per ounce

_____

_____

c. AP cost per cup

_____

_____

31. A ½ gallon of orange juice costs $3.09.

    a. AP cost per quart

_____

_____

    b. AP cost per fluid ounce

_____

_____

    c. AP cost per pint

_____

_____

32. Raisins cost $1.95/pound.

    a. AP cost per ounce.

_____

_____

    b. AP cost per cup.

_____

_____

33. A five-pound container of curry powder costs $11.99.

    a. AP cost per ounce.

_____

_____

    b. AP cost per cup.

_____

_____

34.   Directions: Fill in the blank boxes in the recipe, including total recipe cost and portion cost at the bottom. Use Appendix D for Yield Percents and weight/volume equivalents.

RECIPE: CRAB CAKES

Recipe Yield: 16 servings
Portion Size: Two small cakes (about 2 oz. each)

Ingredient	Recipe Quantity	Recipe Quantity in Purchasing Unit	Quantity to Purchase		AP Cost	Ingredient Cost
			AP Yield %	Quantity		
Crabmeat, frozen	3#				$19.65/#	$
Bread crumbs, fresh	4 oz.				$0.89/#	
Mayonnaise	6 oz.				$15.49/gal	
Eggs	4				$2.45/dzn	
Prepared mustard	2 T				$3.89/gal	
Salt	2 tsp				$0.36/#	
Pepper, white	½ tsp				$8.59/#	
Scallions, chopped fine	1 cup				$1.49/bunch	
Butter	½#				$4.88/#	
Recipe Cost						$
Portion Cost						$

35.   Directions: Fill in the blank boxes in the recipe, including total recipe cost and portion cost at the bottom. Use Appendix D for Yield Percents and weight/volume equivalents.

RECIPE: WALDORF SALAD

Recipe Yield: 24 servings
Portion Size: 3 oz.

Ingredient	Recipe Quantity	Recipe Quantity in Purchasing Unit	Quantity to Purchase		AP Cost	Ingredient Cost
			AP Yield %	Quantity		
Apples, red, crisp, ½" diced	4#				$1.47/#	$
Celery, small diced	1#				$0.89/bunch	
Walnuts, coarsely chopped	6 oz.				$5.29/#	
Romaine lettuce leaves	3 heads (24 leaves)				$1.69/head	
Chantilly dressing	2 cups				$6.76/qt	
Recipe Cost						$
Portion Cost						$

LEARNING OBJECTIVE 6.6 CALCULATE FOOD COST PERCENTAGE

36.   A foodservice had March sales of $238,183 and the food cost for that period was $78,157. What was the food cost percentage for March?

_____

_____

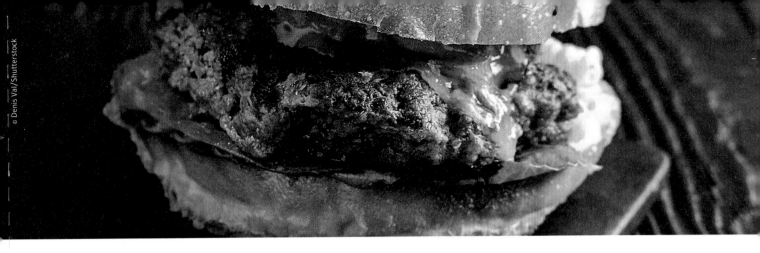

© Denis Val/Shutterstock

APPLICATIONS FOR CHAPTER 7

LEARNING OBJECTIVE 7.1 OUTLINE THE DISTRIBUTION SYSTEM FOR FOOD AND SUPPLIES

1. A chef is planning to open a new restaurant in the town where you live. She needs the following information from you.

   a. The name and location of two national broadline distributors in the area.

   _____

   _____

   _____

   _____

   b. The name and location of a local dairy.

   _____

   _____

   c. The name and location of a cash-and-carry distributor.

   _____

   _____

   d. The name and location of an organic farm that would sell to a restaurant.

   _____

   _____

2. Compare and contrast a central distribution center to a commissary run by a multiunit restaurant chain.

   _____

   _____

   _____

_____

_____

_____

LEARNING OBJECTIVE 7.2 DESCRIBE THE ORGANIZATION AND OBJECTIVES OF A PURCHASING DEPARTMENT

3. Describe two ways in which purchasing is different in an independent foodservice versus a multiunit foodservice.

_____

_____

_____

4. Buyers need to monitor trends and new products on the market that may improve the menu or save time in the kitchen. Describe three new products for foodservices—include two new foods and one new piece of equipment.

_____

_____

_____

_____

_____

_____

5. Why shouldn't a buyer publicly endorse products?

_____

_____

_____

6. As the Beverage Manager, Ben does all the purchasing of alcoholic beverages. Lately, he has noticed that usage of a very expensive whiskey is higher than normal. After observing beverage service for several days, he has discovered that one of the bartenders is giving free drinks of this whiskey to certain people and the bartender is benefiting by getting generous tips. He knows that the bartender really needs the money. If he allows this behavior, which ethics guideline in **Table 7-1** would he be violating? What should Ben do?

_____

_____

_____

_____

_____

_____

LEARNING OBJECTIVE 7.3 EXPLAIN HOW PRE-PURCHASING ACTIVITIES ARE ACCOMPLISHED

7. Letters A–E are a beef specification. Numbers 1–6 list the parts of a specification. Match A–E with the appropriate section of the specification.

  A. 16/10 lb. case, individually wrapped
  B. 10-oz. portion ± 0.5 oz., raw, refrigerated
  C. Entrée, grilled
  D. Surface fat shall not exceed 1/4" at any point.
  E. Strip Loin Steak, center-cut, boneless, IMPS #1180A
  F. U.S. Choice (High)

  1. Name of product:
  2. Intended use:
  3. Description:
  4. Quality indicators:
  5. Packaging/pricing unit:
  6. Other requirements:

8. Do a make-or-buy analysis in which you compare the cost of making meatballs from scratch (recipe given) with buying precooked meatballs at $10.00/pound. Consider costs, quality, and time required. To get costs, go to a supermarket website or use Target's website. Enter the costs for salt, pepper, and Worcestershire sauce as $0.05 each. Would you choose to purchase precooked meatballs or cooking from scratch? Explain your answer.

Recipe: Meatballs

Yield: 1 pound meatballs

1 lb 80/20 ground beef

½ cup bread crumbs

¼ cup milk

½ teaspoon salt

½ teaspoon Worcestershire sauce

¼ teaspoon pepper

1 small onion, finely chopped (¼ cup)

1 egg

_____

_____

_____

_____

_____

_____

_____

_____

9.   In a cooks' meeting, the chef was asked to maintain higher par values on some items, such as hamburgers, that are used frequently. Why are the cooks interested in higher par values and how should the chef respond?

_____

_____

_____

_____

_____

10.   When you purchase foods and beverages, what qualities are you looking for in a company/supplier? Discuss four qualities.

_____

_____

_____

_____

_____

_____

LEARNING OBJECTIVE 7.4 SUMMARIZE FEDERAL FOOD SAFETY LAWS AND AGENCIES INVOLVED

11.   Match the agency with its appropriate responsibility.

Agency Name	Responsibility
_____ 1. U.S. Food and Drug Administration	A. Oversees Seafood Inspection Program
_____ 2. U.S. Public Health Service	B. Inspects meat, poultry, and processed eggs.
_____ 3. U.S. Department of Agriculture Food Safety and Inspection Service	C. Ensures overall safety of food supply, including imported foods, and inspects food plants.
_____ 4. U.S. Department of Commerce NOAA Fisheries	D. Grades fruits, vegetables, meat, poultry, shell eggs, and butter.
_____ 5. U.S. Department of Agriculture Agricultural Marketing Service	E. Along with FDA, sets standards for Grade A fresh milk.

12. Compare and contrast standards of identity with standards of fill and standards of quality.

_____

_____

_____

_____

_____

_____

_____

_____

13. Go to the website of the U.S. Department of Agriculture—Agricultural Marketing Service. Click on "Grades and Standards" in the green bar at the top of the page. Click on Fruits, and then "Apple Grades and Standards." What is the highest grade of apples? *Briefly* describe three characteristics of that grade.

_____

_____

_____

_____

_____

_____

_____

LEARNING OBJECTIVE 7.5 OUTLINE HOW VARIED BUYING METHODS WORK

14. How is a purchase requisition different from a purchase order?

_____

_____

_____

15. Describe the advantages and disadvantages of a prime vendor contract.

_____

_____

_____

_____

16. Read about a group purchasing organization for restaurants at www
     .garcpurchasing.com. Explain the service they offer and how it works to benefit
     both the restaurant and the purchasing group.

     _____

     _____

     _____

     _____

     _____

     _____

17. Chef Connor needs to order several produce items. If he uses line-item pur-
     chasing, how much will this order cost? If he uses bottom-line purchasing, how
     much will this order cost?

     What is the EP cost/box of romaine lettuce if the yield percentage from
     Supplier A is 70% and the yield percentage from Supplier B is 76%?

Product	Amount	Supplier A Price	Supplier B Price
Washington state apples, Size 138, Washington Fancy	2 boxes	$ 15.00/case	$ 14.50/case
Romaine lettuce, whole, 24 ct.	3 boxes	$ 18.50/box	$ 18.90/box
Onions, ¼" sliced, 10 lb.	30 pounds	$ 1.09/pound	$ 0.99/pound

     _____

     _____

     _____

     _____

     _____

EXTRA EXERCISES TO PRACTICE WRITING FOOD SPECIFICATIONS

18. Chef Addison works in an upscale foodservice that provides meals for employ-
     ees of a medium-sized aerospace company. She works with one of the assistant
     managers to order the food. Due to recently changing the menu to add more
     specials and more summer dishes, she has asked you to write specifications for
     the following items. Under "Unit price/Packaging," just enter the packaging
     information.

A. Fresh peaches (as snack)

Name:
Intended Use:
Description:
Quality:
Unit price/Packaging:
Other Requirements:

B. Beef steak cubes (for kabobs)

Name:
Intended Use:
Description:
Quality:
Unit price/Packaging:
Other Requirements:

C. Frozen California blend vegetables (side dish)

Name:
Intended Use:
Description:
Quality:
Unit price/Packaging:
Other Requirements:

D. Fresh Pacific halibut (main dish)

Name:
Intended Use:
Description:
Quality:
Unit price/Packaging:
Other Requirements:

E. Fusilli pasta (for pasta salad)

Name:
Intended Use:
Description:
Quality:
Unit price/Packaging:
Other Requirements:

F. Chocolate ice cream (premium)

Name:
Intended Use:
Description:
Quality:
Unit price/Packaging:
Other Requirements:

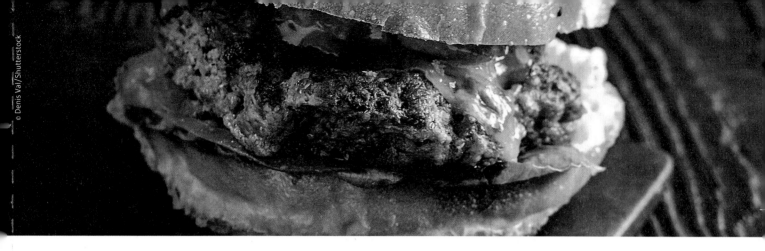

© Denis Val/Shutterstock

APPLICATIONS FOR CHAPTER 8

LEARNING OBJECTIVE 8.1 RECEIVE PRODUCTS

1. Go to the following webpage of the Institute of Child Nutrition:
   https://theicn.org/icn-resources-a-z/produce-safety/

   - Under the heading "Produce Safety Videos," click on "Videos—What Went Right and What Went Wrong."
   - Watch the video titled, "What Went Wrong? Videos—Receiving Produce." Using the form below (box on the left), list all of the *incorrect food safety practices* identified in the video.
   - Watch the video titled, "What Went Right? Videos—Receiving Produce." Using the form below (box on the right), list all of the *correct food safety practices* identified in the video.

Receiving Produce	
What Went Wrong?	**What Went Right?**
_____	_____
_____	_____
_____	_____
_____	_____
_____	_____
_____	_____
_____	_____
_____	_____
_____	_____
_____	_____

2. Using a resource such as the webstaurantstore.com, list five pieces of equipment (including manufacturer, model number, and brief description) that are needed for a receiving clerk.

_____

_____

_____

_____

_____

_____

_____

_____

_____

_____

_____

_____

LEARNING OBJECTIVE 8.2 STORE PRODUCTS SAFELY

3. Go to the following webpage of the Institute of Child Nutrition: https://theicn.org/icn-resources-a-z/produce-safety/

    • Under the heading "Produce Safety Videos," click on "Videos—What Went Right and What Went Wrong."
    • Watch the video titled, "What Went Wrong? Videos—Storing Produce." Using the form below, list all of the *incorrect food safety practices* identified on the video.
    • Watch the video titled, "What Went Right? Videos—Storing Produce." Using the form below, list all of the *correct food safety practices* identified on the video.

Storing Produce	
What Went Wrong?	**What Went Right?**
_____	_____
_____	_____
_____	_____
_____	_____
_____	_____
_____	_____
_____	_____
_____	_____
_____	_____
_____	_____
_____	_____
_____	_____

4. Find the following document online and read Chapter 3 on "Traceability." Write a summary of this chapter.

    Inventory Management and Tracking Reference Guide (2012), by the National Food Service Management Institute and USDA.

    _____

    _____

    _____

    _____

    _____

    _____

    _____

    _____

    _____

    _____

    _____

_____

_____

_____

5. Develop a mini-poster (11" × 17") showing the basics on how to store food products safely.

LEARNING OBJECTIVE 8.3 MANAGE INVENTORY INCLUDING CALCULATING FOOD/BEVERAGE COST

6. Compare and contrast physical and perpetual inventories.

_____

_____

_____

_____

_____

7. Using the information in this chart, calculate the Cost of Goods Sold for each food group. Also, complete the row "Totals" at the bottom of the chart.

Food Group	Beginning Inventory 10/1	Purchases (October)	Ending Inventory 10/31	Cost
Meat	$28,112	$30,161	$27,077	
Dairy	$12,260	$18,300	$15,560	
Baked Goods	------	$14,000	------	
Produce	$ 8,269	$11,624	$ 8,069	
Dry Goods	$25,810	$19,962	$25,772	
Totals				

8. Using data from #7, what was the cost/meal for this foodservice if they served 16,000 meals in October?

_____

_____

_____

9. Using data from #7, calculate the inventory turnover rate for meat, dry goods, and total inventory.

_____

_____

_____

_____

_____

_____

_____

_____

LEARNING OBJECTIVE 8.4 ISSUE PRODUCTS

10. Tomorrow, you have to make 36 meatloaf portions. Following is a recipe for 12 portions. Fill in the first three columns of the Requisition Form with all of the items you will need. Information on units, such as 46 oz. cans of tomato juice or 10 pounds of ground beef, can be found in the Distributor Catalog on the Companion Website. Yield information for vegetables is found in Appendix D.

Meatloaf (Makes 12 4-ounce portions)

8 oz. onions, fine dice

4 oz. celery, fine dice

1 oz. vegetable oil

6 oz. bread crumbs

6 fl. oz. tomato juice

2 pounds ground beef

1¾ pounds ground pork

4 oz. beaten egg (extra large egg contains 2 oz.)

2 teaspoons salt

1½ pints tomato sauce

Requisition Form   **Date: 8/20/2021**   **Number: 2273**

Item/GTIN	Unit	Number of Issue Units	Cost/Issue Unit	Total Cost

You don't need to fill in the last two columns!

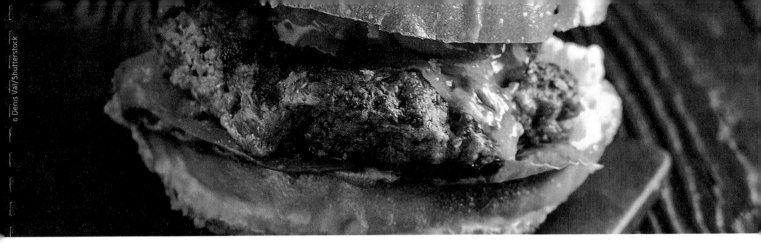

APPLICATIONS FOR CHAPTER 9

LEARNING OBJECTIVE 9.1 CHOOSE APPROPRIATE COOKING METHODS

1. Name one cooking method to cook each of these foods. Do not use the same cooking method more than once.

   A. 10-pound beef rib roast (tender) _____

   B. 10-pound beef chuck roast (not so tender) _____

   C. 8-ounce beef sirloin steak _____

   D. Mongolian beef in a wok _____

   E. 8-ounce salmon fillet _____

   F. 1 cup onions to make caramelized onions _____

   G. Pancakes _____

   H. Spaghetti _____

   I. French fried potatoes _____

   J. Fresh broccoli _____

2. How are these three cooking methods similar and how are they different: dry sauté, sauté, and stir-fry? Why are they listed under healthy cooking methods?

   _____

   _____

   _____

   _____

   _____

   _____

   _____

   _____

3. Find a recipe that uses at least one of the healthy preparation techniques (not cooking methods) such as dry rubs. List the name of the recipe and describe how the technique is used.

_____

_____

_____

_____

_____

_____

LEARNING OBJECTIVE 9.2 FORECAST PRODUCTION QUANTITIES

4. To forecast the *total number of customers* who will come in for a lunch meal at the following foodservices, which type of data would you consult?

   A. Restaurant with table service

   _____

   _____

   B. Quick-service restaurant

   _____

   _____

   C. Hospital (in-patients)

   _____

   _____

   D. College

   _____

   _____

   E. Business and industry foodservice

   _____

   _____

   F. High school

   _____

   _____

5. Give two reasons why underproduction is not desirable and two reasons why overproduction is not desirable.

_____

_____

_____

_____

_____

_____

_____

6. Beef Tacos appear on Day 2 of your 21-day menu cycle for ABC University. The first time the cycle ran was during orientation week when only 420 meal plans had been sold and you served 122 portions of taco meat. Now you are three weeks into the semester with 560 meal plans. For the last week, Taco Tuesday has been featured on the Campus Dining website and on the Menu Boards at the entrance to the dining hall. How many portions and batches of taco meat should you prepare? Explain your answer. Keep these two things in mind: one batch of taco meat makes 35 portions and students were new during the 1st cycle but now read the menu and anticipate menu offerings like Taco Tuesday.

_____

_____

_____

_____

7. The following are the six breakfast entrées for a restaurant along with the percentage of customers who normally order each item. The manager needs to forecast what the cooks will have to produce for Saturday's breakfast when 250 customers are expected. Use percentage forecasting to fill in the third column and then determine what would be an appropriate padding.

Breakfast Menu Items	Percent of Order	Forecast	Padding
Pancakes and sausage/bacon	26% of orders		
French toast with sausage/bacon	12%		
Scrambled eggs with toast	18%		
Cheese omelet with toast	10%		
Egg and cheese on bagel	9%		
Pancakes, sausage/bacon, scrambled eggs	25%		

8. You have been running out of chocolate cake and apple pie on weekend nights so you have decided to check the historical records. Every night, there are five desserts offered at dinner: chocolate cake, apple pie, cheesecake, vanilla ice cream, and carmelized pears with a cookie. Using the following information, determine the average sold as well as the historical high and historical low. Also develop a forecast for each item based on history and servings per cake, pie, or gallon of ice cream. Include some padding in your forecast.

Menu Item	Number Sold for Past Six Saturday Nights	Average Sold	Historical High	Historical Low	Forecast
Chocolate Cake 10 servings/cake	61, 55, 68, 71, 72, 73				
Apple Pie 6 servings/pie	81, 77, 69, 78, 86, 88				
Cheesecake 12 servings/cake	35, 31, 29, 36, 30, 33				
Vanilla Ice Cream 14 servings/gallon	44, 50, 42, 47, 40, 41				
Carmelized Pears with cookie	26, 29, 22, 30, 25, 20				

9. Fill in the five-day moving average in the chart below.

Day	Number of Salmon Sold	5-Day Moving Average
1	96	
2	104	
3	89	
4	110	
5	115	_____
6	99	_____
7	103	_____
8	88	_____
9	108	_____
10	116	_____

LEARNING OBJECTIVE 9.3 WRITE A PRODUCTION SCHEDULE

10. Write up a production schedule for the desserts in question #8.

_____

_____

_____

_____

_____

_____

11. A manager finds that while the cooks used up all 100 portions of turkey with stuffing, the POS system shows that there were only 81 portions sold. List three possible reasons for the discrepancy and what management should do.

_____

_____

_____

_____

_____

_____

_____

_____

12. Develop a prep sheet for a deli station where sandwiches are made to order. In the first column, write in at least eight different sandwich fillings, four cheeses, four toppings such as sliced tomatoes, and condiments. Next, develop par levels based on the forecast that 200 sandwiches will be made during the lunch period.

Deli Station Items	On Hand	Par Level	Comments

LEARNING OBJECTIVE 9.4 USE PORTION CONTROL

13. Recommend the best portion control tool to use for each of the following foods. Include scoop size when appropriate.

    A. 4 ounces turkey for sandwich _____

    B. 1 fresh roll _____

C. 1 cup soup _____

D. ½ cup vegetables _____

E. 1 fluid ounce gravy _____

F. ½ cup mashed potatoes _____

G. Salad greens in salad bar _____

H. Salad dressing in salad bar _____

I. ½ cup cooked rice _____

J. 1 cup ice cream _____

14. What is the difference between a perforated and a slotted spoon? Which situations are better suited for each type of spoon?

_____

_____

_____

_____

_____

_____

Learning Objective 9.5 Monitor Quality of Meals

15. Pick a recipe and write up a Quality Score Card for it using the categories listed.

Name of Recipe: _____

Quality Standards

1. Flavor

_____

_____

_____

2. Appearance

_____

_____

_____

3. Texture

_____

_____

_____

4. <u>Temperature</u>

_____

_____

_____

Learning Objective 9.6 Identify Sustainable Practices

16. At the following EPA website, view any of the first three videos under "Milestone 3" to see how an actual restaurant or college foodservice reduced waste. Write below three ways in which waste was reduced.

https://www.epa.gov/smm/sustainable-materials-management-smm-web-academy-webinar-series-step-step-guide-conducting

_____

_____

_____

_____

_____

_____

_____

17. At the same website listed in #16, under "Milestone 1," view the video that explains how to use the EPA's Spreadsheet Tracking Tool. Write a paragraph about what you learned on how to track waste in a foodservice.

_____

_____

_____

_____

_____

_____

_____

18.   In the town where you live or nearby, try to locate at least two of these:

    a. A food bank or food rescue operation that will take leftover food
    b. A place that accepts donated food to feed animals
    c. A company that would take used fats and oils
    d. A community composter

When researching possibilities, be sure to check the website of the local waste management company to see what services they may offer to make foodservices more sustainable.

_____

_____

_____

_____

_____

_____

_____

_____

_____

_____

_____

19.   With other classmates, find out what your college foodservice is doing to decrease food waste and energy use. Describe here.

_____

_____

_____

_____

_____

_____

_____

_____

_____

_____

_____

_____

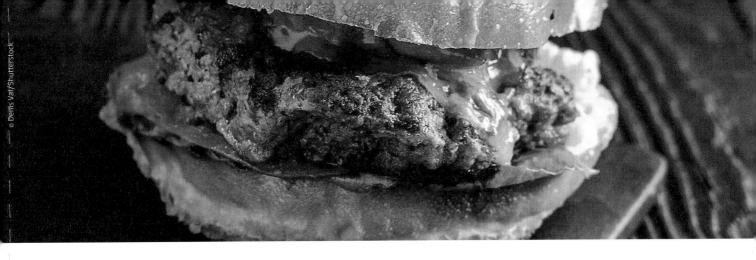

© Denis Val/Shutterstock

APPLICATIONS FOR CHAPTER 10

LEARNING OBJECTIVE 10.1 COMPARE AND CONTRAST DIFFERENT SERVICE STYLES

1. Describe the types of service used in various dining venues at your college or university, including each location on campus.

_____

_____

_____

_____

_____

_____

_____

_____

_____

_____

2. Compare and contrast vending machines to micromarkets.

_____

_____

_____

_____

_____

LEARNING OBJECTIVE 10.2 MANAGE MEAL ASSEMBLY, DISTRIBUTION, AND SERVICE IN HEALTHCARE

3. As the Foodservice Director in a 300-bed hospital outside of Baltimore, Maryland, your administrator is asking for your input. The hospital administration has recently decided to open a rehabilitation hospital across the street from the main hospital. The new facility will include 80 beds and will be about ¾ mile away across a very busy street. The average length of stay will be approximately six days. How would you handle menus, meal assembly, distribution, and service for this new facility? Justify your answers.

    _____

    _____

    _____

    _____

    _____

    _____

    _____

    _____

    _____

    _____

    _____

    _____

    _____

    _____

4. Compare and contrast assisted-living facilities to long-term skilled nursing facilities. Why do assisted living facilities offer more food choices than many skilled nursing facilities?

    _____

    _____

    _____

    _____

    _____

    _____

    _____

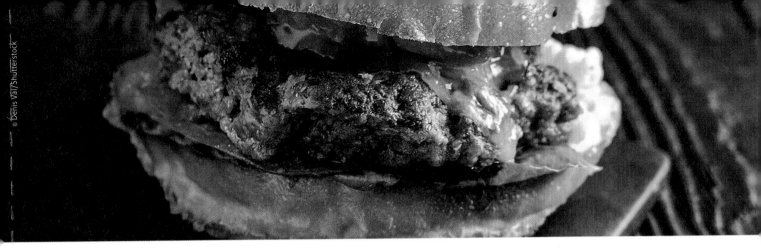

APPLICATIONS FOR CHAPTER 11

11.1 DESCRIBE MANAGEMENT SKILLS, FUNCTIONS, AND ROLES

1. Identify each of the following examples as involving technical, interpersonal, *or* conceptual skills.

   _____ A. After running out of certain menu items almost every day, the manager looks at production records and talks to key people to solve the problem.

   _____ B. Due to more guests coming in to eat than expected, the evening manager tries to persuade a server to stay two hours past the end of her shift.

   _____ C. The production manager completes the Production Sheet for the next day.

   _____ D. The dining room manager talked with the servers about a problem they had brought up.

   _____ E. The general manager had to make a decision about whether to renovate the dining room.

   _____ F. The healthcare supervisor kept a tally of which patient floors had been served lunch.

2. As the manager of a university dining hall, give two examples of how you would perform each of these functions, such as planning four-week cycle menus. Be specific.

   <u>Plan</u>:

   _____

   _____

   _____

   <u>Organize</u>:

   _____

   _____

   _____

Control:

_____

_____

_____

Lead:

_____

_____

_____

3. The key to human skills is emotional intelligence, which includes self-awareness, self-regulation, motivation, empathy, and social skills. Take either of these free, online, self-assessment tools to evaluate your emotional intelligence.

    Mind Tools https://www.mindtools.com/pages/article/ei-quiz.htm

    Institute for Health and Human Potential https://www.ihhp.com/free-eq-quiz/

    Name two things that you learned about your emotional intelligence from doing this self-assessment.

    _____

    _____

    _____

    _____

    _____

4. Think about a supervisor (boss) you have now or have had in the past. Write down three examples of how your supervisor was good at, or not very good at getting along with people, planning, organizing, leading, or controlling. For each of the three examples, include whether it is related to the supervisor's decision-making skills, interpersonal skills, or specific management function.

    _____

    _____

    _____

    _____

    _____

_____

_____

_____

5.   Design an organizational chart for a restaurant with the following positions.

   – General Manager, Chef Manager, Dining Room Manager, Bar Manager, Human Resources/Marketing Manager
   – Hourly employees: six in the kitchen (four cooks and two food preparation workers), eight in the dining area (two hosts, six servers), four in the bar (bartenders).

11.2   COMPARE AND CONTRAST MAJOR APPROACHES TO MANAGEMENT THEORY

6.   Which type of organization would you rather work in: mechanistic or organic? Give three reasons for your choice.

_____

_____

_____

_____

_____

_____

7. Do you see yourself as a Theory X or a Theory Y manager? Explain why.

_____

_____

_____

_____

_____

8. Explain how the quantitative approach and the contingency approach have made managers better at what they do.

_____

_____

_____

_____

_____

_____

11.3   COMMUNICATE EFFECTIVELY

9. For each of the following messages, choose the best form of communication: face-to-face, phone, Email, memo, or poster. In some cases, you may pick more than one form of communication.

_____ **A.** A manager needs to question an employee about an absenteeism problem.

_____ **B.** A manager needs to announce the time for a meeting.

_____ **C.** After having a conversation with an employee, a manager needs to document it.

_____ **D.** After a manager trains a number of employees on how to set up the three-compartment sink using new dispensers and products, she wants to make sure all employees get the information.

_____ **E.** The manager needs a quick answer to a question.

_____ **F.** A manager has been asked to write a reference letter for an employee who is applying to colleges.

_____ **G.** The human resources manager has revised a policy and procedure and wants to communicate it to managers and employees.

10. Assess your listening skills by answering the following questions and checking under "Usually Do" or "Should Do More Often." Which skills do you need to work on?

Listening Skills	Usually Do	Should Do More Often
1. I assume everyone has something worthwhile to say.		
2. I don't assume I know what the speaker is going to say.		
3. I give others my full attention when they speak to me by smiling, nodding, and so forth.		
4. I maintain good eye contact with the speaker.		
5. I concentrate on the whole message even when I am not really interested or agree with the speaker.		
6. I listen without judging or jumping to conclusions. I keep an open mind and try to be patient.		
7. I try not to form a rebuttal in my head while others are talking.		
8. I observe and interpret the speaker's nonverbal messages including tone of voice so I can better understand what the speaker is trying to tell me.		
9. I let the speaker finish speaking before I begin talking. I do not interrupt.		
10. I ask the speaker to clarify or repeat information when I am unsure about what was meant.		
11. I use questions to guide speakers so they will make their message clear to me.		
12. I paraphrase main points in my own words to make sure that I understand them correctly.		
13. As I listen, I figure out how others are feeling and try to see things from their perspective.		
14. I encourage the speaker to share their feelings and vent negative feelings without becoming defensive.		
15. I know which words and phrases I respond to emotionally.		

11. Read the following case study and answer the questions.

You have been asked to head a small working group within your organization. When your group was assembled, you were pleased to see that a colleague named Ron had been assigned to your group. Ron is reputed to be a very bright and creative fellow who was part of another highly successful group in the organization. However, Ron has been arriving late to group meetings and recently showed up halfway through the meeting and was clearly unprepared.

You overheard two members of the group discussing Ron's behavior. One group member, Marsha, was wondering why Ron had not been removed from the group yet; the other team member, Luis, speculated that Ron has been having some problems at home and suggested that everyone should cut him some slack.

Next week, your group is expected to hand in an important project so that the results can be passed along to other members of the organization. Each team member is responsible for a different part of the project, and Ron is responsible for the two most important parts. Your group is scheduled to meet tomorrow to do any last-minute coordination that may be required. Ron emails you today and says he doesn't have his sections finished and probably won't be able to finish them before next week. He says he just needs more time. You are very unhappy with the situation.

A. Which communication channel is best for you to respond? Explain your choice.

_____

_____

_____

_____

_____

B. What is the goal of your communication with Ron?

_____

_____

_____

C. Write up a plan of what you want to discuss with Ron and how you would like this discussion to proceed.

_____

_____

_____

_____

_____

12. As a manager, should you pay attention to the grapevine or not? Explain your answer.

_____

_____

_____

_____

_____

11.4   DISCUSS HOW TO MOTIVATE EMPLOYEES

13. Name three factors that increase your job satisfaction at work and three factors that decrease your job satisfaction.

A. Increase job satisfaction:

_____

_____

B. Decrease job satisfaction:

_____

_____

14. As the director of foodservice in an upscale retirement community, you are find-
    ing it hard to motivate the part-time high school students who come in late in
    the afternoon to serve dinner in the main dining room. They prefer to socialize
    with each other rather than giving attention to the elderly residents. Give an
    example of how you might use each of theories to help motivate them to perform
    their jobs better.

Motivational Theory	Example
Maslow's Hierarchy of Needs Theory	
Herzberg's Two-Factor Theory	
McClelland's Three-Needs Theory	
Locke's Goal-Setting Theory	
Vroom's Expectancy Theory	
Equity Theory	
Reinforcement Theory	

11.5   IDENTIFY EFFECTIVE DECISION-MAKING TECHNIQUES

15.   In a current or past job, give two examples of programmed decisions you had to make. In your personal life, give two examples of nonprogrammed decisions you have made in the past or will have to make in the coming years.

_____

_____

_____

_____

_____

_____

_____

16.   How good are your decision-making skills? Use the inventory at Mindtools and then discuss and interpret the score you got.

https://www.mindtools.com/pages/article/newTED_79.htm

_____

_____

_____

_____

_____

17.   Read the following article from the *Harvard Business Review*: The Seasoned Executive's Decision-Making Style (February 2006). It is available at this website.

https://hbr.org/2006/02/the-seasoned-executives-decision-making-style

Answer the following questions.

A.   Briefly describe the four styles of decision making discussed in this article.

_____

_____

_____

_____

_____

_____

_____

_____

B. Describe how the selection of leadership styles changes as lower-level managers work their way to upper management.

_____

_____

_____

_____

_____

_____

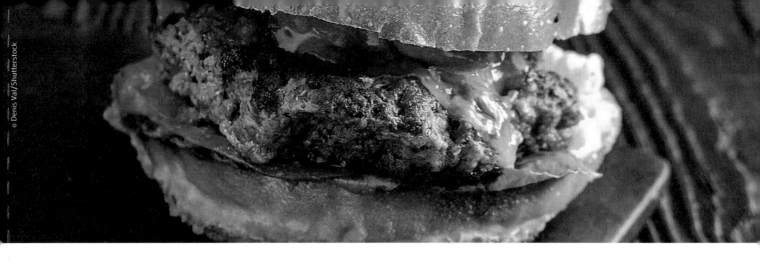

APPLICATIONS FOR CHAPTER 12

LEARNING OBJECTIVE 12.1 USE THE STRATEGIC PLANNING PROCESS

1. Match the type of plan with the correct example. Some examples will have two answers.

   Examples

   _____ A 10-year sales plan

   _____ A policy on storeroom withdrawals

   _____ Plan to open 30 new stores a year globally over 5 years

   _____ Annual budget

   _____ A plan to switch to a new dairy supplier within 3 months

   Types of Plans

   A. Short-term plan

   B. Intermediate-term plan

   C. Long-term plan

   D. Single-use plan

   E. Standing plan

   F. Strategic plan

   G. Operational plan

2. You have worked for three months in the kitchen of a restaurant that two brothers (both chefs) have operated for 10 years after taking it over from their father. They upgraded the kitchen and dining area before reopening. The breakfast and lunch meals continue to include mostly traditional items, several with a modern twist, while the dinner menu shows off their creativity. The chefs change a few menu items on the dinner menu regularly to keep a seasonal menu, and they buy some locally produced foods. Every menu item is made from scratch, including the bread and desserts (even the ice cream), and quality and appearance is very important. Prices are moderate for breakfast and lunch, and higher for dinner. Write a mission statement for this restaurant.

   _____

   _____

   _____

   _____

   _____

   _____

_____

_____

3. You spent last week observing in a retirement community's foodservice department. The facility includes independent living apartments and a nursing home wing. Some of the notes you took include the following.

    1. Health care (especially senior living) is one of the fastest growing areas in the foodservice industry due to an aging population.
    2. The independent-living residents were happy with the variety and quality of their meals in the main dining room. The meals looked great.
    3. The meals for the nursing facility looked okay but were not always hot when served.
    4. Most of the full-time kitchen employees have worked there for a number of years due to good salary and benefits (health insurance, vacation, etc.).
    5. The servers (mostly part-timers) in the dining room are not paid well and often quit after working for just a few months.
    6. The foodservice director said that management is seriously considering building a wing for assisted-living residents. These are residents who need too much help to be considered for independent living but are not yet ready for the nursing home.
    7. The purchasing agent was concerned about serving something like salad greens contaminated with harmful microbes.
    8. The foodservice director constantly feels under pressure to lower costs.
    9. The foodservice director also feels under pressure every time the state health department comes to inspect the nursing home.
    10. A new nursing home is opening down the street.

    Using this information, fill in the SWOT analysis below.

SWOT Analysis

Internal Factors	Strengths	Weaknesses
External Factors	Opportunities	Threats

4.   Rewrite the following objectives to make them SMART objectives.

    A. To have satisfied customers.

    _____

    _____

    B. To maximize sales.

    _____

    _____

    C. To lower food costs.

    _____

    _____

5.   Give an example of a foodservice/restaurant that uses a differentiation strategy and one that uses a low-cost strategy (that were *not* mentioned in the book). Briefly explain why you picked each foodservice as an example.

Differentiation Strategy:

_____

_____

_____

Low-Cost Strategy:

_____

_____

_____

LEARNING OBJECTIVE 12.2 PLAN FOR RISK AND EMERGENCIES/DISASTERS

6.   Develop *part* of a policy and procedure for a pandemic (highly infectious disease) for a continuing care retirement foodservice that feeds 200 independent and 50 assisted living residents. Almost all residents are fed in dining rooms. You are to address how you will change the menu and meal delivery system to ensure that everyone is fed in a safe manner.

_____

_____

_____

_____

_____

_____

_____

_____

_____

_____

_____

_____

_____

_____

LEARNING OBJECTIVE 12.3 PLAN YOUR OWN TIME

7.   Keep track of how you spend your time for two to three days using a Daily Time Log or a mobile phone app. Harvest is one example of a free and easy-to-use app that will help you see how you spend your time. Write down two things you learned about how you spend your time and two changes you could make to be more productive.

_____

_____

_____

_____

_____

_____

_____

_____

LEARNING OBJECTIVE 12.4 INTERPRET ORGANIZATIONAL STRUCTURE

8.   Identify which organizational principle is represented by each of the eight statements below.

   A. Departmentalization
   B. Work specialization (division of labor)
   C. Chain of command
   D. Staff authority
   E. Span of control (span of management)
   F. Centralized authority
   G. Delegation
   H. Coordination

————— **1.** "Jamel, I would like you to be the one in charge of the catering order for the President's luncheon next week."

————— **2.** "I need the receiving clerk to take care of an issue, so I will talk to his boss first."

————— **3.** "The pantry chef prepares all the cold foods except for desserts, which are done by the pastry chef."

————— **4.** "As the human resources director, I agree that Jackson would be a good hire for that position."

————— **5.** "Before we implement any changes like that here in the hospital's foodservice, we need to talk to nursing."

————— **6.** "I have 17 employees who report to me but many of them are part-timers."

————— **7.** "Servers, bussers, and hosts are all part of front-of-the-house staff."

————— **8.** "It doesn't seem like hourly employees are asked for feedback on many questions and that most decisions are made at the top."

9. In what ways are foodservice organizations more mechanistic than organic? Present three ideas using concepts in **Figure 12-5**.

_____

_____

_____

_____

_____

_____

_____

_____

LEARNING OBJECTIVE 12.5 ANALYZE AND DESIGN JOBS

10. Write a job description for a job you have had using these headings.

  1. Job Identification

   Job Title:

   Department:

   Reports to:

   Exempt or Nonexempt:

  2. Job Summary

_____

_____

3. **Responsibilities and Tasks**

_____

_____

_____

_____

_____

_____

_____

4. **Job Setting**

_____

_____

_____

_____

_____

_____

_____

5. **Level of Supervision**

_____

_____

11. Identify which job design principle is represented by each of the four statements given.

   A. Job enlargement
   B. Job enrichment
   C. Job rotation
   D. Job simplification

   _____ **1.** "As a crew member, you work one of three positions each day: counter, drive-thru line, or dining room."

   _____ **2.** "During meal service, your job is to check the meal for accuracy and put the garnish on."

   _____ **3.** "Do you want to also take on ordering the milk each day? It seems that you have the ability and time to do it."

   _____ **4.** "To give you more freedom, you won't have to get my "okay" before starting meal service each day. You can make that decision."

Learning Objective 12.6 Create and Manage Groups and Teams

12. Match the type of group/team with the correct example

<u>Examples</u>

_____ A group that meets weekly to prepare for using new software

_____ A supervisor and his subordinates

_____ A group that meets to solve the problem of frequent broken dishes

_____ The CEO and top executives

_____ The foodservice department in a hospital

_____ A team in charge of using cook/chill technology to prepare the next day's meals

_____ Four employees who eat lunch together daily

<u>Types of Groups/Teams</u>

A. Formal group

B. Self-managed work team

C. Task group

D. Top management team

E. Informal group

F. Problem-solving team

G. Command group

13. Watch the following video (on YouTube) and write a paragraph on the skills the group demonstrated when they successfully worked on the problem.

"Skills for Work: Team-Working Skills" by Macmillan Education ELT.

_____

_____

_____

_____

_____

_____

_____

_____

_____

_____

_____

14. Part of being a good team member is having some skills and characteristics, Listed here are 10 skills needed to be a productive team member. Circle the skills you think you need to work on.

1. Reliable: You can be counted on to get the job done.
2. Effective Communicator: You express your thoughts and ideas clearly and directly, with respect for others.
3. Active Listener: You listen to and respect different points of view. When others offer you constructive feedback, you don't get upset or defensive.
4. Prepared: You do the work required to help the team.
5. Share openly and willingly: You are willing to share information, experience, and knowledge with the group.
6. Cooperative: You work well with other members of the team.
7. Open-minded: You can keep an open mind to different ideas.
8. Committed: You are responsible and dedicated.
9. Problem solver: You focus on solutions.
10. Respectful: You treat other team members with respect and consideration all of the time.

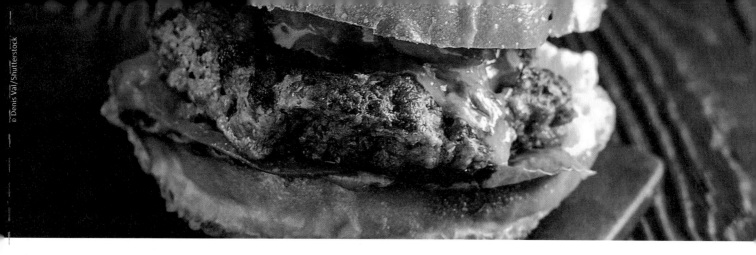

APPLICATIONS FOR CHAPTER 13

LEARNING OBJECTIVE 13.1 APPLY FEDERAL LAWS AFFECTING HUMAN RESOURCES MANAGEMENT

1. For each of the following situations, identify a law/legislation that might apply.

    A. Two employees speak with their supervisor about having to listen to off-color jokes from co-workers.

    _____

    B. A group of female employees file a lawsuit that shows they are being paid less than men.

    _____

    C. A group of black male managers file charges with the Equal Employment Opportunity Commission that they have been discriminated against because of race.

    _____

    D. A disabled applicant needs to request a reasonable accommodation during the employment interview.

    _____

    E. A 60-year-old employee worries that he will be terminated due to his age.

    _____

2. Read the following situations. Then answer the questions.

    Situation 1. Bill has a private office and a computer assigned to him. You are his supervisor. Your IT staff informs you that the office's network management software has detected that Bill's computer has been used to visit explicit sexually oriented websites. Bill admits that he has visited these sites during his personal time before and after work and at lunch.

    a. Is this an example of sexual harassment? Why or why not?

    _____

    _____

b. What if he was printing the pictures on the office printer? Is that sexual harassment? Why or why not?

_____

_____

Situation 2. Carmen works as a pastry chef in a restaurant kitchen. Two male coworkers tell dirty jokes of a sexual nature to her and make lewd remarks. She tried to ignore the comments by walking away. The verbal comments increased, and one coworker began to touch her in sexually suggestive ways. Carmen complained to her boss, the Executive Chef, who said he "would take care of it," but did nothing and the harassment became worse over the next month. Carmen felt forced to look for another job.

a. Is this an example of sexual harassment? Why or why not?

_____

_____

_____

b. If it is sexual harassment, was it quid pro quo harassment (meaning a job benefit is tied to an employee submitting to unwelcome sexual advances) or a hostile work environment? Justify your answer.

_____

_____

_____

_____

3. Three ways to solve safety problems in a foodservice could involve removing or isolating the hazard, improving work practices, and/or providing personal protective equipment. Name one safety hazard in a foodservice and give two possible solutions.

_____

_____

_____

_____

LEARNING OBJECTIVE 13.2 RECRUIT AND SELECT EMPLOYEES

4. Check any of the following questions if they are *allowed* in a job interview.

_____ A. When did you graduate from high school/college?

_____ B. Can you perform the specific duties of this job?

_____ C. Do you have child care arrangements?

     _____ **D.**   What is your maiden name?

     _____ **E.**   Are you a U.S. citizen?

     _____ **F.**   Can you provide proof of your work visa status?

     _____ **G.**   Can you work on Saturdays?

     _____ **H.**   Do you have access to a car or the bus to get to work?

     _____ **I.**   Are you already a member of the union here?

5. As the dining room manager, you need to interview three candidates for a job as host/hostess. You plan to use a structured interview. Develop a list of six questions to use for all candidates.

6. You need to hire a new cook. Give two examples of employment tests that would be the most important to include in the selection process. Explain why you chose them.

LEARNING OBJECTIVE 13.3 TRAIN EMPLOYEES

7. Using the instructional methods listed in **Table 13–7**, which method would work well to teach each of the following topics. You may write in more than one method.

   A. Teach servers how to deal with customer complaints.

B. Teach servers which foods are gluten-free.

_____

_____

C. Teach utility staff to operate the new dish machine.

_____

_____

D. Teach decision-making skills to managers in foodservices across three states.

_____

_____

E. Conduct diversity training.

_____

_____

8. You have been asked to teach an in-service class to production staff on how to use and wash knives safely. Write at least two learning objectives for the class and how you will evaluate each one.

Learning Objectives	Evaluation Method
1.	1.
2.	2.

LEARNING OBJECTIVE 13.4 MANAGE EMPLOYEES' PERFORMANCE

9. You are responsible for completing performance appraisals for each line cook and prep cook. Which appraisal format would work well? Explain why your choice is a good one.

_____

_____

10. As a General Manager, you must do the annual performance appraisals for the three managers who report to you. Which appraisal format(s) would work well? Explain why your choice is a good one.

_____

_____

11.   Develop a behaviorally anchored rating scale for teamwork that will be used in evaluations for servers and bussers (dining room attendants).

12.   Describe an experience in which you were unhappy with either how a supervisor was coaching your performance or how a supervisor reviewed your performance appraisal with you.

_____

_____

_____

_____

13.   Write up a "Description of Incident" in a Disciplinary Action Notice, being as specific and objective as possible. You are allowed to add in additional details.

The offense involves Tom—a foodservice worker in a hospital who delivers trays to patient rooms and then returns them to the kitchen to get washed and put away. He delivered lunch trays late twice this week because Nursing reports that he is talking and texting on his cell phone by the cart of trays instead of delivering them.

Description of Incident

_____

_____

_____

_____

_____

_____

LEARNING OBJECTIVE 13.5 SCHEDULE EMPLOYEES

14.   Use ZoomShift or Google calendar to schedule the following employees.

Restaurant is open 7:00 AM to 2:30 PM for breakfast and lunch every day but is closed on Mondays.

Full-timers (4) who work 6:30 AM to 3:00 PM: Tom, Amira, Katherine, Jade.

Part-timers (2) work as needed to cover part or all of a full-timer's shift (around 20 hours/week): Sean, Selena.

Staffing level is four employees during hours of 6:30 AM to 3:00 PM.

Jade (full-timer) has requested Wednesday off.

LEARNING OBJECTIVE 13.6 WORK WITH UNIONS

15.   Suppose you are a General Manager for a successful foodservice with over 120 employees. You hear that some of your employees have been speaking with representatives of the Service Employees International Union (SEIU) in the parking lot after work. SEIU has worked in the past to seek an increase in wages. What are your (the employer) rights when a union starts the organizing process and what are the union's rights? What steps have to take place before a union is certified?

_____

_____

_____

_____

_____

_____

_____

16.   Watch the following YouTube video: "Managing Unionized Employees—How Hard Is It?" Write down what you learned in a brief paragraph.

_____

_____

_____

_____

_____

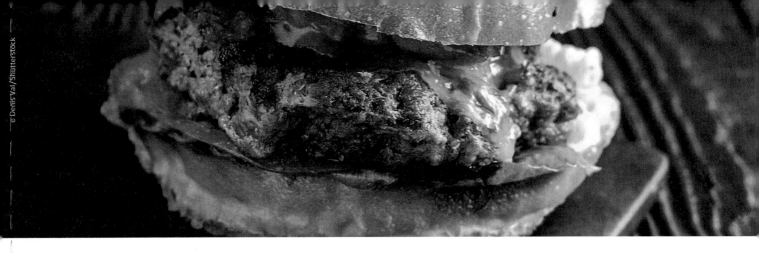

© Denis Val/Shutterstock

APPLICATIONS FOR CHAPTER 14

LEARNING OBJECTIVE 14.1 DESCRIBE APPROACHES TO QUALITY

1. Watch the video "Introduction to DMAIC" on YouTube. DMAIC is Six Sigma's process improvement methodology.

   https://www.youtube.com/watch?v=nG3BoGRZjOc

   Describe one possible opportunity for improvement in a foodservice and give an example of one potential root cause and one solution.

   _____

   _____

   _____

   _____

   _____

   _____

2. Watch the video "How Lean Manufacturing Lets You Eat Mor Chikin at Chick-Fil-A."

   https://www.youtube.com/watch?v=ai12RKbiwUI

   Describe one example of how Lean was used to increase sales and customer satisfaction.

   _____

   _____

   _____

   _____

   _____

LEARNING OBJECTIVE 14.2 USE APPROPRIATE QUALITY TOOLS TO SUPPORT QUALITY MANAGEMENT

3. As the cafeteria manager in a hospital cafeteria that serves patients' families and hospital employees, you have recently noticed that after the dinner meal, there are a lot of leftover hot entrées and hot side dishes. Develop a cause-and-effect diagram showing possible causes of this problem.

4. Draw a flowchart, using appropriate flowchart symbols, that shows the steps an employee uses to make 50 peanut butter and jelly sandwiches. First think through the process.

LEARNING OBJECTIVE 14.3 MANAGE CUSTOMER SATISFACTION

5. Using **Table 14–5**, evaluate a foodservice where you have eaten a number of times. Describe any service failures that occurred there, how they were handled, and if you were satisified.

    _____

    _____

    _____

    _____

    _____

    _____

    _____

6. You have recently taken a position as the Manager of a foodservice serving 500 pharmaceutical employees in Princeton, NJ. You are in charge of several dining venues but the most popular is the food court visited by many employees on a daily basis. You are very interested in knowing how satisfied these customers are with the food court. Design a brief, effective survey for customers to take and also describe how you will get at least 30% of current employees to complete the survey.

    _____

    _____

    _____

    _____

    _____

    _____

    _____

    _____

    _____

    _____

_____

_____

_____

_____

_____

_____

_____

_____

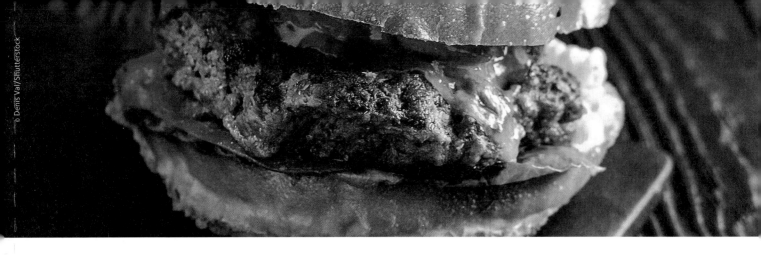

© Denis Val/Shutterstock

APPLICATIONS FOR CHAPTER 15

LEARNING OBJECTIVE 15.1 COMPLETE AND ANALYZE AN INCOME STATEMENT

1. Fill in the blank spaces in this Profit and Loss Statement.

   Profit and Loss Statement (January 1–March 31, 2021)

Sales		
Food	$_____	_____%
Beverage	82,546	_____%
Total Sales	$281,623	100.0%
Cost of Sales		
Food	$ _____	35.1%
Beverage	18,160	_____%
Total Cost of Sales	_____	_____%
Gross Profit	_____	_____%
Controllable Expenses		
Salaries and wages	$ 81,671	_____%
Benefits	18,306	_____%
Employer-paid payroll taxes/W. comp	_____	2.0%
Direct operating expenses	_____	5.8%
Utilities	14,081	_____%
Administrative expenses/fees	10,983	_____%
Repairs & maintenance	_____	2.3%
Marketing and advertising	_____	1.5%
Total Controllable Expenses	$157,708	_____%
Controllable Income	_____	_____%
Non-Controllable Expenses		
Occupancy Costs	$ 25,346	_____%
Depreciation & Interest	_____	_____%
Total Non-Controllable Expenses	$ 31,823	_____%
Net Income/Net Loss Before Taxes	_____	_____%

2. Using the Income Statement in #1, calculate each of the following.

    A. Food cost percentage

    B. Beverage cost percentage

    C. Cost of sales percentage

    D. Labor cost percentage

    E. Prime cost percentage

    F. Profit margin percentage

3. Given the following information for March, calculate the cost of sales, also called cost of goods sold.

Beginning inventory:	$63,650
Ending inventory:	$70.300
Protein purchases:	$37,500
Dairy purchases:	$ 5,000
Fruits and vegetables:	$15,600
All other food purchases:	$ 7,900
Beer and wine purchases:	$ 7,000

LEARNING OBJECTIVE 15.2 COMPLETE AND ANALYZE A BALANCE SHEET

4. The following is information on assets, liabilities, and equity for a business. Create a balance sheet using this information.

Owner's equity	$115,750
Accounts payable	$145,000
Accounts receivable	$5,000
Equipment	$125,000
Inventory	$ 37,500
Cash	$185,250
Accumulated depreciation	($45,000)
Wages & benefits payable	$ 30,000
Lease payments	$ 14,000
Sales tax	$ 3,000

_____

_____

_____

_____

_____

_____

_____

_____

_____

_____

_____

_____

LEARNING OBJECTIVE 15.3 PREPARE AN OPERATING BUDGET AND MONITOR PERFORMANCE

5.

A. Project each line item for the next year's budget (shown in the chart) using this information.

- The management team has agreed that sales will increase 2.5% next year mostly due to price increases.
- Human resources has told you to increase payroll costs by 2.8% and benefits by 1%.
- Food costs will be going up from 1–2% next year. Use 2% for proteins and produce, 1.5% for groceries, and 1% for other items.
- Beverage costs will be going up by 1.5%.
- Operating expenses should be relatively stable, except paper supplies, cleaning supplies, utilities, and credit card fees are expected to increase by about 1%.

Budget Worksheet for FY 2022	FY2021 Budget (A)	Projected % Increase (B)	2022 Budget (C)
1. **Revenue**			
Food	$294,000		
Beverage	70,000		
Total Revenue	364,000		
2. **Food Cost**			
Proteins	51,200		
Dairy/eggs	15,500		
Groceries	9,500		

(continues)

Budget Worksheet for FY 2022	FY2021 Budget (A)	Projected % Increase (B)	2022 Budget (C)
Fruits and vegetables	18,800		
Baked Goods	5,250		
Miscellaneous	4,200		
Total Food Cost	**$104,450**		
Food Cost %	**35.5%**		
3. **Beverage Cost**			
Wine	3,200		
Draft beer	8,000		
Liquor	2,500		
Bar mix, mixers, etc.	1,000		
Total Beverage Cost	**$14,700**		
Beverage Cost %	**21.0%**		
COST OF SALES	**$119,150 (32.7%)**		
GROSS PROFIT	**$244,850 (67.3%)**		
4. **Labor Cost**			
Salaries/wages	128,000		
Benefits	4,000		
Total Labor Cost	**$132,000**		
Labor Cost %	**36.3%**		
5. **Operating Expenses**			
Paper supplies	3,700		
Cleaning supplies	7,500		
Misc. direct expenses	7,000		
Utilities	10,800		
Credit card fees	6,200		
Other administrative expenses	7,200		
Repairs & maintenance	8,100		
Marketing/advertising	2,800		
Rent/lease	30,000		
Property/real estate tax	3,400		
Insurance	2,800		
Depreciation	3,900		
Total Operating Exp	**$93,400**		

B. Using the chart from A, calculate the food cost percentage and labor cost percentage for 2021 and 2022. How do they compare?

_____

_____

C. Once you have projected each line item, allocate the revenue and food costs across all 12 months. Assume that the busiest months are from April to December, with January through March being slower. Explain how you allocated these costs.

_____

_____

_____

_____

_____

Budget Worksheet for FY 2022	Jan	Feb	March	April	May	June	July	Aug	Sept	Oct	Nov	Dec
1. **Revenue**												
Food												
Beverage												
TOTAL REVENUE												
2. **Food Cost**												
Proteins												
Dairy/eggs												
Groceries												
Fruits and vegetables												
Baked goods												
Miscellaneous												
TOTAL FOOD COST												

6. The following is an expense report showing what your foodservice spent for the month of August and what was budgeted.

   A. Complete the final column with the variance, variance percentage, and whether the variance was favorable or unfavorable.

   B. Also complete the bottom line: Net Performance.

   C. Write a short paragraph giving your thoughts on whether one or more of the variances show a potential problem that needs to be looked into and why.

_____

_____

_____

_____

_____

_____

Expense Report for August 2021

Category	August 2021 Actual	Budget	Variance, Variance %, Favorable or Unfavorable
SALES			
Food sales	$189,450	$180,000	
Beverage sales	48,800	50,000	
Total Sales	**$238,250**	**$230,000**	
FOOD & BEVERAGE			
Food	$66,100	$ 54,500	
Beverages	13,600	15,000	
Total food & beverage	**$79,700**	**$69,500**	
LABOR			
Salaries/wages	$80,100	$77,000	
Benefits	4,400	4,600	
Total Labor	**$84,500**	**$81,600**	
EXPENSES			
Direct operating expenses	$14,600	$12,500	
Rent & utilities	20,000	$21,000	
Administrative expenses	13,500	$13,000	
Repairs/maintenance	3,500	$ 4,000	
Marketing	3,500	$ 3,500	
Misc. Expenses	4.800	$ 4,500	
Total Expenses	**59,900**	**$58,500**	
Net performance			

7.

   A. As a hospital foodservice manager, you have just spoken with the head of Human Resources who has told you that they project 110,000 patient days in the next fiscal year. If you serve 2.7 meals/patient day, how many patient meals will you project for next year's budget?

_____

_____

B. In your hospital foodservice, the meal equivalent for cafeteria meals is $5.75. If next year's cafeteria revenue is estimated to be $1,500,000, how many cafeteria meals are planned?

_____

_____

C. If your food cost per meal for the current fiscal year is $4.25, and it is expected to increase by 2% next year, how big will your total food budget (including patient and cafeteria meals) need to be?

_____

_____

_____

_____

_____

LEARNING OBJECTIVE 15.4 PREPARE A CAPITAL BUDGET

8. As the hospital's director of food and nutrition services, your boss has asked you to submit a written request/proposal for a new dish machine since the current one is on its last legs and the repair bills are overwhelming. Even though your boss is on your side, you still need to compete with many other departments who also need equipment and justify this large cost. Give two examples of how you will justify the need for the new dish machine. The cost for the new machine is $29,000 and is supposed to lower your utility costs by 20%.

_____

_____

_____

_____

_____

_____

_____

_____

LEARNING OBJECTIVE 15.5 USE FINANCIAL ANALYSIS TOOLS

9. Take the balance sheet you created in #4 and make it into a common-size balance sheet by expressing each line item as a percentage. Just add a column to the right showing the percentage.

10. If a foodservice has monthly sales of $124,000, fixed costs of $25,000, and variable costs of $77,000, calculate the break-even point in sales.

11. Calculate return on sales using the data from #1.

12. Given the following information, calculate the inventory turnover rate and compare it with foodservice industry averages.

    This month's beginning inventory: $21,254
    This month's ending inventory: $17,894
    Cost of sales: $45,171

13. Use the following information from a one-week period to complete the listed operating ratios.

    Sales: $97,000
    Number of customers (meals) served: 10,800
    Number of seats: 100 seats
    Food cost: $33,610
    Beverage cost: $4,400
    Labor cost: $35,500

A. Average check

_____

_____

B. Sales per seat

_____

_____

C. Food cost per meal

_____

_____

D. Beverage cost per meal

_____

_____

E. Labor cost per meal

_____

_____

F. Prime cost per meal

_____

_____

G. Prime cost percentage—Calculate and compare to industry averages.

_____

_____

_____

_____

LEARNING OBJECTIVE 15.6 MEASURE PRODUCTIVITY

14. Use the following information from a school district's foodservice for a 2-week period to calculate the listed productivity ratios.

Number of meals: 39,456　　　Total labor hours: 2,303

Sales: $167,000　　　Total productive labor hours: 2,165

A. Meals per paid labor hour

_____

_____

B. Meals per productive labor hour

_____

_____

C. Meals per FTE

_____

_____

D. Sales per paid labor hour

_____

_____

E. Paid labor hours per meal

_____

_____

F. Productive labor hours per meal

_____

_____

LEARNING OBJECTIVE 15.7 CONTROL COSTS

15. Interview a restaurant or college foodservice manager and ask for what they consider the most important ways to control food and labor costs. Write a paragraph on what you learned.

_____

_____

_____

_____

_____

_____

_____

_____

_____

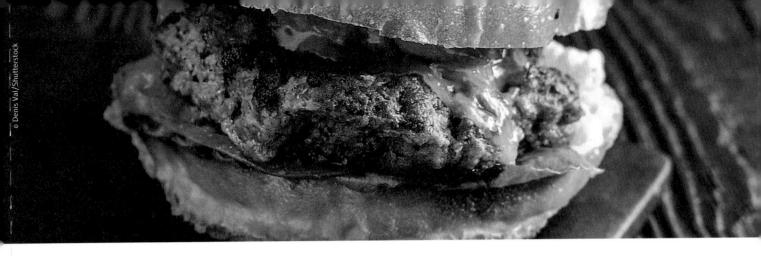

APPLICATIONS FOR CHAPTER 16 MARKETING AND BUSINESS PLANS

16.1 EXPLAIN THE CONSUMER DECISION-MAKING PROCESS AND FACTORS THAT INFLUENCE IT

1. Describe the process you go through when deciding where to eat out or pick up a meal. Use the consumer decision-making process to guide the steps and be sure to list the criteria you use when making your choice.

_____

_____

_____

_____

_____

_____

_____

_____

16.2 DEVELOP THE MARKETING PLAN

2. The Values, Attitudes, and Lifestyles Model (VALS) is a proprietary model used for psychographic market segmentation. It puts American consumers into one of eight segments based on two dimensions: motivation and resources. Take the VALS survey to determine which segment you fit into.

http://www.strategicbusinessinsights.com/vals/presurvey.shtml

What was your result? Describe the segment.

_____

_____

_____

_____

3. As a manager, you are helping to develop a program promoting green initiatives in the moderate-price casual dining restaurant where you work. Some of the initiatives include the use of more local and organic foods, sustainable seafood, eco-friendly take-out containers, and efforts to save water and electricity. Describe how you would use three different forms of promotion to inform and persuade consumers to visit the restaurant.

A.

_____

_____

_____

B.

_____

_____

_____

C.

_____

_____

_____

4. When the American economy is in a slump, consumers usually spend less money, especially on frills such as eating out or going to the movies. At these times, McDonald's finds it useful to offer their Dollar Menu, which lowers prices on certain items. Read about their Dollar Menu online to understand how it works, then answer the following questions.

A. Why are McDonald's favorites (Big Mac, Quarter Pounder with Cheese) not on the Dollar Menu?

_____

_____

B. Why are beverages on the Dollar Menu?

_____

_____

C. Name two benefits of having a Dollar Menu.

_____

_____

5. NPD Group, Inc. continually collects data for the foodservice industry, such as market share information and purchasing trends. On their website, click on "Industries" and then "Foodservice". Read the brief "Reports" and other materials to see which topics they are currently looking at. Briefly describe two things you learned below.

A.

_____

_____

_____

B.

_____

_____

_____

16.3   WRITE A BUSINESS PLAN

6. On the Navigate Companion website, you will find a business plan for the Pier Restaurant. After reading it, give two criticisms of the business plan.

_____

_____

_____

7. Listed below are the major sections and subsections for a business plan. Next, you will see 20 excerpts from a restaurant business plan. Match the excerpt with the subsection where it belongs by putting the number from the excerpt into the correct blank under #2–#6.

1. Executive Summary
2. Business Description

    _____ **A.**   Company Description
    _____ **B.**   Mission Statement
    _____ **C.**   Business History
    _____ **D.**   Management/Key People
    _____ **E.**   Products/Services

3. Operating Plan

   _____ **A.** Location

   _____ **B.** Facilities and Layout

   _____ **C.** Operations

   _____ **D.** Labor/Personnel

   _____ **E.** Quality Control and Customer Service

4. Industry Analysis

   _____ **A.** Industry Description

   _____ **B.** Industry Competition

   _____ **C.** Industry Growth and Sales Projection

5. Market Analysis & Plan

   _____ **A.** Target Market

   _____ **B.** Competition

   _____ **C.** Sales Forecast and Assumptions

   _____ **D.** Marketing Plan

6. Financial Plan

   _____ **A.** Start-Up Costs

   _____ **B.** Pro Forma Statement

   _____ **C.** Cash Flow Statement

EXCERPTS FROM THE MARKETING PLAN

1. The foodservice business is the third-largest industry in the country. It accounts for over $240 billion annually in sales.
2. The initial costs for the restaurant center around the lease payments for the building, remodeling of the kitchen and dining room, purchasing of initial food and supply inventory, and payroll.
3. Beacon's Restaurant will be offering a menu of moderate-priced ethnic and American items with a common theme—healthy, flavorful, and familiar.
4. The quality of our products will constantly be tested by our executive chef and other management personnel.
5. The restaurant will attract three different customer profiles: college students, the health-conscious person, and local business people looking for light, healthy meals.
6. Cando, Inc. will operate Beacon's. Cando, Inc. is a corporation based in Boston, Massachusetts.
7. Beacon's Restaurant is located in the Harvard Square area of Cambridge.
8. There are over 20 restaurants in the Harvard Square area that sell food at similar prices. The restaurants include both independents and chains.
9. Our mission is to maintain a profitable business and provide a healthy menu for our customers.
10. Staffing for the restaurant will require an executive chef, sous chef, six cooks, three dishwashers, and 12 front-of-the-house personnel.
11. Within the restaurant industry, not enough new restaurants are opening every month to keep up with demand.

12. This statement shows how much cash will be coming in each month for the first year, as well as the cash going out to pay the lease, insurance, food and supplies, other expenses, and payroll.

13. The restaurant is a 3,400 square foot space, which needs some minor remodeling.

14. Our sales forecast is based on a check average of $5.60.

15. The President of Cando, Inc. is Fred Binder, a veteran restaurateur.

16. There are four ways in which we will create an advantage over our competitors: fresh food that tastes great, highly trained and enthusiastic waitstaff, service and delivery options, and our emphasis on healthy food.

17. After 18 months of operation, we anticipate reaching our break-even point.

18. Cando, Inc. was founded in 2005.

19. Food production and assembly will take place in the kitchen of the restaurant.

20. The restaurant industry will grow approximately 3% each year.

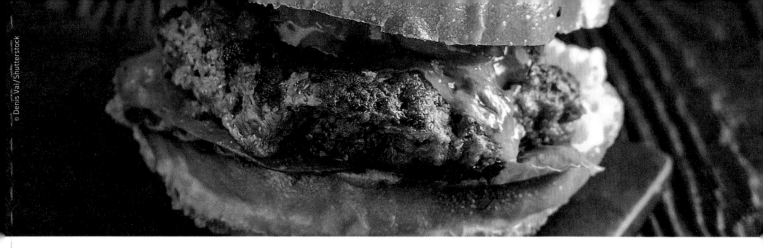

APPLICATIONS FOR CHAPTER 17

LEARNING OBJECTIVE 17.1 EXPLAIN AND CLASSIFY THEORIES OF LEADERSHIP

1. Complete the "What's Your Leadership Style" at this website.

    https://www.mindtools.com/pages/article/leadership-style-quiz.htm

    What were your results? Is your leadership style more authoritarian, democratic, or laissez-faire? Were you surprised by the results?

    _____

    _____

2. To be a leader, you need to be able to use persuasion well to get things done. Listen to the following free podcast (available at Apple Podcasts or Google Podcasts) and write a paragraph about how to persuade others.

    "Mastering the Art of Persuasion" by Jonah Berger (Wharton Professor)

    _____

    _____

    _____

    _____

    _____

    _____

    _____

    _____

    _____

    _____

3. Hamdi Ulukaya came to the United States from Turkey and founded Chobani yogurt. Listen to his TED talk using the link, then answer the questions below.

    https://www.ted.com/speakers/hamdi_ulukaya

    A. List four things Mr. Ulukaya did to make Chobani successful.

    _____

    _____

    _____

    _____

    _____

    B. Which contemporary model of leadership does he fit into? Explain why.

    _____

    _____

    _____

    _____

    _____

    _____

    _____

Learning Objective 17.2 Discuss the Delegation Process

4. Listen to the YouTube Video titled, "Leadership Delegation Skills from Dale Carnegie Training," which shows an example of poor delegating and then much improved delegating. List at least three reasons why the second conversation on delegation went well.

    https://www.youtube.com/watch?v=y4NyD1ovjpQ

    _____

    _____

    _____

    _____

    _____

    _____

LEARNING OBJECTIVE 17.3 MANAGE CHANGE

5. In a hospital foodservice, the final decision to switch from a traditional tray-line system to a room service system was made. A few trayline employees were involved in the discussion and final selection of the room service model, which was chosen to (hopefully) improve the quality of patient meals. As managers start discussing the changes with the employees, there are many employees expressing doubts about why the change is needed and worry about how their jobs will change. Discuss how you would use two methods for dealing with resistance to change to gain commitment to the new system.

_____

_____

_____

_____

_____

_____

_____

_____

LEARNING OBJECTIVE 17.4 DESCRIBE GUIDELINES FOR NEGOTIATING

6. You have likely wanted to be paid more money in a prior or your current job. Suppose you decided to have a meeting with your supervisor (past or present) to ask for a pay raise or improved benefits. Answer the following questions.

A. What is your optimum goal, target goal, and minimum goal? Do you want to use anything as leverage (such as taking on another responsibility) to get what you want?

_____

_____

_____

_____

_____

B. Why should your supervisor agree to increase your salary or other benefits?

_____

_____

_____

_____

_____

_____

C. What is your backup plan (Best Alternative To a Negotiated Agreement, BATNA)?

_____

_____

_____

_____